PHEOCHROMOCYTOMA
First International Symposium

ANNALS OF THE NEW YORK ACADEMY OF SCIENCES
Volume 1073

PHEOCHROMOCYTOMA
First International Symposium

Edited by
Karel Pacak and Graeme Eisenhofer

Published by Blackwell Publishing on behalf of the New York Academy of Sciences
Boston, Massachusetts
2006

Library of Congress Cataloging-in-Publication Data

Pheochromocytoma : first international symposium / edited by Karel Pacak and Graeme Eisenhofer.
p. ; cm. – (Annals of the New York Academy of Sciences, ISSN 0077-8923 ; v. 1073)
Includes bibliographical references.
ISBN-13: 978-1-57331-597-5 (alk. paper)
ISBN-10: 1-57331-597-4 (alk. paper)
1. Pheochromocytoma–Congresses. I. Pacak, Karel. II. Eisenhofer, Graeme. III. New York Academy of Sciences. IV. Series.
[DNLM: 1. Pheochromocytoma–diagnosis–Congresses. 2. Pheochromocytoma–genetics–Congresses. 3. Diagnosis, Differential–Congresses. 4. Pheochromocytoma–therapy–Congresses.
W1 AN626YL v.1073 2006 / QZ 380 P5405 2006]

RC280.A3P4554 2006
616.99'445–dc22

2006019005

The *Annals of the New York Academy of Sciences* (ISSN: 0077-8923 [print]; ISSN: 1749-6632 [online]) is published 28 times a year on behalf of the New York Academy of Sciences by Blackwell Publishing, with offices located at 350 Main Street, Malden, Massachusetts 02148 USA, PO Box 1354, Garsington Road, Oxford OX4 2DQ UK, and PO Box 378 Carlton South, 3053 Victoria Australia.

Information for subscribers: Subscription prices for 2006 are: Premium Institutional: \$3850.00 (US) and £2139.00 (Europe and Rest of World).
Customers in the UK should add VAT at 5%. Customers in the EU should also add VAT at 5% or provide a VAT registration number or evidence of entitlement to exemption. Customers in Canada should add 7% GST or provide evidence of entitlement to exemption. The Premium Institutional price also includes online access to full-text articles from 1997 to present, where available. For other pricing options or more information about online access to Blackwell Publishing journals, including access information and terms and conditions, please visit www.blackwellpublishing.com/nyas.

Membership information: Members may order copies of the *Annals* volumes directly from the Academy by visiting www.nyas.org/annals, emailing membership@nyas.org, faxing 212-888-2894, or calling 800-843-6927 (US only), or +1 212 838 0230, ext. 345 (International). For more information on becoming a member of the New York Academy of Sciences, please visit www.nyas.org/membership.

Journal Customer Services: For ordering information, claims, and any inquiry concerning your institutional subscription, please contact your nearest office:
UK: Email: customerservices@blackwellpublishing.com; Tel: +44 (0) 1865 778315; Fax +44 (0) 1865 471775
US: Email: customerservices@blackwellpublishing.com; Tel: +1 781 388 8599 or 1 800 835 6770 (Toll free in the USA); Fax: +1 781 388 8232
Asia: Email: customerservices@blackwellpublishing.com; Tel: +65 6511 8000; Fax: +61 3 8359 1120
Members: Claims and inquiries on member orders should be directed to the Academy at email: membership@nyas.org or Tel: +1 212 838 0230 (International) or 800-843-6927 (US only).

Printed on acid-free paper.

Mailing: The *Annals of the New York Academy of Sciences* are mailed Standard Rate. **Postmaster:** Send all address changes to *Annals of the New York Academy of Sciences*, Blackwell Publishing, Inc., Journals Subscription Department, 350 Main Street, Malden, MA 01248-5020. Mailing to rest of world by DHL Smart and Global Mail.

Annals are available to subscribers online at the New York Academy of Sciences and also at Blackwell Synergy. Visit www.annalsnyas.org or www.blackwell-synergy.com to search the articles and register for table of contents e-mail alerts. Access to full text and PDF downloads of *Annals* articles are available to nonmembers and subscribers on a pay-per-view basis at www.annalsnyas.org.

The paper used in this publication meets the minimum requirements of the National Standard for Information Sciences Permanence of Paper for Printed Library Materials, ANSI Z39.48_1984.

ISSN: 0077-8923 (print); 1749-6632 (online)
ISBN-10: 1-57331-597-4 (paper); ISBN-13: 978-1-57331-597-5 (paper)

A catalogue record for this title is available from the British Library.

ANNALS OF THE NEW YORK ACADEMY OF SCIENCES

Volume 1073
August 2006

PHEOCHROMOCYTOMA
First International Symposium

Editors

KAREL PACAK AND GRAEME EISENHOFER

This volume is the result of a meeting entitled **First International Symposium on Pheochromocytoma (ISP2005)**, sponsored by the National Institutes of Health and held on October 20–23, 2005 in Bethesda, Maryland.

CONTENTS

Part II. Genetics: Increasing Importance for Clinical Decision Making

Part III. Tumor Biology, Molecular Pathways, and Genotype Phenotype Relationships

Part IV. Biochemical Diagnosis and Tumor Localization

Part V. Management

Part VI. Malignant Pheochromocytoma

Part VII. Pathology

Financial assistance was received from:

- National Institute of Child Health and Human Development, NIH
- Office of Rare Diseases, NIH
- National Cancer Institute, NIH
- National Institute of Neurological Disorders and Stroke, NIH
- National Genome Research Institute, NIH
- Molecular Insight Pharmaceuticals
- GE Healthcare
- Endocrine Technologies, Germany
- German Society of Endocrinology
- Novartis Oncology
- Daiichi Radioisotope Labs., Ltd., Japan

Preface

Pheochromocytomas and paragangliomas are neuroendocrine tumors derived, respectively, from adrenal chromaffin cells and extra-adrenal paraganglia. These catecholamine-producing tumors are rare but important causes of hypertension and have potentially lethal consequences if not diagnosed and treated appropriately. Improvements in diagnosis, localization, management, and treatment of pheochromocytomas and paragangliomas are being heralded by recent leaps in our understanding of these genetics and biology of these tumors coupled with advances in fields such as analytical chemistry, genomics, molecular biology, biotechnology, and nuclear medicine. Ineffective treatments for malignant pheochromocytoma, inadequate methods to distinguish malignant from benign disease, and lack of consensus about how to apply recent scientific and medical advances to improve diagnosis and management of patients with these tumors remain important unresolved problems.

The material in this volume was compiled from the proceedings of the First International Symposium on Pheochromocytoma (ISP2005), held in Bethesda, Maryland, from October 20 to 23, 2005. The incentive for ISP2005 arose from a workshop on malignant pheochromocytoma held at Cold Spring Harbor in the fall of 2003 at the behest of Drs. James Watson and William Manger. The Pheochromocytoma Research Support Organization (PRESSOR) was established from that workshop with the objective of facilitating collaborations and sharing materials, information, and expertise among investigators and clinicians interested in research about pheochromocytoma (for information visit the PRESSOR website, http://www.pressor.org). The venue and organization for ISP2005 were decided on at a PRESSOR work group meeting held in the summer of 2004.

The focus of ISP2005 was to provide an update on recent advances in genetics, biochemical diagnosis, tumor localization, and management and treatment of patients with pheochromocytomas and paragangliomas. Such advances and improvements in our understanding of these tumors are being achieved through the efforts of basic scientists and clinical investigators working in a variety of disparate disciplines, most of whom rarely have the opportunity to meet together in person. This symposium enabled these investigators to meet and share their expertise and knowledge among themselves and with other health care professionals who see the patients, as well as with the patients themselves.

An important feature of the symposium centered around several breakout sessions held to stimulate discussion on issues that could benefit from resolution in the form of recommendations, or, where possible, some form of

Ann. N.Y. Acad. Sci. 1073: xv–xvi (2006). © 2006 New York Academy of Sciences.
doi: 10.1196/annals.1353.061

consensus from leaders in the field. Under the guidance of impartial moderators, participants were asked to formulate recommendations that were subsequently discussed and agreed upon at a final general session of the symposium at which all attendees could be present. The summaries of those sessions, with outlined recommendations, are included at the beginning of five of the seven sections of this volume: Part 2, Genetics; Part 4, Biochemical Diagnosis and Localization; Part 5, Management; Part 6, Malignant Pheochromocytoma; and Part 7, Pathology.

The symposium attracted over 170 participants, including about 30 patients and their family members, with about two-thirds of attendees arriving from overseas and as far away as China, Japan, the Philippines, Australia, and South Africa. The editors are grateful for the time and effort of those who organized and participated in the meeting and for the final contributions of the participants to this volume. We also extend our thanks to Ms. Shiromi Perera, who assisted in compiling the contributions to this volume, and we are grateful to the Office of Rare Diseases at the National Institutes of Health (NIH) and to the many NIH Institutes and private organizations responsible for sponsoring the symposium.

The Second International Symposium on Pheochromocytoma (ISP2008), to be held at Cambridge University, is scheduled for September 17–20, 2008. For information, please contact Professor Morris J. Brown: cm121@medschl.cam.ac.uk.

—Karel Pacak
National Institute of
Child Health and Human Development
National Institutes of Health
Bethesda, Maryland 20892, USA

—Graeme Eisenhofer
National Institute of Neurological
Disorders and Stroke
National Institutes of Health
Bethesda, Maryland 20892, USA

An Overview of Pheochromocytoma

History, Current Concepts, Vagaries, and Diagnostic Challenges

WILLIAM M. MANGER

Chairman, National Hypertension Association, Inc., Clinical Professor of Medicine, New York University Medical Center, New York, New York, USA

ABSTRACT: Tragically as many as 50% of pheochromocytomas are discovered at autopsy, mainly because the diagnosis of this neuroendocrine tumor was not considered. Missing the diagnosis almost invariably results in devastating cardiovascular complications or death. Clinicians must always think of pheochromocytoma whenever evaluating a patient with sustained or paroxysmal hypertension or any manifestations suggesting hypercatecholaminemia. Very rarely, familial pheochromocytomas may cause no hypertension, symptoms, or signs. But biochemical testing can always establish the presence or absence of a pheochromocytoma, and localization with magnetic resonance imaging, computed tomography, or ^{131}I or ^{123}I-MIBG is almost always possible.

KEYWORDS: familial; metanephrine; normetanephrine; imaging; treatment

INTRODUCTION

Common manifestations induced by catecholamines include hypertension, headaches, palpitations, tachycardia, excess sweating, anxiety, tremulousness, pallor, chest and abdominal pain, nausea and vomiting, weight loss, heat intolerance, orthostatic hypotension, constipation, transitory electrocardiographic changes, and hyperglycemia. A number of peptides have been identified in pheochromocytomas, which may contribute to these manifestations when released into the circulation.

Familial pheochromocytomas may occur in patients with multiple endocrine neoplasia (MEN) syndromes and coexist with medullary thyroid carcinoma (MTC) and parathyroid hyperplasia or neoplasia and sometimes with a phenotype consisting of mucosal neuromas, thickened corneal nerves, intestinal ganglioneuromatosis, and marfanoid habitus; it may coexist with

Address for correspondence: William M. Manger, M.D., Ph.D., National Hypertension Association, 324 East 30th Street, New York, NY 10016. Voice: 212-689-0873; fax: 212-447-7032.
e-mail: nathypertension@aol.com

Ann. N.Y. Acad. Sci. 1073: 1–20 (2006). © 2006 New York Academy of Sciences.
doi: 10.1196/annals.1353.001

Von Hippel–Lindau (VHL) disease and with cutaneous neurofibromatosis. MTC releases calcitonin and sometimes serotonin into the blood, which may cause severe diarrhea. Parathyroid hyperplasia or neoplasia may cause hyperparathyroidism, and VHL disease may cause neurological manifestations and visual disturbances. Gene mutations of mitochondrial succinate dehydrogenase (SDHD and SDHB) predispose to pheochromocytomas as well as to neck and head paragangliomas.

The very large variety of symptoms and signs encountered in patients with pheochromocytoma frequently suggests a number of other conditions and may mislead and confuse the physician and cause an erroneous diagnosis. This treacherous tumor has correctly earned the title of the "Great Masquerader."

Above all, it is essential when confronted with any manifestations of these conditions that the clinician be forever alert and *think* of pheochromocytoma!

A brief chronological review of the historical highlights and investigations that have led to an understanding of the pathophysiology, biochemistry, and genetics of pheochromocytoma are worth mentioning at this first international symposium regarding this treacherous neuroendocrine tumor. The historical review was based largely on information contained in the textbook; *Clinical and Experimental Pheochromocytoma.*[1]

IDENTIFICATION OF SPORADIC AND FAMILIAL PHEOCHROMOCYTOMAS AND ASSOCIATED CONDITIONS

In 1886 Frankel first described pheochromocytomas in both adrenal glands of an 18-year-old girl who suddenly collapsed and died. She had a 1-year history of recurrent episodes of palpitations, headaches, vomiting, pallor accompanied by a strong pulse, and "retinitis." Myocardial hypertrophy and arterial changes in her kidneys, characteristic of hypertensive vascular disease, were discovered at autopsy.

In 1896 Manasse demonstrated that a pheochromocytoma developed a brownish color when exposed to chromium salts similar to that occurring in the adrenal medulla.

In 1908 Alezais and Peyron introduced the term *paraganglioma* to designate extra-adrenal chromaffin tumors arising in paraganglia, and in 1912 Pick coined the term *pheochromocytoma*, indicating tumors whose cells had affinity for chromium salts.

In 1922 L'Abbé *et al.* first made the fascinating observation of paroxysmal hypertensive crises in a 28-year-old woman who was found to have a pheochromocytoma at autopsy. This syndrome was established by Vaquez in 1926 and a pheochromocytoma was removed successfully by Roux in Switzerland and by C.H. Mayo at the Mayo Clinic in the United States in 1926.

Pincoffs is credited with first preoperatively recognizing a pheochromocytoma in 1929 that was removed successfully by Shipley. In 1938 sustained hypertension caused by an adrenal pheochromocytoma and a paraganglioma was reported by Binger and Craig, and by Palmer and Castleman, respectively.

Association of pheochromocytoma with neurofibromatosis was reported by Suzuki in 1910 and with retinal angioma (von Hippel's disease) by Glushien *et al.* in 1953. It had been noted previously that about 20% of patients with von Hippel's disease developed hemangioblastoma of the cerebellum (Lindau's disease); this combination of retinal angioma and hemangioblastoma, known as von Hippel–Lindau disease, was reported by Chapman and Diaz-Perez in 1962 and confirmed by others to occasionally coexist with pheochromocytoma. The first familial pheochromocytoma was documented in 1943 by Hyman and Mencher. In 1952 DeCourcy and DeCourcy and in 1961 Sippel reported the association of thyroid carcinoma with pheochromocytoma; also in 1961 Cushman and Manning found parathyroid adenomas in some patients harboring pheochromocytoma and thyroid carcinoma.

In 1968 Steiner *et al.* suggested that familial pheochromocytoma in association with multiple endocrine tumors (i.e., medullary thyroid carcinoma and sometimes parathyroid neoplasia) be designated multiple endocrine neoplasia (MEN) type 2. Also in the 1960s patients with a combination of pheochromocytoma, medullary thyroid carcinoma, and mucosal neuromas and sometimes a marfanoid habitus were identified and designated MEN type 2b or MEN-3 (Carney *et al.* 1976, Chong *et al.* 1975).

Genetic abnormalities responsible for these familial abnormalities have been identified, for example, mutations of the *RET* proto-oncogene on chromosome 10q likely result in MEN 2a (Simpson *et al.* [1987], Mathew *et al.* [1987], Narod *et al.* [1992]); 3p for von Hippel–Lindau disease (Latif *et al.* [1993]), and chromosome 17q for neurofibromatosis (Cawthon *et al.* [1990] and Wallace *et al.* [1990]). Most recently, germline mutations encoding succinate dehydrogenase subunits B (*SDHB*) on chromosome 1p and D (*SDHD*) on chromosome 11q predispose to head and neck paragangliomas as well as pheochromocytomas (Baysal *et al.* 2000, Astuti *et al.* 2001, Neumann *et al.* 2002, Neumann *et al.* 2004). It now appears that 20% to 30% of pheochromocytomas are familial.

HISTOPATHOLOGY AND HEMODYNAMIC CHARACTERISTICS OF PHEOCHROMOCYTOMA

Many investigators have contributed to the histopathologic characterization of pheochromocytomas, for example, Humphrey (1946), Symington and Goodall (1953), Minno *et al.* (1954), Sherwin (1959), Glenner and Grimley (1974), and Melicow (1977). Tannenbaum (1970) and Carmichael and Winkler (1985) investigated the ultrastructure of pheochromocytomas, identifying epinephrine and norepinephrine cellular granules; Lloyd *et al.* (1984), Unger *et al.* (1991), and True (1996) demonstrated the immunohistochemical characteristics of these tumors and some of their protein, peptide, and enzyme contents.

Human hemodynamic studies of pheochromocytomas by Frohlich *et al.* (1969), Levenson *et al.* (1980), and Bravo *et al.* (1990) revealed that the hemodynamics in patients with pheochromocytic hypertension were similar to that of patients with essential hypertension.

BIOCHEMICAL AND DIAGNOSTIC MILESTONES

In 1929 Rabin demonstrated a pressor agent in pheochromocytomas that was greater than that in the normal adrenal medulla, and in 1937 Beer *et al.*, using a bioassay, discovered a pressor substance in plasma during a hypertensive crisis of a patient with pheochromocytoma. In 1939 Strombeck and Hedberg, using a chemical assay, reported a marked increase in plasma epinephrine in a patient with this tumor.

In 1945 Roth and Kvale found that histamine given intravenously could precipitate an attack of marked hypertension and other manifestations in patients with pheochromocytoma. This proved valuable in detecting patients harboring the tumor but who were normotensive. In 1967 Lawrence introduced glucagon, administered intravenously, as a similar provocative test for detecting pheochromocytoma.

Goldenberg *et al.*, in 1947, reported that intravenously administering the adrenergic-blocking agent benzodioxan would dramatically lower the blood pressure of patients with pheochromocytic hypertension but had no effect on the pressure of individuals with essential hypertension or normotension. Subsequently, in 1951, Iseri reported that i.v. administration of the α-adrenergic-blocking agent phentolamine (Regitine) could more reliably lower pheochromocytic hypertension, and it became a popular drug for detecting this tumor.

Although norepinephrine was synthesized by Stolz in 1904, it attracted little attention until 1946, when von Euler reported its occurrence in the body, and that it was the neurotransmitter of sympathetic nerves. It was mainly for this discovery that he shared the Nobel Prize for Physiology or Medicine with J. Axelrod and B. Katz in 1970. In 1947 Holtz and co-workers also reported norepinephrine in the body and that the adrenal medulla contained both epinephrine and norepinephrine.

Holton, in 1949, first demonstrated norepinephrine in a pheochromocytoma and, in 1951, von Euler and Hellner showed that patients with pheochromocytomas excreted increased quantities of epinephrine and/or norepinephrine, and sometimes dopamine. (The presence of dopamine in normal urine had been reported by Holtz and co-workers in 1942.) Lund, in 1952, reported elevations of epinephrine and norepinephrine in the plasma as well as in the urine of patients with pheochromocytoma. In 1954 Goldenberg *et al.* reported results of chemically screening urine for epinephrine and norepinephrine in 16 patients with pheochromocytoma, and, in the same year, Manger *et al.* reported results of fluorometrically quantitating plasma epinephrine and norepinephrine in 13 patients with pheochromocytoma. The latter investigators established the diagnostic value of quantitating plasma catecholamines during a hypertensive episode provoked by i.v. administration of histamine in some patients with pheochromocytoma who had only paroxysmal hypertension; also, they were the first to demonstrate dopamine in the extract of a pheochromocytoma. In 1956 Weil-Malherbe identified not only the presence of dopamine but also of dihydroxyphenylalanine (dopa) in a pheochromocytoma. Subsequently, dopa was demonstrated in one malignant pheochromocytoma by Anton *et al.* in 1967 and in two benign pheochromocytomas in 1972 by Louis *et al.*

Studies by Armstrong *et al.* in 1957 and in 1959 demonstrated increased concentrations of vanilmandelic acid (VMA), a major metabolite of epinephrine and norepinephrine, in the urine of patients with pheochromocytoma. Axelrod *et al.* and La Brosse *et al.* in 1958 established that O-methylation was the principal pathway for the metabolism of epinephrine and norepinephrine in the blood and some tissues, and in the same year La Brosse *et al.* reported increased urinary concentrations of both VMA and normetanephrine in patients with pheochromocytoma. Previously, in 1937, Blaschko *et al.* had demonstrated a major pathway of catecholamine metabolism to be oxidative deamination by monoamine oxidase.

With these discoveries and improvements in methods for measuring catecholamines and their metabolites and the enzymes involved in their metabolism, Sjoerdsma *et al.* (1959), as well as Crout *et al.* (1961, 1964), Gitlow *et al.* (1961), Kopin and Axelrod (1960), and Smith and Winkler (1972) significantly clarified aspects of metabolism, function, and chemical diagnosis of pheochromocytoma.

In 1981 Bravo *et al.* developed the clonidine suppression test, which proved helpful in differentiating pheochromocytic hypertension from neurogenic hypertension; suppression of plasma norepinephrine was relied upon to identify neurogenic hypertension (67% accurate). Subsequently, in 2003, Eisenhofer *et al.* markedly improved the accuracy of the clonidine suppression test by measuring suppression of plasma normetanephrine (96% accurate).[2] The value of measuring plasma normetanephrine in diagnosing pheochromocytoma was first reported by Kobayashi, De Quatro *et al.* in 1970.[3] However, Lenders, Pacak, Eisenhofer *et al.* established that determination of plasma metanephrine and normetanephrine was the best test for excluding or confirming the presence of a pheochromocytoma; measuring these metabolites in the urine was almost as reliable for diagnosing the tumor. The sensitivity of detecting a pheochromocytoma by measuring plasma or fractionated urinary metanephrine and normetanephrine with high-performance liquid chromatography (HPLC) ranged from 97% to 99%.[4]

Especially important advancements in understanding catecholamine metabolism were made by Eisenhofer, Kopin, and Goldstein, who demonstrated that most of the metabolism of catecholamines occurs within the cells where catecholamines are synthesized and converted to normetanephrine and metanephrine.[5,6]

Additional clinicians, scientists, surgeons, and radiologists, who have very significantly improved our knowledge of the clinical characteristics, detection, localization, and management of pheochromocytoma include R.W. Gifford, Jr., G.W. Sizemore, K. Engelman, S.G. Sheps, O. Kuchel, H.R. Keiser, W.H. Remine, S.D. Averbush, J.A. van Heerden, V. De Quattro, J.C. Sisson, B. Shapiro, I.J. Fink, G. A. Deoreo, O.F. Agee, J.V. Zelch, H. Hermann, and R. Mornex.[1] Those who have contributed most significantly to understanding experimental pheochromocytoma include L. Greene, A. Tischler, B. Hoffman, P. Buu, W.M. Manger, S. Warren, R. Chute, O. Kuchel, G. Tsujimoto, and S. Simchon.[1]

CURRENT CONCEPTS OF PHEOCHROMOCYTOMA

Introduction

Think of it! This dictum is key to diagnosing pheochromocytoma. There is no more deceptive and treacherous tumor or cause of hypertension than pheochromocytoma. If not recognized and treated appropriately, it will almost always cause fatal cardiovascular events or devastating complications. The peril of overlooking this "pharmacologic bomb" is strikingly indicated by a Mayo Clinic report of 54 autopsies where pheochromocytoma contributed to 55% of deaths but was not suspected in 75% of cases.[7] Unfortunately, pheochromocytomas continue to be unrecognized and diagnosed only after they have caused the patient's death.[8] Although the exact prevalence of this tumor is uncertain, it may occur in 0.05% to 0.2% of individuals with sustained diastolic hypertension.

Origin and Pathophysiology

Pheochromocytomas occur at any age, but mostly in the fourth and fifth decades. They usually secrete norepinephrine and epinephrine (but predominantly norepinephrine); rarely dopamine and/or dopa is secreted. The following substances, mostly peptides and hormones, have been identified in some pheochromocytomas: vasoactive intestinal peptide (VIP), adrenocorticotropic hormone (ACTH), neuropeptide Y, atrial natriuretic factor, growth hormone-releasing factor, somatostatin, parathyroid hormone-related peptide, calcitonin, serotonin, and others. Some of these substances may be released into the circulation and cause a variety of physiologic, pharmacologic, and clinical manifestations.[1,9]

About 85% of pheochromocytomas arise in adrenal medullary chromaffin cells, and as many as 18% arise in extra-adrenal chromaffin cells in the abdomen, pelvis, and rarely in the chest or neck. These extra-adrenal tumors (sometimes termed paragangliomas) are more frequent in children (30%) than in adults (15%). Why 30% to 40% of extra-adrenal and only 10% of adrenal pheochromocytomas are malignant is unknown. Roughly 50% of patients harboring a pheochromocytoma have sustained but often labile systolic and diastolic hypertension, 45% have paroxysmal hypertension, some (especially those with epinephrine-secreting tumors) have hypertension alternating with hypotension, and 5% (especially patients with familial tumors) have normotension. Hypovolemia often results if hypertension is sustained and may partly account for postural hypotension encountered in many of these patients; however, downregulation of adrenergic receptors caused by excess circulating catecholamines may contribute to the postural hypotension.[1,9]

Since surgical removal of pheochromocytomas usually results in restoration of normotension, one might assume that elevated blood pressure in patients with pheochromocytoma is entirely due to elevated circulating catecholamines; however, orally administered clonidine, a centrally acting α_2-agonist that suppresses the sympathetic nervous system, reduces blood pressure in patients with pheochromocytoma to the same degree as in patients with essential hypertension. These observations suggest that both elevated circulating catecholamines and the sympathetic nervous system participate in maintaining the hypertension, which is due to increased peripheral resistance.

The mechanisms involved in maintaining blood pressure in patients and animals with pheochromocytoma are complex. Downregulation of α- and β-receptors by excess circulating catecholamines can alter cardiovascular reactivity to vasopressor agents and blood pressure responsiveness. It is noteworthy that blood pressure in some patients harboring a pheochromocytoma may be normal or only slightly elevated despite significant elevations of catecholamines.[10]

Familial Pheochromocytoma

Perhaps 20% to 30% of pheochromocytomas are familial on account of germline mutations. Coexistence of pheochromocytomas with medullary thyroid carcinoma (MTC) or c-cell hyperplasia, and parathyroid hyperplasia or neoplasia in 50% of cases constitutes multiple endocrine neoplasia (MEN) type 2a. Coexistence of pheochromocytoma with MTC, mucosal neuromas, thickened corneal nerves, alimentary tract ganglioneuromatosis, and often a marfanoid habitus, but rarely parathyroid disease, constitutes MEN type 2b. MTC may secrete calcitonin, serotonin, and prostaglandin. Pheochromocytomas may also secrete these hormones, and rarely VIP. Hypercalcitonemia suggests MTC or c-cell hyperplasia, but hypercalcitonemia can be caused by other conditions, and occasionally pheochromocytoma. Hypercalcemia may occur in the MEN syndrome or may result from parathyroid hormone secreted by some pheochromocytomas; hence, reevaluation for MEN should be performed after pheochromocytoma removal.[1,9]

Since von Hippel–Lindau disease (i.e., hemangioblastoma of the central nervous system and retinal angioma [VHL]), neurofibromatosis type 1, and carotid body tumors may coexist with familial pheochromocytoma, hypertension in any of these conditions should prompt a search for pheochromocytoma. Pheochromocytoma occurs in about 14% of patients with VHL. Patients with pheochromocytoma should be screened for MTC, VHL, and hyperparathyroidism. If familial disease is established, first-degree relatives should be evaluated for genetic mutations of the *RET* proto-oncogene on chromosome 10q for MEN 2a and 2b, on chromosome 3p for VHL, and on chromosome 17q for familial neurofibromatosis. Gene mutations of the succinate dehydrogenase family, the *SDHD* gene on chromosome 11q[11] and the *SDHB* gene on chromosome 1p,[12] may account for up to 12% of pheochromocytomas. These mutations predispose to pheochromocytomas as well as neck and head paragangliomas.[13,14] Tumors, which are usually benign, are more frequent with *SDHD* mutation carriers, but *SDHB* carriers have an increased frequency of malignancy.

Clinical and Laboratory Presentation

Sustained, labile, or paroxysmal hypertension is almost always present and is due to excess circulating catecholamines. However, very rarely pheochromocytomas, especially familial tumors, may not secrete enough catecholamines to cause hypertension. Also, a few cases of pheochromocytomas have been reported that secreted only dopamine and did not cause hypertension.

Attacks usually occur weekly, but may occur several times daily or once every few months; 80% last less than an hour but rarely they last for several days. Attacks may be precipitated by palpation of the abdomen near the tumor, postural changes, exertion, anxiety, trauma, pain, ingestion of foods or beverages containing tyramine (certain cheeses, beers, and wines), use of certain drugs (histamine, glucagon, tyramine, phenothiazine, metoclopramide, ACTH), intubation, induction of anesthesia, chemotherapy, and micturition or bladder distention (with bladder tumors).[1,9]

Manifestations that result primarily from excess circulating catecholamines and hypertension consist of severe headaches, generalized inappropriate sweating, and palpitations (with tachycardia or occasionally bradycardia), severe anxiety (fear of death), tremulousness, pain in chest and/or abdomen, nausea, vomiting, weakness, fatigue, prostration, weight loss, visual disturbances (rarely acute blindness), severe constipation (rarely pseudo-obstruction), paresthesias, face pallor (rarely flushing), and hypertensive retinopathy when hypertension is severe and sustained. Occasionally seizures occur and very rarely intense mesenteric artery vasoconstriction may cause ischemic enterocolitis with intestinal necrosis and intestinal obstruction. Intense vasoconstriction of cerebral vasculature may suggest cerebral vasculitis. Vasointestinal peptide, serotonin, or calcitonin, secreted by some pheochromocytomas, may cause diarrhea, which, if severe, may be accompanied by hypokalemia and hypochlorhydria or achlorhydria. Children may also experience polyuria, polydipsia, and convulsions.[1,9]

Pheochromocytomas, coexisting endocrine tumors, and VHL may cause abnormal laboratory results. Hypercatecholaminemia (especially elevated epinephrine) can cause hyperglycemia and hypertriglyceridemia. Calcitonin, serotonin, and prostaglandin may be secreted by MTC and pheochromocytomas, and hypercalcemia may be caused by increased secretion of parathyroid hormone from neoplasia or hyperplasia of parathyroid glands, and rarely from pheochromocytomas.[1,9]

Occasionally, a central nervous system hemangioblastoma in VHL can secrete erythropoietin and cause polycythemia. Very rarely, Cushing's syndrome may result from pheochromocytomas secreting ACTH, which elevates plasma cortisol.[1,9]

Severe catecholamine-induced vasoconstriction can cause ischemia in multiple organs and result in lactic acidosis and elevations of pancreatic, hepatic, and cardiac enzymes. Plasma renin, angiotensin II, and aldosterone may be elevated from catecholamine stimulation of renal β_1-adrenergic receptors, or, rarely, from renal artery compression by a pheochromocytoma or coexisting neurofibroma.[1,9]

Electrocardiographic changes representing arrhythmias, changes suggesting myocardial ischemia, damage, or left ventricular strain may develop. Their transient appearance during paroxysmal hypertension suggests pheochromocytoma in the absence of other causes. Permanent ECG changes can result from prolonged hypertension, myocardial ischemia, or catecholamine cardiomyopathy. However, almost any ECG change can occur, and it is not specific for pheochromocytoma.

As mentioned previously, plasma and 24-h urinary metanephrine and normetanephrine are the most sensitive (97% to 99%) biochemical tests for making the diagnosis of pheochromocytoma, and they are equally sensitive for detecting sporadic and familial pheochromocytoma (TABLE 1.) Only rarely will a clonidine suppression test be needed.[9]

TABLE 2 reveals the ranges of concentrations of catecholamines and their metabolites in adults. Urinary concentrations of catecholamines and metanephrines and normetanephrines for different ages, and excretion of catecholamines and their metabolites relative to urinary creatinine excretion (i.e., μg/g creatinine) is recorded elsewhere (see reference at bottom of TABLE 2).

TABLE 1. Sensitivity and specificity of biochemical tests for diagnosing pheochromocytoma

	Sensitivity		Specificity	
	Hereditary (%)	Sporadic (%)	Hereditary (%)	Sporadic (%)
Plasma				
Free metanephrines	98	99	96	82
Catecholamines	68	92	89	72
Urine				
Fractionated metanephrines	97	99	82	45
Catecholamines	76	90	96	75
Total metanephrines	60	88	97	89
Vanillylmandelic acid	43	76	99	86

From W.M. Manger and Eisenhofer G. 2004 Pheochromocytoma: diagnosis and management update. *Current Hypertension Reports* 6:477–484. Reprinted with permission.

Preoperative Localization

Although imaging studies are only justified after biochemical establishment of a pheochromocytoma, imaging may be justified in some patients suspected of having familial pheochromocytoma, even though biochemical tests are normal. Some familial tumors may occasionally be identified by imaging before significant amounts of catecholamines are secreted.

CT can identify 95% of adrenal pheochromocytomas 1 cm or larger, and it can localize 90% of extra-adrenal pheochromocytomas larger than 2 cm;

TABLE 2. Concentrations of catecholamines and metabolites in adults [a]

Plasma (pg/mL)	Free normetanephrine	Free metanephrine	
Normotensives (supine 30 min.)	18–101	12–67	
Hypertensives (supine 30 min.)	24–145	12–72	
	Norepinephrine	Epinephrine	Dopamine
Normotensives (supine 30 min.)	77–467	3–86	<87
Normotensives (sitting 15 min.)	120–680	<60	<87
Hypertensives (supine 30 min.)	101–692	4–125	
	Normetanephrine	Metanephrine	
Urine (μg/24 h)	105–354	74–297	
	Norepinephrine	Epinephrine	Dopamine
	15–80	0.5–20	65–400
	VMA	HVA	
Urine (mg/24 h)	1.4–6.5	1.4–8.8	

Modified from: Rosano, T.G. *et al.* 2005. Catecholamines and serotonin. *In* Tietz Textbook of Clinical Chemistry and Molecular Diagnostics, 4th ed. C.A. Burtis *et al.*, Eds.: 1033–1075. Elsevier Inc. New York. Reprinted with permission.

*VMA = vanilmandelic acid; HVA = homovanillic acid.

[a]Different laboratories may report slightly different concentrations for normal and abnormal catecholamines and their metabolites.

however, MRI is even more sensitive and more specific than CT. MRI signal intensity on T_2-weighted images can be fairly characteristic for pheochromocytoma; only rarely will other benign or malignant lesions resemble pheochromocytoma.[1,15,16] MRI is noninvasive, and CT artifacts caused by surgical clips are not encountered with MRI. Furthermore, some contrast media used with a CT scan may occasionally cause an allergic reaction; this type of reaction is almost never caused by the gadolinium media used for contrast with MRI imaging. MRI is superior to CT in detecting extra-adrenal abdominal and pelvic tumors and some cardiac[17,18] and familial adrenal pheochromocytomas.[1] Liver metastases are best detected by MRI or CT. Metastases frequently involve lymph nodes, liver, lung, and bone but not brain. Since no radiation is involved with MRI, it is ideal for imaging pregnant patients and children suspected of having pheochromocytomas.

Tumor uptake of the radiopharmaceutical agent ^{131}I-metaiodobenzylguanidine (MIBG) occurs in 81% to 85% of pheochromocytomas and is highly specific (95% to 100%) for diagnosis.[19,20] MIBG may be very helpful in detecting adrenal medullary hyperplasia, small and extra-adrenal pheochromocytomas, and metastases, because it scans the entire body. MIBG uptake may also occur in neuroblastomas, MTC, carcinoids, and small-cell lung cancer. Since uptake may be inhibited by labetalol, reserpine, calcium channel blockers, tricyclic antidepressants, sympathomimetics, cocaine, adrenergic neuron blockers, and some tranquilizers, these drugs should be discontinued 1 week before scintigraphy.[1] Most recently 6-[^{18}F]-fluorodopamine ([^{18} F]DA) positron emission tomography (PET) scan was reported to be superior to ^{131}I-MIBG scintigraphy in locating metastatic pheochromocytomas.[21]

If MRI and CT fail to demonstrate pheochromocytomas in the abdomen and pelvis, MRI of the chest, neck, and head is recommended. Whenever available, whole body MIBG scan should be performed to establish that the tumor is a pheochromocytoma and to detect any metastases before operation.

Incidentally recognized adrenal masses (incidentalomas) are encountered in 3% to 4% of patients having abdominal CT examination and, although MRI and MIBG can be especially helpful in determining that these adenomas are pheochromocytomas, plasma and urinary measurement of catecholamines, and/or their metabolites are essential to establish the diagnosis. One large survey indicated that 4.2% of incidentalomas are pheochromocytomas.[22]

Management

Preoperative, operative, and postoperative management of benign and malignant pheochromocytoma are discussed in detail elsewhere.[1,9] With the remarkable improvement of imaging techniques, laparoscopic removal of adrenal and some extra-adrenal pheochromocytomas is usually performed. Open surgical exploration of the abdomen is indicated when tumors are multiple, very large, or difficult to remove laparoscopically.

Pheochromocytoma of the bladder, chest, or neck require special surgical procedures; during pregnancy tumors usually should be removed expeditiously, but if pregnancy is carried to term, cesarean section is advisable to avoid the stress of labor and vaginal delivery.

Resection of as much of malignant pheochromocytomas as possible can be helpful in reducing catecholamines entering the circulation. Radiotherapy with ^{131}I MIBG may reduce tumor size and catecholamine secretion. Intravenous chemotherapy with cyclophosphamide, vincristine, and dacarbazine is usually reserved to treat aggressive metastatic tumors, particularly if they are symptomatic and causing pain or pressure on vital structures. X-ray radiation may be helpful in treating bone metastases. Alpha and beta blockers may control hypertension and symptoms for many years, and metyrosine can markedly inhibit catecholamine synthesis and reduce symptoms. Metyrosine and beta blockers also may prevent catecholamine cardiomyopathy.

Vagaries and Diagnostic Challenges

Pheochromocytoma has been called "the Great Masquerader," since it can mimic so many conditions, such as those listed in TABLE 3. These and other

TABLE 3. Conditions that may suggest the presence of a pheochromocytoma

1. Anxiety, *panic attacks* with labile blood pressure
2. Migraine
3. Paroxysmal atrial tachycardia
4. Hyperdynamic β-adrenergic circulatory state
5. Preeclampsia (*eclampsia with convulsions*)
6. *Unexplained shock*
7. *Unexplained multi-system organ failure and lactic acidosis*
8. Cardiomyopathy (*with failure*)
9. *Baroreflex failure*
10. Familial dysautonomia (Riley–Day syndrome)
11. *Carcinoid*
12. *Neuroblastoma*
13. *Drug-induced hypertension*
14. *Factitiously produced hypertension*
15. Cushing's syndrome
16. *Postural tachycardia syndrome (POTS)*
17. Acute infectious disease
18. *Autonomic hyperreflexia*
19. Hyperthyroidism
20. Menopause
21. Hyperglycemia without diabetes mellitus
22. *Acrodynia ("Pink disease"—mercury poisoning)*
23. Cerebral vasculitis

Modified from Manger W.M. and R.W. Gifford Jr. 1996. *Clinical and Experimental Pheochromocytoma*. Blackwell Science. Cambridge, MA.

NOTE: Conditions in italics may cause increased plasma and/or urinary catecholamines and their metabolites.

less common conditions, which may challenge the diagnostic acumen of the clinician, are discussed in detail elsewhere.[1] However, brief comments about each of the conditions in the table may be helpful in the differential diagnosis. Of course, pheochromocytoma should always be considered in any patient with hypertension of unknown cause. Furthermore, clinicians must always recall that resistance to antihypertensive medications or paroxysmal blood pressure increases during treatment with β-blockers, or marked pressure increases by conditions known to precipitate attacks (mentioned earlier), may indicate that the patient is harboring a pheochromocytoma.

1. *Anxiety* and *panic attacks* are often associated with manifestations suggesting pheochromocytoma and, accompanied by labile blood pressure, may suggest liberation of catecholamines by a pheochromocytoma. Panic attacks may be accompanied by elevations of plasma and urinary catecholamines and their metabolites.[23] However, in the absence of a panic attack, catecholamines and their metabolites are normal. Unlike patients with pheochromocytoma, individuals with anxiety or panic attacks usually have chronic emotional problems, and some may develop phobias to places where panic attacks occur or where help is limited.
2. *Severe headaches* occurring with pheochromocytoma may suggest *migraine*. However, pheochromocytomas usually cause marked blood pressure elevations, whereas migraines are not accompanied by severe elevations of blood pressure; furthermore, these headaches usually occur suddenly and stop suddenly, unlike the gradual onset and prolonged regression of migraine headaches. Sumatriptan and similar drugs generally eliminate migraine headaches, but not those caused by pheochromocytoma. When the differential diagnosis remains uncertain, it is essential to eliminate pheochromocytoma as the cause of the headaches by demonstrating normal plasma or urinary catecholamines and their metabolites.
3. *Paroxysmal atrial tachycardia* (PAT) frequently accompanied by palpitations and breathlessness may recur spontaneously and may be precipitated by use of coffee or tobacco. Tachycardia may be >150 beats per minute and may suggest hypercatecholaminemia. The very abrupt onset and abrupt termination is characteristic. Termination may occur spontaneously or can be induced by pressure on a carotid sinus or the Valsalva maneuver. PAT may be confused with transitory tachycardia suddenly appearing because of release of catecholamines from a pheochromocytoma; however, subsidence of tachycardia is gradual, unlike abrupt cessation with PAT. Headaches and hypertension are not manifestations of PAT, and biochemical tests for pheochromocytoma are not abnormal.
4. *Hyperdynamic β-adrenergic circulatory state* results from a hyperkinetic circulation with β-receptor hyperresponsiveness. Usually mild tachycardia occurs (but it may occasionally reach 170 beats per minute) and may be associated with palpitations, anxiety, chest and abdominal

discomfort, orthostatic hypertension, mild-to-moderate hypertension, and headaches. However, manifestations respond dramatically to β-blockade. Catecholamines and metabolites remain normal.

5. *Pre-eclampsia* (*eclampsia with convulsions*). Unrecognized pheochromocytoma during pregnancy carries a high risk of maternal and fetal mortality.[24] Manifestations may first appear in pregnancy, remit after delivery, and return in a subsequent pregnancy. Pheochromocytoma attacks may be aggravated or subside during pregnancy and can be confused with pre-eclampsia or eclampsia. However, pre-eclampsia usually occurs after 20 weeks of pregnancy and usually is accompanied by modest hypertension, periorbital and ankle edema, proteinuria, and an elevated blood uric acid—manifestations atypical for pheochromocytoma. Patients with pre-eclampsia may develop the HELLP syndrome (hemolysis, elevated liver enzymes, and low platelets). Myocardial infarction has occurred in several pregnant patients, probably due to catechomamine-induced coronary vasoconstriction caused by a pheochromocytoma. Myocardial infarction during pregnancy should suggest pheochromocytoma.

   Shock during labor or after delivery may suggest a ruptured uterus. Catecholamines and their metabolites may be elevated by shock or convulsions occurring with eclampsia, otherwise they remain normal during pregnancy. It is always crucial and may be lifesaving to consider pheochromocytoma as a possible cause of hypertension developing during pregnancy.
6. Pheochromocytoma should be considered in *unexplained shock*, especially if accompanied by abdominal pain, pulmonary edema, and pronounced mydriasis unreactive to light.[25] Rarely, *hemorrhagic necrosis* in a pheochromocytoma presents as an acute abdomen or cardiovascular crisis and shock. Only rarely will prompt recognition and immediate intervention reverse these conditions, which are usually lethal.[1] Shock from any cause can elevate catecholamines and their metabolites.
7. Another rare presentation is *multi-system organ failure* accompanied by severe hypertension or hypotension, encephalopathy, hyperpyrexia, and lactic acidosis (i.e., pheochromocytoma multi-system crisis or PMC).[26] However, any cause of lactic acidosis can elevate catecholamines and their metabolites.
8. It is extremely important for clinicians to appreciate that *congestive heart failure* may be a complication of catecholamine myocarditis and cardiomyopathy caused by a pheochromocytoma. Prompt recognition is crucial since appropriate treatment may return even severely depressed cardiac function to normal. The stress of congestive heart failure from any cause may increase plasma and urinary catecholamines and their metabolites. Therefore, imaging studies are needed to establish the presence of a pheochromocytoma.

9. *Baroreflex failure* and *familial dysautonomia* are conditions caused by impairment of the autonomic nervous system. Clinically they may closely resemble pheochromocytoma manifestations; however, the differential diagnosis is not difficult. Baroreflex failure is an extremely rare condition that is usually attributed to neck irradiation, damage, or section of the glossopharyngeal and/or vagal nerves during neck surgery, or degenerative changes in both nuclei of the solitary tracts of the brain stem. Sometimes no cause is evident. Clinically, baroreflex failure may closely resemble pheochromocytoma. The hallmark of baroreflex failure is marked lability of blood pressure with systolic and diastolic hypertension and tachycardia (usually lasting less than 30 min, but sometimes persisting for several days) alternating at times with hypotension and bradycardia. Some of these patients may have significantly elevated plasma catecholamines.

   The following guidelines should aid in the differential diagnosis.[27]

   a. A history of damage to the glossopharyngeal and vagal nerves or brain stem suggests baroreflex failure.
   b. Hypertension alternating with hypotension is very rare in patients with pheochromocytoma, occurring only in those secreting primarily epinephrine. Baroreflex failure is usually accompanied by periodic hypertension alternating with hypotension.
   c. In baroreflex failure blood pressure elevations may be accompanied by marked increases of plasma norepinephrine but only by slight increases of epinephrine; however, when blood pressure is normal, catecholamines are normal or subnormal. Urinary 24-h catecholamine excretion may be minimally elevated in baroreflex failure, because circulating catecholamines are elevated only during hypertensive periods. Urinary catecholamine excretion is usually elevated in patients with pheochromocytomas, and plasma and urinary metanephrines and/or normetanephrines should be invariably elevated in patients harboring a pheochromocytoma but not in baroreflex failure.
   d. The clonidine suppression test should lower plasma norepinephrine and normetanephrine in baroreflex failure during hypertensive periods (as it does in neurogenic hypertension), but it should not cause a change in norepinephrine and normetanephrine concentrations in patients with pheochromocytoma.

10. *Familial dysautonomia* is a familial disease with manifestations of disturbance of the central nervous system and impaired autonomic function. Of unknown etiology, it is a disease that occurs almost exclusively in Ashkenazi Jews and is probably the expression of an autosomal recessive gene. Anxiety, transient episodes of hypertension (especially precipitated by excitement), orthostatic hypotension, and excessive perspiration are

almost constant findings, and sometimes gagging, vomiting, abdominal pain, and constipation occur. Hence, it is not surprising that dysautonomia has been misdiagnosed as pheochromocytoma.

The diagnosis can be made on a clinical basis, and differentiation from pheochromocytoma should be simple. The following signs are almost invariably present in dysautonomia: reduced lacrimation, disturbed swallowing, poor motor coordination, dysarthria, relative indifference to pain, corneal anesthesia, and markedly decreased taste discrimination with the absence of fungiform papillae (probably pathognomonic). Catecholamines and their metabolites are normal or decreased.

11. The *carcinoid syndrome* may sometimes mimic manifestations of pheochromocytoma; however, usually there is a characteristic intense flushing pattern (pink, red, violacious with white blotches, which may last a few minutes or hours) accompanied by normotension or hypotension, but occasionally there is sustained or episodic hypertension and tachycardia. Wheezing, diarrhea, abdominal pains, intestinal obstruction, and tricuspid and pulmonic valve abnormalities may occur. Hyperserotonemia and increased urinary excretion of 5-hydroxyindole acetic acid and tumor biopsy can establish the diagnosis of carcinoid. False-positive elevations may occur from eating serotonin-rich foods (bananas, pineapples, walnuts, pecans, avocados, etc.) or taking certain medications (acetaminophen, salicylates, L-dopa, some cough syrups). It is noteworthy that elevations of serotonin may occur in some patients with pheochromocytoma, and rarely elevations of catecholamines occur in the carcinoid syndrome. Carcinoids may also secrete kallikrein, bradykinins, tachykinins, histamine, 5-hydroxytryptophan, prostaglandins, insulin, glucagon, gastrin, ACTH, dopamine, and norepinephrine.
12. *Neuroblastoma* must be differentiated from pheochromocytoma in young children. Neuroblastoma is one of the most common malignancies of infancy and childhood, usually occurring under the age of 5 years. Rarely, the tumor is diagnosed in the second decade. Generally, it occurs in an adrenal gland (rarely bilaterally), but it may arise elsewhere in the abdomen, chest, neck, and head. Neuroblastoma is usually functional. Dihydroxyphenyl-alanine (dopa), dopamine, norepinephrine, vanilmandelic acid, and homovanillic acid (HVA) may be increased in the urine, and paroxysmal attacks and manifestations seen in patients with pheochromocytoma may occur. Hypertension occurs in about 50% of cases. Manifestations of tumor malignancy (anorexia, weight loss, metastatic nodules, and neurological abnormalities, etc.) are often present. Concentrations of dopa, dopamine, and HVA are commonly elevated in neuroblastoma but not in patients with pheochromocytoma; furthermore, norepinephrine and normetanephrine may be elevated, but not epinephrine or metanephrine. Biopsy of the tumor or metastatic lesions provides the definitive diagnosis.

13. *Consumption of certain illegal substances* (amphetamines, cocaine, phencyclidine, lysergic acid diethylamide), and *some prescription and nonprescription drugs* containing phenylpropanolamine or ephedrine) may cause manifestations mimicking pheochromocytoma and may elevate catecholamines during the hypertension they cause.
14. *Factitious* production of manifestations suggesting pheochromocytoma (pseudo-pheochromocytoma) should be considered in emotionally disturbed persons who have access to prescription drugs containing catecholamines.[1]
15. Very rarely a patient with a pheochromocytoma may secrete ACTH and present as *Cushing's syndrome* with elevated serum and urine cortisol concentrations.[24] The demonstration of a tumor that is secreting catecholamines and their metabolites and ACTH establishes the diagnosis.
16. Another very rare condition, *chronic orthostatic intolerance with postural tachycardia syndrome (POTS)* may present with some of the manifestations of pheochromocytoma, for example, headache, anxiety, pallor, sweating, tremulousness, nausea, and abdominal pain.[28] However, the absence of hypertension at any time would almost eliminate the diagnosis of pheochromocytoma; furthermore, plasma and urinary catecholamines and their metabolites are elevated in this condition only during periods of orthostatic tachycardia.[29]
17. *Unexplained acute infection* may be simulated by a pheochromocytoma because of catecholamine-induced pyrexia and a marked elevation of the white blood cell count (epinephrine provoked). Infections without accompanying complications do not cause increased catecholamines and their metabolites.
18. *Autonomic hyperreflexia*: Patients with transverse cervical spinal cord lesions frequently (85% of patients) have spontaneous or induced stimulation of the autonomic nervous system accompanied by severe headaches, marked paroxysmal hypertension with sweating and flushing of the head and neck—but pallor and decreased skin temperature elsewhere. During hypertensive attacks, catecholamines and their metabolites may be elevated, but at other times the blood pressure, catecholamines, and metabolites tend to be normal or decreased.
19. *Hyperthyroidism*, with its manifestations of tachycardia, diaphoresis, weight loss, tremor, and hypertension, may suggest the presence of a pheochromocytoma. However, hypertension is usually only systolic on account of increased cardiac output, but diastolic hypertension may also occur. The presence of an enlarged thyroid, exophthalmos, and a lid lag are often present, but a depressed thyroid-stimulating hormone (TSH) is diagnostic. Catecholamines and their metabolites are normal.
20. *Menopause* may be associated with sustained or labile hypertension, and with paroxysms of flushing (hot flashes) and sweating which may awaken the patient at night. There are often some emotional lability and

manifestations of atrophic vaginitis and vulvitis. Signs and symptoms of the menopause are dramatically relieved by estrogen administration, whereas no benefit occurs in patients with pheochromocytoma. Catecholamines and their metabolites remain normal.

21. *Diabetes mellitus*: Hyperglycemia occurs in 65% and 56% of patients with pheochromocytoma and sustained or paroxysmal hypertension, respectively; this results from increased glycogenolysis and inhibition of insulin secretion caused by hypercatecholaminemia. Therefore, it is essential to always consider pheochromocytoma whenever hyperglycemia and hypertension coexist, especially in the absence of diabetes and its complications. Levels of catecholamines and their metabolites are normal in diabetes without complications; however, the development of acidosis can significantly increase catecholamines and their metabolites.
22. *Acrodynia (Pink disease—mercury poisoning)* is usually a disease of infants and young children but rarely affects adults. Mercury poisoning may cause abdominal pain, hypertension, tachycardia, diaphoresis, parethesias, hyperglycemia, weakness, memory loss, and psychic instability. Erythema of fingers, toes, nose, and buttocks, and desquamation of the palms and soles may occur. There may be a history of mercury exposure, but this may not be evident. Severe poisoning from mercury-contaminated seafood can cause neurological manifestations and death. Slight elevations of catecholamines and their metabolites in the blood and urine have been reported, but increased mercury levels in the blood and urine are diagnostic of mercury poisoning.
23. *Cerebral vasculitis* may rarely be simulated by pheochromocytoma. We reported two 33-year-old women who presented with severe headaches, hypertension, blurred vision but normal fundi, paresthesias, muscle weakness, and dysarthria. One developed seizures and expired, and the other became blind, quadriplegic, and with limited ability to verbalize. Both had pheochromocytomas.[1] These tragic cases illustrate the extreme importance of considering pheochromocytoma as the cause of fluctuating neurologic symptoms—especially when associated with hypertensive episodes. Segmental narrowing of cerebral arteries, evident on cerebral angiograms, suggested a vasculopathy to an expert consultant and the radiologists. However, segmental narrowing of the cerebral arteries probably resulted from vasoconstriction due to excess circulating norepinephrine. It is unknown whether cerebral vasculitis has any significant effect on the level of catecholamines and their metabolites.

Many of these conditions can be excluded clinically. It is important to recognize that some of these conditions and many types of stress (e.g., strenuous exercise, myocardial infarction, congestive heart failure, hypoglycemia, increased intracranial pressure, hypoxia, acidosis, surgery, trauma) and certain medications may elevate plasma and urinary catecholamines and their metabolites or interfere with their analysis. However, few conditions increase them to levels occurring with pheochromocytoma.

All of these rare and unusual presentations of pheochromocytoma require clinical acumen and a knowledge of the vagaries of pheochromocytoma; however, above all, *the key to diagnosis, of course, is to first think of this treacherous tumor*. Failure to consider pheochromocytoma in the differential diagnosis may result in the patient's death.

REFERENCES

1. Manger, W.M. & R.W. Gifford, Jr. 1996. Clinical and Experimental Pheochromocytoma. Blackwell Science. Cambridge, MA.
2. Eisenhofer, G., D.S. Goldstein & M.M. Walther. 2003. Biochemical diagnosis of pheochromocytoma: how to distinguish true from false-positive test results. J. Clin. Endocrinol. Metab. **88:** 2656–2666.
3. Kobayashi, K., V. De Quatro , R. Kolloch, *et al.* 1980. A radioenzymatic assay for plasma normetanephrine in man and patients with pheochromocytoma. Life Sci. **26:** 567–573.
4. Lenders, J.W.M., K. Pacak, M.M. Walther, *et al.* 2002. Biochemical diagnosis of pheochromocytoma: which test is best? JAMA **287:** 1427–1434.
5. Eisenhofer, G., I.J. Kopin & D.S. Goldstein. 2004. Catecholamine metabolism: a contemporary view with implications for physiology and medicine. Pharmacol. Rev. **56:** 331–349.
6. Eisenhofer, G., D.S. Goldstein, I.J. Kopin, *et al.* 2003. Pheochromocytoma: rediscovery as a catecholamine-metabolizing tumor. Endocr. Pathol. **14:** 193–212.
7. Sutton, M., S.G. Sheps & J.L. Lie. 1981. Prevalence of clinically unsuspected pheochromocytoma. Mayo Clin. Proc. **56:** 354–360.
8. McNeil, A.R., B.H. Blok, T.D. Koelmeyer, *et al.* 2000. Pheochromocytoma discovered during coronal autopsies in Sydney, Melbourne and Auckland. Aust. N.Z. J. Med. **30:** 648–652.
9. Manger, W.M. & G. Eisenhofer. 2004. Pheochromocytoma: diagnosis and management update. Curr. Hypert. Rep. **6:** 477–484.
10. Bravo, E.L., R.W. Gifford, Jr. & W.M. Manger. 1993. Adrenal medullary tumors: pheochromocytoma. *In* Endocrine Tumors. L.L. Mozzaferri & N.A. Samaan, Eds.: **28:** 426–447. Blackwell Scientific. Boston, MA.
11. Baysal, B.E., R.E. Ferrell, J.E. Willett-Brozick, *et al.* 2000. Mutations in SDHD, a mitochondrial complex II gene, in hereditary paraganglioma. Science **287:** 848–851.
12. Astuti, D., F. Latif, A. Dallol, *et al.* 2001. Gene mutations in the succinate dehydrogenase subunit SDHB cause susceptibility to familial pheochromocytoma and to familial paraganglioma. Am. J. Human Genetics **69:** 49–54.
13. Neumann, H.P.H., B. Bausch, S.R. Whinney, *et al.* 2002. Germ-line mutations in nonsyndromic pheochromocytoma.N. Engl. J. Med. **346:** 1459–1466.
14. Neumann, H.P.H., C. Pawlu, M. Peczkowska, *et al.* 2004. Distinct clinical features of paraganglioma syndromes associated with *SDHB* and *SDHD* gene mutations. JAMA **292:** 943–951.

15. FINK, I.J., J.W. REINIG, A.J. DWYER, *et al.* 1985. J. Comput. Assist. Tomogr. **9:** 454–458.
16. BAKER, E.M., C. SPRITZER, R. BLINDER, *et al.* 1987. Benign adrenal lesions, mimicking malignancy on MR imaging: report of two cases. Radiology **163:** 669–671.
17. JEBARA, V.A., M.S. UVA, A. FARGE, *et al.* 1992. Cardiac pheochromocytomas. Ann. Thorac. Surg. **53:** 356–361.
18. STOWERS, S.A., P. GILMORE, M. STERLING, *et al.* 1987. Cardiac pheochromocytoma involving the left main coronary artery presenting with exertional angina. Am. Heart J. **114:** 423–427.
19. SISSON, J.C., M.S. FRAGER, T.W. VALK, *et al.* 1981. Scintigraphic localization of pheochromocytoma. N. Engl. J. Med. **305:** 12–17.
20. JALIL, N.D., F.N. PATTOU, F. COMBEMALE, *et al.* 1998. Effectiveness and limits of preoperative imaging studies for the localizations of pheochromocytomas and paragangliomas: a review of 282 cases. Eur. J. Surg. **164:** 23–28.
21. ILIAS, I., J. YU, J.A. CARRASQUILLO, *et al.* 2003. Superiority of 6-[18F]-fluorodopamine positron emission tomography versus [^{131}I]-metaiodobenzylguanidine scintigraphy in the localization of metastatic pheochromocytoma. J. Clin. Endocrinol. Metab. **88:** 4083–4087.
22. MANTERO, F., T. MASSIMO, G. ARNOLDI, *et al.* 2000. A survey on adrenal incidentaloma in Italy. J. Clin. Endocrinol. Metab. **85:** 637–644.
23. WILKINSON, D.J.C., J. M. THOMPSON, G. W. LAMBERT, *et al.* 1998. Sympathetic activity in patients with panic disorder at rest, under laboratory mental stress, and during panic attacks. Arch. Gen. Psychiatry **55:** 511–520.
24. MANGER, W.M. 2005. The vagaries of pheochromocytoma. Am. J. Hypertension **18:** 1266–1270.
25. BERGLAND, B.E. 1989. Pheochromocytoma presenting as shock. Am. J. Emerg. Med. **7:** 44–48.
26. NEWELL, K.A., R.A. PRINZ, J. PICKLEMAN, *et al.* 1988. Pheochromocytoma multisystem crisis: a surgical emergency. Arch. Surg. **123:** 956–959.
27. MANGER, W.M. 1993. Baroreflex failure—a diagnostic challenge. N. Engl. J. Med. **329:** 1494–1495.
28. STEWART, J.M. 2004. Chronic orthostatic intolerance and the postural tachycardia syndrome (POTS). J. Pediatr. **145**(6): 725–730.
29. ROBERTSON, D., N. FLATTEM, T. TELLIOGLU, *et al.* 2001. Familial orthostatic tachycardia due to norepinephrine transporter deficiency. Ann. N. Y. Acad. Sci. **940:** 527–543.

Paragangliomas

Clinical Overview

WILLIAM F. YOUNG, JR.

Division of Endocrinology, Diabetes, Metabolism, Nutrition, and Internal Medicine, Mayo Clinic, and Mayo Foundation, Rochester, Minnesota, USA

ABSTRACT: Paragangliomas are rare tumors that arise from extra-adrenal paraganglia. The effective diagnosis and management of the paraganglioma patient involves the close collaboration of endocrinologists, endocrine surgeons, anesthesiologists, geneticists, laboratory specialists, radiologists, oncologists, and pathologists. Paragangliomas are diagnosed in the following clinical settings: signs and symptoms related to catecholamine hypersecretion, mass effect symptoms (e.g., with head and neck paragangliomas), incidental finding on imaging, or family screening for hereditary paraganglioma. Paragangliomas that hypersecrete catecholamines may cause signs and symptoms identical to those in patients with hyperfunctioning adrenal pheochromocytoma. When a catecholamine-secreting tumor is suspected in a patient because of paroxysmal symptoms, biochemical documentation of catecholamine and fractionated metanephrine hypersecretion should precede any form of imaging study. Catecholamine-secreting paragangliomas are found where chromaffin tissue is located (e.g., along the para-aortic sympathetic chain, or within the organs of Zuckerkandl at the origin of the inferior mesenteric artery, the wall of the urinary bladder, and the sympathetic chain in the neck or mediastinum). As many as 50% of paragangliomas are hereditary and may be associated with familial paraganglioma, neurofibromatosis Type 1, von Hippel–Lindau disease, the Carney triad, and, rarely, with multiple endocrine neoplasia Type 2. Genetic testing should be considered in all patients with paraganglioma. The treatment of choice for paraganglioma is surgical resection; most tumors are benign and can be excised totally. Following surgical cure, annual biochemical testing assesses for metastatic disease, tumor recurrence or delayed appearance of multiple primary tumors.

KEYWORDS: paraganglioma; metanephrines; catecholamines

Paraganglia are specialized neural crest-derived cells (chromaffin cells) that are divided into sympathetic and parasympathetic paraganglia.[1,2] The sympathetic

Address for correspondence: William F. Young, Jr., M.D., Mayo Clinic, 200 First Street S.W. Rochester, MN 55905, USA. Voice: 507-284-2191; fax: 507-284-5745.
e-mail: Young.William@Mayo.edu

**Ann. N.Y. Acad. Sci. 1073: 21–29 (2006). © 2006 New York Academy of Sciences.
doi: 10.1196/annals.1353.002**

paraganglia are symmetrically distributed along the paravertebral axis from high in the neck near the superior cervical ganglion to the abdomen and pelvis. Small sympathetic paraganglia can also be associated with organs such as the urinary bladder and prostate gland. The parasympathetic paraganglia are primarily localized to the skull base and neck. Paragangliomas are rare tumors that arise from extra-adrenal paraganglia; they represent 10–18% of all chromaffin tissue–related tumors.[3–5] The diagnosis, localization, and treatment of paragangliomas offer potential cure of symptoms associated with functional tumors, prevention of a lethal hypertensive paroxysm, prevention of morbidity from mass effects, and the early diagnosis of malignant tumors. The effective diagnosis and management of the paraganglioma patient involves the close collaboration of endocrinologists, endocrine surgeons, anesthesiologists, geneticists, laboratory specialists, radiologists, oncologists, and pathologists.

CLINICAL PRESENTATION

Paragangliomas are diagnosed in the following clinical settings: signs and symptoms related to catecholamine hypersecretion, mass effect symptoms (e.g., with head and neck paragangliomas), incidental finding on imaging, or family screening for hereditary paraganglioma. We recently reported our experience with benign paragangliomas diagnosed over a 20-year period at Mayo Clinic.[6] The patient population consisted of 141 females (60%) and 95 males (40%). The mean age at the time of diagnosis was 47 ± 16 years (range: 14–93). Most of the patients presented with mass effect symptoms or an incidental imaging finding; only 20% had documented catecholamine hypersecretion. In the patients with catecholamine hypersecretion, most tumors were localized to the abdomen and pelvis. Only 3.6% of the head and neck paragangliomas were documented to have catecholamine hypersecretion.[6]

Paragangliomas that hypersecrete catecholamines may cause signs and symptoms identical to those in patients with hyperfunctioning adrenal pheochromocytoma. Episodic symptoms may occur in spells, or paroxysms, that can be extremely variable in presentation but typically include forceful heartbeat, pallor, tremor, headache, and diaphoresis. The spell may start with a sensation of a "rush" in the chest and a sense of shortness of breath, followed by a "pounding" heartbeat in the chest that typically progresses to a throbbing headache. Peripheral vasoconstriction with a spell results in cool/cold hands and feet and facial pallor. Increased sense of body heat and sweating are common symptoms that occur toward the end of the spell. Spells may be either spontaneous or precipitated by postural change, anxiety, medications (e.g., metoclopramide, anesthetic agents), exercise, or maneuvers that increase intra-abdominal pressure (e.g., change in position, lifting, defecation, exercise, colonoscopy, pregnancy, trauma). Catecholamine-secreting urinary bladder paragangliomas may be associated with painless hematuria and paroxysmal attacks induced by micturition or bladder distension. Although the types of spells experienced across the patient population are highly variable, spells tend to be stereotypical for each patient. Spells may occur multiple times daily or as infrequently as once in a month. The typical duration of a catecholamine-secreting tumor spell is 15–20 min, but it may be much shorter or last several hours.

DIAGNOSIS

When a catecholamine-secreting tumor is suspected in a patient because of paroxysmal symptoms, biochemical documentation of catecholamine and metanephrine hypersecretion should precede any form of imaging study. Most major reference laboratories in the United States measure fractionated catecholamines by high-pressure liquid chromatography with electrochemical detection and fractionated metanephrines by liquid or gas chromatography tandem mass spectrometry methods. Refined laboratory techniques have overcome the problems associated with fluorometric analysis (e.g., false-positive results caused by α-methyldopa and other drugs with high native fluorescence). Fractionated catecholamines and metanephrines can be measured in the blood or the urine.[7,8] The biochemical documentation of a catecholamine-secreting tumor is reviewed in detail in accompanying articles in this volume.

LOCALIZATION

Catecholamine-secreting paragangliomas are found where chromaffin tissue is located (e.g., along the para-aortic sympathetic chain, or within the organs of Zuckerkandl at the origin of the inferior mesenteric artery,[9] the wall of the urinary bladder, and the sympathetic chain in the neck or mediastinum (FIG. 1).[4,6,10] The imaging characteristics on MRI scanning are quite typical for paraganglioma. If the results of abdominal imaging are negative or if additional sites of disease are sought, scintigraphic localization with ^{123}I-metaiodobenzylguanidine is indicated. In certain cases, ^{18}F-fluorodeoxyglucose (FDG) positron emission tomography (PET) may be indicated to investigate metastatic disease (FIG. 2).[11] The approach to localization of a catecholamine-secreting tumor is reviewed in detail in other articles in this volume.

GENETIC AND SYNDROMIC FORMS OF PARAGANGLIOMA

Overall, 10–50% of paragangliomas are hereditary. Catecholamine-secreting paragangliomas may be associated with familial paraganglioma, neurofibromatosis Type 1, von Hippel-Lindau disease, Carney triad, and, rarely, multiple endocrine neoplasia (MEN) Type 2. From the Mayo Clinic series of

(A)

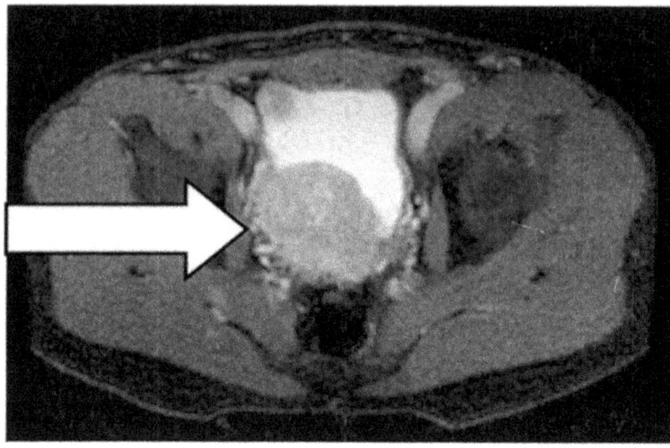

(B)

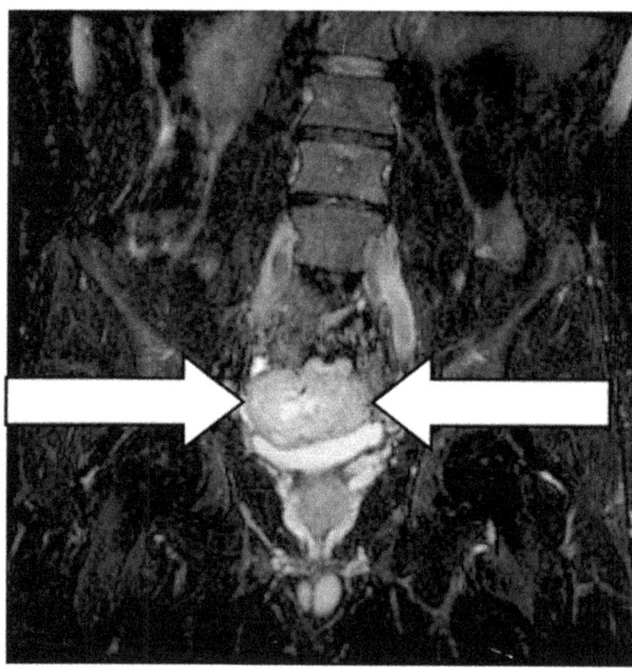

FIGURE 1. Magnetic resonance imaging (MRI) in a 43-year-old man with a catecholamine-secreting paraganglioma arising from the superior/posterior urinary bladder wall and associated with a mutation in *SDHB* (IVS3-1 G > C). (**A**) Axial MRI shows a 6.1 × 3.8 × 6.7-cm vascular mass (*arrows*) intimately associated with the posterior aspect of the urinary bladder. (**B**) Coronal MRI shows the paraganglioma (*arrows*) just superior to the urinary bladder.

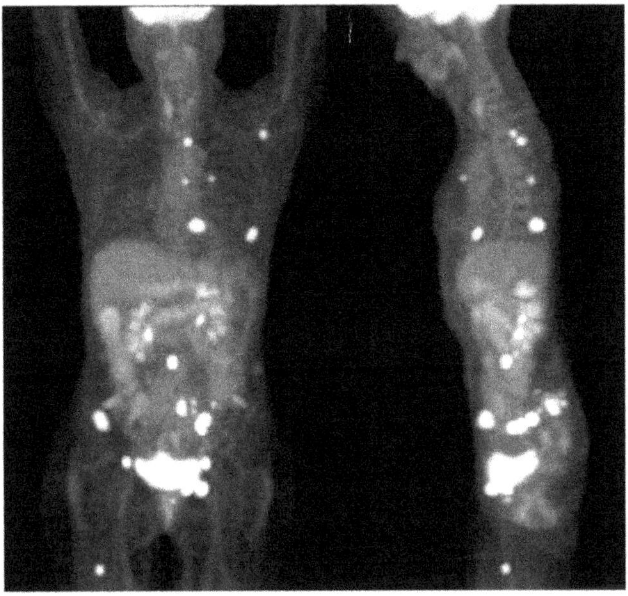

FIGURE 2. F-18 flurodeoxyglucose (FDG) positron emission tomography (PET) scan from a 46-year-old woman, who had a 2.5-cm urinary bladder paraganglioma resected 9 years ago. The patient developed recurrent signs and symptoms of a catecholamine-secreting tumor 4 years after the initial operation, and a 2-cm sacral metastasis and an involved iliac lymph node were removed. Six years after the initial operation, painful bony metastatic disease was treated with radiotherapy to the lumbar spine, iliac crest, and femur. Mutation testing for *SDHB* was positive (c.268 C > T). Nine years after the initial operation, the fractionated plasma-free metanephrines remained abnormal: metanephrines were 0.44 nmol/L (normal <0.5) and normetanephrines 30.0 nmol/L (normal <0.9). The FDG-PET scan shows diffuse skeletal and lymph node metastases on the anterior–posterior (*left panel*) and lateral images (*right panel*).

236 paraganglioma patients, 29 patients (12.3%) had a documented family history of paragangliomas; 19 of these had familial paraganglioma, 5 had von Hippel–Lindau disease, and 1 had MEN Type 2B; 4 patients presented with the Carney triad (paraganglioma, gastric stromal sarcoma, and pulmonary chondroma).[6] The Carney triad or syndrome is a rare disorder that primarily affects young women and includes gastric stromal sarcoma, pulmonary chondroma, paraganglioma, adrenal cortical adenoma, and esophageal leiomyomas.[12] The longest reported interval between detection of the first and second components of the syndrome is 26 years (mean: 8.4 years; median: 6 years).[12] The Carney triad is a chronic, persistent, and indolent disease. Although the disorder may be familial, the responsible gene has yet to be identified.

Familial paraganglioma is a rare disorder characterized by slow-growing tumors derived from paraganglia tissue in the head and neck, thorax, abdomen, and pelvis. Disease-causing mutations in three genes (*SDHB, SDHC,* and

SDHD) encoding subunits of succinate dehydrogenase (SDH), or mitochondrial complex II, are responsible for most cases of familial paraganglioma.[13–16] From December 2001 through October 2005, 42 unrelated patients with paraganglioma completed SDH mutation testing at Mayo Clinic. Six (46%) of 13 patients with head and neck paragangliomas had *SDHD* ($n = 5$) or *SDHC* ($n = 1$) mutations; all 5 of the patients with *SDHD* mutations had a known family history of paraganglioma. Seventeen (59%) of 29 patients with chest or abdominal or pelvic paragangliomas had mutations in *SDHB*; only 3 of the 17 patients with mutations had a known family history of paraganglioma. In 2002, we reported the very interesting association between a mutation in *SHDB* and malignant paraganglioma in a father and a son; the clinical course of metastatic paraganglioma in the father was clinically indolent with a 30-year survival with metastatic disease.[17] Subsequently, the link between malignant paraganglioma and mutations in *SDHB* was confirmed in 5 (63%) of 8 patients with *SDHB* mutations in a report from France[18] and 11 (34%) of 32 patients with *SDHB* mutations in a report from Germany.[16] Twelve (71%) of our 17 patients with mutations in *SDHB* had metastatic paraganglioma; all are alive and have the typical indolent clinical course we reported previously (alive at 10, 10, 11, 20, 31, 33, and 33 years after diagnosis of malignant paraganglioma).

Understanding the relationship between mutations in *SDHB*, *SDHC*, and *SDHD* and the clinical manifestations of familial paraganglioma assists in management, genetic testing, and appropriate genetic counseling. The SDH Mutation Database tool, based on the Leiden Open (source) Variation Database system at http://chromium.liacs.nl/lovd˙sdh/ provides an overview of all known *SDH* mutations and the associated tumor types.[19] Given the considerable cost of genetic testing, using a stepwise approach when evaluating a patient for the presence of an *SDH* mutation is prudent.[20] Thus, when deciding which genetic test to order first, the clinician must consider tumor location, tumor hormonal status, presence of malignancy, existence of multifocal tumors, and family history.[20] The familial and genetic forms of paraganglioma are also discussed in this volume.

TREATMENT

The treatment of choice for paraganglioma is surgical resection; most tumors are benign and can be excised totally. From the Mayo Clinic series, of the 246 resected benign paragangliomas, the average volume was 17.1 cm^3 for head and neck tumors and 94.1 cm^3 for tumors below the neck. If the tumor is catecholamine secreting, the chronic and acute effects of excess circulating catecholamines should be reversed prior to the operation. Combined α- and β-adrenergic blockades are required preoperatively to control blood pressure and to prevent intra-operative hypertensive crises. An α-adrenergic blockade should be started at least 7 days preoperatively to allow for expansion of the contracted blood volume. A liberal salt diet is advised during the preoperative period. Once adequate α-adrenergic blockade is achieved, β-adrenergic blockade is initiated (e.g., 3 days preoperatively). With this approach, only 7% of patients undergoing catecholamine-secreting tumor resection at Mayo Clinic have needed postoperative hemodynamic management.[21] The treatment of patients with pheochromocytoma and paraganglioma are further discussed in this volume.

POSTOPERATIVE AND LONG-TERM FOLLOW-UP

Approximately 1–2 weeks after surgery, 24-h urinary fractionated catecholamines and metanephrines or fractionated plasma metanephrines should be measured. If the levels are normal, the resection of the biochemically active paraganglioma should be considered complete. Increased levels of catecholamines and/or fractionated metanephrines detected postoperatively are consistent with residual tumor due to either a second primary lesion or occult metastases. Twenty-four-hour urinary excretion of fractionated catecholamines and metanephrines or fractionated plasma metanephrines should be checked annually for life. Annual biochemical testing assesses for metastatic disease, tumor recurrence, or delayed appearance of multiple primary tumors. Follow-up imaging (e.g., CT, MRI, ^{123}I-MIBG, FDG-PET) is not needed unless the fractionated metanephrine and/or catecholamine levels become elevated or if the original tumor was associated with no or minimal catecholamine/fractionated metanephrine excess. In addition, all first-degree relatives of a patient with paraganglioma should have biochemical testing (e.g., 24-h urine exammation for fractionated metanephrines and catecholamines).

Genetic testing should be considered in all patients with paraganglioma. A mutation should be confirmed in an affected individual before genetic testing is offered to at-risk asymptomatic relatives. Genetic testing can be complex; testing one family member clearly has implications for related individuals. Genetic counseling is recommended to help families understand the implications of genetic test results, to coordinate testing of at-risk relatives, and to help families work through the psychosocial issues that may arise before, during, or after the testing process. If mutation testing in a patient is positive, first-degree relatives (patient's parents, siblings, and children) should offered genetic testing.

REFERENCES

1. Lack, E.E. 2000. Tumours of adrenal and extra-adrenal paraganglia. *In* Histological Typing of Endocrine Tumors, 2nd. ed. Solae, G. Kloppel & L.H. Sobin, Eds.: 38–48. Springer. Berlin.
2. Fries, J.G. & J.A. Chamberlin. 1968. Extra-adrenal pheochromocytoma: literature review and report of a cervical pheochromocytoma. Surgery **63**: 268–279.

3. Lloyd, R.V., A.S. Tischer, N. Kimura, *et al.* 2004. Adrenal tumors: introduction. *In* World Health Organization Classification of Tumours: Pathology and Genetics of Tumours of Endocrine Organs. R.A. DeLellis, R.V. Lloyd, P.U. Heitz & C. Eng, Eds.: 136–138. IARC Press. Lyon, France.
4. Whalen, R.K., A.F. Althausen & G.H. Daniels. 1992. Extra-adrenal pheochromocytoma. J. Urol. **147**: 1–10.
5. Beard, C.M., S.G. Sheps, L.T. Kurland, *et al.* 1983. Occurrence of pheochromocytoma in Rochester, Minnesota, 1950 through 1979. Mayo Clin. Proc. **58**: 802–804.
6. Erickson, D., Y.C. Kudva, M.J. Ebersold, *et al.* 2001. Benign paragangliomas: clinical presentation and treatment outcomes in 236 patients. J. Clin. Endocrinol. Metab. **86**: 5210–5216.
7. Lenders, J.W., K. Pacak, M.M. Walther, *et al.* 2002. Biochemical diagnosis of pheochromocytoma: which test is best? JAMA. **287**: 1427–1434.
8. Kudva, Y.C., A.M. Sawka & W.F. Young Jr. 2003. Clinical review 164: the laboratory diagnosis of adrenal pheochromocytoma: the Mayo clinic experience. J. Clin. Endocrinol. Metab. **88**: 4533–4539.
9. Brantigan, C.O. & R.Y. Katase. 1969. Clinical and pathologic features of paragangliomas of the organ of Zuckerkandl. Surgery **65**: 898–905.
10. O'Riordain, D.S., W.F. YoungJr & C.S. Grant, *et al.* 1996. Clinical spectrum and outcome of functional extra-adrenal paraganglioma. World J. Surg. **20**: 916–921.
11. Ilias, I., J. Yu, J.A. Carrasquillo, *et al.* 2003. Superiority of 6-[(18)F]-fluorodopamine positron emission tomography versus [(131)I]-metaiodobenzylguanidine scintigraphy in the localization of metastatic pheochromocytoma. J. Clin. Endocrinol. Metab. **88**: 4083–4087.
12. Carney, J.A. 1999. Gastric stromal sarcoma, pulmonary chondroma, and extra-adrenal paraganglioma (Carney triad): natural history, adrenocortical component, and possible familial occurrence. Mayo Clin. Proc. **74**: 543–552.
13. Baysal, B.E., R.E. Ferrell, J.E. Willett-Brozick, *et al.* 2000. Mutations in SDHD, a mitochondrial complex II gene, in hereditary paraganglioma. Science **287**: 848–851.
14. Benn, D.E., A.-P. Gimenez-Roqueplo, J.R. Reilly, *et al.* 2006. Clinical presentation and penetrance of pheochromocytoma/paraganglioma syndromes. J. Clin. Endocrinol. Metab. **91**: In press.
15. Schiavi, F., C.C. Boedeker, B. Bausch, *et al.* 2005. Predictors and prevalence of paraganglioma syndrome associated with mutations of the SDHC gene. JAMA **294**: 2057–2063.
16. Neumann, H.P., C. Pawlu, M. Peczkowska, *et al.* 2004. Distinct clinical features of paraganglioma syndromes associated with SDHB and SDHD gene mutations. JAMA **292**: 943–951.
17. Young, A.L., B.E. Baysal, A. Deb & W.F. YoungJr. 2002. Familial malignant catecholamine-secreting paraganglioma with prolonged survival associated with mutation in the succinate dehydrogenase B gene. J. Clin. Endocrinol. Metab. **87**: 4101–4105.
18. Gimenez-Roqueplo, A.P., J. Favier, P. Rustin, *et al.* 2003. Mutations in SDHB gene are associated with extra-adrenal and/or malignant phaeochromocytomas. Cancer Res. **63**: 5615–5621.
19. Bayley, J.P., P. Devilee & P.E. Taschner. 2005. The SDH mutation database: an online resource for succinate dehydrogenase sequence variants involved in

pheochromocytoma, paraganglioma and mitochondrial complex II deficiency. BMC Med. Genet. **6**: 39.
20. Young, W.F. Jr. & A.L. Abboud. 2006. Paraganglioma: all in the family. J. Clin. Endocrinol. Metab. **91**: 790–792.
21. Kinney, M.A., M.E. Warner, J.A. vanHeerden, *et al.* 2000. Perianesthetic risks and outcomes of pheochromocytoma and paraganglioma resection. Anesth. Analg. **91**: 1118–1123.

Characteristics of Pheochromocytoma in a 4- to 20-Year-Old Population

MARTA BARONTINI, GLORIA LEVIN, AND GABRIELA SANSO

Centro de Investigaciones Endocrinológicas (CONICET), Hospital de Niños Ricardo Gutiérrez, 1425 Buenos Aires, Argentina

ABSTRACT: Hypertension in children and adolescents has become a major health problem recently recognized, and in a significant number of patients it is due to an endocrine tumor. The aim of this study was to establish the characteristics of pheochromocytoma in a population of 58 patients between 4 and 20 years of age studied at our Center. They represented a 23% of the total population of 255 pheochromocytoma patients studied. In the younger group (under 20 years of age), there was a marked predominance of severe sustained hypertension (93%), only 7% presented paroxysmal hypertension and none of them was normotensive. The youngsters studied showed a higher incidence of bilateral adrenal pheochromocytoma (34%) and extra-adrenal pheochromocytoma (22%). Malignancy was found in 12% of these patients. In addition, the incidence of familial pheochromocytoma was elevated in these patients (39%). Surprisingly, in contrast with the adult population where the most frequent familial pheochromocytomas were multiple endocrine neoplasia (MEN) type 2A (15%), the younger population showed a higher predominance of von Hippel–Lindau (VHL) (28%) and lower incidence of MEN 2A, MEN 2B, neurofibromatosis (NF), and succinate dehydrogenase subunit B (SDHB). In the VHL group, only two patients belonging to one family, showed the R167W mutation, while the others showed novel mutations in conserved amino acids. It may be speculated that the high incidence of VHL in youngsters may account for the biochemical and clinical features they usually present.

KEYWORDS: children; pheochromocytoma; VHL; MEN 2; hypertension; catecholamines

Hypertension in children and adolescents has become a major health problem recently recognized, and in an increasing number of patients it is due to an endocrine tumor. Pheochromocytoma is a somewhat rare but important cause of secondary hypertension in children. This tumor is responsible for approximately 1% of the cases of childhood hypertension.[1,2]

Address for correspondence: Marta Barontini, M.D., Ph.D., Centro de Investigaciones Endocrinológicas, Hospital de Niños Ricardo Gutiérrez, Gallo 1360, (1425) Buenos Aires, Argentina. Voice: 054-11-4963-5931; fax: 054-114963-5930.
e-mail: mbarontini@cedie.org.ar

Ann. N.Y. Acad. Sci. 1073: 30–37 (2006). © 2006 New York Academy of Sciences.
doi: 10.1196/annals.1353.003

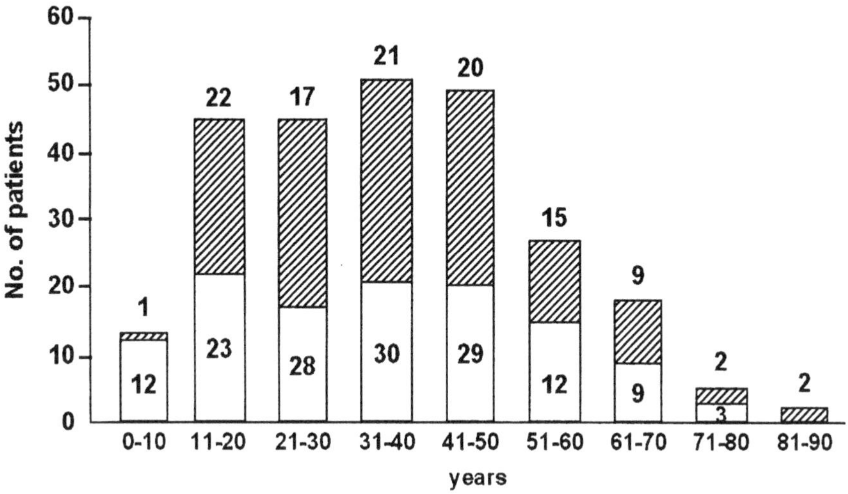

FIGURE 1. This figure depicts the frequency of pheochromocytoma according to sex and age. Total $n = 255$: males ▭ $n = 146$; females ▨ $n = 109$.

The aim of this study was to establish the characteristics of pheochromocytoma in a population of 58 patients between 4 and 20 years of age studied at our Hospital. They represent a 23% of the total population of 255 patients, aged 4–86 years, studied over a period of 40 years. Pheochromocytoma was diagnosed by determinations of urinary and plasma catecholamines (epinephrine [E], norepinephrine [NE], and dopamine).[3] Urinary vanillylmandelic acid (VMA) was also measured as well as urinary normetanephrine (NMN) and metanephrine [MN], when available.[4,5] The diagnosis was confirmed at surgery.

FIGURE 1 shows the distribution of pheochromocytoma according to sex and age. Although no clear sexual differences were found in the whole population studied, a predominance of males under 10 years of age is evident. A much greater incidence of the disease was found in both males and females as of prepuberty, decreasing after age of 50 years. The predominance of females over males during the reproductive period suggests that hormones may influence the development of the disease and also that pregnancy can activate a pheochromocytoma that had been silent so far.[6]

The clinical features of pheochromocytoma are on account of an excessive release of catecholamines produced by the tumor.[7] The diverse symptomatology is related to the relative proportions of NE and E secreted by the tumor, their pattern of release, and individual differences in catecholamines sensitivity.

Elevation of blood pressure is the most consistent manifestation of pheochromocytoma (TABLE 1). In contrast to adults, hypertension is more likely to

TABLE 1. Pheochromocytoma: Clinical findings according to age

	<20	>20
Hypertension		
Sustained	93%	68%
Without paroxysms	63%	58%
With paroxysms	37%	42%
Paroxysmal	7%	26%
Normotension	0	5%
Other symptoms		
Headache	95%	90%
Sweating	90%	92%
Visual disturbances	80%	47%
Neurologic signs	65%	57%
Tachycardia, dysrhythmias	35%	72%
Weight loss	15%	72%

be sustained in children, with or without paroxysmal crisis superimposed. Hypertension is paroxysmal in a low percentage of patients. Headaches and sweating are the most common symptoms associated with hypertension experienced by children with this disorder.

Other frequent symptoms are visual disturbances and neurologic signs. Vision may be blurred by hypertensive retinitis and convulsions and stupor may result from hypertensive encephalopathy. Tachycardia, dysrhythmias, and alterations in mood and character are also present, but they are 50% less frequent than in adults. In our population, weight loss was found in a smaller number of patients than previously reported.[2] It is noticeable that in contradistinction with adults, elevated fasting blood sugar levels were only occasionally found.

Once pheochromocytoma is suspected, biochemical testing must be done to confirm the diagnosis.[2] Since pheochromocytomas are a heterogeneous group of catecholamine-secreting tumors no biochemical test has 100% sensitivity.[6,8–10]

However, available measurements of urine and plasma catecholamines often confirm the diagnosis in a relatively easy way. Nevertheless, to evaluate correctly the results in children some important considerations must be taken in account: (*a*) there is a progressive increase in the daily output of each catecholamine and its metabolites (as μg-24 h) as age increases from birth to adulthood.[11,12] This means that a normal value for an adult may be high for a child. On the other hand, catecholamine excretion per gram of urinary creatinine decreases with age, as a consequence of the increment in creatinine excretion resulting from an increase in muscle mass; (*b*) interference from various medications and dietary compounds has to be considered depending on the assay performed; and (*c*) it is essential that patients are in a relaxed supine position while blood samples for measurement of plasma catecholamines are

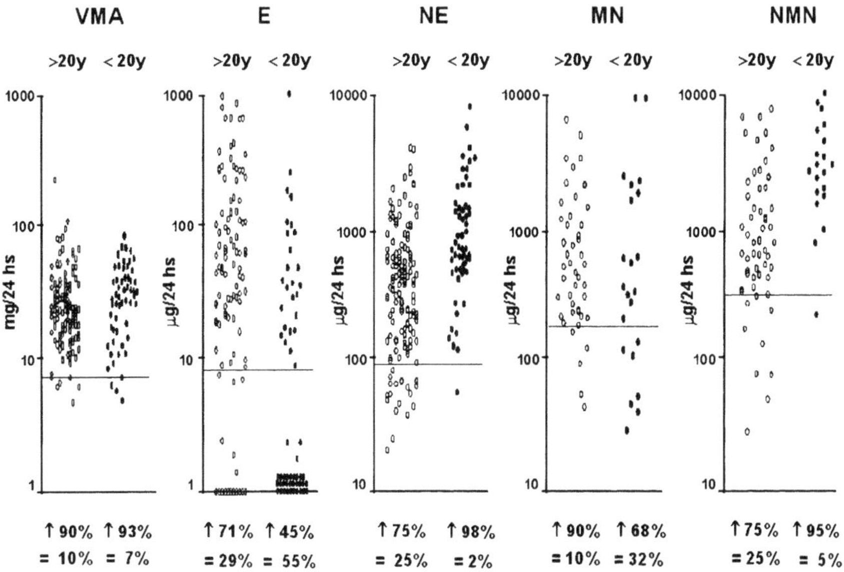

FIGURE 2. The 24-h urinary excretion of VMA, E, NE, MN, and NMN in pheochromocytoma patients over >20 years (open dots) and under <20 years of age (dark dots), each point corresponds to one patient. The horizontal lines represent the upper normal limits. ↑ represents the percentage of increased values. = represents the percentage of normal values.

obtained. These basal conditions required can be difficult to achieve in young children.

In patients with paroxysmal hypertension, it is mandatory to register blood pressure during sampling since plasma catecholamines may be normal during the normotensive interval. Thus, certain circumstances may produce spurious measurements leading to either false negative or false positive test results that are of clinical relevance. The most commonly used diagnostic tests in children are 24-h collections of urine for free catecholamines, VMA, and MN.[2] When plasma samples can be obtained under optimal conditions, results from urinary and plasma assays are often coincident.

Urinary NE was increased in 98% of our young patients (FIG. 2). It was elevated in all but one patient who had multiple endocrine neoplasia (MEN) type 2A. Urinary E showed the lowest sensitivity. It was normal in more than half of the patients (32) and increased in 26. MN and NMN were assessed when available. For that reason, they were measured in only 22 patients. There was some correspondence between MN excretion and E excretion: when MN excretion was normal, E excretion was also normal. However, when E values were increased, MN values were sharply incremented. This proved to be particularly useful in those patients whose E values were borderline (a little over cutoff values). The only patient with normal urine NE values presented a high increase in NMN excretion. We have observed this behavior also in adults, although not in all of them. The noradrenergic profile found in the young patients may account for the obvious clinical features they present. Regarding VMA, urinary excretion has been highly sensitive. Three out of the four patients with normal urinary VMA showed diagnostic increases in urinary E and slight increments in NE urinary excretion. In the remaining patient only urinary NE was moderately increased. These results are in contrast with most results in the literature.[13,14] Differences in the methodology and/or the cutoff values used may account for these contradictory results.

Biochemical confirmation of the presence of a pheochromocytoma should be complemented by means of an assessment through imaging studies to locate the tumor. Most pheochromocytomas may be located through nonspecific methods for the detection of abdominal tumors. Imaging studies, such as CT scan, MRI imaging together with scintigraphy with ^{123}I-meta-iodobenzylguanidine and ^{131}I MIBG render important anatomic and functional information. Scintigraphy with ^{131}I and ^{123}I MIBG is a valuable technique to detect whether they are adrenal or extra-adrenal pheochromocytomas, or they are metastasis of malignant pheochromocytomas. However, results may be falsely negative in 15% of the patients.[15]

If results from the different imaging studies are compared, it can be concluded that they are complementary since results tend to coincide, but one technique may disclose a tumor that went unseen to others, even in the same patient. Presurgery localization is particularly critical in children considering the high incidence of extra-adrenal, multiple, and bilateral adrenal tumors in childhood.[7,16–18]

In our patients tumor localization showed a high incidence of bilaterality (34%), particularly in patients under 10 years of age (62%) (TABLE 2). In this subgroup five were bilateral at diagnosis. Three patients with unilateral disease developed a second pheochromocytoma in the contralateral adrenal gland in a period ranging from 1 to 3 years. Extra-adrenal pheochromocytoma was observed in only one patient aged 10 years.

In the over 10-year-old group, unilateral adrenal pheochromocytoma was predominant, followed by bilateral adrenal pheochromocytoma. In these patients when the disease started as unilateral, bilaterality appeared within a period of 5 years. One of these patients presented adrenal medullary hyperplasia. When extra-adrenal, sites were abdominal paraganglia in 4, abdominal pelvic paraganglia in 2, bladder in 2, thorax in 1, and organ of Zuckerkandl in 1.

TABLE 2. Localization of pheochromocytoma according to age

	<10 years	>10 years
Adrenal bilateral	8 (62%)	13 (29%)
Adrenal unilateral	4 (31%)	23 (51%)
Extra-adrenal	1 (7%)	10 (22%)

Seven patients with sporadic pheochromocytomas had malignant tumors. The multiple recurrences appeared at different periods of time independently of the primary site. In a youngster of 16 years, the adrenal unilateral tumor was irresectable and the patient died few months after surgery. Three other patients presented multiple recurrences and died at periods ranging from 8 to 18 years. Three are still alive, one of them after a follow-up of 21 years. During her third relapse all imaging studies performed (CT, MRI, scintigraphy with ^{131}I MIBG) failed to localize the site of the tumor. Venous sampling obtained at various levels in the inferior and superior cava vein for plasma catecholamine concentrations succeeded in localizing multiple abdominal tumor sites. At present, she has sustained hypertension treated with four drugs, multiple bone metastasis, high levels of catecholamines and their metabolites, but, surprisingly, she has a normal quality of life. Studies conducted to disclose malignancy in the primary tumor were negative.

It is a widespread assumption that most pheochromocytomas are sporadic and only about 10% are hereditary.[19,20] Nevertheless, there is increasing evidence that familial pheochromocytomas are found much more often than traditionally assumed. Familial pheochromocytoma is inherited as an autosomal dominant trait alone or as a component of the MEN type 2 syndromes (MEN 2A and 2B), von Hippel–Lindau disease (VHL) or, less frequently, in neurofibromatosis type 1 (NF 1) or paraganglioma of the neck.[21–24]

Thirty-nine percent of our children with pheochromocytoma had a familial disease, almost two times the frequency found in adults (22%).

Besides, they showed the greatest incidence of VHL, 28%, while MEN 2A was found in a small percentage (2%). NF1, MEN 2B, and succinate dehydrogenase subunit B (SDHB) were also observed in a few cases.

On the contrary, in the over 20-year-old group, there was a clear predominance of MEN 2A (15%); only 2% had VHL.

It is remarkable that pheochromocytoma was the first manifestation of VHL disease in all but one of the younger population. Two children belonging to the same family had VHL type 2A and presented the frequent mutation R167W. Another affected youngster had VHL type 2B and presented the new P138R mutation. The other affected children belonged to five families that have presented pheochromocytoma as the only manifestation of the disease to date (followed from 3 to 40 years).[25,26] They showed novel mutations in conserved amino acids.

Advances in genetics, biochemical measurements, and imaging make early detection and precise localization of pheochromocytomas possible.

This study shows that pheochromocytomas in children are heterogenous and display important molecular and biochemical differences. It also emphasized the importance of molecular diagnosis to disclose a familial disease at earlier stages allowing more effective treatment of these tumors as well as the identification of family members at risk.

ACKNOWLEDGMENTS

This work was supported in part by grants: PICT 05–8658 from Agencia de Promoción Científica y Tecnológica and PIP 2867 from CONICET, Buenos Aires. Argentina.

Marta Barontini and Gloria Levin are Senior Investigators from CONICET.

REFERENCES

1. Ciftci, A.O. *et al.* 2001. Pheochromocytoma in children. J. Pediatr. Surg. **36:** 447–452.
2. Fonkalsrud, E.W. 1991. Pheochromocytoma in childhood. Prog. Pediatr. Surg. **26:** 103–111.
3. Einsenhofer, G. 1986. Simultaneous liquid-chromatographic determination of 3, 4-dihydroxyphenylglycol, catecholamines, and 3,4dihydroxyphenylalanine in plasma and their responses to inhibition of monoamine oxidase. Clin. Chem. **32:** 2030–2033.
4. Pisano, J., J. Crout & P. Abraham. 1962. Determination of 3-methoxy-4hydroxymandelic acid in urine. Clin. Chim. Acta. **7:** 285–291.
5. Lenders, J.W. *et al.* 1993. Determination of metanephrines in plasma by liquid chromatography with electrochemical detection. Clin. Chem. **39:** 97–103.
6. Ross, J.H. 2000. Pheochromocytoma. Special considerations in children. Urol. Clin. North Am. **27:** 393–402.
7. Newman, K.D. & T. Ponsky. 2002. The diagnosis and management of endocrine tumors causing hypertension in children. Ann. N. Y. Acad. Sci. **970:** 155–158.
8. Goldstein, R.E. *et al.* 1999. Clinical experience over 48 years with pheochromocytoma. Ann. Surg. **229:** 755–766.
9. Barontini, M. & G. Levin. 2004. Diagnóstico y tratamiento del feocromocitoma: nuevos conceptos. Rev. Hosp. Niños BAires. **46:** 45–49.
10. Bravo, E.L. 2004. Pheochromocytoma: current perspectives in the patogénesis, diagnosis, and management. Arq. Bras. Endocrinol. Metab. **48:** 746–750.
11. Levin, G., I. Armando & M. Barontini.1994. Características del feocromocitoma en niños. Rev. Hosp. Niños BAires. **36:** 98–100.
12. Parra, A. *et al.* 1980. Urinary excretion of catecholamines in healthy subjects in relation to body growth. Acta. Endocrinol. **94:** 546–551.
13. Lenders, J.W. *et al.* 2002. Biochemical diagnosis of pheochromocytoma: which test is best? JAMA **287:** 1427–1434.
14. Pacak, K. *et al.* 2005. Biochemical diagnosis, localization and management of pheochromocytoma: focus on multiple endocrine neoplasia type 2 in relation to other hereditary syndromes and sporadic forms of the tumour. J. Intern. Med. **257:** 60–68.
15. Bravo, E.L. & R. Tagle. 2003. Pheochromocytoma: state-of-the-art and future prospects. Endocr. Rev. **24:** 539–553.
16. Levine, C., J. Skimming & E. Levine. 1992. Familial pheochromocytomas with unusual associations. J. Pediatr. Surg. **27:** 447–451.
17. Reddy, V.S. *et al.* 2000. Twenty-five-year surgical experience with pheochromocytoma in children. Am. Surg. **66:** 1085–1091.

18. KAUFMAN, B.H. *et al.* 1983. Pheochromocytoma in the pediatric age group: current status. J. Pediatr. Surg. **18:** 879–884.
19. KOCH, C.A. *et al.* 2001. Genetic aspects of pheochromocytoma. Endocr. Regul. **35:** 43–52.
20. GIMM, O. 2005. Pheochromocytoma-associated syndromes: genes proteins and functions of RET, VHL and SDHx. Fam. Cancer **4:** 17–23.
21. OPOCHER, G. *et al.* 2003. Clinical and genetic aspects of phaeochromocytoma. Horm. Res. **59:** 56–61.
22. MULLER, U., C. TROIDL & S. NIEMANN. 2005. SDHC mutations in hereditary paraganglioma/pheochromocytoma. Fam. Cancer **4:** 9–12.
23. OPOCHER, G. *et al.* 2005. Pheochromocytoma in von Hippel-Lindau disease and neurofibromatosis type1. Fam. Cancer **4:** 13–16
24. PAWLU, C., B. BAUSCH & H.P. NEUMANN. 2005. Mutations of the SDHB and SDHD genes. Fam. Cancer **4:** 49–54
25. SANSÓ, G. *et al.* 2004. Familial isolated pheochromocytoma presenting a new mutation in the von Hippel-Lindau gene. Am. J. Hypertens. **17:** 1107–1111.
26. SANSÓ, G. *et al.* 2004. Early development of pheochromocytoma as initial manifestation of VHL disease [abstract]. J. Pediatr. Endocrinol. Metab. **17:** 1342.

1,111 Patients with Adrenal Incidentalomas Observed at a Single Endocrinological Center

Incidence of Chromaffin Tumors

ANNA A. KASPERLIK-ZALUSKA,[a] ELŻBIETA ROSLONOWSKA,[a] JADWIGA SLOWINSKA-SRZEDNICKA,[a] MACIEJ OTTO,[b] ANDRZEJ CICHOCKI,[c] JAROSLAW CWIKLA,[d] RAFAL SLAPA[e] AND GRAEME EISENHOFER[f]

[a]*Department of Endocrinology, Centre for Postgraduate Medical Education, Warsaw, Poland*

[b]*Department of Vascular Surgery, Warsaw University of Medicine, Warsaw, Poland*

[c]*Department of Surgery, Institute of Oncology, Warsaw, Poland*

[d]*Department of Imaging, MSW&A Hospital, Warsaw, Poland*

[e]*Department of Imaging, Warsaw University of Medicine, Warsaw, Poland*

[f]*Clinical Neurocardiology Section, National Institute of Neurological Disorders and Stroke, National Institutes of Health, Bethesda, USA*

ABSTRACT: A majority of incidentally found adrenal tumors derive from the adrenal cortex. The aim of our study was evaluation of the incidence of chromaffin tumors in a group of 1,111 patients with adrenal incidentalomas. In this group there were 803 women and 308 men, aged 10–87 years. Clinical examination, imaging studies (ultrasound scans, CT, and MRI if necessary), and hormonal determinations (cortisol, ACTH and androgens in the blood, dexamethasone suppression test, urinary excretion of 17-OHCS, aldosterone and 17-KS, as well as PRA/aldosterone stimulation test and metanephrines in hypertensive patients and those with density in CT over 20 HU) were used. In 380 patients treated by surgery (mainly by laparoscopic approach), histological and immunocytochemical examinations were performed. Clinical examination revealed hypertension in 25% of the patients under study. Chromaffin tumors were detected in 43 patients, 33 women, and 10 men aged 20–75 years: pheochromocytoma in 36 (malignant in 3); chromaffin cells hyperplasia in 2; paraganglioma in 3; ganglioneuroblastoma in 1; ganglioneuroma in 1; and schwannoma in 2. The tumors' diameter ranged between 1.1 and

Address for correspondence: Anna A. Kasperlik-Zaluska, Centre for Postgraduate Medical Education, Ceglowska 80, 01-809 Warsaw, Poland. Voice: +48-22-8343131; fax +48-22-8343131.
e-mail: anna@ultima.neostrada.pl

**Ann. N.Y. Acad. Sci. 1073: 38–46 (2006). © 2006 New York Academy of Sciences.
doi: 10.1196/annals.1353.004**

20.0 cm, density = 25 Hounsfield units (HU) or more before contrast medium injection. Hypertension was present in 53% of these patients. The urinary metanephrines excretion was elevated in 31 of 38 patients, in whom the determinations were done. Chromaffin tumors were detected in 4% (pheochromocytomas in 3%) of 1,111 patients with adrenal incidentalomas. Malignancy was present in 9% of 43 patients with chromaffin tumors. High density in CT was a very important diagnostic finding in the incidentally found medullary tumors.

KEYWORDS: **adrenal incidentaloma; pheochromocytoma; paraganglioma; chromaffin tumors; metanephrines; hypertension**

INTRODUCTION

Most of incidentally found adrenal tumors (adrenal incidentaloma) derive from adrenal cortex.[1,2] Tumors derived from the adrenal medulla comprise mainly chromaffin as well as neural and mixed tumors. In the WHO classification both types of the tumors are distinguished on the basis of different embryonal origins. The cortex derives from mesoderm while medulla derives from neural crest.

In this study we evaluated the incidence of the adrenal medulla–derived tumors in a group of over 1,100 patients with adrenal incidentalomas observed at the Department of Endocrinology (Centre for Postgraduate Medical Education) in Warsaw in the last 15 years.

MATERIAL AND METHODS

Subjects included 1,111 patients—803 women and 308 men, aged 10–87 years. Thirty-eight percent of patients were over 60 years of age, while only 4% were below 30 years of age. Tumor size ranged between 1.0 and 23 cm (63% had size of 1.0–3.0 cm). Fifty percent were localized to the right side, 32% to the left, and 18% were bilateral.

Our analysis of the clinical data accounted for the frequency of hypertension, diabetes mellitus, and other features of adrenal hyperfunction.

Imaging techniques included ultrasound scans, computed tomography (CT), and magnetic resonance imaging (MRI), mainly for differentiation of adenomas from nonadenomas. The size of the tumors and imaging phenotype were evaluated in these studies.

Adrenocortical activity was assayed by the measurement of serum levels of cortisol (circadian rhythm), dehydroepiandrosterone sulfate (DHEAS), androstendione, 17-hydroxy progesterone (17-OH progesterone), ACTH and urinary excretion of 17-hydroxycorticosteroids (17-OHCS), and 17-ketosteroids (17-KS). Cortisol levels were determined by radioimmunoassay (RIA) and during the last 5 years by LIA (Immulite 2000 – DPC); DHEA-S, androstendione, and 17-OH progesterone levels by RIA; and ACTH concentration by a radioimmunometric method. Urinary 17-OHCS and 17-KS contents were measured by routine methods (Silber and Porter and Zimmerman method, respectively). In patients with high normal cortisol levels and in those with tumors exceeding 3.0 cm of size, an overnight low-dose (1 mg) dexamethasone test was performed. In obese patients with hypertension and/or diabetes mellitus and in those with tumors >4.0 cm of diameter, a 2-day or 4-day dexamethasone suppression test was performed. In hypertensive patients with low normal potassium levels, urinary excretion of aldosterone and plasma aldosterone/plasma renin activity (PRA) stimulation tests were performed. In hypertensive patients with high unenhanced CT attenuation (exceeding 10 HU) of the adrenal tumor, the content of urinary metanephrines was determined. In 54 nonselected patients, referred to the Department of Endocrinology between 15 September 1998 and 15 March 1999, plasma-free and total normetanephrine and metanephrine as well as norepinephrine and epinephrine levels were measured.

Histological and immunocytochemical studies were performed in 381 patients treated by surgery, including all the patients with chromaffin tumors. Although there is no sound histopathological method for determining malignancy or malignant potential of pheochromocytomas, in this article pheochromocytomas were defined as benign if there was no evidence of metastases and any remaining disease in the postoperative period. Most patients (with tumors up to 5.0–6.0 cm of diameter) were operated on through laparoscopy, and selected patients underwent open surgery by laparotomy or lumbotomy. In cases with suspected malignancy, laparoscopy was avoided. The patients with suspected chromaffin tumors were treated with phenoxybenzamine before surgery.

RESULTS

Clinical Examination

Hypertension was the most frequent clinical sign, present in 283 patients (25%). Obesity was found in 165 patients (15%). Diabetes mellitus was diagnosed in 60 patients (5%). Supraclavicular fat pads and facial telangiectasia were present in rare cases, and combined with the results of cortisol determinations were interpreted as signs of pre-Cushing's syndrome.

Imaging Techniques

Ultrasound scan was the most frequent screening method revealing incidental adrenal masses; it was also a routine method for control examinations during long-term observation in the patients not treated by surgery. Ultrasound findings were always verified by CT or MRI. CT was the main imaging method to evaluate the size, shape, borders, unenhanced attenuation values (density) of the adrenal tumors, and washout of the contrast medium. For differentiation of adenoma/nonadenoma, MRI was performed to evaluate intensity on T-2 scans and thus to reveal tissue without lipid content. All of the foregoing imaging characteristics are helpful for evaluating malignant potential of adrenal tumors. Imaging phenotypes of chromaffin tumors were characterized by high unenhanced CT attenuation (25 HU or more) and high enhancement with i.v. contrast medium, inhomogeneous structure (frequently cystic or hemorrhagic), and high signal intensity on T-2 weighted MRI.

Hormonal Assays

Slightly elevated cortisol levels and excretion of cortisol metabolites in basal conditions and insufficient decrease of cortisol concentrations in the evening (in the circadian rhythm), and after dexamethasone administration[3]were characteristic for pre-Cushing's syndrome (70 cases = 6.5%) The highest DHEA-S and androstendione levels were found in some adrenocortical carcinomas. Moderately elevated serum androgen levels were due not only to benign adrenal tumors but, probably, also to coexisting polycystic ovary syndrome. Subclinical androgen secretion of noncarcinomatous origin was found in 11 adrenocortical tumors (1%). Elevated 17-OH progesterone values were observed in rather rare cases of nonclassic congenital adrenal hyperplasia and in some patients with adrenal cancer. The excretion of 17-KS in most cases was similar to serum androgen levels. Increased aldosterone excretion and/or positive aldosterone/PRA ratios were detected only in six cases (0.5%). Increased urinary outputs of metanephrines (> 1,000 μg/24 h) were found in 31 patients. High plasma catecholamines were detected in only 1 (a 41-year-old man) of 54 patients where these were measured: NE, 4,476 pg/mL (upper limit = 498 pg/mL); fNMN, 3,596 pg/mL (upper limit = 112 pg/mL); tNMN, 82,553 pg/mL (upper limit = 3,170 pg/mL); epinephrine, 915 pg/mL (upper limit = 83 pg/mL); fMN, 1,663 pg/mL (upper limit = 61; pg/ml); tMN, 69,608 pg/mL (upper limit = 1,706 pg/mL).[4]

Taking into account the results described above as well as the results of histological and immunocytochemical examinations of the 380 surgically removed tumors we defined three groups of tumors

(a) nonmalignant tumors:957 = 86%
(b) primary malignant tumors:108 = 10% (in this number carcinoma: 98 = 9%)
(c) metastatic tumors:46 = 4%

Among the patients with primary malignant tumors, 98 had adrenal carcinomas, 5 had lymphoma, 3 patients had malignant pheochromocytoma, 2 had

(A)

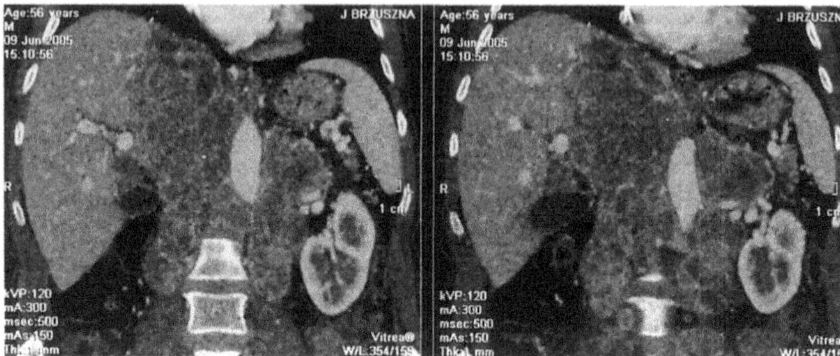

(B)

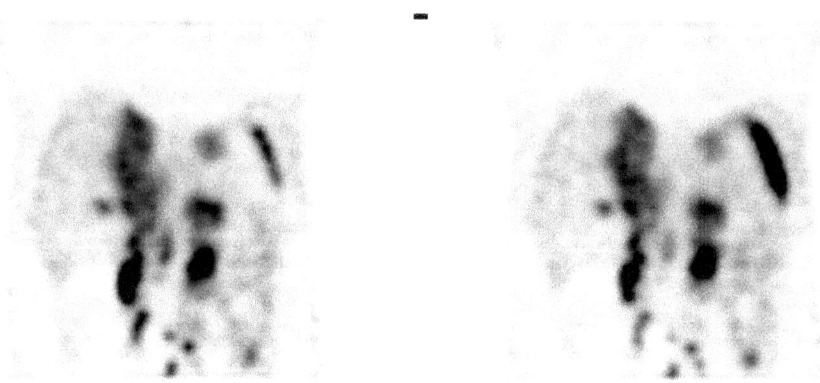

FIGURE 1. A 56-year-old patient with mixed type of tumor: malignant pheochromocytoma and adrenocortical carcinoma, after surgery, chemotherapy and ^{131}I mIBG treatment. Before start of ^{90}Y DOTA TATE therapy, clinically and radiological disease progression (RECIST-DP). (**A**) Standard CT after i.v. contrast enhancement, before radionuclide treatment (coronal view), large tumor mass involved liver and retroperitoneal space; (**B**) somatostatin receptor scintigraphy (SRS ^{99m}Tc HYNIC TATE), high uptake of radiotracer, confirmation of large tumor avid mass with heterogeneous uptake of radiotracer.

sarcoma, and 1 had ganglioneuroblastoma. The three patients with malignant pheochromocytoma included two men (53 and 64 years of age) and one woman (45 years of age). Metastatic lymph nodes and regional invasion were found in all of them. In the female patient, treated three times because of recurrent abdominal masses, pulmonary metastases developed in the late period of observation. All three patients received chemotherapy. However, two patients (the female patient and the 64-year-old man) died within 4 and 7 months of this treatment, respectively. The remaining patient, with large metastatic infiltration in the lungs, liver, and retroperitoneal space (FIG. 1), received therapy with a radioactive somatostatin analogue[5] to treat recurrent invasive masses (total time of survival 3.5 years). An adrenal tumor, diagnosed microscopically as ganglioneuroblastoma, was found in a 20-year-old pregnant woman on ultrasound scan. Three-dimensional ultrasound scans were performed during pregnancy,[6] while MRI was performed after labor, just before surgery.

Thirty-nine patients were determined to have chromaffin tumors (without evidence of metastases) based on the imaging phenotype, the results of biochemical testing (metanephrines), and the results of histologic and immunocytochemical studies. These 39 patients included 31 women and 8 men, aged 20–75 years, with pheochromocytoma in 33 patients, adrenal medullary hyperplasia (with typical, tumorous-like image in CT) in 2 patients, and ganglioneuroma in 1 patient. In three patients the masses incidentally found in close vicinity to the adrenal gland were initially mistakenly described as adrenal tumors during imaging studies. On surgical resection it became clear that these tumors had no connection with the adrenal gland and they were reclassified as extra-adrenal paragangliomas. This diagnosis was confirmed by microscopic and immunocytochemical studies. Schwannoma was diagnosed in two women, 53 and 68 years of age. The age of patients with pheochromocytoma ranged between 20 and 40 years in 10 cases, between 41 and 60 years in 16 cases, and over 60 years in 7 patients. Multiple endocrine neoplasia (MEN), Type 2, was diagnosed in two patients, in a 27-year-old man and a 46-year-old woman. In both patients pheochromocytoma was the first, incidentally found abnormality. Adrenalectomies in these patients were followed by thyroidectomies for medullary carcinoma. In the male patient, two tumors of the contralateral adrenal gland developed 13 years later.

Hypertension was present in 53% of the patients with chromaffin tumors. Paroxysmal hypertension was observed in four patients, including two men with pheochromocytomas, without evidence of metastases (both with elevated catecholamines and metanephrines) and in two patients with malignant pheochromocytoma, occurring as hypertensive crisis in the late period of observation (after two operations).

In the patients with malignant pheochromocytoma, diameters of primary tumors were 7.0, 10.0, and 13.3 cm. In the patient with a ganglioneuroblastoma, the diameter was 20.0 cm. Diameters of the other pheochromocytomas ranged between 1.1 and 10.0 cm: between 1.1 and 3.0 cm in 12 patients; 3.1 and 5.0 cm in 18 patients; and 5.1 and 10.0 cm in 12 cases (in sum 41 tumors in 32 patients, in two patients three tumors were found). Diameters of paragangliomas were 6.2, 12.0, and 12.5 cm. In the patients with schwannomas the diameter was 3.1 and 7.0 cm. The abnormal adrenal masses identified as adrenal medullary hyperplasia were diagnosed on CT as adrenal tumors sized 3.0 and 5.5 cm in diameter.

Thirty-two tumors were localized on the right side, six on the left, and seven were bilateral. Coexistence of chromaffin tumors with adrenal adenomas was found in three cases.

DISCUSSION

Progress in imaging techniques has resulted in a growing number of incidentally detected adrenal tumors. From our first presentation of 208 patients with adrenal incidentalomas in 1997,[1] we registered more than 900 new cases. Although a majority of them appear to be adrenal adenomas, a real challenge is their malignancy or hormonal hyperactivity, especially in so-called clinically silent pheochromocytoma. In our experience such tumors do not always remain dormant and many become activated (e.g., by anesthesia, childbirth) sometimes resulting in life-threatening paroxysmal hypertension. As the number of adrenal incidentalomas observed in our department seems to be representative of this new clinical entity, we tried to analyze the frequency of chromaffin tumors, mainly of pheochromocytomas.

Among the group of 1,111 patients we found 43 chromaffin tumors (4%), among them 36 cases of pheochromocytoma (3%), and 2 cases of schwannoma, a tumor of neural origin, deriving from adrenal medullary cells (WHO classification). Findings of other groups have indicated that about 5% of adrenal incidentalomas are pheochromocytomas.[7,8] We are not sure why such a discrepancy concerning the incidence of pheochromocytomas appeared. Maybe it was due to our very rigorous criteria concerning the incidental character of findings on imaging. A rather rare pathologic form, chromaffin cell hyperplasia, was present in two hypertensive women, while paragangliomas were found in three patients (7%).

An evident prevalence of female patients was found in our material (F/M ratio = 3.4). Nearly one-third of the patients with pheochromocytomas and no evidence of metastases were aged 20–40 years, while the malignant pheochromocytomas, paragangliomas, ganglioneuroma, and schwannomas were detected in the patients over 40 years of age.

In our experience the imaging phenotype was a very valuable diagnostic finding for incidentally detected chromaffin tumors. In the group of 98 patients with incidentally found adrenal carcinomas there were two women with lipid-rich tumors, while a high unenhanced CT attenuation was characteristic for all chromaffin tumors and schwannomas. Heterogeneous structure was also a characteristic feature cited in the literature.[9] Bilateral tumors were present in 15% of the patients, similar to the whole group of adrenal incidentalomas (18%), where the most frequent were bilateral adenomas.

Hypertension was present in 53% of patients with chromaffin tumors, twice as frequent as in the combined group of all incidentalomas (25%). In all patients, including both patients with chromaffin cell hyperplasia, hypertension improved or resolved following adrenalectomy. In a 27-year-old, normotensive woman with bilateral pheochromocytomas (up to 10.0 cm of diameter) cardiac arrhythmia was the single complaint. A nonobese somatic type was characteristic of all patients with incidentally found pheochromocytoma.

Determination of urinary metanephrine excretion is the most widely used chemical screening test for pheochromocytoma in Poland. According to Krakoff[10] its sensitivity ranges from 80 to 85%, and its specificity is in excess of 90%. In our group of patients with chromaffin tumors, urinary metanephrine excretion was increased in 31 of 38 patients under study (82% sensitivity). Measurements of urinary fractionated metanephrines and plasma-free metanephrines offer higher diagnostic sensitivity than measurements of urinary total metanephrines,[11–13] but are not yet available in Poland.

In summary, in our experience, high unenhanced CT attenuation has been the most valuable characteristic of pheochromocytoma when measurements of plasma-free or urinary fractionated metanephrines were unavailable. However it should be kept in mind that such a finding is also typical for adrenal carcinoma and metastatic tumors. An analysis of clinical picture and imaging phenotype together with determination of metanephrine levels are necessary to establish a precise preoperative diagnosis of pheochromocytoma.

CONCLUSIONS

(*a*) Chromaffin cell–derived tumors were found in 4% of a group of 1,111 patients with adrenal incidentalomas (including pheochromocytomas in 3%).
(*b*) Malignancies were detected in 9% of 43 chromaffin tumors.
(*c*) Imaging phenotype, especially high unenhanced CT attenuation (25 HU or more), was very important finding in chromaffin tumors.
(*d*) More than half (73%) of the incidentally found chromaffin tumors had a diameter of at least 4.0 cm.

ACKNOWLEDGMENTS

This work was supported by CMKP Grant 501-2-2-07-45/01.

REFERENCES

1. Kasperlik-Zaluska, A.A. *et al.* 1997. Incidentally found adrenal mass (incidentaloma): investigation and management of 208 patients. Clin. Endocrinol. **46:** 29–37.
2. Barzon, L. *et al.* 2002. Prevalence and the natural course of adrenal incidentaloma. NIH-State-of-the-Science Conference of the Clinically Inapparent Adrenal Mass ("Incidentaloma"). Feb. 4–6, Bethesda, Maryland: 25–30.
3. Arnaldi, G. *et al.* 2003. Diagnosis and complications of Cushing's syndrome: a consensus statement. J. Clin. Endocrinol. Metab. **88:** 5593–5602.
4. Kasperlik-Zaluska, A.A. *et al.* 2002. Utility of plasma metanephrines in the diagnosis of adrenal incidentalomas. Endokrynol. Pol. **53:** 549–556.

5. Cwikla, J.B. *et al.* 2005. Using ^{90}Y Dota Tate treatment in patients with malignant pheochromocytoma[abstract]. pp. 160–161. First International Symposium on Pheochromocytoma, Oct. 20–23, Bethesda, Maryland.
6. Slapa, R.Z. *et al.* 2002. Adrenal ganglioneuroblastoma in pregnant woman: diagnosis with three-dimensional ultrasound. Eur. Radiol. **12:** S121–S126.
7. Young, W.F. Jr. 2000. Management approaches to adrenal incidentalomas: a view from Rochester, Minnesota. Endocrinol. Metab. Clin. North Am. **29:** 207–214.
8. Lenders, J.W.M. *et al.* 2005. Phaeochromocytoma. Lancet **366:** 665–675.
9. Young, W.F. Jr. 2004. Adrenal incidentaloma MTP. ENDO 2004, New Orleans, 7–15.
10. Krakoff, L.R. 1995. Searching for pheochromocytoma: a new and better test? Ann. Intern. Med. **123:** 150–151.
11. Eisenhofer, G. *et al.* 1998. Plasma metanephrines are markers of pheochromocytoma produced by catechol-O-methyltransferase within tumors. J. Clin. Endocrinol. Metab. **83:** 2175–2185.
12. Eisenhofer, G. 2001. Free or total metanephrines for diagnosis of pheochromocytoma: what is the difference? Clin. Chem. **47:** 988–989.
13. Eisenhofer, G. *et al.* 2003. Biochemical diagnosis of pheochromocytoma: how to distinguish true- from false-positive test results. J. Clin. Endocrinol. Metab. **88:** 2656–2666.

Lack of Symptoms in Patients with Histologic Evidence of Pheochromocytoma

A Diagnostic Challenge

DEBBIE L. COHEN,[a] DOUGLAS FRAKER,[b]
AND RAYMOND R. TOWNSEND[a]

[a]*Renal Electrolyte and Hypertension Division, University of Pennsylvania, Philadelphia, Pennsylvania 19104, USA*

[b]*Department of Surgery, University of Pennsylvania, Philadelphia, Pennsylvania 19104, USA*

ABSTRACT: Pheochromocytoma (Pheo) is a rare cause of hypertension (HTN). Classically, a triad of symptoms includes sweating, palpitations, and headache. HTN is often present and labile. Although a triad of symptoms is cited as the most frequent presenting complaints, our clinical experience leads us to question how often these are present. Thirty-two patients with histologically proven pheo or paraganglionoma were evaluated. Around 84.4% patients had adrenal pheos and 15.6% had extra-adrenal pheos. Two patients had bilateral adrenal tumors, two had a history of prior pheos, and four had a family history of pheo. There were 19 (59.4%) female and 13 (40.6%) male patients. Six (18.7%) patients were black and 26 (81.3%) were white. The mean age at presentation was 43.2 $\pm$ 13.9 years. Two patients were known to have neurofibromatosis type 1, two had von Hippel–Lindau disease, one had multiple endocrine neoplasia 2A, and one PGL/SDHD genetic mutation. Twenty-six patients had sporadic tumors or had not had genetic testing. Biochemical diagnosis was confirmed with 24-h urine measurements. Urine catecholamine measurements were elevated at least 2 to 4 times above normal levels. Mean SBP readings at presentation were 128 $\pm$ 19 mmHg. Mean DBP readings were 81 $\pm$ 13 mmHg. Around 65.6% patients were hypertensive at presentation. Fifty percent of the patients had palpitations, 40.6% had tachycardia, 34.4% had sweating, and 31.3% had headaches. Initial presenting symptoms were diverse. Pheo is a rare clinical entity and remains a huge diagnostic challenge for all clinicians.

KEYWORDS: pheochromocytoma; diagnosis; symptoms

Address for correspondence: Debbie Cohen, M.D., University of Pennsylvania, 210 White Building, 3400 Spruce Street, Philadelphia, PA, 19104, Voice: 215-615-0794; fax: 215-615-0349.
e-mail: cohendl@mail.med.upenn.edu

Ann. N.Y. Acad. Sci. 1073: 47–51 (2006).
doi: 10.1196/annals.1353.005

INTRODUCTION

Pheochromocytoma is a rare cause of hypertension.[1] Clinical presentation can be highly variable but classically patients present with a triad of symptoms including sweating, palpitations, and headache.[1,2] This is often accompanied by hypertension, which may be labile.[2] Although the classic triad of symptoms is commonly cited as the most frequent presenting complaints, our clinical experience leads us to question how frequently patients present with these classic symptoms.

METHODS

A retrospective study was performed to evaluate the presenting symptoms and demographics of 32 patients with histologic evidence of pheochromocytoma or paraganglionoma. All patients were seen for preoperative evaluation at the University of Pennsylvania in the last 2.5 years. All patients were evaluated by the same team of physicians; this evaluation included a thorough history and examination specifically asking for a history of the presence or absence of sweating, palpitations, headache, and hypertension. Data are presented as mean ± SD.

RESULTS

All 32 patients had histologically confirmed chromaffin cell tumors. Twenty-seven (84.4%) patients had adrenal pheochromocytomas and 5 (15.6%) patients had extra-adrenal pheochromocytomas. Two (6.3%) patients presented with bilateral adrenal tumors. Two (6.3%) patients had a history of prior pheochromocytomas. Four (12.5%) patients had a family history of pheochromocytoma.

TABLE 1. Patient demographics

Adrenal pheo (%)	27 (84.4)
Bilateral adrenal pheo	2 (6.3)
Extra-adrenal pheo (%)	5 (6.3)
Sex	
Female (%)	19 (59.4)
Male (%)	13 (40.6)
Race	
White (%)	26 (81.3)
Black (%)	6 (18.7)
Age (years)	43.2 ± 13.9
MEN 2	1
VHL	2
NF1	2
SDHD/PGL	1
Spontaneous mutation/unknown	26

TABLE 2. Mean 24-h urine catecholamine measurements (normal range)

Norepinephrine mcg/day (0–100)	1471 ± 2511
Epinephrine mcg/day (0–25)	345 ± 402
Normetanephrine mcg/day (50–650)	11435 ± 24326
Metanephrine mcg/day (30–350)	2425 ± 2379
VMA mg/day (0–7)	93.8 ± 16

The demographics are shown in TABLE 1. There were 19 (59.4%) female and 13 (40.6%) male patients. Six (18.7%) patients were black and 26 (81.3%) were white. The mean age of patients at presentation was 43.2 ± 13.9 years. Two patients were known to have neurofibromatosis type 1, two patients had von Hippel–Lindau disease, one patient had multiple endocrine neoplasia (MEN) 2A, and one patient had PGL/SDHD genetic mutation. Twenty-six patients had sporadic tumors or had not had genetic testing.

Biochemical diagnosis was confirmed with 24-h urine measurements for catecholamines, metanephrines, and vanillylmandelic acid (VMA). The mean catecholamine and metabolite measurements are shown in TABLE 2. Urine catecholamine measurements were elevated at least two to four times above normal levels.

Mean systolic blood pressure (SBP) readings at presentation were 129 ± 19 mmHg and mean diastolic blood pressure readings were (DBP) 81 ± 13 mmHg. Twenty-one (65.6%) patients were hypertensive at presentation. Mean number of medications required to control BP prior to surgery was 1.06 ± 0.9. Postoperatively 28.1% of patients were hypertensive. Mean SBP postsurgery was 113 ± 9 mmHg and mean DBP postsurgery was 73 ± 7. These results are shown in TABLE 3.

Most patients did not have the classic presenting symptoms associated with pheochromocytoma. Fifty percent of the patients had palpitations, 40.6% had

TABLE 3. Blood pressure measurements and presence of hypertension pre- and postoperatively

SBP at presentation (mmHg)	128 ± 19
DBP at presentation (mmHg)	81 ± 13
Number of BP medications prior to surgery	1.06 ± 0.9
SBP post surgery (mmHg)	113 ± 9
DBP post surgery (mmHg)	73 ± 7
Preoperative HTN	
Present (%)	21 (65.6)
Postoperative HTN	
Present (%)	9 (28.1)

TABLE 4. Classic pheochromocytoma symptoms

	Present	Absent
Headaches (%)	6 (18.7)	26 (81.3)
Sweating (%)	11 (34.4)	21 (65.6)
Palpitations (%)	16 (50.0)	16 (50.0)
Tachycardia (%)	13 (40.6)	19 (59.4)

TABLE 5. Initial presenting symptoms

Hypertension = 13	Seizures = 1
Family history = 1	Abdominal pain = 3
Syncope = 1	Elevated LFTs = 2
GI bleeding = 1	ARF = 2
Weight loss = 1	CHF = 2
Sweating = 1	Incidentaloma = 2
Atypical chest pain = 1	Fatigue = 1
Diarrhea = 1	Agitation = 1
Palpitations = 1	Diabetes and HTN = 1

tachycardia, 34.4% had sweating, and 31.3% had headaches. The presence of these symptoms is shown in TABLE 4.

Patients' initial presenting symptoms were diverse and are listed in TABLE 5.

DISCUSSION

Pheochromocytoma is a rare cause of secondary hypertension.[1] Pheochromocytoma occurs in about 1–2 per 100,000 adults per year in the United States.[3] The University of Pennsylvania is a referral center for preoperative and operative care in the Delaware Valley of the northeastern United States. We describe the demographics and initial symptoms at presentation of 32 patients with histologic confirmation of a pheochromocytoma.

As expected,[1,2,3] most tumors were located within the adrenal gland. The biochemical diagnosis was made with 24-h urine measurements and these levels were extremely elevated in most patients.

In our experience many patients did not present with the classic symptoms of headaches, palpitations, tachycardia, and sweating. A recent review on pheochromocytomas[1] based on prior studies[4–6] showed headaches to be present in 60–90% of patients, palpitations in 50–70% of patients, sweating in 55–75% of patients, and sustained hypertension in 50–60% of patients. Approximately, 66% of patients in this study were hypertensive on presentation. It is documented in the literature that between 5% and 13% of patients are normotensive.[3] Some patients only have episodic hypertension. The percentage of patients presenting with headache, palpitations, and sweating was slightly lower in our study population than is reported in the literature. The exact reason for this is unclear. It should be noted that none of the patients in our study were seen for pheochromocytoma evaluation as a result of screening in patients with known genetic predisposition. One would obviously expect this type of patient to be less symptomatic if picked up entirely on the basis of screening. Another explanation for the apparent lack of symptoms in some of our patients may be due to lack of recognition by the patients themselves of the symptoms. Often symptoms have been present for an extended period of time and patients become adjusted to living with these symptoms and do not recognize them as being abnormal.

Pheochromocytoma is referred to as the great mimic,[1] as presenting features have been reported to be diverse. This is confirmed by the widely varied presentations seen in our patients. The fact that pheochromocytoma can present in many ways explains why these tumors are often not considered in the differential diagnosis.[3] These data emphasize the importance of maintaining a high index of suspicion in a variety of patients. It is a diagnosis that is easily missed and autopsy studies show that the diagnosis is often not suspected during the patient's life.[7] It is difficult to determine those patients that should be screened for pheochromocytoma and although these tumors are frequently searched for, they are rarely found.[1] It is obviously easier to entertain the diagnosis when patients do present with at least some of the classic symptoms. Pheochromocytoma remains a rare clinical entity but poses a huge diagnostic challenge for all clinicians. Our experience indicates that while its triad of symptoms are often present, they are usually not the presenting or primary complaint, and seeking their confirmatory presence requires clinical vigilance.

REFERENCES

1. LENDERS, T.J., G. EISENHOFER, M. MANNELLI & K. PACAK. 2005. Phaeochromocytoma. Lancet **366:** 665–675.
2. WALTHER, M.M., H.R. KEISER & W.M. LINEHAN. 1999. Pheochromocytoma: evaluation, diagnosis and treatment. World J. Urol. **17:** 35–39.
3. BRAVO, E.L. & R. TAGLE. Pheochromocytoma: state-of-the-art and future prospects. 2002. Endocrinol Rev. **24:** 539–553.
4. MANGER, W.M. & R.W. GIFFORD. 1996. Clinical and Experimental Pheochromocytoma 2nd ed. Blackwell Science. Cambridge, MA.
5. WERBEL, S.S. & K.P. OBER. 1995. Pheochromocytoma. Update on diagnosis, localization, and management. Med. Clin. N. Amer. **765 :** 131–153.
6. KEBEBEW, E. & Q.Y. DUH. 1998. Benign and malignant pheochromocytoma: diagnosis, treatment, and follow-up. Surg. Oncol. Clin. N. Amer. **7:** 765–789.
7. SUTTON, M.G., S.G. SHEPS & J.T. LIE. 1981. Prevalence of clinically suspected pheochromocytoma: review of a 50-year autopsy series. Mayo Clin. Proc. **56:** 354–360.

A Case of Catecholamine and Glucocorticoid Excess Syndrome Due to a Corticotropin-Secreting Paraganglioma

HOLGER S. WILLENBERG,[a] JOACHIM FELDKAMP,[b] REINER LEHMANN,[c] MATTHIAS SCHOTT,[a] PETER E. GORETZKI,[d] AND WERNER A. SCHERBAUM[a]

[a]*Department of Endocrinology, Diabetes and Rheumatology, University Hospital of Duesseldorf, Duesseldorf, Germany*

[b]*1st Medical Clinic, Hospital Bielefeld-Mitte, Bielefeld, Germany*

[c]*Hospital Porz, Cologne, Germany*

[d]*Department of Surgery I, Lukas Hospital, Neuss, Germany*

ABSTRACT: We present a case of a 61-year-old female patient with ectopic corticotropin (ACTH) syndrome, hypopituitarism, and catecholamine excess due to a paraganglioma at the inferior pole of the left kidney. In this article we discuss the hormonal findings in the patient and its consequences, the pitfalls of the endocrine workup, and the results of our immunohistological and molecular studies in more detail.

KEYWORDS: ectopic hormone secretion; corticotropin; Cushing's syndrome; pheochromocytoma; paraganglioma

INTRODUCTION

Catecholamine excess and Cushing's syndrome are potentially life-threatening conditions. Fortunately, a combination thereof is rare. This condition may be due to the co-existence of a pheochromocytoma and an adrenocortical adenoma or a chromaffin tumor secreting corticotropin (ACTH).[1] Ectopic secretion of ACTH by an adrenal paraganglioma was first described by Schteingart *et al.* in 1972,[2] 10 years after the first descriptions of ectopic ACTH syndrome (EAS).[3,4] Since then only a small number of case reports on that issue have been published. However, histopathological studies showed that production of ACTH peptides occur in 5–28% of paragangliomas.[5,6] It was

Address for correspondence: Holger S. Willenberg, M.D., Department of Endocrinology, Diabetes and Rheumatology, University Hospital Düsseldorf, Moorenstr. 5, D-40225 Düsseldorf, Germany. Voice: +49-211-811-7810; fax: +49-211-811-7860
e-mail: Holger.Willenberg@uni-duesseldorf.de

Ann. N.Y. Acad. Sci. 1073: 52–58 (2006). © 2006 New York Academy of Sciences.
doi: 10.1196/annals.1353.006

found that certain tumor cells may secrete pro-opiomelanocortin and precursors of ACTH and that these peptides correlated with cortisol levels and were markedly elevated in patients with EAS, in contrast to patients with Cushing's disease.[7,8]

In this article we present a case that illustrates the typical hormonal findings and clinical problems associated with EAS and catecholamine excess.

CASE REPORT

After returning from vacation at the Mediterranean Sea, a 61-year-old female patient presented to her family doctor with ongoing sweating, weakness, and facial plethora. Physical examination revealed a seated blood pressure of 230/130 mmHg. The heart rate was 139 bpm. Because serum potassium was low (3.1 mmol/L), antihypertensive treatment with lisinopril was initiated. Two days later, the patient developed facial swelling and was admitted to a hospital under the suspicion of an angiotensin-converting enzyme (ACE) inhibitor-induced angioedema.

On questioning, she admitted ankle edema and hypertensive episodes for about 7 years, and a recent increase in facial hair. A 24-h blood pressure monitoring showed a mean blood pressure of 147/87 mmHg during the day, 196/105 mmHg at night, and a mean heart rate of 102 bpm. The combination of hypertension, hypokalemia, sweating, and hirsutism pointed to an endocrine disorder.

Further work-up revealed highly elevated serum cortisol levels with loss of diurnal rhythm (171.0 μg/dL at 8:00 AM, 173.0 μg/dL at 1:00 PM, 156.5 μg/dL at 6:00 PM, 162.0 μg/dL 11:00 PM). Twenty-four-hour urinary free cortisol values were markedly raised (TABLE 1). The diagnosis of hypercortisolism was established.

Since post-menopausal gonadotropin levels were low, an MRI study of the pituitary gland was performed and revealed no abnormalities except for enlarged adrenals. This investigation was followed by a CT scan of the chest that gave no hint for a tumorous mass. A CT scan of the abdomen showed no signs of a tumor but a bilateral adrenal hyperplasia and a mass at the inferior lobe of the left kidney with a size of 2.5 × 2.0 × 3.0 cm that initially was believed to be a lymph node (FIG. 1 A). The patient was referred to our hospital.

We continued to characterize the patient's glucocorticoid excess. Although high cortisol levels suggested EAS, the differentiation between ACTH-dependent and ACTH-independent forms of hypercortisolism was not yet complete. ACTH was found to be strongly elevated and ACTH and cortisol failed to be suppressed with dexamethasone (TABLE 1). In addition, both hormones showed no response to CRH (TABLE 1). Thus, these test results proved EAS and we started again to search for a suspicious lesion.

Since CT studies were interpreted as being normal, octreotide scanning was performed, but was found negative. Therefore, we returned to the lymph node that was initially described in the CT of the abdomen. Doppler/Duplex

TABLE 1. Results of hormonal studies, in patient with ectopic ACTH syndrome[a]

Urinary free cortisol and catecholamines					
Hormone	Cortisol	Metanephrines	Adrenalin	Noradrenalin	Dopamine
Normal range	<110 μg/day	<1.0 mg/day	<20 μg/day	<100 μg/day	<500 μg/day
Before surgery	10,948.0	8.5	122.8	1,108.4	537.5
1 month after surgery	72.8	0.1	<5.0	14.8	45.9
3 months after surgery	36.0	0.5	<5.0	13.0	197.4

2 mg overnight-dexamethasone suppression tests			
Hormone/date	Prior to surgery	1 month after surgery	3 months after surgery
ACTH (pg/mL)	1,078.0	<1.0	<1.0
Cortisol (μg/dL)	176.0	3.3	1.5

Pituitary hormone challenge tests before surgery			
Test	Hormones	Basal	Maximum
CRH (100 μg i.v.)	ACTH (pg/mL)	1,151.0	1,057.0
	Cortisol (μg/dL)	171.0	195.0
TRH (200 μg i.v.)	TSH (μU/mL)	<0.1	0.12
	Prolactin (pg/mL)	13.0	18.0
LH-RH (100 μg i.v.)	LH (mU/mL)	0.19	0.98
	FSH (mU/mL)	<0.1	2.2
GH-RH (50 μg i.v.)	GH (ng/mL)	<0.5	<0.5

[a]These studies include urinary excretion of cortisol and of catecholamines, values of ACTH and cortisol following overnight suppression with 2 mg of dexamethasone, and hormone levels after challenge with hypothalamic releasing hormones

ultrasound revealed the abdominal lesion as a sharp-bordered para-aortal mass (30 × 25 mm in size) without any connection to the aorta (FIG. 2 A). We employed MRI and found that the abdominal tumor was localized para-aortally and adjacent to the sympathetic trunk (FIG. 1 B and C). There were no signs of either metastasis or infiltration of any abdominal structure. Since the lesion was reported to be adjacent to the sympathetic trunk, and since the patient suffered from episodes of tachycardia, we needed to exclude the possibility of a catecholamine-producing paraganglioma prior to biopsy of the lesion. Surprisingly, we found strongly elevated urinary catecholamine levels (TABLE 1) and an uptake of ^{123}I-metaiodobenzylguanidine by the para-aortic mass, indicating the presence of a catecholamine-producing paraganglioma (FIG. 2 B). Additional laboratory testing revealed an increase in neuro-endocrine tumor-related markers (chromogranin A, 302 μg/L ([normal: <110]) and neuron-specific enolase, 63.0 ng/mL ([normal: <12.0])). In addition, we found strong suppression of pituitary hormone secretion and other abnormalities consistent with ACTH-driven hypercortisolism: androstendione, 11.4 ng/mL (normal: <1.5); albumin, 2.4 g/dL (normal: 3.5–5.0); serum protein, 4.4 g/dL (normal: 6.2–8.2); free T_4, 0.9 ng/dL (normal: 0.8–2.0); free T3, 1.1 pg/mL (normal: 1.5–3.5); and diabetes mellitus (TABLE 1).

Meanwhile, the patient developed severe insulin resistance and osteoporosis with multiple vertebral fractures (T/Z scores: spine, –4.37/–2.9; left femur neck: –2.3/–1.89). In addition, the patient had multiple urinary tract infections and pneumonia. She was treated with multiple compounds, including phenoxybenzamine (180 mg/day), metoprolol, amlodipin, ketokonazole, spironolactone, i.v. potassium infusion, vitamin D and calcium, insulin, multiple antibiotics, and omeprazole. We removed the paraganglioma. Fortunately, after surgical intervention neither glucocorticoid nor catecholamine excesses were present and the patient recovered slowly. Immunohistological studies showed that the tumor tissue could be stained with antibodies against chromogranin A, tyrosine hydroxylase, neuron-specific enolase, and ACTH (FIG. 3). In addition, we found presence of POMC messenger RNA in material obtained from the paraganglioma (data not shown).

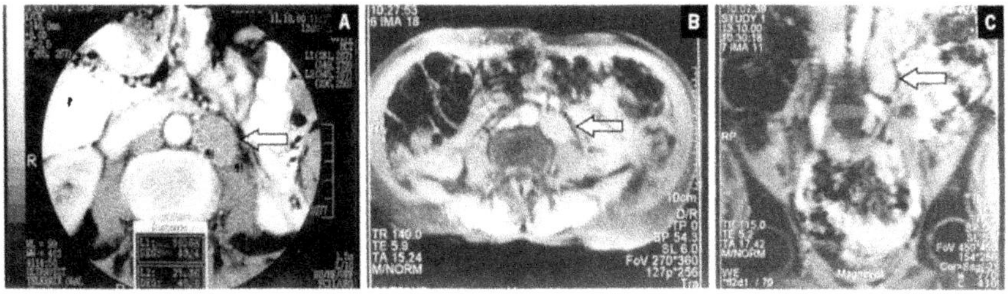

FIGURE 1. (**A**) CT scan of the abdomen with the patient's tumor. (**B**) The equivalent of an contrasted T1 MRI study with a transversal scan while (**C**) shows the same study in a coronary view. *Arrows* point to the mass.

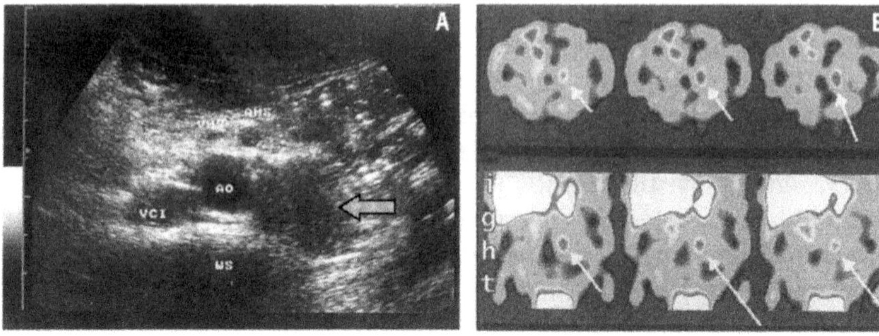

FIGURE 2. (**A**) Ultrasound image of the para-aortal lesion (*arrow*) and its distance to the abdominal aorta (AO), the lower vena cava (VCI), the spine (WS), and other vessels. (**B**) Summary findings in the ^{123}J-MIBG scan of the abdomen; *upper panel* transversal scans; *lower panel*, lower part coronary scans (*white arrows* indicate the lesion).

After being operated upon, the patient suffered initially from severe thrombocytosis (>800,000/μL) over a period of 3 months. She needed more than 60 mg of hydrocortisone per day. Fortunately, hypertension and diabetes no longer needed to be treated. Though she initially recovered well, this patient died from pulminary bleeding of unknown cause 6 months after the operation.

DISCUSSION

Hormonal, molecular and immunohistological studies suggest that our patient suffered from a paraganglioma with excess catecholamine and ACTH secretion. Although hypertension and tachycardia were present, our patient seemed to suffer most from the sequelae of hypercortisolism. Noncorticotrophs

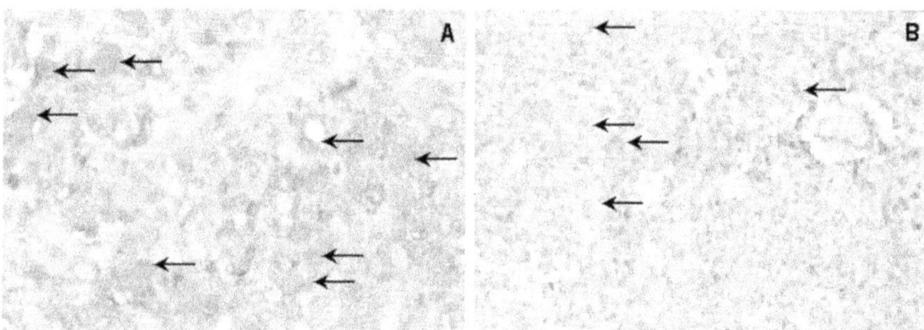

FIGURE 3. Immunohistological studies demonstrated that the patient's tumor tissue could be stained with antibodies against ACTH (polyclonal rabbit, dilution 1:100; DakoCytomation, Hamburg, Germany (**A**) and chromogranin A (monoclonal mouse, dilution 1:200; DakoCytomation (**B**); magnification 40× and 20×, respectively. Linked-streptavidin biotin-method with DAB (dark; *arrows*) as chromogen.

may gain the power to aberrantly produce ACTH, but usually not acquire mechanisms to control secretion of ACTH via classic negative feedback loops.[9] Consequently, the glucocorticoid excess in EAS is frequently more severe than in cases of Cushing's disease. In addition, coexistence of excess catecholamine and ACTH secretion drives adrenal steroidogenesis via different pathways. ACTH leads to the expression of steroidogenic enzymes and peptides, and catecholamines also stimulate expression of steroidogenic enzymes and peptides, thus adding to the effect of ACTH.[10] Moreover, catecholamines increase renin activity and, therefore, also intensify hyperaldosteronism. All these effects may lead to severe hypertension, hypokalemia, and hyperglycemia in addition to the suppression of the immune system and hypophyseal hormone secretion by glucocorticoids.[11] Relief from hypercortisolism is the therapy of choice to overcome suppression of the pituitary gland and there is little, if any, benefit from substitution of decreased hormones except cortisol in critically ill patients.[12] However, there are only few and old data for substitution therapy in hypercortisolism.

However, the presence of hypokalemic hypertension was an indication for further endocrine work-up. In addition, laboratory results have to be interpreted with caution. For example, excess glucocorticoid secretion can explain suppression of hypophyseal hormone secretion. Later, the results of the dexamethasone suppression test and of the CRH challenge showed that EAS was a proven diagnosis.[13,14] Thus, there was no indication for the performance of an MRI scan of the pituitary gland.

Our case underscores the need for further characterization of hypertensive patients with low potassium and for heeding the patient's specific complaints. Furthermore, the case tells us to characterize hormone excess syndromes thoroughly before performing unnecessary and misleading imaging studies. In addition, we learned to take a closer look at structures that could be lymph nodes, metastases or other masses in imaging studies, and we see that more than 70 years after the first description of Cushing's disease and more than 40 years after the definition of EAS we are still far from understanding these disorders.

ACKNOWLEDGMENTS

This work was supported by a grant from the University of Düsseldorf and by the Eberhard-Igler-Stiftung Düsseldorf, Germany to H.S.W.

REFERENCES

1. WOLF, A., H.S. WILLENBERG, K. CUPISTI, *et al.* 2005. Adrenal pheochromocytoma with contralateral cortisol-producing adrenal adenoma: diagnostic and therapeutic management. Horm. Metab. Res. **37:** 391–395.

2. SCHTEINGART, D.E., J.W. CONN, D.N. ORTH, *et al.* 1972. Secretion of ACTH and MSH by an adrenal medullary paraganglioma. J. Clin. Endocrinol. Metab. **34:** 676–683.
3. MEADOR, C.K., G.W. LIDDLE, D.P. ISLAND, *et al.* 1962. Cause of Cushing's syndrome in patients with tumors arising from "nonendocrine" tissue. J. Clin. Endocrinol. Metab. **22:** 693–703.
4. LIDDLE, G.W., D.P. ISLAND, R.L. NEY, *et al.* 1963. Nonpituitary neoplasms and Cushing's syndrome: ectopic "adrenocorticotropin" produced by nonpituitary neoplasms as a cause of Cushing's syndrome. Arch. Intern. Med. **111:** 471–475.
5. MORAN, C.A., W. RUSH & H. MENA. 1977. Primary spinal paragangliomas: a clinicopathological and immunohistochemical study of 30 cases. Histopathology **31:** 167–173.
6. LINNOILA, R.I., E.E. LACK, S.M. STEINBERG, *et al.* 1988. Decreased expression of neuropeptides in malignant paragangliomas: an immunohistochemical study. Hum. Pathol. **19:** 41–50.
7. WHITE, A. & S. GIBSON. 1998. ACTH precursors: biological significance and clinical relevance. Clin. Endocrinol. **48:** 251–255.
8. STEWART, P.M., S. GIBSON, S.R. CROSBY, *et al.* 1994. ACTH precursors characterize the ectopic ACTH syndrome. Clin. Endocrinol. **40:** 199–204.
9. CLARK, A.J.L., M.F. STEWART, P.M. LAVENDER, *et al.* 1990. Defective glucocorticoid regulation of proopiomelanocortin gene expression and peptide secretion in a small cell lung cancer cell line. J. Clin. Endocrinol. Metab. **70:** 485–490.
10. HAIDAN. A., S.R. BORNSTEIN, A. GLASOW, *et al.* 1998. Basal steroidogenic activity of adrenocortical cells is increased 10-fold by coculture with chromaffin cells. Endocrinology **139:** 772–780.
11. VREZAS, I., H.S. WILLENBERG, G. MANSMANN, *et al.* 2003. Ectopic adrenocorticotropin (ACTH) and corticotropin-releasing hormone (CRH) production in the adrenal gland: basic and clinical aspects. Microsc. Res. Tech. **61:** 308–314.
12. LIGTENBERG, J.J.M., A.R.J. GIRBES, J.A.M. BEENTJES, *et al.* 2001. Hormones in the critically ill patient: to intervene or not to intervene? Intensive Care Med. **27:** 1567–1577.
13. ILIAS, I., D.J. TORPY, K. PACAK, *et al.* 2005. Cushing's syndrome due to ectopic corticotropin secretion: twenty years' experience at the National Institutes of Health. J. Clin. Endocrinol. Metab. **90:** 4955–4962.
14. ORTH, D.N. 1995. Cushing's syndrome. N. Engl. J. Med. **332:** 791–803.

Catecholamine-Secreting Metastatic Carcinoid as Differential Diagnosis in Pheochromocytoma

Clinical, Laboratory, and Imaging Clues in the Search for the Lurking Neuroendocrine Tumor (NET)

HENDRICKS H. WHITMAN III,[a,b,c] ELLIOT K. FISHMAN,[d]
KJELL ÖBERG,[e] JOSEPH M. WILDMAN,[f,g] AND ANDREA L. LONG[h]

[a]*Summit Medical Group, Berkeley Heights, New Jersey 07922, USA*

[b]*Rheumatology Division of the Hospital for Special Surgery, New York, New York 10021, USA*

[c]*Hypertension Center of New York Presbyterian Hospital-Weill Cornell Medical Center, New York, New York 10021, USA*

[d]*Radiology and Oncology and Director, Diagnostic Radiology and Body CT, The Russell H. Morgan Department of Radiology and Radiological Science, The Johns Hopkins University School of Medicine, Baltimore, Maryland 21287, USA*

[e]*Endocrine Oncology and Dean, Medical Faculty, Uppsala University Hospital, Uppsala, Sweden*

[f]*Summit Medical Group, Oncology Department, Berkeley Heights, New Jersey 07922, USA*

[g]*New York University School of Medicine, New York, New York 10016, USA*

[h]*R&D, Bell Laboratories Holmdel (Ret.), Warren, New Jersey 07059 USA*

ABSTRACT: Catecholamine-secreting metastatic carcinoid should be considered in differential diagnosis of malignant pheochromocytoma. Paroxysmal functioning or hormonally silent gastroenteropancreatic neuroendocrine tumors (GEP NETs) require repeat biochemical measurements and sensitive anatomic and functional imaging studies overlapping those for malignant pheochromocytoma. This report presents clinical, laboratory, and radiologic findings in a patient presenting with heart rate variability; vasoactive headaches reactive to ethanol, tyramine and tryptophan; labile blood pressure; diaphoresis; diarrhea;

Address for correspondence: Hendricks H. Whitman III, M.D., Summit Medical Group. One Diamond Hill Road, Berkeley Heights, NJ 07922, USA. Voice: +1-908-769-2521; fax: +1-908-769-2530.
e-mail: whitmanh@hss.edu

Ann. N.Y. Acad. Sci. 1073: 59–78 (2006). © 2006 New York Academy of Sciences.
doi: 10.1196/annals.1353.007

abdominal pain; unexplained pancreatitis; joint pain; and paroxysmal flushing with pallor. GI studies (including endoscopic ultrasound) and multiple imaging modalities (including 2D CT, MRI with gadolinium, [^{18}]FDG PET/CT, [^{123}I]MIBG, and SRS [^{111}In]Octreotide [OctreoScan]) were not diagnostic. 24-h BP, Holter and 30-day cardiac event monitors plus urinary biochemical studies consistently suggested catecholamine-synthesizing NET. NIH plasma metanephrines studies and [6]-[^{18}F]Fluorodopamine PET ruled out malignant pheochromocytoma (pheo). Repeated studies showed persistently abnormal GEP NET biomarkers and urinary catecholamines. Capsule endoscopy revealed suspicious submucosal lesions throughout the small intestine. Dual-phase 64-slice multidetector computed tomography (MDCT) with 3D volumetric reconstruction of the abdomen and pelvis revealed multiple diffuse liver metastases and three extrahepatic lesions consistent with metastatic carcinoid. In combination, intensive biochemical testing repeated over time, dual-phase 64-slice MDCT with 3D image reconstruction and volume-rendering (VR) technique, and advanced radionuclide imaging are required to detect NETs' sporadic or paroxysmal functioning, rule out extra-adrenal pheochromocytoma, and localize and characterize metastatic carcinoid. If pheochromocytoma is ruled out, yet symptoms and biochemical markers for catecholamine excess are present, then carcinoid and other amine-precursor-uptake decarboxylation (APUD) tumors must remain in the differential diagnosis.

KEYWORDS: **carcinoid; imaging; multidetector CT (MDCT); catecholamines; tumor markers; pheochromocytoma**

INTRODUCTION

Requiring consideration in differential diagnosis of malignant pheochromocytoma, both catecholamine-secreting metastatic carcinoid and endocrine pancreatic tumor (subclasses of GEP NET) are uncommon but heterogeneous neuroendocrine neoplasms that exhibit variable patterns of hormone secretion and growth in the course of the disease.[1,2] Problems in diagnosis and localization of GEP NET when lesions are 3 cm or smaller (since 70–90% already may have metastasized by the time they are 1 cm) arise from amine-precursor-uptake-decarboxylation (APUD) characteristics common to the etiology and behavior of pheochromocytoma and GEP NET, despite heterogeneity in embryology between and within neuroendocrine tumor types.[3–5]

In this case report, APUD characteristics and their risks, common to GEP NET and pheochromocytoma, suggest that (1) the process for diagnosis and localization of catecholamine-producing NET must consider both pheochromocytoma and GEP NET and (2) the work-up can be concluded only when *both* pheochromocytoma and GEP NET with sporadic or paroxysmal function are ruled out.

CASE REPORT

This patient presented with abdominal and pelvic pain and history of vasoactive attacks for over twenty years following a lengthy systemic infection probably with *Staphylococcus aureus*. The attacks (increasingly awakening the patient between 4 and 6 A.M.) consisted of severe vasoactive headaches consistently reactive to ethanol, tyramine, and tryptophan; palpitations; sweating; tachycardia; labile hypertension; severe muscle rigidity across neck, back and arms; edema; sweating; ice-cold hands and feet; hyperglycemia; paroxysmal hypotension; diaphoresis; polyuria; and diarrhea. Over an 8- to 32-hour attack cycle, edema followed by polyuria led to water gain and loss in excess of 12 percent of body weight. Flushing alternated with pallor during the attacks. Retrospectively, the patient suffered vasoactive attacks consistent with excessive catecholamine secretion after injection with [^{123}I]MIBG tracer; after anesthetic for a GI study; after tilt-table positioning and 1-gram glucagon stimulation during barium enema study; and after physical activity following supine rest (even without food ingestion).

Review of clinical history, physical examination, and historical medical records as far back as 15 years earlier suggested the possibility of neuroendocrine tumor with paroxysmal functioning and excessive hormonal release. Ten years earlier, renal ultrasound and CT of abdomen/pelvis showed one 1.5-cm lesion in the left hepatic lobe. Two and four years earlier, pelvic ultrasound revealed a right adnexal cyst possibly containing a solid nodule suggesting neoplasm; and CT (abdomen/pelvis) reported three small hypodensities in the dome of the liver that were too small to characterize.

Follow-up abdominal ultrasounds and CTs of abdomen/pelvis showed soft-tissue density in the left adrenal. Subsequent MRI showed nodularity in the left adrenal gland but visualized no definite adrenal nodule. Initial Octreoscan revealed no uptake. Gastrointestinal studies (including upper GI with small bowel follow-through, endoscopy, colonoscopy, and glucagon-stimulated barium enema) were all non-diagnostic. Occurring both while fasting and after meals, pancreatitis developed during the period of intensive GI studies. Gadolinium-enhanced MRI reported finding no occult primary neuroendocrine tumor. That study did report a non-aggressive hypervascular lesion within the dome of the liver not revealed on T2-weighted image favoring benign cyst or hemangioma with marked hypervascular enhancement on arterial phase, favoring focal nodular hyperplasia.

Subsequent dual-phase CT reported one smaller hepatic lesion and one indeterminate lesion with hypervascular blush in its anterior two-thirds that was conceivably an atypical hemangioma or possibly a lesion of focal nodular hyperplasia. Endoscopic ultrasound (EUS) revealed thickened left adrenal gland without obvious masses, pancreas in a more cephalad position than normal (perhaps pushed by the thickened adrenal), multiple punctuate gastric erosions ranging from 2 to 3 mm, and a linear gastric ulcer 4 mm × 1 cm with gastrin output in the 200–300 range. EUS as well as endoscopy 10 years earlier confirmed *H. pylori*-negative gastric ulcer.

METHODS AND RESULTS

TABLE 1 shows the marked similarity between clinical characteristics classically associated with pheochromocytoma[5] and characteristics seen in this patient (distinguishing continuous, sporadic [S] or paroxysmal [P]) and in other GEP NET patients. Biochemical tests reconfirmed 5-HIAA elevated four to five times above normal (TABLE 2). Although the patient's normal diet avoided serotonin-intensive foods, tyramine- and tryptophan-containing meals preceding two 5-HIAA collections inadvertently provoked severe vasoactive attacks aborted by the patient with a 6-mg injection of the serotonin antagonist sumatriptan. Serotonin antagonist injection during two collections was the probable cause of false-negative 5-HIAA.[6] Chromogranin A repeatedly tested normal. Notably, urinary studies' 24-h volumes ranged from 6.0 to 12.9 L/24 h despite normal fluid intake and foods failing to account for more than 40–50% of this volume. Initial local plasma tests [dated 10/21/03; TABLE 2] showed epinephrine 283 pg/mL* (0–110 pg/mL), norepinephrine 444 (70–750) pg/mL, and dopamine 30 pg/mL (0–30 pg/mL).

Multiple imaging modalities and GI studies had not definitively identified neuroendocrine tumors. 2D CT studies had shown a possible left adrenal lesion; MRI of the pituitary gland suggested equivocal findings; and [^{123}I]MIBG showed bilateral uptake in the adrenals. Endoscopic ultrasound had shown a thickened adrenal gland but a normal pancreas. 2D dual-phase CT studies indicating multiple hypervascular liver lesions ruled out hemangioma or cysts, but were unable to characterize them or to visualize extra-hepatic tumors. Imaging with [^{18}F]fluorodeoxyglucose (FDG) PET, [^{123}I]MIBG, and a second somatostatin receptor scintigraphy with [^{111}]Indium pentetreotide (Octreoscan) revealed tracer uptake in multiple endocrine sites not considered diagnostic by the interpreting radiologists.

Methods resolving diagnosis were the following. Despite a normal ECG, 24-h Holter monitor and 30-day cardiac event recorder demonstrated paroxysmal heart rate variability (HRV) and cardiovascular events compatible with neuroendocrine tumor.[7] As observed among pheochromocytoma patients, this patient exhibits a diurnal pattern of hypertension even during sleep; an absence of correlation between heart rate and blood pressures; and correlation between headache, low pulse, high heart rate variability, and high blood pressure lability. During two paroxysms, clinical monitoring of 24-h blood pressure and pulse, serum GEP NET markers, urinary catecholamines, and plasma metanephrines (before, during, and after the paroxysm for some measures) revealed patterns of hypersecretion over the spell. Over many months' observations and in the absence of medication, self-monitored blood pressures and pulse repeatedly exhibited hypertensive and hypotensive patterns (e.g., 157/100 and 94/65 mmHg) within a few hours.

TABLE 1. Clinical signs

Category	Possible indicators of BP changes and catecholamine excess of pheo patients[a]	Incidence in this patient with metastatic carcinoid (P = paroxysmal, S = sporadic, + = increased, ++ = increased)		Incidence in GI carcinoid/ GEP NET population
Blood pressure	Hypertension ± wide fluctuations	P+	Diurnal patterns; paroxysmal spikes provoked by eating; alternating with hypotension	Medium
	Hypotension, paroxysmal	P+	Diurnal patterns; paroxysmal spikes provoked by eating, physical activity; alternating with hypertension	High
Cardiovascular	Arrhythmia	S+	During severe vasoactive attacks only	Medium
	Bradycardia	P+	Paroxysmal, provoked by eating, physical activity	High
	Palpitations	P+	Diurnal patterns; paroxysmal, provoked by eating, physical activity	High
	Tachycardia, very forceful heart beat	P+	Paroxysmal, provoked by eating, physical activity, posture change	High
Catecholamines	Dilated pupils	0	No	No
	Dyspnea	S+	Sporadic nocturnal, high CO_2	
	Fever (occasionally very elevated)	0	Subnormal temperature	Low
	Hypertensive retinopathy	0	No	No
	Nervousness, depression	0	No	Medium
	Numbness, cold in extremities	P+	Paroxysmal	Medium
	Polyuria (children with pheo)	P++	High nonparoxysmal (4 ×UL); higher paroxysmal (5–8×UL))	Low
	Raynaud's syndrome	P+	Severe, hands and feet	Medium
	Red, cyanotic hands or face	+	High (including before skin metastasis in hand)	High
	Sweating, generalized	P+	Paroxysmal; drenching; provoked by eating	High
	Warmth ± heat intolerance	+	Sustained	High
	Weakness, fatigue	+	High	High

[a]Adapted from Tables 4.1, 6.1, and 6.4 from MANGER, W.M. & R.W. GIFFORD, JR. 1996. *Clinical and Experimental Pheochromocytoma*, 2nd ed. Blackwell. Cambridge, MA.

(*Continued.*)

TABLE 1. ***Continued.***

Category	Possible indicators of BP changes and catecholamine excess of pheo patients[a]	Incidence in this patient with metastatic carcinoid (P = paroxysmal, S = sporadic, + = increased, ++ = increased)		Incidence in GI carcinoid/ GEP NET population
Gut-hormonal	Constipation	S+	Paroxysmal	Medium
	Diarrhea	P++	Daily, sometimes explosive	High
	Hyper/hypoglycemia	++	Diurnal; cyclic in vasoactive attacks; hyper/hypotension correlation; vasoconstriction/vasodilation correlation. Glucose 55–60 mg% (stage I), 126–136 (stage II)	High
	Nausea ± vomiting	0	Infrequent except severe vasoactive attacks	Medium
	Pain in abdomen, epigastrium	++	High; provoked by eating, physical activity, physical position	High
	Weight loss, unexplained	++	10% loss, 8 months	High
Vasoactive (gut-hormonal)	Flushing (uncommon in pheo patients)	P++	Paroxysmal; provoked by eating, physical activity; hypotension troughs	High
	Headaches, severe vasoactive	P++	High, paroxysmal, provoked by eating, physical activity	Medium
	Pallor	P+	Paroxysmal; in hypertension peaks of severe vasoactive attacks	Low
	Paroxysmal reaction to glucagon stimulation	P++	Severe vasoactive attack	Low
	Reaction to induction of some anesthesia	++	Severe vasoactive attack	Low
	Vasoactive reactions induced by ethanol, tyramine, glucagon, tryptophan-rich foods	++	Diurnal; attacks wave-like; alternating hypotension and hypertension	High
Other	Hyperamylasemia	++	High amylase, lipase, trypsin, low c-peptide, low insulin, low conversion of proinsulin to insulin, high proinsulin, high somatostatin (1×). EPT?	Depends on GI carcinoid vs. EPT subgroup
	Impaired glucose tolerance	++	Dizzy, hot spell if ingest sugar	Medium
	Hypokalemia	++	Low K+, low Na, low Cl	Medium
	N.A.	++	Hyperperistalsis, steatorrhea, dyspnea, diaphoresis, enlarged liver, excess salivation	Medium

[a]Adapted from Tables 4.1, 6.1, and 6.4 from MANGER, W.M. & R.W. GIFFORD, JR. 1996. *Clinical and Experimental Pheochromocytoma*, 2nd ed. Blackwell. Cambridge, MA.

Urinary biochemical studies showing elevations of metanephrines, epinephrines, dopamine, vanillymandelic acid (VMA), and homovanillic acid (HVA) consistently suggested the presence of catecholamine-synthesizing neuroendocrine tumor, possibly pheochromocytoma or paraganglioma (TABLE 2). Urinary dopamine exceeded the sum of norepinephrines and epinephrines in five of six studies; and exceeded the Mayo Clinic limit 4571 nmol/day[8,9] in five of six studies. The ratios of urinary dopamine/creatinine were 0.373, 0.403, and 0.380 compared with upper normal ratio of 0.28.[5]

However, highly controlled and specific plasma metanephrine studies and [6]-[^{18}F]fluorodopamine PET both performed at the NIH definitively ruled out malignant pheochromocytoma.[10–17] Highly controlled plasma O-methylated metabolite measurement also performed at NIH ruled out dopamine-producing paraganglioma.[18] The patient's urinary dopamine values in six of six studies fell between the 10th and 45th percentile of nine patients with dopamine-producing paragangliomas studied at NIH.[18,19]

Persistently abnormal GEP NET biomarkers (TABLE 3)[1–3,20–24] and urinary catecholamine elevations[19] both were consistent with neuroendocrine tumor because both carcinoids and pheochromocytomas have the ability to decarboxylate amine precursors.[3,5,21,25,26] Nearly 100% specificity of 5-HIAA (TABLE 2) and other biochemical measures associated with gastrointestinal carcinoid and endocrine pancreatic tumor (TABLE 3) consistently indicated the presence of nonlocalized GEP NET, either gastrointestinal carcinoid or endocrine pancreatic tumor or both.[1,2,21]

In addition to 5-HIAA, plasma serotonin was repeatedly elevated, with higher values seen at those times when other biomarkers suggested tumor functioning (TABLE 3).[27,28] Carcinoembryonic antigen values were also elevated. TABLE 3 shows repeated elevations of amylase, lipase and trypsin suggestive of but not specific for islet cell damage. Chromogranin A, gastrin, vasoactive intestinal polypeptide (VIP), neuron-specific enolase (NSE), calcitonin, prolactin, histamine, insulin-like growth factors I and II were normal in repeated tests. Other normal tests in test periods shown in Table include calcitonin, histamine, ferratin (low), TIBC (low), vasoactive intestinal peptide, neuron-specific enolase, creatinine kinase, Insulin antibodies RIA, HGC total, niacin (serum), CA 19–9, erythropoietin, CA-125, CA 27, 29, calcium (total, serum), ionized calcium, PTH intact, prolactin, thyroid peroxidase AB, thyroglobulin AB, cortisol, aldosterone, and ESR (Westergren). With patterns suggesting NF-1 mutation, the patient was found to have at least two café-au-lait spots and reported maternal family members with cutaneous neurofibroma, spinal-cord malignant tumor, and high penetrance of congenital heart defects.[5,29,30] However, tumors' hormonal activity in this patient contradicts NF1 casuality.

As soon as malignant pheochromocytoma and dopamine-producing paraganglioma were definitely ruled out by the controlled studies of plasma metanephrines and imaging with [6]-[^{18}F]fluorodopamine PET at NIH,[12]

TABLE 2. Urinary biochemical tests in chronological order in a patient with catecholamine-secreting enzymes from metastatic carcinoid

Date	Ur 24 hr Volume (mL/24 h) (500–1600) if extrap to 24 h	Ur catecholamines total (mcg/24 h)	Ur metanephrines total (mcg/24 h)	Ur metanephrines (mcg/24 h)	Ur normetaneprhines (mcg/24 h)	Ur norepinephrines (mcg/24 h)	Ur epinephrines (mcg/24 h)	Ur dopamine (mcg/24 h)	Ur creatinine (mg/24 h)	Ur VMA (mg/24 h)	Ur dopamine: Ur creatinine ratio (mcg/mcg)	Ur 5HIAA (mg/24 h)	Ur Cortisol (mcg/dL)	HVA w/ creatinine
3/28/93	6,000	48 (0–100)	0.42 (0.1–0.9)									**29.4 (0–9)**		
8/27/03	6,200		620 (0–1300)	**500 (0–400)**	120 (0–900)	55.8 (12.1–85.5)	12.4 (1.7–22.4)	341 (65–400)		2.5 (1.4–6.5)			6.7 (4–22)	
8/30/03	4,950											**11.9 (0–6)**	1.4 (4–22)	
10/7/03	7,290											**24.1 (0–6)**		
11/27/03	9,300											(x5HT) 7.0 (0–15)		
12/10/03	7,300											(x5HT) 12.0 (0–15)		
6/14/04	9,975								1416 (800–1800)					
8/17/04	7,150								1,494 (800–1,800)					
8/27/04	12,300		**750 (95–475)**	**664 (19–140)**	86 (52–310)	49.0 (15.0–100.0)	**25.0 (2.0–24.0)**	480 (52–480)		3.7 (1.4–6.5)				
9/29/04	6,000		**600 (95–475)**	**414 (19–140)**	176 (52–310)	42.0 (15.0–1,00.0)	12.0 (2.0–24.0)	476 (52–480)	1,180 (630–2,500)	5.4 (< 6.0)	**0.4034 (< 0.28)**			
10/1/04	1,200 (2h) = 14400*					**192* (15.0–100.0)**	**72.0* (2.0–24.0)**	**2424* (52–480)**						
10/3/04	6,000		**1,362 (95–475)**	**1,098 (19–140)**	264 (52–310)	66 (15.0–100.0)	18.0 (2.0–24.0)	**630 (52–480)**	1,690 (630–2,500)	**6.6 (<6.0)**	**0.3728 (< 0.28)**			
10/5/04	600 (4 h) = 3600*					**264* (15.0–100.0)**	**48.0* (2.0–24.0)**	**1384* (52–480)**						
10/7/04	5,100 (9.5 h) = 12,900*		1,87.3* (95–475)	10.1* (19–140)	187.3* (52–310)	**127.6* (15.0–100.0)**	**38.5* (2.0–24.0)**	**872.3* (52–480)**		**9.5* (<6.0)**				
12/21/04	5,100												**100 (5.0–50.0)**	
12/23/04	8,300								1670 (630–2,500)			**12.5 (0–6)**		
12/27/04	3,550		383 (95–475)	**241 (19–140)**	142 (52–310)	53 (15.0–1,00.0)	14 (2.0–24.0)		1,210 (630–2,500)					5.0 (1.6–7.5)
1/28/05	2,150* (12 h)= 4,300			**142* (19–140)**	246* (52–310)	90* (15.0–1,00.0)	**26* (2.0–24.0)**	370* (52–480)		**6.4* (<6.0)**				**9.0 (1.6–7.5)**
6/05												**10.0 (0–6)**		
7/05												**13.8 (0–6)**		

Shaded boldface = Abnormal; x5HT = interfered by serotonin antagonist injection, 6 mg, 5HT 1B/1D. *Extrapolated to 24–h volume and concentration from spot collections < 24–h collections.

TABLE 3. GEP NET biochemical tests in chronological order in a patient with catecholamine–secreting enzymes from metastatic carcinoid

Date	U–5HIAA (mg/24 h)	p–Serotonin (ng/mL)	Chromogranin A (ng/mL)	Amylase (u/L)	Lipase (u/L)	Trypsin (ng/mL)	Pancreatic polypeptide (pg/mL)	Gastrin (ng/L)	Carcinogenic antigen (ng/mL)	Insulin (mIU/mL)	Proinsulin (pmol/L)	Glucagon (pg/mL)	C-Peptide (ng/mL)
3/93	**29.4 (0.0–9.0)**												
2/95		290 (46–319)											
8/03	**11.9 (0–6)**												
10/03	**24.1 (0–6)**	**203 (22–180)**	14.6 (6.0–39.0)						**3.25 (0.00–2.50)**				
11/03	x5HT 7.0 (0–15)		22 (0.0–51.0)										
2/04	x5HT 12.0 (0–15.0)			**164 (25–115)**	274 (114–286)								
3/04(a)				**123 (25–115)**	193 (114–286)		164 (100–780)	23 (0–90)	**3.21 (0.00–2.50)**	8.0 (<17.0)	**12.5 (<8.8)**	47 (20–100)	2.6 (0.8–3.1)
3/04(b)							**75 (100–780)**	24 (0–90)		invalid tests (2)	**12.5 (<8.8)**	**<20 (20–100)**	**0.6 (0.8–3.1)**
3/04(c)													1.1 (0.8–3.1)
4/04		**261 (22–180)**						200–300 (EUS)		5.0 (<17.0)	8.2 (<8.8)	**<20 (20–100)**	1.8 (0.8–3.1)
5/04		invalid test		**108 (21–101)**	29 (7–60)		**65 (100–780)**			9.1 (<17.0)	**13.1 (<8.8)**	***<50 (<60)**	2.7 (0.8–3.1)
6/04(a)		**378 (22–180)**						22 (0–90)		6.0 (<17.0)	**10.4 (8.8)**	***<50 (<60)**	2.1 (0.8–3.1)
7/04				**140 (21–101)**	**74 (7–60)**								
8/04(a)		**309 (22–180)**		**366 (21–101)**	**344 (114–286)**			26 (0–90)	**3.34 (0.00–2.50)**			***<50 (<60)**	**7.3 (0.8–3.1)**
8/04(b)				**194 (25–115)**									
9/04		**333 (22–180)**		**133 (21–101)**		**32 (7–30)**			**3.35 (0.00–2.50)**				1.0 (0.8–3.1)
10/04(a)		**265 (22–180)**		98 (21–101)	**69 (7–60)**	**45 (7–30)**							
10/04(b)		**419 (22–180)**											
11/04(a)		**254 (22–180)**		**210 (21–101)**	**65 (7–60)**	**36 (7–30)**	106 (100–780)						1.1 (0.8–3.1)
11/04(b)		**298 (22–180)**		**182 (21–101)**	49 (7–60)	**37 (7–30)**							
1/05(a)			12.7 (6.00–39.0)	**225 (25–115)**	284 (114–286)				**2.90 (0.00–2.50)**				
1/05(b)				**153 (21–101)**	57 (7–60)								
2/05		**200 (22–180)**	12.5 (6.0–39.0)	**146 (21–101)**	**64 (7–60)**	**57 (7–30)**	**<50 (100–780)**	15 (< 100)		<2 (<17.0)	8.2 (8.8)		0.9 (0.8–3.1)

Shaded boldface = Abnormal; x5HT = interfered by serotonin antagonist injection, 6 mg, 5 HT 1B/1D.

the patient was started therapeutically on long-acting somatostatin analogue 6 weeks before localization of tumors, and reported the first good night's rest without early-morning palpitations and start of vasoactive paroxysm.[1,3] Treatment with slow-release intramuscular (i.m.) formulation of octreotide (Sandostatin LAR®) achieved significant symptom control; including sharp reduction in the frequency and severity of vasoactive attacks described previously.[31]

Tumor localization remained incomplete. Subsequently, capsule endoscopy (FIG. 1E and 1F) revealed multiple possible submucosal lesions at four segments throughout the small intestine, consistent with gastrointestinal carcinoid.

MDCT imaging of abdomen/pelvis and thoracic/chest on a 64-slice multidetector CT (MDCT) (Siemens Sensation 64; Leonardo Workstation) with 3D volumetric reconstruction revealed multiple liver metastases, including all four largest hepatic lesions characterized as hypervascular on dual-phase CT.[32,33] MDCT interpretation readily imaged three extrahepatic lesions 1.0 to 1.5 cm in size, consistent with metastatic carcinoid (FIG. 1A through D), located in the right-lower-quadrant abdomen superficial to the retroperitoneum, center lower pelvis, and gastric antrum. Notably, *all* previous equivocal abnormal sites of radionuclide uptake subsequently were localized as potential carcinoid tumor sites using 3D volumetric reconstruction of dual-phase MDCT images on the 64-slice MDCT scanner. However, MDCT additionally imaged two extrahepatic sites that no previous radionuclide study had shown, despite significant patient pain at those sites at the time of those studies. As for purported anomalies visible on reportedly negative [^{123}]IMIBG, dual-phase CT and [^{18}]FDG-PET, respectively, MDCT imaging (FIG. 1) reconfirmed benign thymic hyperplasia and benign adenoma on the left adrenal gland. Shortly after the NIH plasma metanephrine study, dual-phase CT using sequential contrast enhancement on 10-min delayed CT images estimated the adrenal nodule having dynamic attenuation (123HU) and 10-min delay attenuation (50HU), indicating relative and absolute percentage washouts both exceeding 50% and characteristic of adrenal adenoma. Those values are substantially higher than those in adrenocortical carcinoma or pheochromocytoma.[34–36]

In preparation for surgery, the patient's hypertension was successfully controlled pre-operatively and post-recurrence with phenoxybenzamine. The patient's carcinoid crisis was blocked with increased dose (40 mg) of octreotide. Pre-operative single-phase CT failed to discriminate between hemangioma and liver metastases; and it failed to visualize extra- and intrahepatic tumors because the critical time interval between bolus injection and image acquisition may not have been optimally controlled.

DISCUSSION

Systematic patterns of severe headache in predictable paroxysms, caused by neuroendocrine disease years before tumors are detectable radiologically, suggest that NET hormones' hypersecretion may be causing a patient's sudden transient elevation or rapid rate of change of blood pressure (rather than sustained hypertension or stable high blood pressure level) and triggering headache.[37,38] Serial measurements of urinary catecholamines and 5-HIAA during and after paroxysms are necessary. Dopamine production by the tumor cells, acting as both a natriuretic and vasodilator, explains edema followed by polyuria among patients with catecholamine-producing neuroendocrine tumors.[5] Compared with migraine- and cluster-headache patients, carcinoid patients' vascular headaches uniquely are accompanied by increases in plasma serotonin[38] (40% in this patient during a paroxysm), lagged hypersecretions of 5-HIAA, and lagged releases of urinary dopamine and often other urinary catecholamines as well.

Catecholamine-synthesizing enzyme production by GEP NET exhibits blood pressure variability in the patient that is comparable *out* of paroxysms to that of normotensive patients (BP coefficient of variability [(0.06 systolic)/(0.07 diastolic)]) and *in* paroxysms comparable to that of pheochromocytoma patients (BP coefficient of variability [(0.06–0.10 systolic)/(0.12–0.15 diastolic)]).[39] Less characteristic for GEP NET than reported for pheochromocytoma is heart rate variability (HRV).[7]

Chromogranin A (CgA)—previously considered the "gold standard" for diagnosing carcinoid, but reported elevated also in malignant pheochromocytoma—was repeatedly normal despite increases in tumor burden in this polyuric patient over the period of diagnosis. Benchmark studies of CgA, collected by Eriksson and published by the Nordic Neuroendocrine Tumor Group, show that CgA is elevated in 87%, 79%, and 100% of midgut, foregut, and hindgut carcinoid tumors, respectively; and CgA-CgB, in 94% of endocrine pancreatic tumors.[21] Excessive renal clearance caused by polyuria reported among some GEP NET and pheochromocytoma patients may be associated with *false-negative* CgA.

Given that aromatic-L-amino acid decarboxylase enzyme (AADC) can metabolize 5-hydroxytryptophan to 5-hydroxytryptamine (serotonin) and also metabolize dihydroxyphenylalamine (DOPA) to dopamine, analysis of biochemical markers in patients with pheo-like symptoms should comprise not only dopamine, norepinephrine and epinephrine measurements from the catecholamine pathway, but also serotonin and 5-HIAA from the serotonin synthesis pathway. Biochemical markers recommended for GEP NET and EPT[1,2,21] should be measured among patients strongly suspected of a GEP NET, EPT, or malignant pheochromocytoma with *a priori* unknown functioning or hormonal patterns

Most critically, these biochemical markers should be measured at random times; measured after overnight ingestion of tryptophan, tyrosine or tyramine; measured after provocation/stimulation (but safeguarding against catecholamine- or carcinoid-crisis) using standardized test protocols; *and* repeated over the course of a symptomatic paroxysm. Biomarkers' abnormal patterns may advance NET diagnosis 5 to 10 years before tumors reach radiologic limits of detection.

A

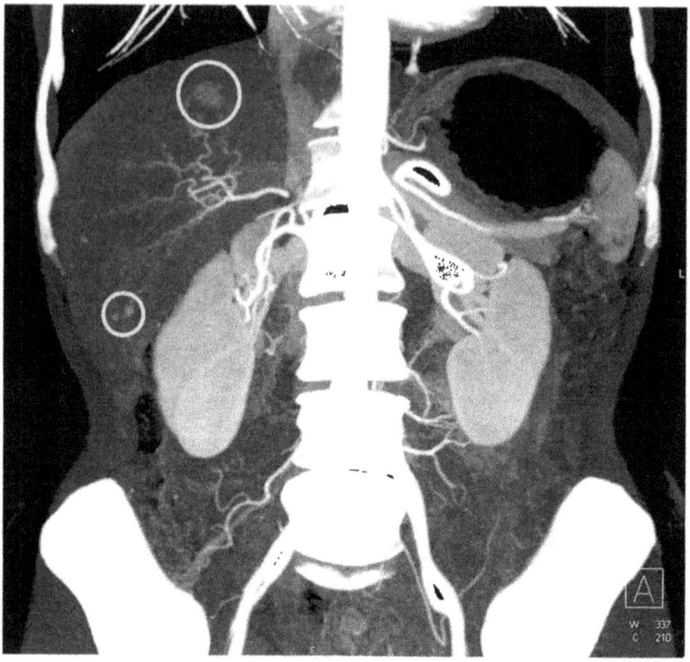

B

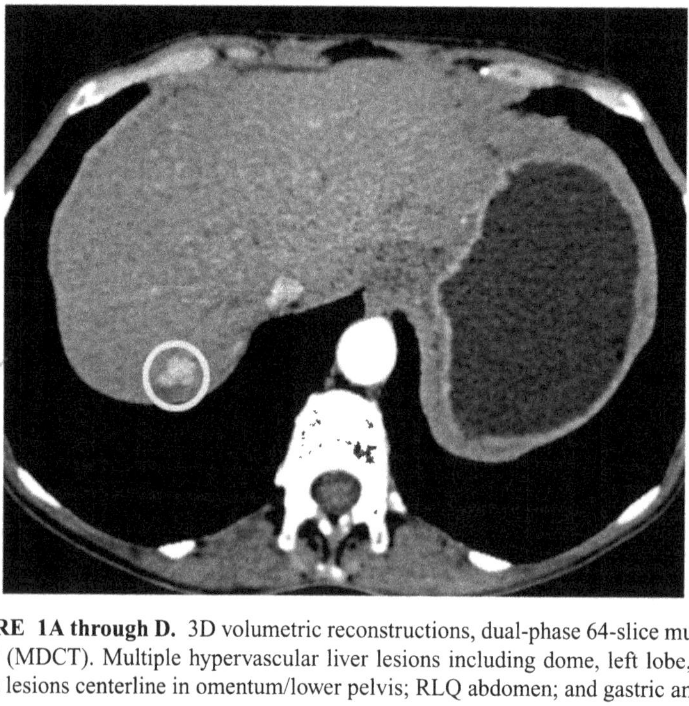

FIGURE 1A through D. 3D volumetric reconstructions, dual-phase 64-slice multidetector CT (MDCT). Multiple hypervascular liver lesions including dome, left lobe, right lobe; plus lesions centerline in omentum/lower pelvis; RLQ abdomen; and gastric antrum.

C

D

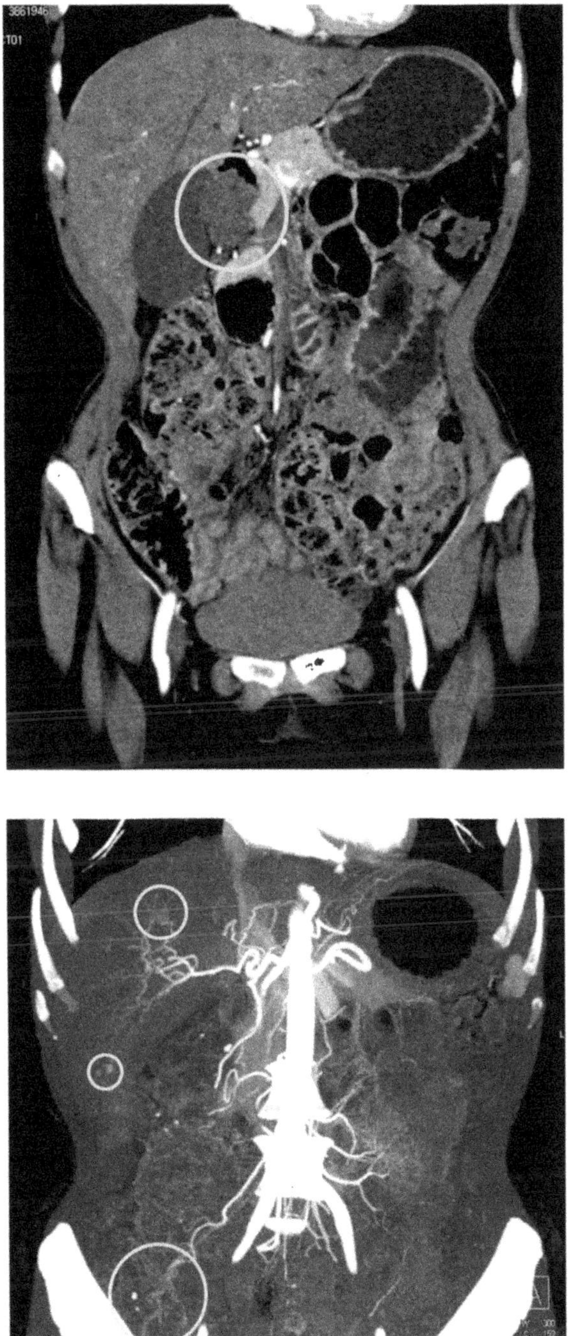

FIGURE 1. *Continued.*

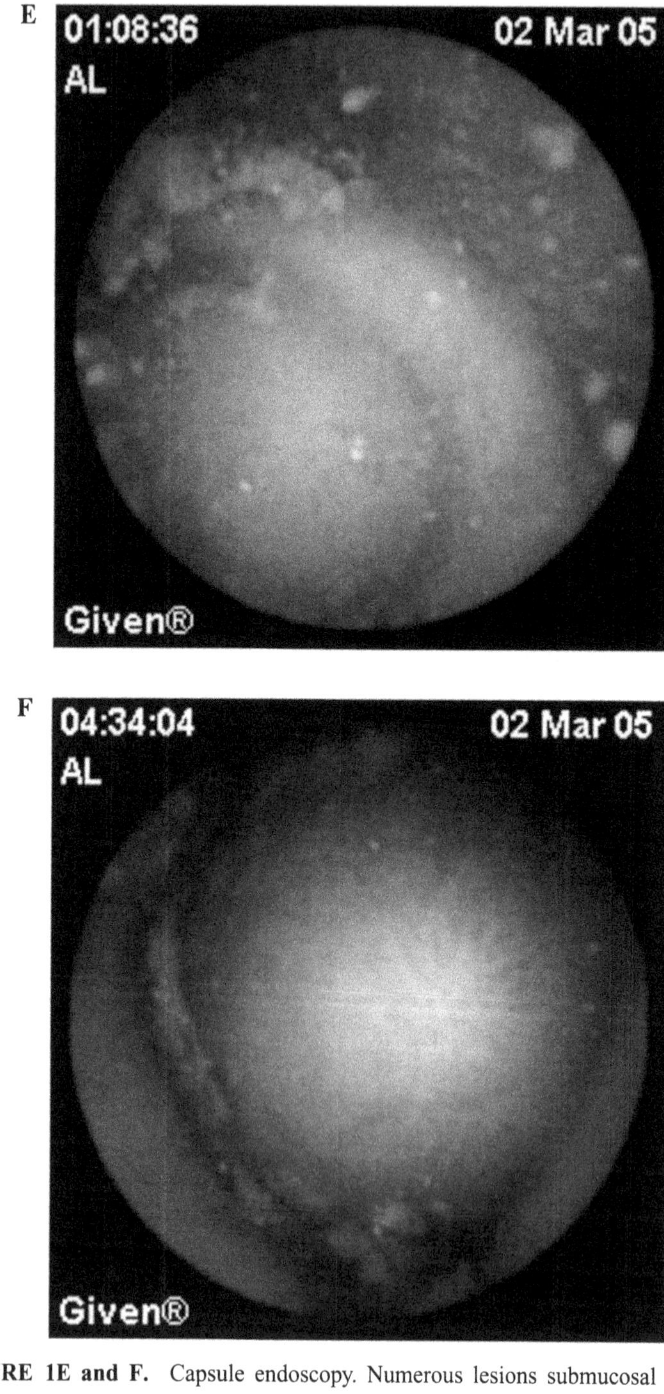

FIGURE 1E and F. Capsule endoscopy. Numerous lesions submucosal off small intestine were seen.

"Clusters" of tumor markers advisable to test jointly and paroxysmally include, but are not limited to, the following: (1) amylase, lipase, trypsin, glucagon, insulin, proinsulin, pancreatic polypeptide, pancreastatin, substance P, somatostatin, plasma metanephrines, plasma CgA, plasma serotonin, calcitonin, prolactin, neuron-specific enolase, histamine, gastrin, vasoactive endothelial growth factor, angiotensin, and insulin-like growth factors I and II; (2) creatinine kinase, carcinoembryonic antigen (CEA) and related discriminatory markers such as CA19-9 as nonspecific serum monitoring parameters, since some may fluctuate significantly with the patient's specific markers in the first group; and (3) urinary catecholamines/metanephrines, HVA, VMA, 5-HIAA, plus creatinine, and urinary total volume as urinary monitoring parameters. To characterize as well as discriminate organs possibly involved in metastases,[40] both serum/plasma and urinary NET markers should be measured in the patient both when asymptomatic and when symptomatic (especially before, during and after a paroxysm if possible). Plasma values of those biochemical markers that are ever significant when symptomatic should be repeated whenever urinary markers are collected in strongly suspected paroxysmally functioning GEP NET.[21]

For imaging, PET with advanced radionuclides designed specifically for APUD uptake in serotonin or catecholamine synthesis pathways has received widespread attention for the GEP NET[41–47] and pheochromocytoma[12,48–50] sensitivity and specificity achieved. However, in the absence of widespread availability of $[^{11}C]$5HTP PET/CT (with or without Carbidopa pretreatment), $[^{11}C]$L-DOPA or $[^{18}F]$DOPA, $[^{18}F]$-Fluorodopamine, $[^{18}F]$Fluorohydroxyphenylalanine, $[^{11}C]$Epinephrine or $[^{11}C]$Hydroxyephedrine, radiologic imaging studies are difficult to put in diagnostic order when an APUD is strongly suspected but when its functioning behavior and hormonal "mix" are unknown. Traditionally, 2DCT, MRI, $[^{18}F]$DG-PET, $[^{123}I]$MIBG, and $[^{111}In]$Octreotide (indium-pentetreotide or OctreoScan) were considered adequate to rule out malignant pheochromocytoma and carcinoid that had grown large enough to threaten or obstruct organ function, with mainly palliative surgical intervention offered for carcinoid formerly thought to have an "indolent" growth course. Liver metastases from carcinoid tumors on portal venous phase CT imaging or delayed imaging through the liver may become isodense, showing why, as in this case report, pre-operative single-phase CT fails to enhance subtle hypervascular liver metastases and small vascular extrahepatic lesions.[32,51]

This case report illustrates that 64-slice multidetector CT (MDCT) with 3D volumetric reconstruction and volumetric rendering may diagnose some cases that are missed on the other studies. Further, MDCT with 3D volumetric rendering and advanced image processing may be the *first* imaging modality to choose in the cases where more specific knowledge of APUD characteristics in a patient is initially absent, and where more than one tumor site is hypothesized. A 64-detector CT allows thinner (0.60 mm) collimation *and* smaller

(0.6 mm) slice thickness *and* smaller (0.5 mm) reconstruction interval, resulting in true volumetric datasets and superior 3D image reconstruction and volume-rendering technique.[52,53] With MDCT, scanning is faster, resulting in better CT angiography images of the mesenteric arteries and veins and other vascular lesions such as carcinoid that enhance after bolus injection and then wash out rapidly.[54] Timing the delivery of contrast in imaging carcinoid is critical in the accumulation of data images because the lesions blush and wash out quickly.[55] The ability to accumulate volumes of data (i.e., 192 images/sec), at the optimal time after bolus injection, is one MDCT diagnostic advantage.[32] Ordinary CT with contrast is too slow to image enhancement with washout of vascular GEP NET lesions occurring rapidly.[52,55]

CONCLUSION

This case report confirms that GEP NET can exhibit the pheochromocytoma "symptom triad" and can produce impressive urinary catecholamines in rising concentrations over the distinctive cyclical course of a single paroxysm caused by the same provocative substances as in pheochromocytoma (tyramine and tyrosine load); but also by tryptophan and other adrenergic substances such as glucagon. If urinary catecholamines are positive and/or pheochromocytoma-like symptoms are clinically present, but plasma metanephrines are negative, then carcinoid and/or other GEP NET including predominantly dopamine-secreting paraganglioma must remain in the differential diagnosis. The combination of intensive biochemical testing repeated over time, dual-phase 64-slice multidetector CT (MDCT) with 3D image reconstruction and the volume-rendering (VR) technique, and advanced radionuclide imaging are required to detect NETs' sporadic or paroxysmal functioning, rule out extra-adrenal pheochromocytoma, and localize and characterize metastatic carcinoid and/or endocrine pancreatic tumor. Detection before metastasis of both carcinoid, as well as malignant pheochromocytoma sized 1 cm or less, requires both advanced multimodal imaging technologies *plus* an astute neuroendocrine-tumor imaging radiologist. Imaging should include both MDCT and fused PET/CT with advanced radionuclides designed specifically for NET uptake. This case report illustrates the usefulness of 3D volumetric reconstruction of dual-phase 64-slice multidetector in characterizing small vascular lesions. If pheochromocytoma is ruled out, yet symptoms and biochemical markers for catecholamine excess are present, then carcinoid and other amine-precursor-uptake decarboxylation (APUD) tumors must remain in the differential diagnosis.

ACKNOWLEDGMENTS

The authors gratefully acknowledge the following: Dr. Karel Pacak, Dr. Graeme Eisenhofer, and Karen T. Adams, NIH-NICHD for expert testing;

Dr. Charles Gelber, Summit Medical Group, for BP testing; Dr. William Manger, National Hypertension Association for permission to adapt tables, from his book with the late Dr. Ray Gifford[5]; Dr. Ravinder Singh, Department of Pathology, Mayo Clinic, for aid in plasma calculations; Dr. Michael Blake, Department of Radiology, Massachusetts General Hospital; Dr. Ash Thabet, Massachusetts General Hospital; Sue Loomis, Radiology Media Education Services, Massachusetts General Hospital, for image conversion; Dr. Stanley Goldsmith, Department of Nuclear Medicine, New York Presbyterian Hospital-Weill Cornell Medical Center; Doug Ricci, Tricia Janitzky, and Beatrice Mudge, Department of Radiology, Johns Hopkins Hospital; and Deno Bokas, Nat Denkin, and Laurence Johnson for graphics assistance.

REFERENCES

1. Öberg, K. 2005. Neuroendocrine tumors of the gastrointestinal tract: recent advances in molecular genetics, diagnosis, and treatment. Curr. Opin. Oncol. **17:** 386–391.
2. Öberg, K. & B. Eriksson. 2005. Endocrine tumours of the pancreas. Best Pract. Res. Clin. Gastroenterol. **19:** 753–781.
3. Öberg, K., L. Astrump, B. Eriksson, *et al.* 2004. Guidelines for the management of gastroenteropancreatic neuroendocrine tumours (including brochopulmonary and thymic neoplasms). Part I—General overview. Acta Oncol. **43:** 617–625.
4. Öberg, K., L. Astrup, B. Eriksson, *et al.* Nordic NE Tumour Group. 2004. Guidelines for the management of gastroenteropancreatic neuroendocrine tumours (including bronchopulmonary and thymic neoplasms). Part II–Specific NE tumour types. Acta Oncol. **43:** 626–636.
5. Manger, W.M. & R.W. Gifford Jr. 1996. Clinical and Experimental Pheochromocytoma, 2nd ed. Blackwell Science. Cambridge, MA.
6. O'Dorisio, T. Private communication, April 20, 2004.
7. Meijer, W.C., D.J. van Veldhuisen, I.P. Kema, *et al.* 2002. Cardiovascular abnormalities in patients with a carcinoid syndrome. Neth. J. Med. **60:** 10–16.
8. Sawka, A.M., R. Jaeschke, R.J. Singh, *et al.* 2003. A comparison of biochemical tests for pheochromocytoma: measurement of fractionated plasma metanephrines compared with the combination of 24-hour urinary metanephrines and catecholamines. J. Clin. Endocrinol. Metab. **88:** 553–558.
9. Kudva, Y.C., A.M. Sawka, W.F. Young, Jr., 2003. Clinical review 164: the laboratory diagnosis of adrenal pheochromocytoma: the Mayo Clinic experience. J. Clin. Endocrinol. Metab. **88:** 4533–4539.
10. Pacak, K., D.S. Goldstein, J.L. Doppman, *et al.* 2001. A "pheo" lurks: novel approaches for locating occult pheochromocytoma. J. Clin. Endocrinol. Metab. **86:** 3641–3646.
11. Goldstein, D.S., G. Eisenhofer J.A. Flynn, *et al.* 2004. Diagnosis and localization of pheochromocytoma. Hypertension **43:** 907–910.
12. Ilias, I., J. Yu, J.A. Carrasquillo, *et al.* 2003. Superiority of 6-[18F]-fluorodopamine positron emission tomography versus [131I]-metaiodobenzylguanidine scintigraphy in the localization of metastatic pheochromocytoma. J. Clin. Endocrinol. Metab. **88:** 4083–4087.

13. EISENHOFER, G., D.S. GOLDSTEIN, M.M. WALTHER. 2003. Biochemical diagnosis of pheochromocytoma: how to distinguish true from false-positive test results. J. Clin. Endocrinol. Metab. **88:** 2656–2666.
14. EISENHOFER, G., D.S. GOLDSTEIN, M.M. WALTHER, *et al.* 2003. Biochemical diagnosis of pheochromocytoma: how to distinguish true- from false-positive test results. J. Clin. Endocrinol. Metab. **88:** 2656–2666.
15. LENDERS, J.W., G. EISENHOFER, M. MANNELLI, *et al.* 2005. Phaeochromocytoma. Lancet **366:** 665–675.
16. J.W.M. LENDERS, K. PACAK, M.M. WALTHER, *et al.* 2002. Biochemical diagnosis of pheochromocytoma: which test is best? JAMA. **287:** 1427–1434.
17. LENDERS, J.W., K. PACAK, G. EISENHOFER. 2002. New advances in the biochemical diagnosis of pheochromocytoma: moving beyond catecholamines. Ann. N.Y. Acad. Sci. **970:** 29–40.
18. EISENHOFER, G., D.S. GOLDSTEIN, P. SULLIVAN, *et al.* 2005. Biochemical and clinical manifestations of dopamine-producing paragangliomas: utility of plasma methoxytyramine. J. Clin. Endocrinol. Metab. **20:** 2068–2075.
19. MEIJER, W.G., S.C.V.M. COPRAY, H. HOLLEMA, *et al.* 2003. Catecholamine-synthesizing enzymes in carcinoid tumors and pheochromocytomas. Clin. Chem.**49:** 586–593.
20. OBERG, K. & B. SKOGSEID. 1998. The ultimate biochemical diagnosis of endocrine pancreatic tumours in MEN-1. J. Intern. Med. **243:** 471–476.
21. NORDIC NEUROENDOCRINE TUMOUR GROUP. 2004. First guidelines for the management of neuroendocrine tumours: Nordic meeting on the management of gastroenteropancreatic neuroendocrine tumours. Helsinki, May 27, 2004. E-pub.
22. ERIKSSON, B., K. OBERG & M. STRIDSBERG. 2000. Tumor markers in neuroendocrine tumors. Digestion. **62:** 33–38.
23. OBERG, K. 1996. The ultimate biochemical diagnosis of gastroenteropancreatic tumours. Digestion **57:** 45–47.
24. ÖBERG, K. 2002. Carcinoid tumors: molecular genetics; tumor biology; and update of diagnosis and treatment. Curr. Opin. Oncol. **14:** 38–45.
25. AHLUND, L., L.G. KINDBLOM, O. NILSSON, *et al.* 1989. Clinical and experimental studies on a midgut carcinoid tumor. J. Surg. Oncol. **41:** 86–92.
26. AHLUND, L., O. NILSSON, T. KLING-PETERSEN, *et al.* 1989. Serotonin-producing carcinoid tumour cells in long-term culture: studies on serotonin release and morphological features. Acta Oncol. **28:** 341–346.
27. HOLDCROFT, A. 2000. Hormones and the gut. Br. J. Anaesth. **85:** 58–68.
28. MATUCHANSKY, C. & J.J. LAUNAY. 1995. Serotonin, catecholamines, and spontaneous midgut carcinoid flush: plasma studies from flushing and nonflushing sites. Gastroenterology **108:** 743–751.
29. LEOTLELA, P.D., A. JAUCH, H. HOLTGREVE-GREZ, *et al.* 2003. Genetics of neuroendocrine and carcinoid tumours. Endocrine-Related Cancer. **10:** 437–450.
30. HIRSCH, N.P., A. MURPHY, J.J. RADCLIFFE. 2001. Neurofibromatosis: clinical presentations and anaesthetic implications. Br. J. Anaesth. **86:** 555–564.
31. OBERG, K., L. KVOLS, M. CAPLIN, *et al.* 2004. Consensus report on the use of somatostatin analogs for the management of neuroendocrine tumors of the gastroenteropancreatic system. Ann. Oncol. **15:** 966–973.
32. KAMEL, I.R., E. LIAPI, E.K. FISHMAN. 2005. Liver and biliary system: evaluation by multidetector CT. Radiol. Clin. N. Am. **43:** 977–997.
33. KIM, Y.H., S. SAINI, M.A. BLAKE, *et al.* 2005. Distinguishing hepatic metastases from hemangiomas: qualitative and quantitative diagnostic performance through

dual echo respiratory-triggered fast spin echo magnetic resonance imaging. J. Comput. Assist. Tomogr. **29:** 571–579.

34. KAWASHIMA, A., C.M. SANDLER, E.K. FISHMAN, *et al.* 1998. Spectrum of CT findings in nonmalignant disease of the adrenal gland. Radiographics **18:** 393–412.
35. BLAKE, M.A., M.K. KALRA, M.M. MAHER, *et al.* 2004. Pheochromocytoma: an imaging chameleon. Radiographics **24:** S87–S89.
36. BLAKE, M.A., S.K. KRISHNAMOORTHY, G.W. BOLAND, *et al.* 2003. Low-density pheochromocytoma on CT: a mimicker of adrenal adenoma. Am. J. Roentgenol. **181:** 1663–1668.
37. LANCE, J.W., H. HINTERBERGER. 1976. Symptoms of pheochromocytoma, with particular reference to headache, correlated with catecholamine production. Arch. Neurol. **33:** 281–28.
38. SALMON, S., M. BONCIANI, M. FANCIULLACCI, *et al.* 1982. A putative 5-HT central feedback in migraine and cluster headache attacks. Adv. Neurol. **33:** 265–274.
39. ZELINKA, T., B. STRAUCH, O. PETRAK, *et al.* 2005. Increased blood pressure variability in pheochromocytoma compared to essential hypertension patients. J. Hypertens. **23:** 2033–2039.
40. ZUETENHORST, J.M., C.M. KORSE, J.M. BONFRER, *et al.* 2004. Daily cyclic changes in the urinary excretion of 5-hydroxyindoleacetic acid in patients with carcinoid tumors. Clin. Chem. **50:** 1634–1639.
41. OBERG, K. & B. ERIKSSON. 2005. Nuclear medicine in the detection, staging and treatment of gastrointestinal carcinoid tumours. Best Pract. Res. Clin. Endocrinol. Metab. **19:** 265–276.
42. ERIKSSON, B., H. ORLEFORS, K. OBERG. 2005. Developments in PET for the detection of endocrine tumours. Best Pract. Res. Clin. Endocrinol. Metab. **19:** 311–324.
43. HOEGERLE, S., C. ALTEHOEFER, N. GHANEM, *et al.* 2001. Whole-body 18F-DOPA PET for detection of gastrointestinal carcinoid tumors. Radiology **220:** 373–380.
44. HOEGERLE, S., B. SCHNEIDER, A. KRAFT, *et al.* 1999. Imaging of a metastatic gastrointestinal carciinoid by F-18-DOPA positron emission tomography. Nuklearmedizin **38:** 127–130.
45. ÖBERG, K. & B. ERIKSSON. 2005. Nuclear medicine in the detection, staging and treatment of gastrointestinal carcinoid tumours. Best Pract. Res. Clin. Endocrinol. Metab. **19:** 265–276.
46. SUNDIN, A., B. ERIKSSON, M. BERGSTROM, *et al.* 2004. PET in the diagnosis of neuroendocrine tumors. Ann. N. Y. Acad. Sci. **1014:** 246–257.
47. ILIAS, I., B. SHULKIN, K. PACAK. 2005. New functional imaging modalities for chromaffin tumors, neuroblastomas and ganglioneuromas. Trends Endocrinol. Metab. **16:** 66–72.
48. PACAK, K., G. EISENHOFER & D.S. GOLDSTEIN. 2004. Functional imaging of endocrine tumors: role of positron emission tomography. Endocr. Rev. **25:** 568–580.
49. ILIAS, I. & K. PACAK. 2004. Anatomical and functional imaging of metastatic pheochromocytoma. Ann. N. Y. Acad. Sci. **1018:** 495–504.
50. ILIAS, I., S. ALESCI, K. PACAK. 2004. Current views on imaging of adrenal tumors. Horm. Metab. Res. **36:** 430–435.
51. KAMEL, I.R. L.P. LAWLER, E.K. FISHMAN. 2004. Comprehensive analysis of hypervascular liver lesions using 16-MDCT and advanced image processing. Am. J. Roentgenol. **183:** 443–452.

52. HORTON, K.M. & E.K. FISHMAN. 2004. Multidetector-row computed tomography and 3-dimensional computed tomography imaging of small bowel neoplasms: current concepts in diagnosis. J. Comput. Assist. Tomogr. **28:** 106–116.
53. HORTON, K.M. & E.K. FISHMAN. 2003. The current status of multidetector row CT and three-dimensional imaging of the small bowel. Radiol. Clin. N. Am. **41:** 199–212.
54. HORTON, K. & E.K. FISHMAN. 2002. Volume-rendered 3D CT of the mesenteric vasculature: normal anatomy; anatomic variants; and pathologic conditions. Radiographics **22:** 161–172.
55. HORTON, K.M., I. KAMEL, L. HOFMANN, *et al.* 2004. Carcinoid tumors of the small bowel: a multitechnique imaging approach. Am. J. Roentgenol. **182:** 559–567.

Catecholamine Excretion and Circadian Blood Pressure Profile in Patients with Pheochromocytoma

ELZBIETA DABROWSKA, JACEK LEWANDOWSKI, PIOTR JEDRUSIK, BARTOSZ SYMONIDES, BOZENA WOCIAL, MARIUSZ LAPINSKI, AND ZBIGNIEW GACIONG

Department of Internal Medicine, Hypertension, and Angiology, The Medical University of Warsaw, 02-097 Warsaw, Poland

ABSTRACT: Circadian blood pressure (BP) rhythm is often disturbed in patients with secondary forms of hypertension. The aim of the present article was to investigate changes in circadian BP profile parameters using two-step statistical approach by Fourier analysis in relation to day and night urinary catecholamine excretion in 35 patients with pheochromocytoma (mean age 42 ± 19 years). Twenty-four-hour ambulatory BP measurements (ABPM) were obtained using the SpaceLabs 90,207 monitor. Daytime and night-time urine collection was obtained in all patients to determine circadian catecholamine excretion. Fourier analysis was applied to estimate measures of BP circadian rhythm in ABPM, including the highest (Max) and lowest (Min) systolic (SBP) and diastolic (DBP) BP values, norad (ampSBP, ampDBP), and early acrophase (APSBP, APDBP). The Fourier indices of circadian BP rhythm were: MaxSBP 153 ± 28 mm Hg, MaxDBP 99 ± 16 mm Hg, MinSBP 117 ± 17 mm Hg, MinDBP 69 ± 11 mm Hg, ampSBP 18 ± 8 mm Hg, ampDBP 14 ± 5 mm Hg, APSBP 10 ± 5 (h), and APDBP 11 ± 3 (h). Urine noradrenaline (NA), adrenaline (A), and dopamine (DA) excretion during the day (d) and night (n) were: dNA 103.5 ± 89.8 μg/14 h, nNA 52 ± 70.8 μg/10 h, dA 13.2 ± 17.9 μg/14 h; nA 6.13 ± 9.6 μg/10 h, dD 181.8 ± 87.3 μg/14 h, and nD 89.3 ± 59.8 μg/10 h. A positive correlation was observed between urine dNa excretion and MaxDBP ($r = 0.37$, $P < 0.05$), and urine nNA and urine dA excretion were correlated with APDBP ($r = 0.47$, $r = 0.35$, respectively, both $P < 0.05$). Thus, in addition to the effect on mean 24-h BP values, catecholamines released by tumor may also disturb circadian BP rhythm in patients with pheochromocytoma.

KEYWORDS: pheochromocytoma; circadian rhythm; ambulatory blood pressure monitoring; Fourier analysis

Address for correspondence: Zbigniew Gaciong, M.D., Ph.D., Department of Internal Medicine, Hypertension, and Angiology, The Medical University of Warsaw, 1A Banacha Street, 02-097 Warsaw, Poland. Voice: +4822-6597506; fax: +4822-6593373.
e-mail: zgaciong@amwaw.edu.pl

Ann. N.Y. Acad. Sci. 1073: 79–85 (2006).
doi: 10.1196/annals.1353.008

INTRODUCTION

The sympathoadrenal system is pivotal for the short-term regulation of blood pressure (BP) and may also contribute to sustained forms of hypertension. Numerous evidences, including data on sympathetic neural activity in hypertension and lessons learned from patients with autonomic failure,[1–3] demonstrate that catecholamines affect the circadian variation of BP in both physiological and pathological conditions. Circadian BP rhythm is often disturbed in patients with secondary forms of hypertension, including catecholamine excess states, such as pheochromocytoma.[4] Nocturnal BP fall in patients with pheochromocytoma was found to be attenuated compared to patients with essential hypertension.[5] Also, spectral analysis of the systolic blood pressure (SBP) signal in pheochromocytoma showed significant differences compared to other etiologies of hypertension.[6]

The aim of the study was to investigate changes in circadian BP profile parameters in patients with pheochromocytoma using two-step statistical approach by Fourier analysis in relation to day and night urinary catecholamine excretion.

MATERIALS AND METHODS

We studied 35 patients with pheochromocytoma (25 women and 10 men, mean age 42 ± 19 years) hospitalized in the Department of Internal Medicine, Hypertension, and Angiology at the Warsaw Medical University, Poland. All patients but two had a unilateral adrenal catecholamine-producing tumor, and in the remaining two patients pheochromocytoma was found in both adrenals. The diagnosis of pheochromocytoma was on the basis of clinical presentation, elevated urinary excretion of catecholamines and/or metanephrines, and the results of imaging studies. All patients were subsequently referred for the surgical resection of the catecholamine-producing tumor and the diagnosis of pheochromocytoma was confirmed histopathologically. During the initial assessment including 24-h ambulatory blood pressure measurements (ABPM) and urinary collections patients were not receiving antihypertensive drugs and other drugs or substances that might affect catecholamine excretion. Exclusion criteria included severe target organ damage, malignant hypertension, overt heart failure, and history of myocardial infarction or cerebrovascular event.

Daytime (14 h) and night-time (10 h) urine collection was obtained in all patients to determine circadian catecholamine excretion. Urinary noradrenaline (NA), adrenaline (A), and dopamine (DA) excretion were measured using fluorimetric method. Twenty-four-hour ABPM were obtained using the Space-Labs 90,207 monitor (Redmond, Washington, USA), with measurements every 15 min during the day (6.01–22.00 h) and every 20 min during the night (22.01–6.00 h). Mean 24-h, daytime, and night-time SBP and diastolic blood pressure (DBP) values were calculated. Dipper versus nondipper status was determined as the difference of ≥10% or <10%, respectively, between the mean daytime and night-time BP values.

Fourier Analysis

The Fourier analysis was applied to estimate measures of BP circadian rhythm in ABPM. The first four harmonics were used with the periods of 24, 12, 8, and 6 h. The approximated circadian SBP and DBP profiles were then analyzed to determine indices of circadian BP rhythm including the highest (MaxSBP, MaxDBP) and lowest (MinSBP, MinDBP) BP values (in mm Hg), amplitude (ampSBP, ampDBP; in mm Hg) defined as the half of the difference between MaxSBP and MinSBP or between MaxDBP and MinDBP, respectively, and early acrophase (APSBP, APDBP; h) defined as the time of the first global maximum. The circadian BP profile was approximated using the equation $BP(t) = M + C_k \cos(2\pi kt/24 - \varphi_k)$, where $BP(t)$ is BP at the time t (in hours), M is the weighted mean 24-h BP, C_k is the amplitude of the kth harmonic of frequency, and φ_k is the phase of the kth harmonic of frequency, with $k = 1,2,3,4$, and C and φ estimated using multivariate weighted linear regression.

Statistical Analysis

Linear correlation coefficients were calculated to investigate the relationship between the Fourier indices of circadian BP rhythm and daytime and night-time urinary NA, A, and DA excretion. Results are expressed as mean ± SD and also graphically as regression lines with 95% confidence intervals. Statistical significance was set at the 5% level.

RESULTS

TABLE 1 summarizes mean 24-h daytime and night-time SBP and DBP values in the study group. Overall, 23/35 (65.7%) patients were nondippers, and 12/35 (34.3%) patients were dippers. The indices of circadian BP rhythm in the Fourier analysis were as follows: MaxSBP 153 ± 28 mm Hg, MaxDBP 99 ± 16 mm Hg, MinSBP 117 ± 17 mm Hg, MinDBP 69 ± 11 mm Hg, ampSBP 18 ± 8 mm Hg, ampDBP 14 ± 5 mm Hg, APSBP 10 ± 5 (h), and APDBP 11 ± 3 (h).

Urinary NA, A, and DA excretion during the day and night is presented in TABLE 1. We found a significant positive correlation between urinary NA excretion during the day and MaxSBP ($r = 0.37$, $P < 0.05$) (FIG. 1). In addition, urinary NA excretion during the night and urinary A excretion during the day were significantly correlated with APDBP ($r = 0.47$ and $r = 0.35$, respectively, both $P < 0.05$) (FIGS. 2 and 3).

TABLE 1. Mean BP values in ABPM and urinary NA, A, and D excretion during the day and night in patients with pheochromocytoma

	Mean BP values in ABPM (mm Hg)	Urinary catecholamine excretion		
		NA	A	DA
24 h	134 ± 19/82 ± 12			
Daytime	135 ± 19/84 ± 13	103.5 ± 89.8 μg/14 h	13.2 ± 17.9 μg/14 h	181.8 ± 87.3 μg/14 h
Night-time	129 ± 21/76 ± 12	52.0 ± 70.8 μg/10 h	6.13 ± 9.6 μg/10 h	89.3 ± 59.8 μg/10 h

DISCUSSION

In the present study we found abnormal circadian BP rhythm in 65% of patients with pheochromocytoma. Lack of nocturnal fall in BP in the majority

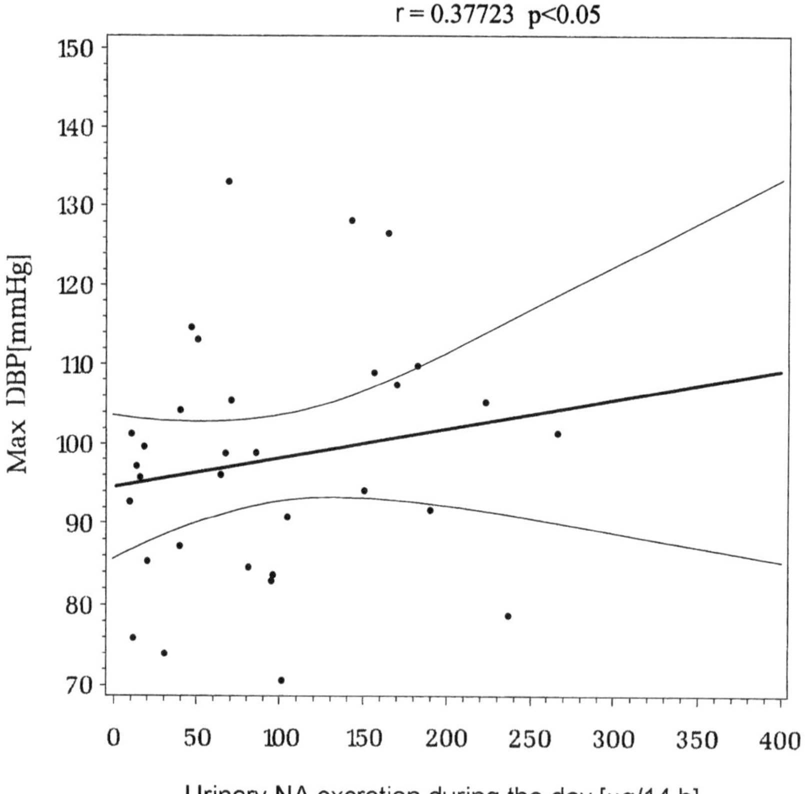

FIGURE 1. Relationship between urinary NA excretion during the day and the highest daytime DBP values (Max DBP) in patients with pheochromocytoma.

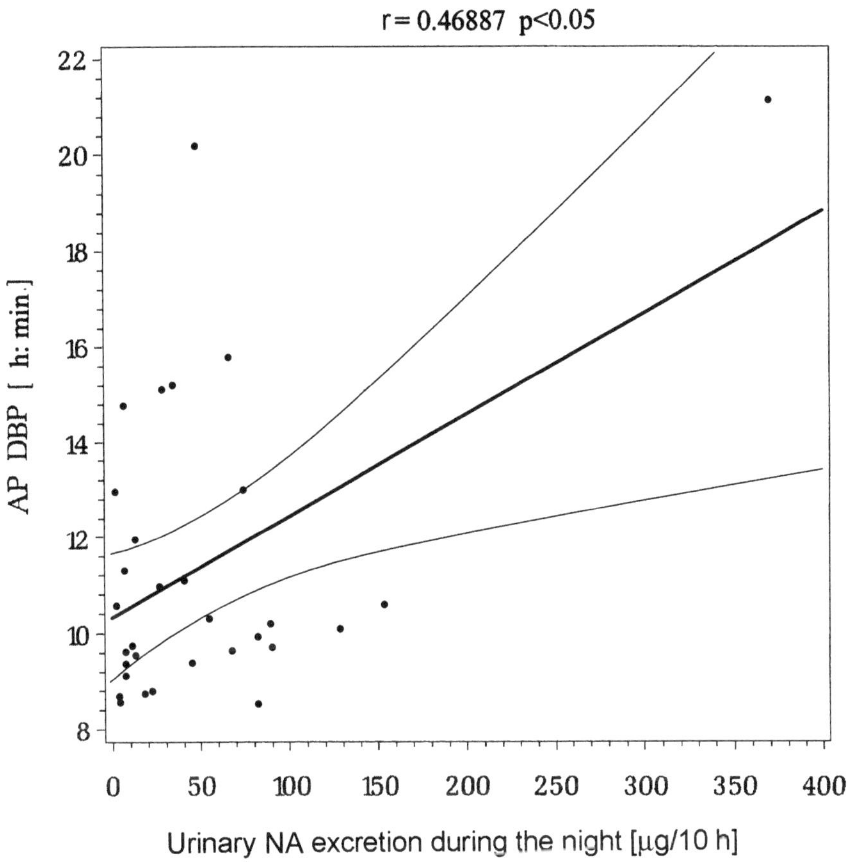

FIGURE 2. Relationship between urinary NA excretion during the night and DBP acrophase (AP DBP) in patients with pheochromocytoma.

of patients with pheochromocytoma was previously found in most[4,7–9] but not all[5,10] studies employing either invasive or noninvasive BP monitoring. These conflicting data are further confounded by the fact that some patients in those studies were receiving alpha- and/or beta-blockers. In addition, patients with pheochromocytoma often have only episodic hypertension with normal average BP values. On the other hand, accumulated evidence demonstrate the prognostic value of not only mean BP, but also BP variability.[11,12] Thus, further characterization of BP circadian rhythm in these patients using Fourier analysis seems promising. Notably, Fourier analysis gives information not only on absolute and relative (i.e., amplitude) BP values throughout the day, but also on the timing of highest BP values (i.e., acrophase).

Although catecholamine excess is a well-established cause of hypertension in pheochromocytoma, relationship between catecholamines released by the

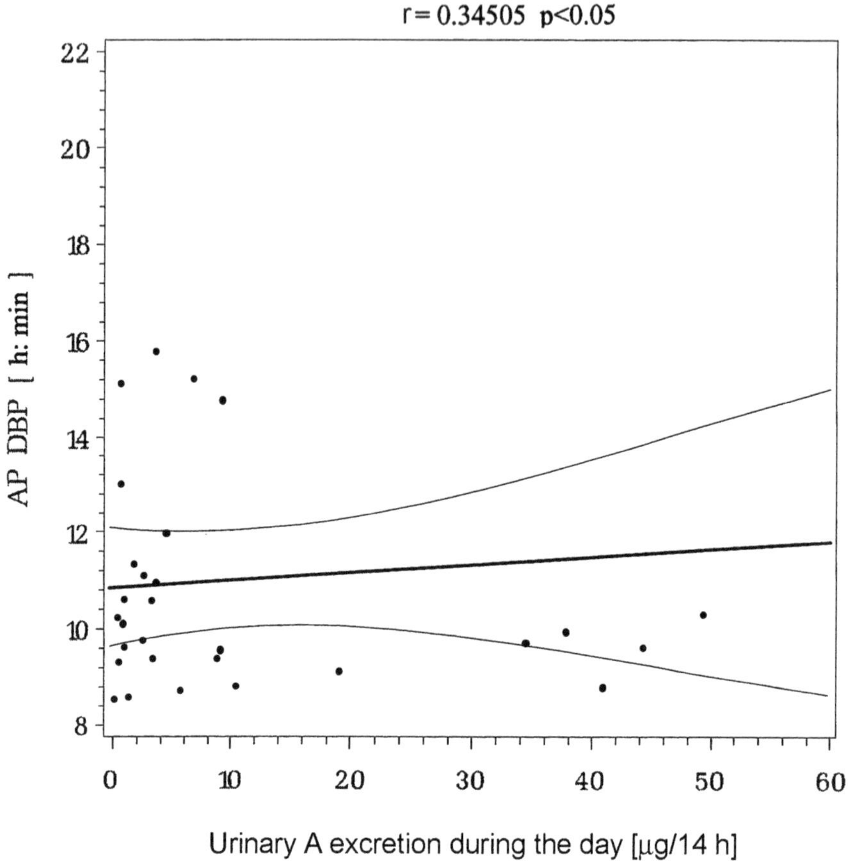

FIGURE 3. Relationship between urinary A excretion during the day and DBP acrophase (AP DBP) in patients with pheochromocytoma.

tumor and BP values is less clear.[13,14] In particular, the pressor effect of chronically elevated catecholamines in pheochromocytoma seems to be attenuated, likely by mechanisms, such as reduced activation of the adrenergic receptors and changes in sympathetic tone, and it has been proposed that episodic BP elevation is more dependent on NA released from sympathetic nerve endings.[5] Overall, this often results in normal average BP values but disturbed circadian BP rhythm in these patients. In spectral analysis, SBP variability in patients with pheochromocytoma was characterized by high-amplitude, low-frequency oscillations and was significantly different from other etiologies of hypertension.[6] In our study, we found a positive correlation between the highest daytime DBP values and urinary NA excretion during the day, and the timing of highest DBP values during the day was related to both urinary A excretion during the day and urinary NA excretion during the night. These data suggest the NA and

A released by the tumor not only affect average BP values but also result in abnormal circadian BP rhythm in these patients. Fourier analysis is a useful tool to assess circadian BP patterns in patients with pheochromocytoma on the basis of ABPM.

REFERENCES

1. MANCIA, G. 1997. The sympathetic nervous system in hypertension. J. Hypertens. **15:** 1553–1565.
2. NARKIEWICZ, K. *et al.* 2002. Relationship between muscle sympathetic nerve activity and diurnal blood pressure profile. Hypertension **39:** 168–172.
3. DIEDRICH, A. *et al.* 2003. The sympathetic nervous system in hypertension: assessment by blood pressure variability and ganglionic blockade. J. Hypertens. **21:** 1677–1686.
4. DABROWSKA, B. *et al.* 1990. Effect of removal of pheochromocytoma on diurnal variability of blood pressure, heart rhythm and excretion of catecholamines. J. Hum. Hypertens. **4:** 397–399.
5. IMAI, Y. *et al.* 1988. Hypertensive episodes and circadian fluctuations of blood pressure in patients with pheochromocytoma: studies by long-term monitoring based on volume oscillometric method. J. Hypertens. **6:** 9–15.
6. MEISEL, S.R. *et al.* 1994. Spectral analysis of the systolic blood pressure signal in secondary hypertension: method for identification of pheochromocytoma. J. Hypertens. **12:** 269–276.
7. LITTLER, W.A. & A.J. HONOUR. 1974. Direct atrial pressure, heart rate and electrocardiogram in unrestrained patients before and after removal of pheochromocytoma. Q. J. Med. **43:** 441–449.
8. PADFIELD, P.L. & M.J. STEWART. 1991. Ambulatory blood pressure monitoring in secondary hypertension. J. Hypertens. **9**(Suppl 8)**:** S69–S71.
9. VAN EPS, R.G.S. *et al.* 1994. Diurnal variation of blood pressure in patients with catecholamine-producing tumors. Am. J. Hypertens. **7:** 492–497.
10. SPIEKER, C. *et al.* 1993. Circadian blood pressure variation in endocrine disorders. Blood Pressure **1:** 35–39.
11. FRATTOLA, A. *et al.* 1993. Prognostic value of 24-hour blood pressure variability. J. Hypertens. **11:** 1133–1137.
12. VERDECCHIA, P. *et al.* 1996. Prognostic significance of blood pressure variability in essential hypertension. Blood Press. Monit. **1:** 3–11.
13. BRAVO, E.L. 1994. Evolving concepts in the pathophysiology, diagnosis, and treatment of pheochromocytoma. Endocr. Rev. **15:** 356–368.
14. BRAVO, E. *et al.* 1990. A reevaluation of the hemodynamics of pheochromocytoma. Hypertension **15**(Suppl 1)**:** I128–I131.

Characteristics of Blood Pressure in Pheochromocytoma

TOMÁŠ ZELINKA,[a] KAREL PACÁK,[a,b] AND JIŘÍ WIDIMSKÝ, JR.[a]

[a]*Third Department of Medicine, General Faculty Hospital, CZ 128 08 Prague 2, Czech Republic*

[b]*Reproductive Biology and Medicine Branch, National Institute of Child Health and Human Development, National Institutes of Health, Bethesda, Maryland 20892–1109, USA*

ABSTRACT: Pheochromocytomas are catecholamine-producing tumors arising from chromaffin cells. One of the most typical symptoms of the catecholamine-excess state is hypertension either in the sustained or paroxysmal form, and its severity does not depend on the level of circulating catecholamines. On the other hand, hypertension in pheochromocytoma is very often characterized by the amelioration or even inversion of the circadian blood pressure rhythm. In some subjects, high circulating levels of catecholamines lead to the enhanced blood pressure variability. One possible explanation for such blood pressure variability is the desensitization of the catecholamine receptors due to high levels of circulating catecholamines.

KEYWORDS: pheochromocytoma; blood pressure; circadian blood pressure rhythm; blood pressure variability

INTRODUCTION

Hypertension in pheochromocytoma occurs in up to 80–90% of the subjects. High blood pressure exists either in the sustained or in the paroxysmal form which may occur superimposed.[1] On the other hand, in up to 10–20% of the subjects with pheochromocytoma, high circulating catecholamines may also lead to the orthostatic hypotension mostly in combination with sustained hypertension.[1,2] Contrasting to other forms of secondary hypertension, where only one circulating hormone is responsible for the development of hypertension, pheochromocytoma may by characterized by the overproduction of three circulating catecholamines—norepinephrine, epinephrine and, also in the minority

Address for correspondence: Tomáš Zelinka, Center for Hypertension, Third Department of Medicine, General Faculty Hospital, U nemocnice 1, CZ 128 08, Prague 2, Czech Republic. Voice: +420224962945; fax: +420224919780.
e-mail: tzeli@lf1.cuni.cz

Ann. N.Y. Acad. Sci. 1073: 86–93 (2006).
doi: 10.1196/annals.1353.009

of cases, dopamine.[3] These catecholamines exhibit different effects on different catecholamine receptors— typically norepinephrine-mediated stimulation of α-receptors leads to vasoconstriction accompanied with diastolic hypertension, and epinephrine-mediated stimulation of β-receptors causes predominantly systolic hypertension with other symptoms such as tachycardia, sweating, and flushing.[1,4] Predominantly dopamine-producing tumors are relatively rare and often present with normotension.[3] In sporadic pheochromocytomas arising from adrenal medulla, the overproduction of both catecholamines (norepinephrine and epinephrine) may also be seen which makes the evaluation of hemodynamics of these patients difficult.

STUDIES ON HEMODYNAMICS IN PHEOCHROMOCYTOMA

Hemodynamic studies performed in subjects with pheochromocytoma have suggested a possible role of the sympathetic nervous system in the development of hypertension. Bravo *et al.* described that hypertension in pheochromocytoma is related only to increased sympathetic activity and that the long-term exposure to high circulating catecholamines does not produce hemodynamic responses typical for acute administration of catecholamines.[5,6] Similar results were found in the other study concerning the hemodynamics in pheochromocytoma.[7] Interestingly, there is also a lack of correlation between blood pressure and plasma catecholamines.[8,9] As mentioned above, for pheochromocytoma is also typical the occurence of orthostatic hypotension[2] perhaps due to the tendency to hypovolemia.[10,11] Studies about the baroreflex function in subjects with pheochromocytoma have shown controversial results but the majority of them have demonstrated the intact baroreflex arc with appropriate increases in heart rate and increases or unchanged diastolic blood pressure after tilting.[5,12–14] Direct or indirect assessments of sympathetic nervous system in pheochromocytoma by means of the measurement of the muscle sympathetic nervous activity or the analysis of the heart rate variability showed depressed central sympathetic outflow.[15–17]

24-H BLOOD PRESSURE MONITORING IN PHEOCHROMOCYTOMA

Blood pressure and heart rate in some patients with pheochromocytoma may be also characterized by a labile blood pressure and heart rate—this phenomenon was first described by Littler and colleagues, who reported three subjects with pheochromocytoma in whom blood pressure was recorded invasively.[18] In one of these patients, attacks of palpitations and tachycardia were accompanied by hypotension; in other patients from this series attacks of fear were associated with blood pressure elevations. All three subjects also demonstrated the absence of diurnal blood pressure variation.[18] In the later study that focused on direct blood pressure measurement in subjects with pheochromocytoma, labile blood pressure was found in only a minority of the subjects whereas the majority of subjects exhibited normal blood pressure recordings also with preserved diurnal blood pressure variation.[19] In some case reports or hemodynamic studies, a cycling character of blood pressure and heart rate fluctuations was also observed in subjects with pheochromocytoma.[19–21]

Studies focused on assessing the circadian blood pressure rhythm performed with 24-h ambulatory blood pressure measurement have also revealed conflicting results—some reports have reported the absence of the nighttime blood pressure falls[18,22–26] and others referred to preserved blood pressure falls during the night.[19,27] All these studies were performed in a relatively small number of patients with pheochromocytoma.

To find out if previously published conflicting results about the circadian blood pressure variation were affected by incidental findings due to the small number of studied subjects, we compared diurnal blood pressure variation in a larger series of subjects with endocrine hypertension, especially pheochromocytoma (45 subjects) and primary aldosteronism (78 subjects). Subjects with primary aldosteronism had significantly higher 24-h blood pressure values in comparison with subjects with pheochromocytoma (systolic/diastolic BP: 151/96 $\pm$ 17/12 mmHg versus 135/85 $\pm$ 18/13 mmHg, $P < 0.001/<0.001$). On the other hand, patients with pheochromocytoma showed more profound amelioration of the circadian blood pressure rhythm (expressed as a relative nighttime blood pressure decline: [daytime BP − nighttime BP/daytime BP $\times$ 100%]) than subjects with primary aldosteronism (systolic/diastolic BP: $-1/1 \pm 10/10$% versus 3/6 $\pm$ 6/6%, $P = 0.01/<0.001$) although these subjects also had diminished circadian blood pressure rhythm compared to the control group with essential hypertension. One half of the subjects with pheochromocytoma exhibited an increase of the nighttime blood pressure.[28] On the other hand, normotensive subjects with pheochromocytoma also demonstrated blunted diurnal blood pressure variation compared to normotensive controls.[29]

BLOOD PRESSURE VARIABILITY IN PHEOCHROMOCYTOMA

Blood pressure variability may also serve as one of the factors contributing to the higher cardiovascular morbidity in subjects with hypertension.[30,31] Concerning blood pressure variability in pheochromocytoma where short- and long-lasting blood pressure changes typically occur, only a small study (on five subjects) was published.[26] In this study, higher blood pressure variability compared to subjects with essential or renovascular hypertension was reported.[26] In our present study, we searched for the differences in blood pressure variability in 54 subjects with pheochromocytoma compared to subjects with essential hypertension. For evaluating blood pressure variability, we used 24-h ambulatory blood pressure monitoring and from the obtained data, the coefficient of blood pressure variation was calculated, standard deviation (SD) of average BP/average BP. As expected, subjects with essential hypertension had significantly higher blood pressure values and on the contrary, patients with pheochromocytoma had significantly lower nighttime blood pressure decline. In the pheochromocytoma group, blood pressure variability was predominantly higher during the daytime in comparison with the group of subjects with essential hypertension (the groups were examined separately according to the treatment with or without α-receptor blockers: without treatment: coefficient of systolic/diastolic BP: 0.11/0.13 ± 0.04/0.03 versus 0.09/0.11 ± 0.03/0.04, $P =$ 0.007/0.006 and in the treated groups: 0.12/0.13 ± 0.04/0.04 versus 0.09/0.12 ± 0.04/0.02, $P < 0.001/0.01$). Surgical removal of pheochromocytoma resulted not only in the expected decline in blood pressure values, but also in the decrease in previously elevated blood pressure variability (coefficient of daytime blood pressure variation: 0.11/0.13 ± 0.03/0.03 versus 0.09/0.12 ± 0.03/0.02, $P = 0.03/0.11$). Interestingly, subjects with nighttime blood pressure increase also had significantly higher coefficient of daytime blood pressure variation (0.13/0.15 ± 0.04/0.03 versus 0.09/0.12 ± 0.02/0.02, $P < 0.001/<0.001$). Patients with isolated norepinephrine-producing pheochromocytomas demonstrated significantly higher blood pressure values than subjects with either isolated epinephrine or epinephrine- and norepinephrine-producing pheochromocytomas.[32] In some subjects with malignant pheochromocytoma, repeated 24-h blood pressure monitorings were also performed. As shown in the FIGURE 1, 24-h blood pressure monitoring was performed in one subject with malignant pheochromocytoma immediately after a debulking operation for malignant pheochromocytoma. We found normal average blood pressure values and the absence of circadian blood pressure rhythm. The progression of the disease was accompanied not only with further blood pressure increase during the night but also with the development of the typical posture-induced complaints due to the rapid blood pressure drops (FIG. 2). On the other hand, diurnal heart rate variation was preserved similar to the other subjects with pheochromocytoma, in whom we noticed only slightly higher heart rate compared to subjects with essential hypertension.[32] These results fit very well into the variety of performed studies focused on blood pressure regulation in subjects with pheochromocytoma. In contrary to the subjects with primary aldosteronism in whom the excess of aldosterone leads to moderate or severe hypertension in the vast majority of patients, each subject with pheochromocytoma is quite unique due to the different presentation of pheochromocytoma-related symptoms (more than 80 manifestations of pheochromocytoma were described[33]). The mechanism that probably leads to these differences in clinical presentation is the desensitization of both catecholamine receptors due to the long-lasting catecholamine elevations.[6,34,35]

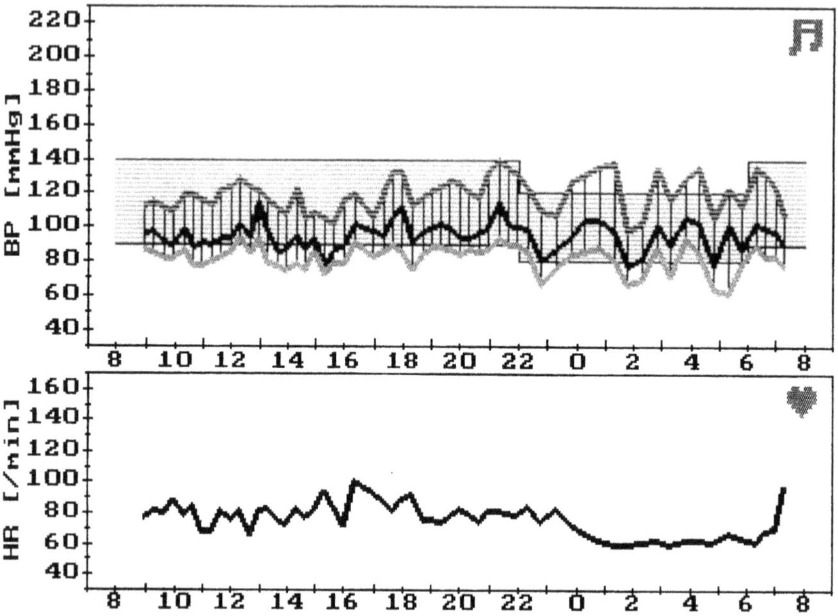

FIGURE 1. A 24-h ambulatory blood pressure monitoring in subject with malignant pheochromocytoma immediately after the debulking operation. BP, blood pressure; HR, heart rate.

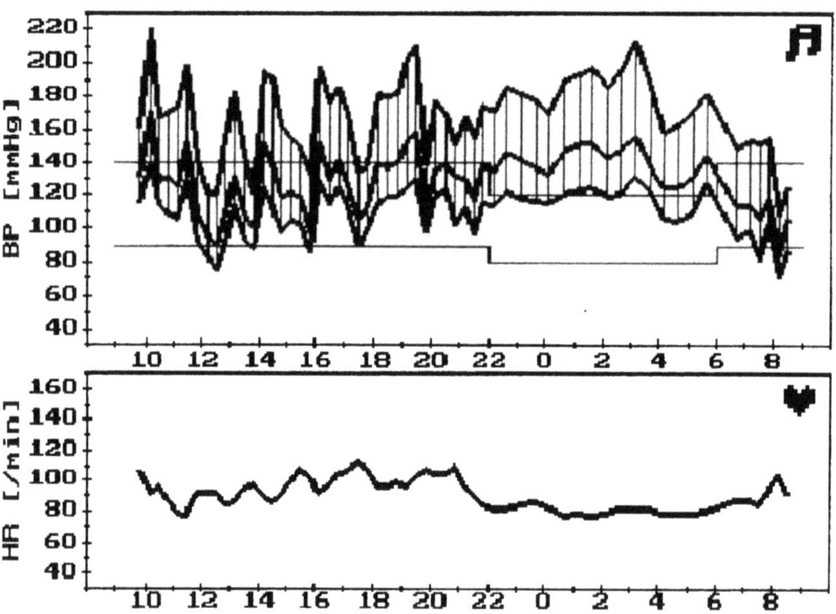

FIGURE 2. A 24-h ambulatory blood pressure monitoring in the same subject with malignant pheochromocytoma after 9 months. BP, blood pressure; HR, heart rate.

SUMMARY

In conclusion, hypertension in pheochromocytoma is very complex with various presentations perhaps due to the desensitization of catecholamine receptors often leading to normotension. In many subjects, hypertension is characterized by the higher daytime blood pressure variability caused not only by blood pressure elevations, but also by posture-induced blood pressure falls and also by the absence or the inversion of circadian blood pressure variation. On the other hand, circadian heart rate variation often remains unchanged. As a higher cardiovascular mortality was reported in subjects with pheochromocytoma,[36] increased blood pressure variability might be another contributing factor of the enhanced cardiovascular morbidity and mortality in this rare disease besides the known risk factors such as hypertension, arrhythmia, and disturbances of glucose metabolism typical for pheochromocytoma.

ACKNOWLEDGMENTS

This study is supported by the research project of the Ministry of Education, J 13/98 111100002–1, 0021620807, 0021620808, and 0021620817.

REFERENCES

1. KAPLAN, N.M. 2002. Pheochromocytoma (with a preface about incidental adrenal masses). *In* Kaplan's Clinical Hypertension. N.M. Kaplan, Ed.: 434–454. Lippincott Williams & Wilkins. Philadelpia.
2. STREETEN, D.H.P. & G.H. ANDERSON, JR. 1996. Mechanisms of orthostatic hypotension and tachycardia in patients with pheochromocytoma. Am. J. Hypertens. **9:** 760–769.
3. PROYE, C., P. FOSATI, P. FONTAINE, *et al.* 1986. Dopamine-secreting pheochromocytoma: an unrecognized entity? Classification of pheochromocytomas according their type of secretion. Surgery **100:** 1155–1162.
4. ITO, Y., Y. FUJIMOTO & T. OBARA 1992. The role of epinephrine, norepinephrine, and dopamine in blood pressure disturbances in patients with pheochromocytoma. World J. Surg. **16:** 759–764.
5. BRAVO, E.L., R.C. TARAZI, M.F. FOUAD, *et al.* 1982. Blood pressure regulation in pheochromocytoma. Hypertension **4**(Suppl II): II-193–II-199.
6. BRAVO, E., F. FOUAD-TARAZ, G.P. ROSSI, *et al.* 1991. A reevaluation of the hemodynamics of pheochromocytoma. Hypertension **15**(Suppl I): I-128–I-131.
7. LEVENSON, J.A., M.E. SAFAR, G.M. LONDON & A.C.H. SIMON. 1980. Haemodynamics in patients with phaeochromocytoma. Clin. Sci. **58:** 349–356.
8. BRAVO, E.L., R.C. TARAZI, R.W. GIFFORD JR. & D.H. STEWART. 1979. Circulating and urinary catecholamines in pheochromocytoma: diagnostic and pathophysiologic implications. N. Engl. J. Med. **15:** 623–626.
9. GRÖNDAL, S., B. HAMBERGER & M. TELENIUS-BERG. 1986. Secretory pattern and blood pressure in pheochromocytoma. World J. Surg. **10:** 724–728.

10. Stenström, G. & J. Kutti. 1985. The blood volume in pheochromocytoma patients before and during treatment with phenoxybenzamin. Acta Med. Scand. **218:** 381–387.
11. Deoreo, G.A. Jr., B.H. Stewart, R.C. Tarazi & R.W. Gifford Jr. 1974. Preoperative blood transfusions in the safe surgical management of pheochromocytoma. A review of 46 cases. J. Urol. **111:** 715–721.
12. Cat Genova, G., F. Veglio, F. Rabbia, *et al.* 2001. Baroreflex sensitivity in secondary hypertension. Clin. Exp. Hypertens. **21:** 89–99.
13. Hamada, M., Y. Shigematsu, M. Mukai, *et al.* 1995. Blood pressure response to the Valsalva maneuver in pheochromocytoma and pseudopheochromocytoma. Hypertension **25:** 266–271.
14. Munakata, M., A. Aihara, Y. Imai, *et al.* 1999. Altered sympathetic and vagal modulations of the cardiovascular system in patients with pheochromocytoma. Am. J. Hypertens. **12:** 572–580.
15. Grassi, G., G. Seravalle, C. Turri & G. Mancia. 1999. Sympathetic nerve traffic responses to surgical removal of pheochromocytoma. Hypertension **34:** 461–465.
16. Dabrowska, B., A. Dabrowski, P. Pruszczyk, *et al.* 1995. Heart rate variability in pheochromocytoma. Am. J. Cardiol. **76:** 1202–1204.
17. Minami, J., M. Todoraki, T. Ishimitsu & H. Matsuoka. 2004. Changes in heart rate variability before and after surgery in patients with pheochromocytoma. Auton. Neurosci. **111:** 144–146.
18. Littler, W.A. & A.J. Honour. 1974. Direct arterial pressure, heart rate, and electrocardiogram in unrestricted patients before and removal of pheaochromocytoma. Q. J. Med. **63:** 441–449.
19. van Eps, R.G.S., A.H. van den Meiracker, F. Boomsma, *et al.* 1994. Diurnal variation of blood pressure in patients with catecholamine-producing tumors. Am. J. Hypertens. **7:** 492–497.
20. Magnano, A.R., D. Bai & D.M. Bloomield. 2002. Cyclic tachycardia and hypotension. Circulation **106:** e1–e2.
21. Guzik, P., A. Wykretowicz, K.H. Wesseling & H. Wysocki. 2005. Adrenal pheochromocytoma associated with dramatic cyclic hemodynamic fluctuations. Int. J. Cardiol. **2005:** 351–353.
22. Dabrowska, B., T. Feltynowski, B. Wocial, *et al.* 1990. Effect of removal of pheochromcytoma on diurnal variability of blood pressure, heart rhythm and excretion of catecholamines. J. Hum. Hypertens. **4:** 397–399.
23. Padfield, P.L., S.G. Jyothinagaram, I.M. McGinley & D.M. Watson. 1991. Reversal of the relationship between heart rate and blood pressure in pheochromocytoma: a non-invasive diagnostic approach? J. Hum. Hypertens. **5:** 501–504.
24. Spieker, C., M. Barenbrock, K.H. Rahn & W. Zidek. 1993. Circadian blood pressure variations in endocrine disorders. Blood Press. **2:** 35–39.
25. Middeke, M. & J. Schrader. 1994. Nocturnal blood pressure in normotensive subjects and those with white coat, primary and secondary hypertension. Br. Med. J. **308:** 630–632.
26. Meisel, S.R., V. Mor-Avi, T. Rosenthal & S. Akselrod. 1994. Spectral analysis of the systolic blood pressure signal in secondary hypertension: a method for the identification of pheochromocytoma. J. Hypertens. **12:** 269–275.
27. Imai, Y., K. Abe, Y. Miura, *et al.* 1988. Hypertensive episodes and circadian fluctuations of blood pressure in patients with pheochromocytoma: studies by

long-term blood pressure monitoring based on a volume-oscillometric method. J. Hypertens. **6:** 9–15.

28. ZELINKA, T., B. ŠTRAUCH, L. PECEN & J. WIDIMSKÝ JR. 2004. Diurnal blood pressure variation in pheochromocytoma, primary aldosteronism and Cushing's syndrome. J. Hum. Hypertens. **18:** 107–111.
29. ZELINKA, T., J. WIDIMSKÝ & J. WEISSEROVÁ. 2001. Diminished circadian blood pressure rhythm in patients with asymptomatic normotensive pheochromocytoma. Physiol. Res. **50:** 631–634.
30. FRATTOLA, A., G. PARATI, C. CUSPIDI, *et al.* 1993. Prognostic value of 24-hour blood pressure variability. J. Hypertens. **11:** 1133–1137.
31. KIKUYA, M., T. HOZAWA, T. OHKUBO, *et al.* 2000. Prognostic significance of blood pressure and heart rate variabilities. The Ohasama study. Hypertension **36:** 901–906.
32. ZELINKA, T., B. ŠTRAUCH, O. PETRÁK, *et al.* 2005. Increased blood pressure variability in pheochromocytoma compared to essential hypertension patients. J. Hypertens. **23:** 2033–2039.
33. MANGER, W.M. 2005. The vagaries of pheochromocytoma. Am. J. Hypertens. **18:** 1266–1270.
34. TSUJIMOTO, G., V.M. MANGER & B.B. HOFFMAN. 1984. Desensitization of β-adrenergic receptors by pheochromocytoma. Endocrinology **114:** 1272–1278.
35. SNAVELY, M.D., M.G. ZIEGLER & P. INSEL. 1985. Subtype-selective down-regulation of rat renal cortical α- and β-adrenergic receptors by catecholamines. Endocrinology **117:** 2182–2189.
36. KHORRAM-MANESH, A., O. AHLMAN, O. NILSSON, *et al.* 2005. Long-term outcome of a large series of patients surgically treated for pheochromocytoma. J. Intern. Med. **258:** 55–66.

Genetic Testing in Pheochromocytoma

Increasing Importance for Clinical Decision Making

STEFAN R. BORNSTEIN[a] AND ANNE-PAULE GIMENEZ-ROQUEPLO[b]

[a]*Carl Gustav Carus University Hospital, Department of Medicine, 01307 Dresden, Germany*

[b]*Université René Descartes, Faculté de Médecine, Département de Génétique, Hôpital Européen Georges Pompidou, Paris, France*

ABSTRACT: Hereditary pheochromocytomas and paragangliomas are caused by germline mutations in syndrome-associated genes. This includes multiple endocrine neoplasia Type 2 (MEN 2) caused by mutations in the *RET* proto-oncogene, von Hippel–Lindau (VHL) syndrome due to mutations of the *VHL* gene, neurofibromatosis Type I (NF1) caused by mutations of the *NF1* gene, and pheochromocytoma/paraganglioma syndromes due to mutations in genes encoding the succinate dehydrogenase subunits D (*SDHD*) and B (*SDHB*). At the First International Symposium on Pheochromocytoma (ISP2005) organized by the National Institutes of Health, a panel of specialist clinicians and scientists from around the world addressed the topic of genetic testing in pheochromocytoma patients. This review summarizes the discussions and conclusions of the panel and provides a recommendation for evidence-based management of genetic testing in these patients and their families. A pragmatic algorithm is presented, taking into account patient age, tumor location (extra-adrenal, intra-adrenal, unilateral, and bilateral), biochemical presentation, and financial costs. This was based on cumulative frequencies ranging from 7.5% to 29% for germline mutations in four genes (*RET, VHL, SDHB,* and *SDHD)* in patients with apparently sporadic pheochromocytomas. This algorithm will need to be validated by further genetic analysis, multicenter studies, and long-term observations.

KEYWORDS: genetics; pheochromocytoma; RET; VHL; SDH

The unraveling of the human genome has given us novel and powerful tools for the identification of disease-associated germline and somatic mutations, deletions, and polymorphisms. Consequently, our knowledge on the genetic

Address for correspondence: Stefan R. Bornstein, Department of Medicine, Technical University of Dresden, Fetscherstrasse 74, 01307 Dresden, Germany. Voice: +49/3514585955; fax: +49/3514586398

e-mail: Stefan.Bornstein@uniklinikum-dresden.de

Ann. N.Y. Acad. Sci. 1073: 94–103 (2006). © 2006 New York Academy of Sciences. doi: 10.1196/annals.1353.010

basis of human disease is expanding at an ever-increasing rate, allowing major progress in early diagnosis, screening, and monitoring of both common and rare disorders. This, however, is not without subsequent implications for patients and physicians, these ranging from cost–benefit issues to ethical and psychological burdens.[1–3]

The genetic factors involved in pheochromocytoma/paraganglioma syndromes represent a perfect example for these exciting advances in modern biomedicine.[4–7] Until recently, more than 90% of these rare but clinically important catecholamine-producing tumors were thought to occur as sporadic nonhereditary entities not requiring genetic screening unless there was a family history of a certain form of MEN.[8,9] The last 3 years, however, have seen mounting evidence that a substantial proportion of patients with these tumors have a definable genetic defect with potentially important clinical implications.

Pheochromocytoma has often been referred to as the "10% tumor," suggesting that 10% are bilateral, 10% malignant, 10% extra-adrenal, and 10% familial. The latter figure refers to a proportion of tumors arising from familial syndromes, including MEN 2, von Hippel–Lindau (VHL) syndrome,[10] and neurofibromatosis Type I (NF1). Germline mutations in these diseases have now been identified in the proto-oncogene *RET* located on chromosome 10, and in *VHL* and *NF1* tumor-suppressor genes. VHL is a dominantly inherited syndrome associated with germline mutations in the *VHL* gene located on chromosome 3. Mutations in this tumor-suppressor gene lead to the development of vascular tumors of the central nervous system and retina. Pheochromocytomas may also occur in a small percentage of people with *NF1* mutations, a syndrome that includes multiple tumors of the skin (neurofibromas), pigmented spots, tumors of the optic nerve of the eye, and bone lesions. More recently, germline mutations in the genes encoding succinate dehydrogenase subunit D (*SDHD*) and subunit B (*SDHB*) have been described in patients with pheochromocytomas and functional paragangliomas.[11] These genes encode three mitochondrial complex II subunits, but the mechanisms by which these mutations cause tumors still remain to be elucidated. Potential mechanisms include mitochondrially mediated failure of apoptosis, or even activation of the angiogenic pathway. Altogether, five different pheochromocytoma susceptibility genes are now under discussion.[12] The first comprehensive study on this topic so far was performed in the year 2002. This investigation included 271 nonsyndromic (sporadic) patients and demonstrated that 24% were carrying a previously unrecognized germline mutation either in *RET*, *VHL*, *SDHD* or *SDHB* genes. Furthermore, these patients were more likely to present at a younger age than those lacking any of the mutations (mean, 25 versus 44 years), and were also more likely to exhibit multifocal disease and extra-adrenal tumors. Thus, germline mutations are more often responsible for pheochromocytomas than previously recognized.[13,14] However, the overall benefits of genetic testing of all patients with apparently sporadic presentation of pheochromocytoma have not been determined.

In light of the above advances and associated issues a moderator-led breakout session was held during the First International Symposium on Pheochromocytoma (ISP2005) to address the following questions:

1. How should paragangliomas and pheochromocytomas best be defined?
2. Should all patients with pheochromocytomas undergo genetic testing for possible disease-causing mutations, or should this be confined to patients where there is a suspicion of an existing syndrome or only to young patients?
3. What are cost–benefit factors to be taken into account when genetic testing is considered?

Specialist clinicians and scientists from around the world working in the field of genetics and pheochromocytomas presented their data at ISP2005, including three speakers chosen to lead discussion on the above issues at the special breakout session on Genetics of Pheochromocytoma/Paraganglioma Syndromes.

The following review is based on comprehensive analysis of the existing data published on these issues, new results provided and updated by the experts in the field, concerns raised by patients and family members present at the meeting, the extensive discussions of the entire panel of experts during the breakout session, and the final general discussion on the last day of the meeting.

Furthermore, the review will present the conclusions and algorithms developed by the panel of experts on the basis of the given evidence. However, we must emphasize that these statements were not intended as binding consensus or guidelines by the organizers or participants of this meeting. Rather, they form a pragmatic and well-balanced recommendation for the time being that requires continuous modification as new data and follow-up studies emerge to create a clearer picture of the value and requirements for genetic testing.

The group of experts agreed upon the use of the WHO classification of 2004[15] for the definition of the terms for pheochromocytoma and paraganglioma as outlined below:

> Pheochromocytomas are rare tumors of the adrenal gland that arise from chromaffin cells in the adrenal medulla. Pheochromocytoma is the term given to a functional paraganglioma arising in the adrenal medulla. Paragangliomas arise from extra-adrenal chromaffin cells and can originate in either the sympathetic nervous system or parasympathetic ganglia.

Although the recommendation was to remain with these simplified definitions for the sake of international standardization, the panel acknowledged that other classifications using the term of thoracic or abdominal extra-adrenal pheochromocytomas distinct from the head and neck paragangliomas or intra-adrenal pheochromocytoma may be used in clinical studies. As long as the histopathological and clinical entities are well defined and accounted for, there was no strong tendency toward the necessity for uniform nomenclature.

The primary question of a genetic testing requirement in patients with pheochromocytoma and/or paragangliomas was addressed from different perspectives in the breakout session. The first speaker, Joyce Graff, representing the VHL Family Alliance patient support group, provided a strong case in favor of more widespread genetic analysis. Availability of earlier genetic testing would have made a difference to the management of her own family history and that of many patients in the VHL Family Alliance support group. She suggested that patients and their families need to know that they might suffer from a genetic disease that may have severe long-term consequences—"You need to know your enemy by name." Joyce Graff stated that this is even more important for these diseases since knowledge about pheochromocytoma and paraganglioma syndromes is limited among the vast majority of physicians and health practitioners. Consequently there is a need to improve information available to patients and their families affected as well as to their doctors.

It was concluded that there was also a need for recommendations and updated treatment guidelines as well as a listing of centers with appropriate experience in treating pheochromocytoma patients. Such a listing might be best provided at a suitable website.

Professor Robert Gagel, a leading expert in the treatment of patients with MEN at the M.D. Anderson Cancer Center in Houston, stressed the need for more information on the long-term consequences of generalized genetic testing for these syndromes. He pointed out that many confounding factors, including a strong bias of ascertainment and selection of patients in those centers that have published studies on the frequency of mutations in patients with pheochromocytoma might not reflect the true picture within the general population.

In reviewing the literature up to 2004, Professor Gagel estimated the cumulative frequency of mutations mounted up to be 20.1%, RET (2.5%), VHL (8.4%), SDHB (4.8%), and SDHD (4.4%). However, taking into account some of the major confounding factors, including possible evidence of familial disease, a revised percentage around 14.2% seemed more likely, including RET 1.7%, VHL 5.3%, SDHB 2.8%, and SDHD 4.4%. This would still be higher than 10% required by the earlier guidelines of the American College of Clinical Oncologists for a general recommendation for genetic testing in tumors.

However, the updated guidelines are more focused on the potential benefit rather than on any statistical cutoff value. Dr. Gagel discussed both the advantages and disadvantages of genetic analysis. Current costs in the United States are around $2,000–4,000 for analysis of all four major susceptibility genes for pheochromocytoma. Issues affecting genetic discrimination are still not settled, and a positive test may trigger uncontrolled, overzealous treatment as a consequence. While early identification of a disease-relevant mutation for MEN 2 and VHL will present clear-cut benefit for the patients on the basis of high penetrance, this remains unclear for the *SDHD* and *SDHB* mutations at this point. Therefore, Professor Gagel stressed the need for more long-term studies on genetic testing with emphasis at this time on increasing awareness among affected patients, families, and their physicians of the possibility and potential implications of genetic disease in patients with an apparently sporadic form of pheochromocytoma.

Members of the panel were concerned that there is already strong evidence that *SDHB* mutation carriers are more likely to develop extra-adrenal pheochromocytomas and malignancy, implying knowledge of such genetic risk in a carrier would therefore be very important for affected families.[16] Existing knowledge about the penetrance of the *SDHB* mutations seems, however, to be incomplete. An Italian study[17] presented at ISP2005 demonstrated that no evidence of pheochromocytoma or paraganglioma was found in 16 relatives (mean age: 49 years, range: 18–83) carrying the R230G *SDHB* mutation so far. On the other hand, the International SDH Consortium reported that in families with *SDHB* or *SDHD* mutations,[18] 5 of 38 asymptomatic mutation-positive carriers were diagnosed with underlying disease. Four of these five carriers were *SDHB* mutation carriers.

Finally, Professor Hartmut Neumann from the University of Freiburg, who performed major studies on the genetic basis of pheochromocytoma/paraganglioma syndromes, provided his perspective on this topic. Like the other speakers, he made it clear that the benefit of genetic testing for the patient must be the primary concern. Diagnosis and treatment of patients with pheochromocytoma requires the concerted team effort of experienced endocrinologists, pediatricians, ENT specialists, and visceral surgeons. There is clearly a need for more basic research and long-term clinical studies. Current data provided by the Prof. Neumann's group have also demonstrated that a substantial percentage of patients with apparently sporadic pheochromocytomas have a germline mutation in one of the four genes.

The moderator of the session, Professor Bornstein, suggested that in summarizing the data presented during ISP2005, there are evidently substantial regional differences in the prevalence of germline mutations in apparently sporadic presentations of pheochromocytoma. European centers other than the Freiburg/Polish group have also analyzed the frequency of germline mutations in patients with apparently sporadic pheochromocytomas (FIG. 1).

In addition to the difference in cumulative frequency of all four genes ranging from 7.5 to 24%, he observed substantial differences in the relative frequency of mutations in each gene in the different centers (TABLE 1). This discrepancy could be explained by a difference in the size of the series, in the clinical work-up and follow-up evaluations of the patients, and in the sources of recruitment between the different European centers. This may also underline the influence of a founder effect in different regions. As yet, little is known about the frequency of these mutations (cumulative and/or relative) throughout other regions in the world.

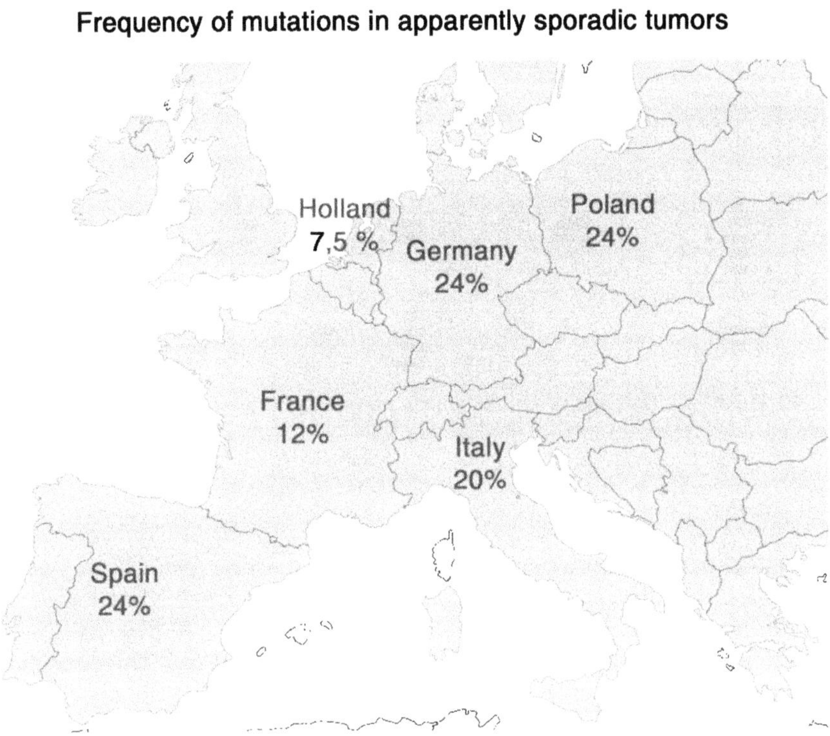

FIGURE 1. Mutation frequency of apparently sporadic pheochromocytoma in other European countries.

Basing their conclusions on the extensive discussions during the entire meeting and the breakout session as well as on the evidence published, the panel of experts agreed upon an algorithm. This algorithm should be appropriate for the time being, but will need to be adjusted as more data become available. We tested this algorithm after the meeting on the recently published French pheochromocytoma/paraganglioma cohort (FIG. 2). This cohort contained 314 patients, 86 of whom had an inherited pheochromocytoma/paraganglioma (13 with a NF1 and 73 with a germline mutation on *VHL*, *RET*, *SDHB* or *SDHD*).

TABLE 1. Relative frequency of genetic mutations from different groups published and presented in this meeting[13,23–25]

	Germany/Poland	Holland	France	Spain
VHL (%)	11	4.4	3.5	6
SDHB (%)	4	1.5	7	10
SDHD (%)	4	1.6	0.8	10
RET (%)	5	0	0.4	1

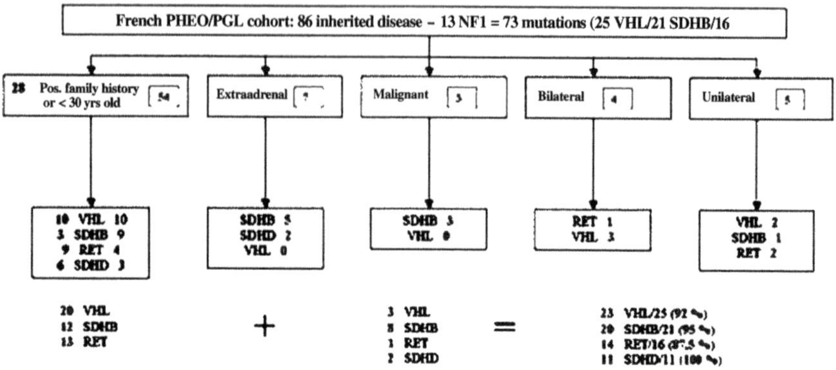

FIGURE 2. Data analysis of the French pheochromocytoma or functional paraganglioma cohort using the PRESSOR algorithm.[24]

Fifty-four patients with a causative mutation had a positive family history or an age of less than 30 years (74%). Among the 19 others patients, 5 did not have an extra-adrenal, malignant or a bilateral tumor and could not be diagnosed with the algorithm (6.8% of the total of patients with a mutation). Three patients harbored phenotypic clues of a specific genetic disease (medullary thyroid carcinoma for the two patients with a *RET* mutation and hemangioblastoma of the retina for one of the two patients with a *VHL* mutation). The two other patients with an apparently adrenal pheochromocytoma, one with a VHL disease Type 2C and one with a *SDHB* mutation, were 34 and 31 years of age. The data suggest that the age limit should be extended to 35 years and that medical work-up before genetic testing should contain plasma thyrocalcitonin measurement and retinal examination. Therefore, based on current evidence, a practical flowchart for genetic testing is depicted in FIGURE 3. Furthermore, the expert panel underlined the importance of a specialized genetic consultation to collect the family history as well as the signed informed consent and of a complete work-up before the genetic testing. The panel also agreed that the following issues should be addressed: (a) the need for design and conduct of large prospective studies, including centers outside Europe; and (b) further genetic analyses, including deletions for SDHD and SDHB genes and long-term monitoring of patients and family members.

Up to now, mutations leading to pheochromocytomas have been defined in at least five independent genes encoding distinct functions.[19] In addition, other genes causing hereditary pheochromocytoma/paraganglioma disease should also be considered.[20] This includes the EgIN3 gene as an important downstream enzyme in the pathway leading to VHL.[21] Finally, a comprehensive database and the future use of the PRESSOR website[22] for recommendations for screening and monitoring should be established.

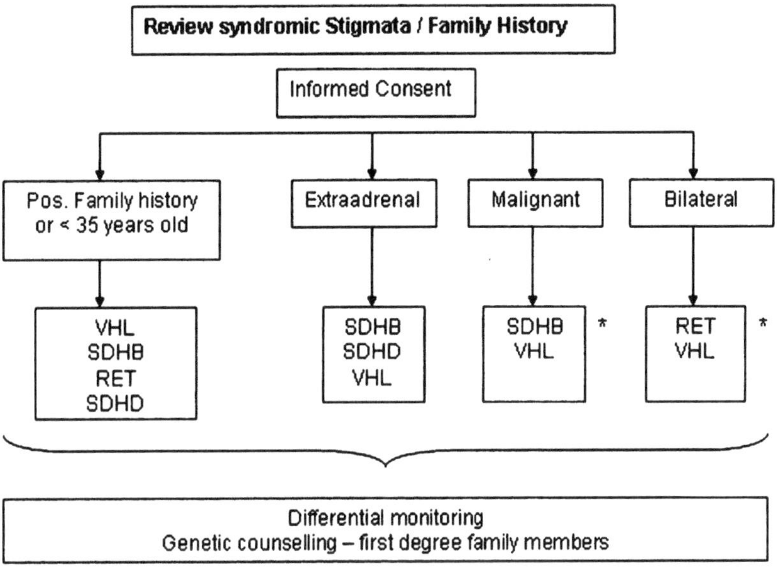

FIGURE 3. Current recommendations for a cost-effective genetic testing approach in sporadic pheochromocytoma. This algorithm requires previous extensive clinical workup of a patient including appropriate neurochemical analysis followed by imaging. The neurochemical pattern may also help to differentiate between VHL- (predominantly normetanephrines/norepinephrines) and MEN 2- (predominantly metanephrine/epinephrine) producing tumors.[7] *It should be noted that there are some exceptions and in some patients further genetic testing is needed. For example, in malignant pheochromocytoma if *SDHB* and *VHL* mutations are negative, patients could be tested for the presence of *SDHD* and *MEN* 2 mutations. Similar, in patients with bilateral pheochromocytomas if *VHL* and *MEN* 2 mutations are negative, patients could be tested for the presence of *SDHB* mutation.

ACKNOWLEDGEMENT

We would like to thank all members of the PRESSOR Group and participants of the ISP2005 for their valuable discussions and input for this summary. Particularly we would like to thank Dr. Karel Pacak and Dr. Diana Benn for their editing of the manuscript and Joyce Graff, Dr. Robert Gagel, and Dr. Hartmut Neumann for their presentation during the breakout session on this topic. We would like to thank Dr. Christian Ziegler and Dr. Flavie Sicard for technical support. This work was also supported by a grant from the DFG (SFB 655/1-05) to S.R.B.

REFERENCES

1. Kievit, J. & H.R. Haak. 2000. Diagnosis and treatment of adrenal incident alone: a cost-effectiveness analysis. Endocrinol. Metab. Clin. North. Am. **29:** 69–90, viii-ix.

2. PACAK, K. *et al.* 2001. Recent advances in genetics, diagnoses, and treatment of pheochromocytoma. Ann. Intern. Med. **134:** 315–329.
3. SAWKA, A.M. *et al.* 2004. The economic implications of three biochemical screening algorithms for pheochromocytomas. J. Clin. Endocrinol. Metab. **89:** 2859–2866.
4. BRAVO, E.L. & R. TAGLE. Pheochromocytoma: state-of-the-art and future prospects. 2003. Endocr. Rev. **24:** 539–553.
5. MANSMANN, G. *et al.* 2004. The clinically inapparent adrenal mass: update in diagnosis and management. Endocr. Rev. **25:** 309–340.
6. LENDERS, J.W. *et al.* 2005. Pheochromocytoma. Lancet **366:** 665–675.
7. EISENHOFER, G. *et al.* 2001. Pheochromocytomas in von Hippel–Lindau syndrome and multiple endocrine heoplasia type 2 display distinct biochemical and clinical phenotypes. J. Clin. Endocrinol. Metab. **86:** 1999–2008.
8. DLUHY, R.G. 2002. Pheochromocytoma: death of an axiom. N. Engl. J. Med. **346:**1486–1488.
9. MANGER, W.M. & R.W. GIFFORD. 1977. Pheochromocytoma. Springer-Verlag. New York.
10. EISENHOFER, G. *et al.* 2004. Malignant pheochromocytoma: current status and initiatives for future progress. Endocr. Relat. Cancer. **11:** 423–436.
11. BAUTERS, C. *et al.* 2003. Hereditary pheochromocytomas and paragangliomas: a study of five susceptability genes. J. Med. Genet. **40:** e75.
12. BERTHERAT, J. & A.P. GIMENEZ-ROQUEPLO. 2005. New insights in the genetics of adrenocertical tumors, pheochromocytomas, and paragangliomas. Horm. Metab. Res. **37:** 384–390.
13. NEUMANN, H.P. *et al.* 2002. Germ-line mutations in nonsyndromic pheochromocytoma. N. Engl. J. Med. **346:** 1459–1466.
14. BRYANT, J. *et al.* 2003. Pheochromocytomas: the expanding genetic differential diagnosis. J. Natl. Cancer. Inst. **95:** 1196–1204.
15. WHO classification: www.who.int/classifications/committees/ICD10Updates_2004.pdf.
16. GIMENEZ-ROQUEPLO, A.P. *et al.* 2003. Mutations in the SDHB gene are associated with extraadrenal and/or malignant phaeochhromocytomas. Cancer Res. **63:** 5615—5621.
17. CASTELLANO, M. *et al.* 2005. Genetic mutation screening in an Italian cohort of non-syndromic pheochromocytoma/paraganglioma patients. Presented at the first International Symposium on Pheochromocytoma, Bethesda, MD, October 2005.
18. BENN, D.E. 2005. SDHD, SDHB mutations: different phenotype and penetrance. Presented at the first International Symposium on Pheochromocytoma, Bethesda, MD, October 2005.
19. DAHIA, P.L. 2005. Linking hypoxia and redox signals in pheochromocytoma: transcription association of VHL and SDH mutations, Presented at the first International Symposium on Pheochromocytoma, Bethesda, MD, October 2005.
20. OPOCHER, G. *et al.* 2005. Familial non-syndromic pheochromocytoma. Presented at the first International Symposium on Pheochromocytoma, Bethesda, MD, October 2005.
21. LEE, S. *et al.* 2005. Neuronal apoptosis linked to EglN3 prolyl hydroxylase and familial pheochromocytoma genes: developmental culling and cancer. first International Symposium on Pheochromocytomas, Bethesda, MD, October 2005.
22. PRESSOR homepage: www.pressor.org/

23. DINJENS. *et al.* 2005. Genetic analysis of pheochromocytomas: the Rotterdam experience. First International Symposium on Pheochromocytoma, Bethesda, MD, October 2005.
24. AMAR, L. *et al.* 2005. Genetic testing in pheochromocytoma or functional paraganglioma. J. Clin. Oncol. **23:** 8812–8818.
25. CASCON. *et al.* 2005. Gross deletions affecting the SDH genes increase the percentage of germline mutations in Spanish pheochromoytoma/Paraganglioma patients. Presented at the first International Symposium on Pheochromocytoma, Bethesda, MD, October 2005..

Genetic Testing in Pheochromocytoma- and Paraganglioma-Associated Syndromes

DIANA E. BENN, ANNE LOUISE RICHARDSON, DEBORAH J. MARSH, AND BRUCE G. ROBINSON

Cancer Genetics, Kolling Institute of Medical Research, Royal North Shore Hospital and University of Sydney, Sydney, NSW, Australia

ABSTRACT: Genetic understanding of pheochromocytoma (PHEO) and paraganglioma (PGL) syndromes has recently expanded with the identification of the involvement of the mitochondrial complex II peptides, namely the succinate dehydrogenase subunit B (SDHB), subunit C (SDHC), and subunit D (SDHD). In patients with PHEO and/or PGL genetic testing for germline mutations in *SDHD* and *SDHB* has been recommended, in addition to the PHEO susceptibility genes *VHL* and *RET*. After careful clinical assessment of the patient, suspected familial disease may direct the clinician to the appropriate gene for testing. In the absence of obvious features of familial disease, the decision regarding the appropriate gene for testing is more difficult. Such testing can be costly and time consuming, but a rational prioritization of gene testing can streamline the process. Therefore in order to achieve this for apparently sporadic cases we propose a decision matrix based on site of tumor, functionality, and age at presentation.

KEYWORDS: **pheochromocytoma; paraganglioma; SDHD; SDHB; SDHC**

INTRODUCTION

The genetic basis for formation of many endocrine tumors is becoming clearer, leading to better classification of the hereditary nature of many of these tumors and stronger genotype–phenotype correlations. This has recently been exemplified in PHEOs, tumors of the sympathoadrenal neuroendocrine system originating in the neural crest–derived chromaffin cells of the adrenal medulla. Generally PHEOs are functionally active, as indicated by the excess secretion of catecholamines. The term PHEO is also frequently applied to extra-adrenal paragangliomas in the abdomen (urinary bladder, filum terminale) and

Address for correspondence: B.G. Robinson, Cancer Genetics, Kolling Institute of Medical Research, Royal North Shore Hospital, St Leonards, NSW 2065, Australia. Voice: +61 2 9926 7267; fax: +61 2 9926 8523.
e-mail: bgr@med.usyd.edu.au

**Ann. N.Y. Acad. Sci. 1073: 104–111 (2006). © 2006 New York Academy of Sciences.
doi: 10.1196/annals.1353.011**

the thorax. Related tumors, PGLs of the neural crest–derived chief cells of the parasympathetic-associated ganglia are, however, generally nonsecretory.[1]

PHEOs and PGLs are now known to be linked genetically. Currently four genes (*RET, VHL, SDHB,* and *SDHD*) are considered for testing in individuals with these tumors,[2] yet testing can be costly, and prioritizing the order of gene testing can partially relieve the financial burden. This review describes clinical features of the major familial syndromes with PHEO and/or PGL as a component tumor and genotype–phenotype correlations with relevance to genetic testing. In addition, based on the literature, a decision matrix for prioritizing gene testing is proposed.

PHEOCHROMOCYTOMA-ASSOCIATED SYNDROMES

Multiple Endocrine Neoplasia Type 2 (MEN2)

PHEOs are component tumors of the MEN2 autosomal dominant syndrome caused by activating germline mutations in the *RET* proto-oncogene.[3] By definition PHEOs are associated with MEN2A (frequently bilateral) and MEN2B (FIG. 1) and are diagnosed as the first manifestation of MEN2A in only 9–27% of cases.[4] It has been shown that MEN2 patients may have a high plasma metanephrine, whereas VHL patients have a high normetanephrine, and this may have a discriminating value.[5]

Testing for *RET* mutations is suggested for the following: exon 10 (codons 609, 611, 618, 620), exon 11 (codon 630, 634), exon 13 (codons 768, 790, 791), exon 14 (codon 804), exon 15 (codons 883, 891), exon 16 (codon 918) as all have been associated with syndromic PHEO.[6] The occurrence of germline *RET* mutations in apparently sporadic cases of PHEO has been estimated as 2.5%.

Von Hippel–Lindau Disease

Von Hippel–Lindau (VHL) disease is a hereditary cancer syndrome (FIG. 1) caused by heterozygous mutations in the *VHL* gene and subsequent somatic loss of the wild-type allele in tumor tissue.[7] Clinically, VHL families can be subdivided on the basis of absence (Type 1) or presence (Type 2) of PHEO, with Type 2c families developing PHEOs only. Germline *VHL* mutations can be detected in virtually 100% of VHL families tested, using complete gene sequencing (to detect point mutation, small intragenic insertions and deletions), in addition to Southern blotting for detection of large-scale deletion.[8] Genotype–phenotype correlations indicate that more than 96% of Type 2 patients harbor missense mutations.[9] The detection rate of germline *VHL* mutations in patients with apparently sporadic PHEO has been reported to be as high as 8.5% in patients younger than 20 years.[2]

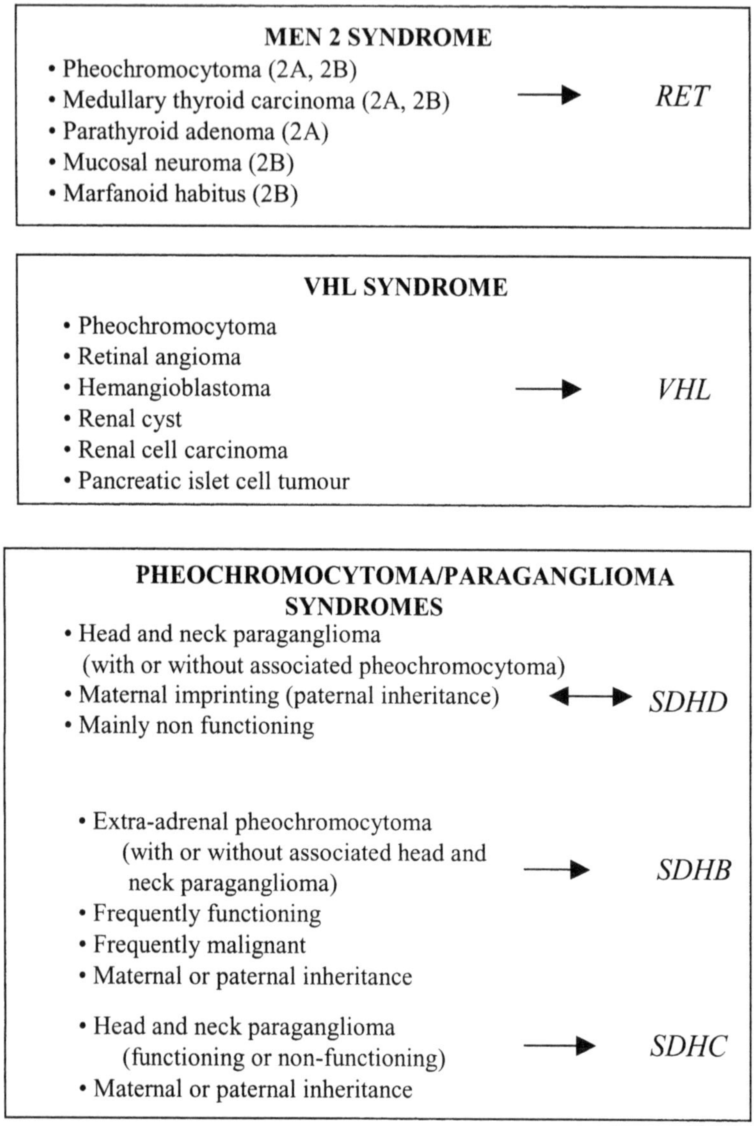

FIGURE 1. Pheochromocytoma and paraganglioma-associated familial syndromes. The most common presentations of the familial syndromes are shown with the respective disease-associated genes. Tumor site, functionality, and pattern of inheritance all assist in prioritizing the genes to be tested.

PHEOCHROMOCYTOMA/PARAGANGLIOMA SYNDROMES

Recent advances have identified three of the four mitochondrial complex II subunits (SDHB, SDHC, and SDHD) as having a role in the development of PHEOs and PGLs. Mitochondrial complex II is involved in the mitochondrial electron transport chain and as the enzyme succinate dehydrogenase that oxidizes succinate to fumarate in the Krebs cycle.

SDHD Linked

PHEOs and PGLs were not known to be linked genetically, until 2000, with the discovery of *SDHD* mutations as causative in familial head and neck PGL (*PGL1* syndrome) and subsequently in PHEOS also.[10,11] The *PGL1*-associated "only paternal transmission of disease" has been borne out in *SDHD*-associated families.

Genotype–phenotype correlations show very strong association between *SDHD* mutations and the development of familial head and neck PGL with or without the presence of PHEOs.[12] In addition, it has been suggested that papillary thyroid carcinoma may be a component tumor of *SDHD* mutation-positive families.[13] Mutations have been identified across the four exons of *SDHD,* with mutation type of missense, nonsense, frameshift, and, rarely, splice site.[14] Also a 96-kb deletion spanning *SDHD* was identified in a family with nonfunctioning carotid body tumors with assumed paternal inheritance.[15] The interpretation of the clinical significance of missense mutations and polymorphisms may be difficult without functional studies,[16] as evidenced by the G12S and H50R variants.[17]

SDHC Linked

SDHC is one of two peptides anchoring mitochondrial complex II in the inner mitochondrial membrane, with the prediction of *SDHC* mutations leading to cellular oxidative stress.[18] Only four *SDHC* mutations have been reported worldwide; one in a family with head and neck PGLs and maternal transmission of disease; the second in a patient with a catecholamine-producing PGL in the carotid bifurcation; the third causing carotid body tumors; and the fourth a large-scale *SDHC* deletion in a family with head and neck PGLs.[13,19] Therefore, routine screening for germline *SDHC* mutations has not yet been recommended. Clearly maternal imprinting is not operating in *SDHC*-linked disease.

SDHB Linked

SDHB in association with SDHA forms the catalytic portion of the enzyme succinate dehydrogenase. Mutations have been reported in *SDHB* exons 1, 2, 3, 4, 5, 6, 7, in addition to a 1-kb deletion at the 5′ end of *SDHB* in a family with functioning PHEO.[15] While germline mutations in *SDHB* coupled with loss of the wild-type allele are predicted to cause constitutive activation of hypoxic pathways, the mechanisms whereby these events lead to tumorigenesis have not been confirmed.[20,21] *SDHB* mutations have been strongly associated with extra-adrenal PHEOs particularly in the abdomen and with malignancy.[22] Head and neck PGLs have been observed less frequently.[23] Interestingly papillary thyroid carcinoma has been diagnosed in one family with an *SDHB* mutation, as has clear cell renal carcinoma in another family.[13]

OTHER PHEOCHROMOCYTOMA OR PARAGANGLIOMA-ASSOCIATED SYNDROMES

PHEOs are a recognized tumor of three other syndromes: multiple endocrine neoplasia Type 1 (MEN1), neurofibromatosis Type 1 (NF1), and the Carney triad.

MEN1 describes a genetic predisposition to neoplasia of the pancreatic islet cells, parathyroid glands, anterior pituitary gland, and rarely PHEO.[24] *MEN1* (11q13) consists of 10 exons, the first of which is not translated. Mutations span the entire gene with the exception of exon 1, and no robust genotype–phenotype correlations have been identified.[24] Currently MEN1 mutation analysis is undertaken in many centers, but to date no guidelines have been published in this regard.[25]

NF1 is an autosomal dominant disorder due to mutations in the *NF1* gene (chromosome 17q11.2) and defined by benign fibromatous tumors of the skin and café-au-lait spots.[26] PHEOs occur in up to 5% of patients with NF1, but diagnosis of syndromic disease is usually made on clinical grounds rather than on genetic testing of this large gene consisting of 59 exons.

The Carney triad is characterized by gastric sarcomas, pulmonary chondromas, and extra-adrenal PGLs.[27] To date a causative gene has not been identified, although it has been suggested that Carney triad and familial PGL may be genetically linked.

CLINICAL ASSESSMENT OF PATIENTS WITH PHEOCHROMOCYTOMA OR PARGANGLIOMA

At the time of initial presentation for a family or individual, it is important to identify clinical features that will assist with diagnosing a particular familial syndrome and confirmation by genetic testing of the appropriate gene. A critical component of the index case assessment involves obtaining a detailed family history and a thorough physical examination including blood pressure, pulse, and careful palpation of the neck and abdomen. Neurological examination including fundoscopic examination for retinal angiomas and examination of the skin for "café au lait" lesions should also be undertaken.[9,26] Urinalysis for evidence of hematuria, and serum calcium and calcitonin levels should be measured in all PHEO patients to ascertain occult VHL and MEN2, respectively. Further investigations of patients with PHEO for evidence of multiple tumors should include scanning with I^{123} meta-iodo-benzylguanidine (MIBG) scintigraphy and computed tomography (CT), scanning from the angle of the jaw to the base of the bladder. The presence of multiple tumors must be identified preoperatively and the finding significantly increases the likelihood of familial disease. Presentation at a young age, bilateral disease, extra-adrenal disease, and other features as described in FIGURE 1 are all suggestive of possible familial disease.

PROPOSED DECISION MATRIX

Targeted gene testing is clearly indicated when familial disease is suspected (FIG. 1). Since up to 25% of apparently sporadic cases of PHEO have germline mutations,[13] a compelling case exists for performing genetic testing in all patients with apparently sporadic PHEO and/or PGL. In order to prioritize the testing of these genes we have developed a decision matrix that utilizes site of tumor, age of presentation, and functional status (FIG. 2).

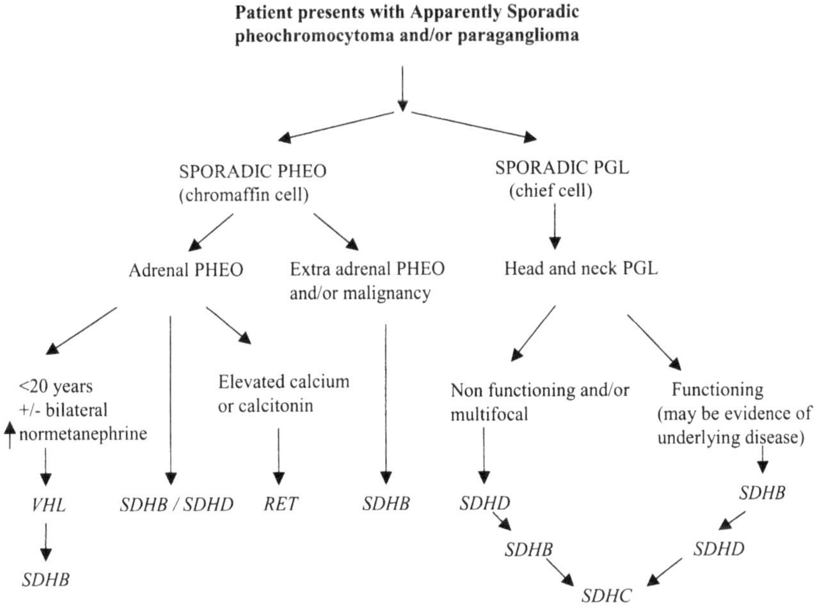

FIGURE 2. Decision matrix for apparently sporadic cases. The first decision is based on the tumor type—pheochromocytoma (PHEO) or paraganglioma (PGL).

CONCLUSIONS

The identification of a causative mutation has far-reaching implications for index cases and their families. As genotype–phenotype correlations become evident, identifying a particular gene mutation can direct the clinical management of the patient, particularly in assessing the risk of development of associated tumors and recurrences.[28] There are additional consequences for other family members who should be offered predictive testing as they may also be at risk of disease. Early detection of at-risk gene carriers should reduce morbidity and mortality, as has been shown with the MEN 2 syndrome.[29] In families where a mutation has been identified, individuals who do not carry this mutation are relieved from the need for further clinical, biochemical, and radiological screening.

In summary, genetic screening and counseling should be offered to all patients with PHEO and or PGL, whether familial or sporadic presentation, and to all first-degree relatives of mutation carriers. This decision matrix will be of benefit in the process of prioritizing the genes to be tested.

REFERENCES

1. SOLCIA, E. *et al.* eds.: 2000. Histological typing of endocrine tumours. *In* World Health Organization International Histological Classification of Tumours, 2nd ed.:38. Springer. London.
2. NEUMANN, H.P.H. *et al.* 2002. Germ-line mutations in non-syndromic pheochromocytoma. N. Engl. J. Med. **346:** 1459–1466.
3. MULLIGAN, L.M. *et al.* 1995. Genotype–phenotype correlation in multiple endocrine neoplasia type 2: report of the International RET Mutation Consortium. J. Intern. Med. **238:** 343–346.
4. BRYANT, J. *et al.* 2003. Pheochromocytoma: the expanding genetic differential diagnosis. J. Natl. Cancer Inst. **95:** 1196–204.
5. EISENHOFER, G. *et al.* 2001. Pheochromocytomas in von Hippel-Lindau syndrome and multiple endocrine neoplasia type 2 display distinct biochemical and clinical phenotypes. J. Clin. Endocrinol. Metab. **86:** 1999–2008.
6. MACHENS, A. *et al.* 2005. Codon-specific development of pheochromocytoma in multiple endocrine neoplasia type 2. J. Clin. Endocrinol. Metab. **90:** 3999–4003.
7. LATIF, F. *et al.* 1993. Identification of the von Hippel-Lindau disease tumor suppressor gene. Science **260:** 1317–1320.
8. STOLLE, C. *et al.* 1998. Improved detection of germline mutations in the von Hippel-Lindau disease tumor suppressor gene. Hum. Mutat. **12:** 417–423.
9. ILIOPOULOS, O. 2001. Von Hippel-Lindau disease: genetic and clinical observations. *In* Genetic Disorders of Endocrine Neoplasia. Frontiers in Hormone Research P.L.M. Dahia & C. Eng, Eds.: 131–166. Karger. Basel, Switzerland.
10. BAYSAL, B.E. *et al.* 2000. Mutations in SDHD, a mitochondrial complex II gene in hereditary paraganglioma. Science **287:** 848–851.
11. GIMM, O. *et al.* 2000. Somatic and occult germ-line mutations in *SDHD*, a mitochondrial complex II gene, in nonfamilial pheochromocytoma. Cancer Res. **60:** 6822–6825.

12. TASCHNER, P.E.M. *et al.* 2001. Nearly all hereditary paragangliomas in the Netherlands are caused by two founder mutations in the *SDHD* gene. Genes Chromosomes Cancer **31:** 274–281.
13. NEUMANN, H.P.H. *et al.* 2004. Distinct clinical features of paraganglioma syndromes associated with *SDHB* and *SDHD* gene mutations. JAMA **292:** 943–951.
14. PAWLU, C. *et al.* 2005. Mutations of the SDHB and SDHD genes. Fam. Cancer **4:** 49–54.
15. MCWHINNEY, S.R. *et al.* 2004. Large germline deletions of mitochondrial complex II subunits SDHB and SDHD in hereditary paraganglioma. J. Clin. Endocrinol. Metab. **89:** 5694–5699.
16. GIMENEZ-ROQUEPLO, A.P. *et al.* 2001. The R22X mutation of the *SDHD* gene in hereditary paraganglioma abolishes the enzymatic activity of complex II in the mitochondrial respiratory chain and activates the hypoxia pathway. Am. J. Hum. Genet. **69:** 1186–1197.
17. CASCON, A. *et al.* 2003. G12S and H50R variations are polymorphisms in the SDHD gene. Genes Chromosomes Cancer **37:** 220–221.
18. ISHII, N. *et al.* 1998. A mutation in succinate dehydrogenase cytochrome B causes oxidative stress and ageing in nematodes. Nature **394:** 694–697.
19. MULLER, U. *et al.* 2005. SDHC mutations in hereditary paraganglioma-pheochromocytoma. Fam. Cancer **4:** 9–12.
20. GIMENEZ-ROQUEPLO, A.P. *et al.* 2002. Functional consequences of a *SDHB* gene mutation in an apparently sporadic pheochromocytoma. J. Clin. Endocrinol. Metab. **87:** 4771–4774.
21. ASTROM, K. *et al.* 2003. Altitude is a phenotypic modifier in hereditary paraganglioma type 1: evidence for an oxygen-sensing defect. Hum. Genet. **113:** 228–237.
22. GIMENEZ-ROQUEPLO, A.P. *et al.* 2003. Mutations in the SDHB gene are associated with extra-adrenal and/or malignant pheochromocytoma. Cancer Res. **63:** 5615–5621.
23. ASTUTI, D. *et al.* 2001. Gene mutations in the succinate dehydrogenase subunit SDHB cause susceptibility to familial pheochromocytoma and to familial paraganglioma. Am. J. Hum. Genet. **69:** 49–54.
24. WAUTOT, V. *et al.* 2002. Germline mutation profile of MEN1 in multiple endocrine neoplasia type 1: search for correlation between phenotype and the functional domains of the MEN1 protein. Hum. Mutat. **20:** 35–47.
25. ELLARD, S. *et al.* 2005. Detection of an MEN1 gene mutation depends on clinical features and supports current referral criteria for diagnostic molecular genetic testing. Clin. Endocrinol **62:** 169–175.
26. ZHU, Y. & L.F. PARADA. 2001. Neurofibromin, a tumor suppressor in the nervous system. Exp. Cell. Res. **264:** 19–28.
27. CARNEY, J.A. 1999. Gastric stromal sarcoma, pulmonary chondroma, and extra-adrenal paraganglioma (Carney triad): natural history, adrenocortical component, and possible familial occurrence. Mayo Clin. Pro. **74:** 543–552.
28. LENDERS, J.W.M. *et al.* 2005. Phaeochromocytoma. Lancet **366:** 665–675.
29. SKINNER, M.A. 2005. Prophylactic thyroidectomy in multiple endocrine neoplasia type 2A. N. Engl. J. Med. **353:** 1105–1113.

New Advances in the Genetics of Pheochromocytoma and Paraganglioma Syndromes

ANNE-PAULE GIMENEZ-ROQUEPLO

Département de Génétique, Hôpital Européen Georges Pompidou, Assistance Publique-Hôpitaux de Paris
Université Paris Descartes, Faculté de Médecine; INSERM U772, Collège de France, Paris, France

ABSTRACT: The discovery of the *SDH* genes in 2000/2001 dramatically changed the genetics of pheochromocytoma (PHEO) and paraganglioma (PGL). Five years on, it is widely accepted that all patients with PHEO/PGL, whatever their age, should undergo genetic testing, because 25–30% of PHEOs are caused by a germline mutation in one of the five PHEO susceptibility genes. However, genetic testing should be targeted according to family and clinical history. The identification of a causal mutation modifies the management and follow-up of the patient and provides an opportunity for presymptomatic genetic testing for other family members. Moreover, the demonstration that the *SDH* genes, are tumor suppressor genes and that their inactivation is involved in the hypoxia-angiogenic pathway activating the transcription factor hypoxia-inducible factor (HIF) by inhibiting prolyl hydroxylases (PHDs) may lead to the identification of new therapeutic targets for these rare diseases. We discuss here these recent findings and their clinical consequences for the management of PHEO/PGL families and the future of research in this field.

KEYWORDS: pheochromocytoma; paraganglioma; SDHD; SDHB; mitochondria

INTRODUCTION

Paragangliomas (PGLs) are highly vascularized tumors that generally arise from the parasympathetic system in the head and neck, sympathetic ganglia in the thorax and abdomen, and the adrenal medulla. These tumors may be functional, secreting catecholamines (pheochromocytoma [PHEO]). The recent

Address for correspondence: Anne-Paule Gimenez-Roqueplo, M.D., Ph.D., Département de Génétique, Hôpital Européen Georges Pompidou, 20-40 rue Leblanc, 75015 Paris, France. Voice: 33-1-56-09-38-81; fax: 33-1-56-09-38-84.
e-mail: Anne-Paule.GIMENEZ@hop.egp.ap-hop-paris.fr

Ann. N.Y. Acad. Sci. 1073: 112–121 (2006).
doi: 10.1196/annals.1353.012

demonstration (2000–2001) that three genes encoding three succinate dehydrogenase subunits belonging to the mitochondrial complex II are involved in the genetics of familial and especially in apparently sporadic PGL and/or PHEO has led to changes in the genetic counselling.

IDENTIFICATION OF THE *SDHS* GENES AND THE FUNCTIONS OF SUCCINATE DEHYDROGENASE

Before 2000, PGLs were known to be highly vascularized, generally benign tumors, preferentially located in the carotid body, in association with other neural-crest-derived tumors (such as PHEOs) in some cases. The association of PGLs and PHEOs in a single syndrome is accounted for by the migration of neural crest cells in the fifth week of embryogenesis, resulting in the distribution of paraganglionic ganglia, including the adrenal medulla, from the base of the skull to the pelvic floor. The leading sites of PGL are a chemoreceptor—the carotid body—in the head and neck and a vestigial chromaffin ganglion—the Zuckerkandl organ—in the abdomen.[1]

Several cases of hereditary PGL (MIM 168000) have been published and it was thought that 10–30% of PGL were inherited. The first locus associated with hereditary PGL (MIM 168000) was identified on 11q23 by genetic linkage analysis in several large families (*PGL1*).[2] Transmission was found to be autosomal dominant via the paternal branch. No disease phenotype is observed in cases of maternal transmission, consistent with maternal genomic imprinting.[3] Three other loci without maternal imprinting were identified on 11q13.1 (*PGL2*),[4] 1q21–q23 (*PGL3*),[5] and 1p35–36 (*PGL4*).[6] In 2000, Bora Baysal *et al.* demonstrated that *PGL1* corresponded to the *SDHD* gene in a genetic linkage analysis study of American and Dutch families.[7] Candidate gene studies rapidly showed that *PGL3* and *PGL4* corresponded to the *SDHC* and *SDHB* genes, respectively.[6,8]

Surprisingly, these three genes encode three subunits of complex II of the respiratory chain, also known as succinate ubiquinone oxidoreductase. Succinate dehydrogenase is a mitochondrial enzyme linking the respiratory chain and Krebs cycle which oxidizes succinate to fumarate.[9] It consists of four subunits. Subunits A and B protrude into the mitochondrial matrix and form the catalytic complex of the enzyme. Subunits C and D anchor the complex to the inner mitochondrial membrane. No *SDHA* mutation has been identified in PHEO/PGL patients but recessive *SDHA* mutations have been associated with a rare type of encephalomyopathy in children—Leigh syndrome.[10] This discrepancy may be accounted for by the recent identification of two different forms of SDHA proteins (type I and type II) encoded by two different *SDHA* genes.[11] In human PGLs, both genes are expressed (as shown by reverse transciption polymerase chain reaction [RT-PCR]) whereas only type I SDHA is found in skin fibroblasts and Hela cells and type II in Raji cells.[12] The presence of both forms of SDHA in PGL tissues suggests that PHEO/PGL is unlikely to result from the inactivation of SDHA. Indeed, two different mutations in two different genes, associated with two somatic events at two different loci, would be required to generate a tumor phenotype in paraganglia tissue in this way.

The *SDH* genes are tumor suppressor genes. We have demonstrated that a heterozygous germline *SDH* mutation is generally associated with somatic loss of the wild-type allele in the tumor tissue—classical loss of heterozygosity. This *SDH* gene inactivation induces the selective and complete loss of succinate dehydrogenase activity regardless of the gene mutated, whether that gene encodes an anchorage subunit (*SDHD*) or a catalytic subunit (*SDHB*).[13,14]

THE *SDHS* GENES: PHENOTYPE–GENOTYPE CORRELATIONS

Several large international cohorts, such as the PGL.NET and COMETE networks (France), the International SDH Consortium, and the large studies (worldwide) published by Hartmut Neumann and Charis Eng, have demonstrated several *SDH* phenotype–genotype correlations. Nonsense and missense mutations, insertions, small and large deletions have been reported in the *SDH* genes of patients with PHEO or PGL.[15,16] Carriers of *SDH* mutations are usually younger and have a more severe phenotype than those with no such mutations. Only four families with a history of head and neck PGL harboring *SDHC* mutations have been reported to date. *SDHD* gene mutations are most frequently identified in families with nonfunctional head and neck PGLs.[17] However, patients with *SDHD* mutations may also develop PHEO or functional PGL.[18] *SDHD* truncating mutations seem to be associated with a more severe phenotype.[19]

SDHB gene mutations are usually associated with abdominal PGLs, which may or may not secrete catecholamines.[17] *SDHB* mutations are often identified in patients with no family history whereas patients with *SDHD* mutations often have a paternal family history. *SDHB* disease seems to have a lower penetrance than *SDHD* disease. In 2003, we reported a high level of malignant *SDHB* PHEOs in a series of 84 patients.[20] Several studies have since confirmed that *SDHB* gene mutation is associated with a high risk of malignancy, identifying such mutations as one of the first prognosis factors for PHEO.[17]

THE NEW INDICATIONS FOR GENETIC TESTING IN PHEO/PGL SYNDROME

Before 2000, three different familial and syndromic diseases were known to result in PHEO and/or PGL: (*a*) multiple endocrine neoplasia type 2 (MEN 2) caused by germline activating mutations in the *RET* proto-oncogene; (*b*) von

Hippel–Lindau (VHL) disease, due to loss-of-function mutations in the *VHL* tumor suppressor gene; and (*c*) neurofibromatosis type 1 (NF1), caused by mutations in the *NF1* gene.[21,22] In 2000/2001, the identification of mutations in the *SDH* (*SDHD, SDHB, SDHC*) genes in patients with hereditary PGL led to changes in genetic counseling and the work-up for affected patients.

The genetic testing of PHEO was challenged by an article published in the New England Journal of Medicine, showing that 24% of a population of 271 nonsyndromic PHEO cases presented with mutations in the *RET*, *VHL*, and *SDH* genes.[23] We recently carried out a retrospective study of 84 apparently sporadic PHEO or functional PGL cases collected by the COMETE network and followed at a single center. We excluded from the study population of all patients with syndromic disease or a family history. We identified mutations in 12% of the patients. Ten percent of the 84 patients had a mutation on the *SDHB* gene. This study demonstrated that *SDHB* gene mutation was a risk factor for extra-adrenal tumors and for malignant disease, in this population followed-up for about 9 years.[20] We recently extended this study to a large cohort including 314 French subjects recruited by different clinical teams in France.[24] The presentation was syndromic or familial in 17.8% of the cases. This series contained 15% malignant PHEOs defined by the presence of extra paraganglionic metastases in bones, liver, lymph nodes, or lung. We identified 86 (27.4%) hereditary PHEOs in this series. An analysis of the distribution of mutations by presentation showed that the disease was inheritable in only 11.6% of the 258 patients with a PHEO or functional PGL with apparently sporadic presentation confirming our previous data in a much larger, multicenter study (TABLE 1). Mutation carriers were younger and more likely to have bilateral or extra-adrenal tumors. Subjects with *RET* mutations frequently had adrenal, mostly bilateral tumors. In patients with *SDHD* mutations, a family history and head and neck PGLs were frequently associated with PHEO. The presentation was apparently sporadic in 30% of the patients with *VHL* mutations and in more that 85% of the *SDHB* mutation carriers. Patients with *SDHB* mutations frequently had large, malignant,

TABLE 1. Genotyping of PHEO/PGL susceptibility genes in large patient cohorts

Patient number[a] Presentation	271[23] Nonsyndromic	84[20] Sporadic	258[24] Sporadic	56[24] Familial	314[24] *Total*
RET mutations	13 (5%)	0	1 (0.4%)	15 (26.8%)	26 (5.1%)
VHL mutations	30 (11%)	2 (2%)	9 (3.5%)	13 (28.6%)	25 (8%)
SDHB mutations	11 (4%)	8 (10%)	18 (7%)	3 (5.4%)	21 (6.7%)
SDHD mutations	12 (4%)	0	2 (0.8%)	9 (16.1%)	11 (3.5%)
SDHC mutations	n.d.	n.d.	0	0	0
Neurofibromatosis type 1	n.d.	n.d.	0	13 (23.2%)	13 (4.1%)
Total	66 (24%)	10 (12%)	30 (11.6%)	56 (100%)	86 (27.4%)

NOTE: n.d: not determined.
[a]Superscript numbers are references.

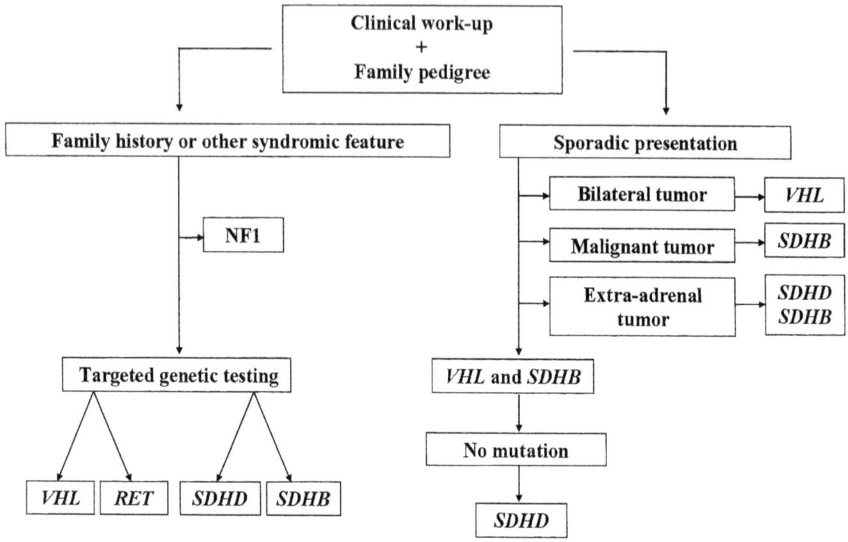

FIGURE 1. The organization of genetic testing in patients with PHEO or functional PGL, after extensive clinical evaluation of the affected patients.

extra-adrenal tumors. We found that 18 of the 52 patients with a malignant tumor harbored a mutation, and *SDHB* is the gene concerned in 15 of these patients, confirming that *SDHB* mutation is a predictive factor for malignancy.

Overall, these data suggest that PHEO is inherited in about a quarter of all patients. About 10–15% of familial cases of PHEO could be diagnosed by clinical criteria and about 12% on the basis of genetic testing for *SDHB* and *VHL* mutations. It is now clear that genetic testing should be offered to all patients with PHEO and/or functional PGL, regardless of tumor location and patient age, but there is no point in screening for all the PHEO susceptibility genes. Genetic testing can be targeted effectively based on the patient's clinical work-up and the drawing of the family pedigree (FIG. 1). Before genetic testing, clinicians and geneticists should look for clinical clues evocative of syndromic disease or family history. Targeted genetic testing should then be offered to patients with phenotypic criteria and/or a family history of NF1 (e.g., café au lait pigmented spots, neurofibromas), MEN 2 (medullary thyroid cancer, hyperparathyoidism), VHL disease (hemangioblastoma, renal, or pancreatic tumors), or hereditary PGL (head and neck PGL, family history in the paternal branch). Genetic testing should also be guided by family pedigree. All the PHEO susceptibility genes display autosomal dominant inheritance but, in families with *SDHD* mutations, the disease is transmitted only by the father, due to maternal genomic imprinting. In cases of a nonsyndromic disease with an apparently sporadic presentation, *VHL*, *SDHB*, and *SDHD* should be analyzed. If the tumor is malignant, *SDHB* should be the first gene to be analyzed. If the tumor is extra-adrenal, then screening for *SDHD* or *SDHB* should be carried out. If the tumor is bilateral, screening should be carried out for *VHL*. If there are no clinical clues, *VHL* and *SDHB* should be analyzed first, followed by *SDHD*.

The identification of a causal mutation in an affected patient should lead to strict, specific follow-up. Physicians should be aware of the malignant potential of *SDHB*-related PHEO/PGL, which should be treated surgically as soon as possible. Presymptomatic genetic testing should be offered to all first-degree relatives if a causal mutation is detected in the index case. The early detection of small tumors in individuals identified as at-risk (mutation carriers) would facilitate surgical treatment and reduce morbidity.[1] The PGL.NET network recommends clinical testing, including head and neck MRI and metanephrine determination. If metanephrine levels are normal, octreotide scintigraphy should be performed to search for nonfunctional PGL. If metanephrine levels are high, ^{123}I-MIBG scintigraphy should be performed to detect functional PGL or PHEO. An abdominal CT scan should also be carried out for patients with *SDHB* mutations. However, all these guidelines remain empriric, and require validation in large prospective studies.

THE MOLECULAR LINK BETWEEN SUCCINATE DEHYDROGENASE INACTIVATION AND HIF ACTIVATION

The mechanisms by which succinate dehydrogenase inactivation induces tumor formation are beginning to become clear. Hypoxia-inducible genes display a higher level of activation in tumors with *SDHB* or *SDHD* mutations than in noninherited PHEO and PGL, probably accounting for the hypervascularization of these tumors.[13,14] The discovery in 2002 that the inactivation of fumarate hydratase, which oxidizes fumarate to generate malate, caused another form of inherited cancer associating cutaneous, uterine, and renal tumors (MCUL or HLRCC syndrome) suggested that the Krebs cycle plays a crucial role in tumorigenesis.[25] However the link between loss-of-function mutation in *SDH* or *FH* genes and angiogenesis remained unclear.[26]

The discovery of hypoxia-inducible factor (HIF) hydroxylation has provided fundamental clues.[27] In VHL disease, another autosomal dominant form of cancer associating hemangioblastoma, renal cancer, and/or PHEO/PGL, HIF is activated because it is not degraded in the absence of functional VHL protein. However, it was recently shown that HIF can be ubiquitinated only after hydroxylation by prolyl hydroxylases. These enzymes are iron- and 2-oxoglutarate-dependent oxygenases and the reaction they catalyse involves succinate and oxoglutarate.[28]

Selak *et al.* showed that the inactivation of *SDHD* gene *in vitro* by siRNA induces succinate accumulation, impairing HIF hydroxylation in HEK 293 cells.[29] Brière *et al.* demonstrated that the accumulation of much larger

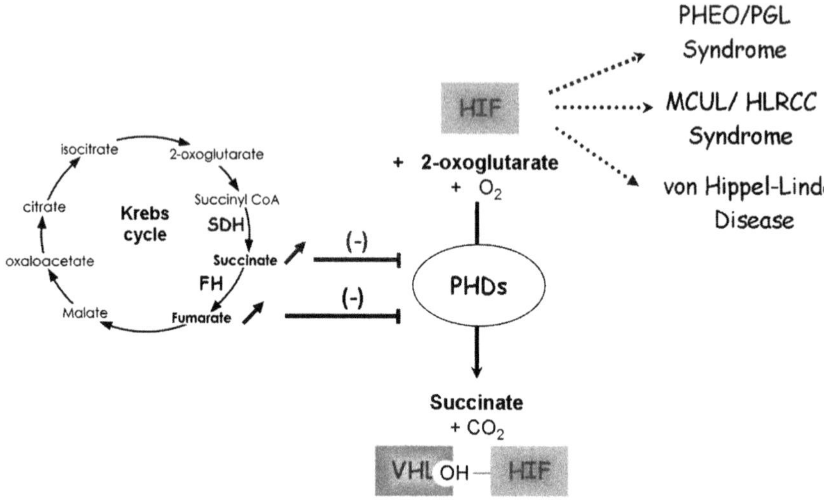

FIGURE 2. Schematic diagram of the link between the tricarboxylic acid cycle (Krebs cycle) and the hypoxia-angiogenesis pathway. In normoxia, HIF in normoxia is ubiquitinated by the VHL protein, eamarking it for degradation. In von Hippel Lindau disease, no normal VHL protein is produced and HIF is stabilized. Stabilisation also occurs in cases of succinate deficiency—causing PHEO/PGL syndrome—or of fumarate hydratase deficiency—causing MCUL/ HLRCC syndrome—due to loss-of-function mutations in the *SDH* and *FH* genes, respectively. Indeed, HIF must be hydroxylated by prolyl hydroxylases (PHDs) before it can be ubiquitinated. Succinate accumulation due to the inactivation of SDH or FH inhibits PHDs, thereby stabilizing HIF.

amounts of succinate in *SDH*-PHEO/PGL than in PHEO induced by a *RET* mutation *in vivo*. They also demonstrated a significant nuclear translocation of HIF1α in SDH-deficient fibroblasts, antagonized by excess oxoglutarate.[9] In cases of fumarate hydratase deficiency, similar levels of fumarate and succinate accumulation have been observed, together with the overproduction of HIF in HLRCC renal tumors due to the inhibition of HIF prolyl hydroxylation.[30,31] These data suggest that there is a link between HIF nuclear translocation and succinate accumulation that may be reversed by oxoglutarate, indicating that substrate (oxoglutarate)/ product (succinate) plays a key role in controlling the prolyl hydroxylation of HIF (FIG. 2). Studies are now required to clarify the role of HIF and/or of other known or unknown targets in tumorigenesis that may account for the specificities of these different autosomal dominant forms of cancers.[32,33]

CONCLUSIONS

Five years after the identification of the *SDH* genes, several important progress has been made towards understanding PHEO/PGL syndrome. The clinical indications for *SDH* genetic testing have been defined and the main genotype–phenotype correlations and the prognosis value of *SDHB* genetic testing are well known. These recent genetic advances should help clinicians to improve patient management, thereby decreasing the morbidity of these inherited cancers and the mortality of *SDHB*-related PHEO/PGL. A fundamental molecular link between the inactivation of succinate dehydrogenase and activation of the hypoxia pathway has been established, highlighting a new role for tricarboxylic acid in cancer. These advances will provide researchers with an opportunity to identify new therapeutic targets and to find original curative and preventive protocols for *SDH* mutation carriers.

ACKNOWLEDGMENTS

I am grateful to Pierre-François Plouin (Unité d'hypertension artérielle, HEGP, Paris) and Xavier Jeunemaitre (Département de Génétique, HEGP, Paris) for their confidence and strong support. I thank my main collaborators; the clinician members of PGL.NET and COMETE networks as well as of the Groupe des Tumeurs Endocrines involved in the clinical studies, Valérie Nau, Isabelle Roncelin, Valérie Boccio, Laurence Strompf, Laurence Amar for genotyping studies (Département de Génétique, HEGP, Paris), and Judith Favier (INSERM U36, Collège de France, Paris), Pierre Rustin, and Jean-Jacques Brière (INSERM U676, Hôpital Robert Debré, Paris) for the fundamental research studies. This study was supported by the Institut National de la Santé et de la Recherche Médicale and by PHRC grant COMETE 2 for the COMETE Network, by GIS-Institut des Maladies Rares for the PGL.NET network. The English text was edited by Julie Sappa.

REFERENCES

1. Favier, J. *et al.* 2005. Hereditary paraganglioma/pheochromocytoma and inherited succinate dehydrogenase deficiency. Horm. Res. **63:** 171–179.
2. Heutink, P. *et al.* 1992. A gene subject to genomic imprinting and responsible for hereditary paragangliomas maps to chromosome 11q23-qter. Hum. Mol. Genet. **1:** 7–10.
3. van der Mey, A.G. *et al.* 1989. Genomic imprinting in hereditary glomus tumours: evidence for new genetic theory. Lancet **2:** 1291–1294.
4. Mariman, E.C. *et al.* 1995. Fine mapping of a putatively imprinted gene for familial non-chromaffin paragangliomas to chromosome 11q13.1: evidence for genetic heterogeneity. Hum. Genet. **1:** 56–62.
5. Niemann, S. *et al.* 1999. PGL3, a third, not maternally imprinted locus in autosomal dominant paraganglioma. Neurogenetics **3:** 167–170.
6. Astuti, D. *et al.* 2001. Gene mutations in the succinate dehydrogenase subunit SDHB cause susceptibility to familial pheochromocytoma and to familial paraganglioma. Am. J. Hum. Genet. **69:** 49–54.

7. BAYSAL, B.E. *et al.* 2000. Mutations in SDHD, a mitochondrial complex II gene, in hereditary paraganglioma. Science **287:** 848–851.
8. NIEMANN, S. & U. MULLER. 2000. Mutations in SDHC cause autosomal dominant paraganglioma, type 3. Nat. Genet. **26:** 268–270.
9. BRIÈRE, J.J. *et al.* 2005. Succinate dehydrogenase deficiency in human. Cell. Mol. Life Sci. **62:** 2137–2324.
10. BOURGERON, T. *et al.* 1995. Mutation of a nuclear succinate dehydrogenase gene results in mitochondrial respiratory chain deficiency. Nat. Genet. **2:** 144–149.
11. TOMITSUKA, E. *et al.* 2003. Direct evidence for two distinct forms of the flavoprotein subunit of human mitochondrial complex II (succinate-ubiquinone reductase). J. Biochem. **134:** 191–195.
12. BRIÈRE, J.J. *et al.* 2005. Mitochondrial succinate is instrumental for HIF1{alpha} nuclear translocation in SDHA-mutant fibroblasts under normoxic conditions. Hum. Mol. Genet. **14:** 3263–3269.
13. GIMENEZ-ROQUEPLO, A.P. *et al.* 2001. The R22X mutation of the SDHD gene in hereditary paraganglioma abolishes the enzymatic activity of complex II in the mitochondrial respiratory chain and activates the hypoxia pathway. Am. J. Hum. Genet. **69:** 1186–1197.
14. GIMENEZ-ROQUEPLO, A.P. *et al.* 2002. Functional consequences of a SDHB gene mutation in an apparently sporadic pheochromocytoma. J. Clin. Endocrinol. Metab. **87:** 4771–4774.
15. BAYSAL, B.E. 2002. Hereditary paraganglioma targets diverse paraganglia. J. Med. Genet. **9:** 617–622.
16. BERTHERAT, J. & A.P. GIMENEZ-ROQUEPLO. 2005. New insights in the genetics of adrenocortical tumors, pheochromocytomas and paragangliomas. Horm. Metab. Res. **6:** 384–390.
17. NEUMANN, H.P. *et al.* 2004. Distinct clinical features of paraganglioma syndromes associated with SDHB and SDHD gene mutations. JAMA **292:** 943–951.
18. DANNENBERG, H. *et al.* 2005. Clinical characteristics of pheochromocytoma patients with germline mutations in SDHD. J. Clin. Oncol. **23:** 1894–1901.
19. ASTROM, K. *et al.* 2003. Altitude is a phenotypic modifier in hereditary paraganglioma type 1: evidence for an oxygen-sensing defect. Hum. Genet. **3:** 228–237.
20. GIMENEZ-ROQUEPLO, A.P. *et al.* 2003. Mutations in the SDHB gene are associated with extra-adrenal and/or malignant phaeochromocytomas. Cancer Res. **63:** 5615–5621.
21. MAHER, E.R. & C. ENG. 2002. The pressure rises: update on the genetics of phaeochromocytoma. Hum. Mol. Genet. **11:** 2347–2354.
22. LENDERS, J.W. *et al.* 2005. Phaeochromocytoma. Lancet **366:** 665–675.
23. NEUMANN, H.P. *et al.* 2002. Germ-line mutations in nonsyndromic pheochromocytoma. N. Engl. J. Med. **346:** 1459–1466.
24. AMAR, *et al.* 2005. Genetic testing in pheochromocytoma and functional paraganglioma. J. Clin. Oncol. **23:** 8812–8818.
25. TOMLINSSON, I.P. *et al.* 2002. Germline mutations in FH predispose to dominantly inherited uterine fibroids, skin leiomyomata and papillary renal cell cancer. Nat. Genet. **30:** 406–410.
26. POLLARD, P.J. *et al.* 2003. The TCA cycle and tumorigenesis: the examples of fumarate hydratase and succinate dehydrogenase. Ann. Med. **5:** 632–639.
27. PUGH, C.W. & P.J. RATCLIFFE. 2003. Regulation of angiogenesis by hypoxia: role of the HIF system. Nat. Med. **9:** 677–684.

28. KAELIN, W.G., JR. 2005. The von Hippel-Lindau protein, HIF hydroxylation, and oxygen sensing. Biochem. Biophys. Res. Commun. **338:** 627–638.
29. SELAK, M.A. *et al.* 2005. Succinate links TCA cycle dysfunction to oncogenesis by inhibiting HIF-alpha prolyl hydroxylase. Cancer Cell **7:** 77–85.
30. POLLARD, P.J. *et al.* 2005. Accumulation of Krebs cycle intermediates and over-expression of HIF1 alpha in tumours which result from germline FH and SDH mutations. Hum. Mol. Genet. **14:** 2231–2239.
31. ISAACS, J.S. *et al.* 2005. HIF overexpression correlates with biallelic loss of fumarate hydratase in renal cancer: novel role of fumarate in regulation of HIF stability. Cancer Cell **8:** 143–153.
32. LEE, S. *et al.* 2005. Neuronal apoptosis linked to EglN3 prolyl hydroxylase and familial pheochromocytoma genes: developmental culling and cancer. Cancer Cell **8:** 155–67.
33. ESTEBAN, M.E. & P.H. MAXWELL. 2005. HIF, a missing link between metabolism and cancer. Nature Med. **11:** 1047–1048.

Genetic and Clinical Investigation of Pheochromocytoma

A 22-Year Experience, from Freiburg, Germany to International Effort

BIRKE BAUSCH,[a] CARSTEN C. BOEDEKER,[b] ANSGAR BERLIS,[c] INGO BRINK,[d] MARKUS CYBULLA,[a] MARTIN K. WALZ,[e] ANDRZEJ JANUSZEWICZ,[f] CLAUDIO LETIZIA,[g] GIUSEPPE OPOCHER,[h] CHARIS ENG,[i] AND HARTMUT P.H. NEUMANN[a]

[a]Department of Nephrology, [b]Department of Otorhinolaryngology, [c]Department of Neuroradiology, and [d]Department of Nuclear Medicine, Albert-Ludwigs-University, D79106 Freiburg, Germany

[e]Department of Surgery, Kliniken Essen-Mitte, Essen, Germany

[f]Department of Hypertension, Institute of Cardiology, Warsaw, Poland

[g]Department of Clinical Sciences, University of Rome, La Sapienza, Italy

[h]Department of Endocrinology, University of Padova, Italy

[i]Genomic Medicine Institute, Cleveland Clinic Foundation, and Department of Genetics, Case Western Reserve University School of Medicine, Cleveland, Ohio, USA

ABSTRACT: Although deceptively simple, the etio-pathogenesis of pheochromocytoma represents a clinical and molecular genetic investigative challenge. Here, we summarize, from a historical point of view, the 22-year-long studies initiated at the University of Freiburg, which developed from a local experience to a national and finally an international effort. All research activities are translational and clinical and hence, registry based and intended to improve the outcome of the patients, whether by improved detection, prevention, or treatment. Major clinical steps are the prospective study on hormone tests and imaging techniques for adrenal and extra-adrenal abdominal tumors as well as the concept of organ sparing and endoscopic tumor resection. Further, we introduced 18-fluoro-dopa positron emission tomography. Population-based registries were used in order to identify germline mutations in the susceptibility genes *VHL*, *RET*, *SDHB*, and *SDHD* in non-syndromic pheochromocytoma. We differentiated distinct clinical features of paraganglioma syndromes associated with *SDHB* and *SDHD* gene mutations. Finally,

Address for correspondence: Dr. Hartmut P.H. Neumann, Medizinische Universitätsklinik, Hugstetter Straße 55, D 79106 Freiburg, Germany. Voice: +49-761-270-3363; fax: +49-761-270-3778.
e-mail: neumann@med1.ukl.uni-freiburg.de

**Ann. N.Y. Acad. Sci. 1073: 122–137 (2006). © 2006 New York Academy of Sciences.
doi: 10.1196/annals.1353.013**

we identified predictors and prevalence of paraganglioma syndromes associated with mutations of the *SDHC* gene.

KEYWORDS: **pheochromocytoma; paraganglioma; VHL; MEN; RET; PGL; SDHB; SDHC; SDHD; registry-based research; guidelines for clinical management**

INTRODUCTION AND KEY CASE REPORT

Pheochromocytoma and paraganglioma are tumors of similar embryogenesis and histology. However, this group of neoplasias displays important molecular differences and are heterogeneous in their natural history, prognosis, and response to treatment. Terminology in science and practice is divergent. Herein the term *pheochromocytoma* is used for location in the adrenal glands, extra-adrenal, abdominal, and thoracic locations. Nearly all pheochromocytomas are endocrinologically active, releasing catecholamines. The symptoms and signs of pheochromocytoma are mainly on account of hypercatecholaminemia with paroxysmal or persistent hypertension. On account of this, headaches, excessive sweating, and palpitations with or without tachycardia occur as only a few of the cardinal clinical features. In contrast, the term *paraganglioma* is used for non-catecholamine-releasing tumors in the head and neck area. The intercarotic, tympanic, intravagal, and jugular paraganglia are the typical locations. Paraganglioma of the head and neck commonly presents as an asymptomatic tumor mass or with symptoms on account of compression and damage of surrounding structures. Different cranial nerve deficits, bradycardia, hoarsness of voice, and hearing loss are typical symptoms patients report on. More than 25% of pheochromocytomas are hereditary. The classic inherited pheochromocytoma associated syndromes are multiple endocrine neoplasia type 2 (MEN 2) on account of mutations of the *RET* gene, von Hippel–Lindau disease (VHL) on account of mutations of the *VHL* gene, neurofibromatosis type 1 (NF 1) caused by mutations of the *NF 1* gene and the recently defined paraganglioma syndromes type 1 (PGL 1) and type 4 (PGL 4) caused by mutations of the *SDHD* and *SDHB* genes, respectively.

The Freiburg Pheochromocytoma study was initiated in June 1983 following findings of a 7-cm right adrenal pheochromocytoma in a 46-year-old normotensive male patient seen by one of the authors (HPHN). The patient's sister had undergone surgery for a hemiangioblastoma 4 years earlier and had a son presenting with bilateral metachronous pheochromocytomas of the right adrenal at 13 years of age, and of the left adrenal at 16 years. Two and 5 years before, the disease presentations in the sister and her son were not recognized as hereditary. The findings in our patient, the second male family member with a pheochromocytoma, clearly suggested a hereditary pattern. Abdominal exploration in our patient during surgery revealed a second 1.5-cm left-adrenal pheochromocytoma, not seen in the computerized axial tomography (CT) scan. Both adrenals were resected. Subcutaneous implantation of normal adrenal cortical tissue in the upper thigh provided ineffective steroid hormone production. However, not believing in lifelong need of steroid medication, the patient induced a nearly life-threatening Addisonian crisis. With appropriate steroid replacement therapy, our patient has remained in good health for the subsequent 22 years. The presence of multiple pheochromocytomas and a hemangioblastoma in this family allowed us to diagnose the autosomal dominantly inherited VHL disease. VHL illustrates many of the facets of pheochromocytoma and associated syndromes, including the circumstances of diagnosis, outcomes of surgical treatment, and requirements for adequate surveillance and follow-up. This case led us to set up our first local registry in Freiburg. New concepts and research activities over the course of the subsequent 22 years were initiated as summarized below.

PHEOCHROMOCYTOMA IN THE CONTEXT OF VHL AND MEN 2

In the 1980s, the two known heritable syndromes containing pheochromocytoma as component tumors were VHL and MEN 2. VHL is an autosomal dominant syndrome occurring in 2.72/100,000 (1/36,000) live births and is characterized by hemangiomas/blastomas, retinal angiomas, pheochromocytomas, and renal cell carcinoma.[1] MEN 2, occurring in 1:200,000 live births, is an autosomal dominant disorder characterized by medullary thyroid carcinoma (MTC), pheochromocytoma, and hyperparathyroidism.[1] Depending on clinical subtype, pheochromocytoma occurs on average in 50% of those affected by MEN 2.

Our first Freiburg study begun with a review of the existing literature in order to formulate the minimal clinical criteria for diagnosis and counseling of patients with VHL, which was important, since the identification of the VHL susceptibility gene was almost 10 years away at that time. In this literature review, we included 239 reported cases and 48 cases from Freiburg resulting in a prevalence of 14% of patients with VHL and associated pheochromocytoma.[2] We performed the first rigorous clinical epidemiological study of VHL in Freiburg and catchment areas and noted that the prevalence was 1:39,000 inhabitants in southwestern Germany (also known as the Black Forest region).[3] Remarkably, unlike the existing literature from elsewhere in the world, we found that the co-occurrence of pheochromocytoma and renal cell carcinoma in the same VHL patient was rare, and that indeed pheochromocytoma predominated in this part of Germany.[3] The latter observation formed the basis of the important concept, described later, of the Black Forest founder mutation in *VHL*.[4] A founder mutation is a particular gene mutation present in a population at increased frequency. The mutation occurred in a small isolated group of "founders," ancestors who gave rise to most of the individuals in the present day population. Further, our meticulous clinical phenotyping led to the later phenotypic classification of VHL type 1 (predominantly with renal clear cell carcinoma) and type 2 (predominantly with pheochromocytoma).

That other non-VHL pheochromocytoma-associated syndromes existed in southwest Germany was soon evident. We were able to clinically screen two families with MEN 2 and detected several asymptomatic tumors including pheochromocytoma.[5]

PROSPECTIVE STUDY FOR THE CLINICAL DIAGNOSIS AND EARLY DETECTION OF PHEOCHROMOCYTOMA

Because the two major pheochromocytoma susceptibility genes, *RET* for MEN 2 and *VHL* for VHL disease were not to be identified until 1993, we decided to collect and update annually clinical phenotypic data for several purposes, which ultimately would lead to improved early detection, diagnosis, and treatment of pheochromocytoma. Such a registry would not only be invaluable for a "gene hunt" but also would help phenotypic characterization after the genes would be identified.

By the time the Freiburg registry reached 19 index cases of familial pheochromocytoma-associated syndromes, MEN 2, and VHL, we were able to perform a unique prospective study for evaluation of diagnostic means for pheochromocytoma. We clinically screened these registrants and their families by comparing various imaging methods, namely, ultrasonography, CT scan, magnetic resonance imaging (MRI), and 131- or 123-iodine-metaiodobenzylgaunidine scintigraphy (MIBG) as well as the hormone analyses for 24-h collection of urine for adrenaline, noradrenaline, and vanillylmandelic acid (VMA) levels, as well as plasma adrenaline, noradrenaline, and chromogranin A levels. The results, published in 1993 in the New England Journal of Medicine,[6] showed a total of 42 new diagnoses of pheochromocytomas found 36 out of 79 participating index cases and relatives. We found that the sensitivity of ultrasonography was 40%, CT scan 76%, MRI 95%, and MIBG scintigraphy 95% and specificities of 95% and higher for all modalities. Sensitivities of hormone analyses were 53% for urine epinephrine, 86% urinary norepinephrine, 64% for urinary VMA, 52% plasma chromogranin A, 33% plasma epinephrine, and 58% plasma norepinephrine. Remarkably, these sensitivity figures remained until recently improved by the group of Graeme Eisenhofer and Karel Pacak, in 1999, by using assays for urinary and plasma metanephrines.[7]

ORGAN SPARING AND ENDOSCOPIC TREATMENT OF PHEOCHROMOCYTOMA

Because our index case (see "Introduction") underwent bilateral adrenalectomy and had a very common side effect of this operation, an Addisonian crisis, self-induced by stopping his replacement steroids, we needed to reconsider alternatives to the then standard-of-care operation. This is particularly germane for all heritable pheochromocytomas that tend to be bilateral and multifocal. Thus, in 1985, we inaugurated adrenal-sparing surgery as the standard operation. Between 1985 and 1998, 39 patients underwent this procedure in Freiburg. Of these 39, 7 cases had lost the contralateral adrenal gland and 6 additional cases had operation of bilateral pheochromocytoma in one session. Only one of the patients became steroid dependent. Pheochromocytoma relapse was only seen in one case after 6 years.[8]

While adrenal-sparing surgery had good outcomes, it was still an open procedure and considered a major surgery. The door to the next step was opened by the Canadians M. Gagner and co-workers who reported in 1992[9] laparoscopic ("key hole") resection of a pheochromocytoma for the first time. The Austrian urologic surgeon Günter Janetschek was the first who agreed to our suggestion for laparoscopic adrenal-sparing surgery and operated on three patients who were diagnosed in Freiburg with VHL-associated pheochromocytoma, all of whom had bilateral adrenal pheochromocytoma as well as extra-adrenal tumors. The first operation was performed in Innsbruck in August 1997.[10] Reinvestigation with ACTH tests resulted in prompt response of the remnent adrenal tissue in all three cases.[8] In parallel in Essen, the German surgeon Martin Walz independently introduced the technique with retroperitoneal laparoscopic access and included the adrenal-sparing concept. He performed the first adrenal-sparing laparoscopic pheochromocytoma operation in January 1996.[11] The Essen series currently comprises 126 cases (including several diagnosed in Freiburg) with 160 pheochromocytomas and abdominal paragangliomas. Operation time, blood loss, and complication rates are comparable or even superior to open procedures, and cosmetic results are optimal.[12]

18-FLUORO-DOPA AND DOPAMINE PET

Noninvasive assessment of tumors is a mainstay in the clinical management of all pheochromocytomas but are particularly important in heritable cases, especially with the possibility of multiple tumors and the timing of laparoscopic adrenal-sparing surgery. The improvement for imaging of pheochromocytoma was achieved in parallel in Freiburg by Stefan Hoegerle and in Bethesda by Karel Pacak, by using 18-fluoro-dopa (Freiburg) or 18-fluoro-dopamine (Bethesda) positron emission tomography (PET), a method superior to MIBG, for abdominal tumors.[13,14] For head and neck paragangliomas, the same advantage of PET scanning over MIBG was demonstrated soon afterward.[15]

MOLECULAR GENETIC STUDIES OF PHEOCHROMOCYTOMA AND PARAGANGLIOMA PATIENTS

While improvements in clinical surveillance, clinical detection, and surgical treatment are important in improving the well-being of pheochromocytoma patients, we believed that the earliest detection, or even the predisease detection, of pheochromocytoma would be the most effective. Thus, finding the susceptibility genes for heritable pheochromocytoma would be vital.

Because of our meticulously clinically documented VHL families, we were able to contribute these families to the group at the Massachusetts General Hospital, Boston, to help map the gene to the short arm of chromosome 3 (i.e., 3p).[16] The collaborative groups led by Berton Zbar from Bethesda and Eamonn Maher then at the University of Cambridge, UK, identified the *VHL* gene, a gene which, at that time, had no known function and did not show homology to other genes.[17] Subsequently in another collaboration, a founder effect was detected in the Black Forest VHL families who displayed predominantly pheochromocytomas, all associated with the identical germline mutation *VHL* c. 505 T>C.[4] This mutation was later shown to be associated with a good prognosis similar to that of the general population, the explanation why pheochromocytomas are relatively frequent in the area around Freiburg.[18]

The Freiburg group and others were fortunate to be able to provide clinically well-documented MEN 2 families to the group led by Bruce Ponder at the University of Cambridge, which ultimately identified germline mutations in the *RET* proto-oncogene in MEN 2 (acknowledgment in Mulligan *et al.*[19]). The Freiburg and other families also contributed to the first suggestion that specific *RET* mutations (genotype) were associated with certain clinical features (phenotype).[20] A seminal finding led to the formation of the International *RET* Mutation Consortium led by Charis Eng and Lois M. Mulligan. The Consortium study accrued over 300 MEN 2 families from around the world and were able to definitively observe specific *RET* genotype–clinical phenotype associations.[21] Specifically, *RET* codon 634 mutations were associated with the development of pheochromocytoma. These data also formed the scientific bases for the subsequent practice of clinical cancer genetics.[22,23]

Since 1994, a very fruitful collaboration and friendship was cultured between Hartmut Neumann and Charis Eng, starting when she was a postdoctoral fellow at the University of Cambridge and continuing during her subsequent independent scientific career in Boston, Columbus, Ohio, and recently, Cleveland. In a serendipitous moment when Hartmut Neumann invited Charis Eng to Freiburg to give a lecture as she was completing her postdoctoral fellowship near the end of 1995, both pledged lifelong collegial collaboration on neuroendocrine, including pheochromocytoma, genetics in order to improve the diagnosis, detection, and management of these patients. In these last 11 years, the major focus was to characterize the clinical relevance of mutations in the genes *RET, VHL, SDHB,* and *SDHD*. The autosomal genes encoding the mitochondrial complex II, succinate dehydrogenase, *SDHB, SDHC,* and *SDHD* were shown to be the susceptibility genes for another set of pheochromocytoma syndromes, which we have termed *pheochromocytoma–paraganglioma* (PGL) syndrome.[24–26] Another serendipitous moment occurred in 1995 when Andrzej Januszewicz from Warsaw met Hartmut Neumann in the home of the prominent nephrologist Friedrich Luft in Berlin. It was then decided that the pheochromocytoma registries of Warsaw and Freiburg become a "joint venture." As of 2005, the registry comprises 570 cases with pheochromocytoma and/or paraganglioma. Of these cases, 60% are German, 35% are Polish, and the remainder from other countries, such as Italy and France. The formation of these joint, mainly population-based, registries have proven extremely helpful in defining specific clinical features associated with mutations in one of several genes associated with pheochromocytoma.

GERMLINE MUTATIONS IN NON-SYNDROMIC PHEOCHROMOCYTOMA

Using clinically well-documented sporadic (not inherited, no family history) pheochromocytoma cases originating from the Freiburg registry, we showed in a pilot study that there was an unexpectedly high frequency of germline mutations in *SDHD* in these sporadic cases.[27] These promising pilot data led us to systematic examination of the entire joint registries for the frequency of unexpected germline *SDH* mutations among non-syndromic pheochromocytomas, a question which is pertinent in clinical cancer genetics practice, including counselling.

In 2002, we reported on 271 unrelated subjects with clinical presentations of adrenal or extra-adrenal abdominal or thoracic pheochromocytoma without evidence of syndromic disease and without a family history.[28] All 8 exons of the *SDHB* gene, all 4 exons of the *SDHD* gene, all 3 exons of the *VHL* gene and exons 10, 11, and 13–16 of the *RET* gene were analyzed for germline mutations in DNA of blood of these patients. Clinical evaluation was performed at presentation and updated. Mutation positive subjects underwent a clinical screening program adjusted to the given disease. Among others, four major findings were obtained. First, we found that 24% of study subjects had an heritable pheochromocytoma disorder, 11% had mutations in *VHL*, 5% *RET,* and 4% each in *SDHB* and *SDHD*. This is a significantly high frequency in apparently sporadic presentations of isolated pheochromocytoma, high enough that one could suggest that all pheochromocytoma patients should be offered genetic testing in the setting of genetic counseling.[29] Second, although mutation frequency decreased steadily by age from 70% in the first decade to 18% in the fifth decade, it is important to note that there were first-time presentations even after the fourth decade, especially associated with *SDHD*. Third, heritable pheochromocytoma, that is, finding a germline mutation, occurred more commonly in patients with multifocal tumors and in those with extra-adrenal pheochromocytoma. However, it should be noted that solitary pheochromocytomas occurred quite commonly at presentation and so, solitary tumors do not necessarily exclude heritability. Finally, during follow-up, only about one-third of the patients developed other syndrome-specific tumors (TABLES 1 and 2).

TABLE 1. Age of the patients and type of tumor at presentation according to genetic status

Variable	MEN 2 ($N = 13$)	*VHL* disease	*SDHD* mutation-associated pheochromocytoma–paraganglioma syndrome ($N = 11$)	*SDHB* mutation-associated pheochromocytoma–paraganglioma syndrome ($N = 12$)	Hereditary disease ($N = 66$)	Non-syndromic disease ($N = 205$)	Total (N = 271)	*P* value*
Age at presentation (year)								
Mean	36.4	18.3	28.7	25.6	24.9	43.9	39.3	<0.001
Range	21–50	5–49	5–59	12–48	5–59	4–81	4–81	
Age at onset $\leq$ 18 years (no.)	0	20	3	4	27	21	48	<0.001
Type of tumor (no.)								
Multifocal	5	12	4	0	21	5	26	<0.001
Extra-adrenal	0	4	4	6	14	16	30	0.006

*The *P* values are for the comparison of hereditary disease with non-syndromic diseases.
From Neumann *et al.* N. Engl. J. Med. 2002[28]

TABLE 2. Age at presentation of patients with mutations of sporadic disease

		Mutated gene (number of mutations)					
Age (Years)	*N* =	*VHL*	*RET*	*SDHD*	*SDHB*	Number	Hereditary disease (%)*
0–10	10	6	0	1	0	3	70
11–20	47	17	0	2	5	23	51
21–30	31	2	4	3	3	19	39
31–40	44	3	4	3	2	32	27
41–50	56	2	5	1	2	46	18
51–60	51	0	0	1	0	50	2
61–80	32	0	0	0	0	32	0

*Values are the percentages of hereditary cases found by molecular genetic methods.
From Neumann *et al.* N. Engl. J. Med. 2002[28]

DISTINCT CLINICAL FEATURES OF PARAGANGLIOMA SYNDROMES ASSOCIATED WITH *SDHB* AND *SDHD* GENE MUTATIONS

Once we established that germline mutations in one of at least four genes occurred to a significant frequency, we decided that it would be impractical and quite expensive to offer gene testing of all these genes to all presentations of pheochromocytoma. In order to help prioritize gene testing order as well as to facilitate clinical management, we characterized in detail the clinical features (FIG. 1) of those with *SDHB* and *SDHD* mutations. As reported in 2004,[30] using the pheochromocytoma/PGL registry and the newly established head and neck PGL registry, we conducted a study that included 417 patients, 334 with pheochromocytomas and 83 with paragangliomas after exclusion of patients with VHL, MEN 2, and NF 1. In this series, 10% were found to have a germline mutation, 5% each in the *SDHB* gene and *SDHD* gene. Including relatives diagnosed by genetic screening, 100 mutation carriers, 53 of the *SDHB* gene and 47 of the *SDHD* gene, were included for clinical characterization. Age at diagnosis of a first tumor was similar for both genes, 29.8 (SD 15.2) versus 30.6 (14.3) years. Overall, penetrance was similar, 50% by 35 years and 31 years for *SDHB* and *SDHD* mutations, respectively. Head and neck paragangliomas and multifocal tumors were statistically more frequent in *SDHD* mutation carriers. *SDHD* mutation carriers had statistically more intra-adrenal tumors and an earlier onset of HNPs compared to *SDHB* mutation carriers. Malignant pheochromocytoma or paraganglioma occurred in 11 *SDHB* mutation carriers but not in *SDHD* mutation carriers, confirming results of the French study (TABLE 3).[31] Astonishingly, two *SDHB* mutation carriers had renal cell carcinoma, which were added later to a collaborative study with Finnish researchers led by Lauri Aaltonen[32] and one mutation carrier each of both genes had a papillary thyroid cancer.

(A)

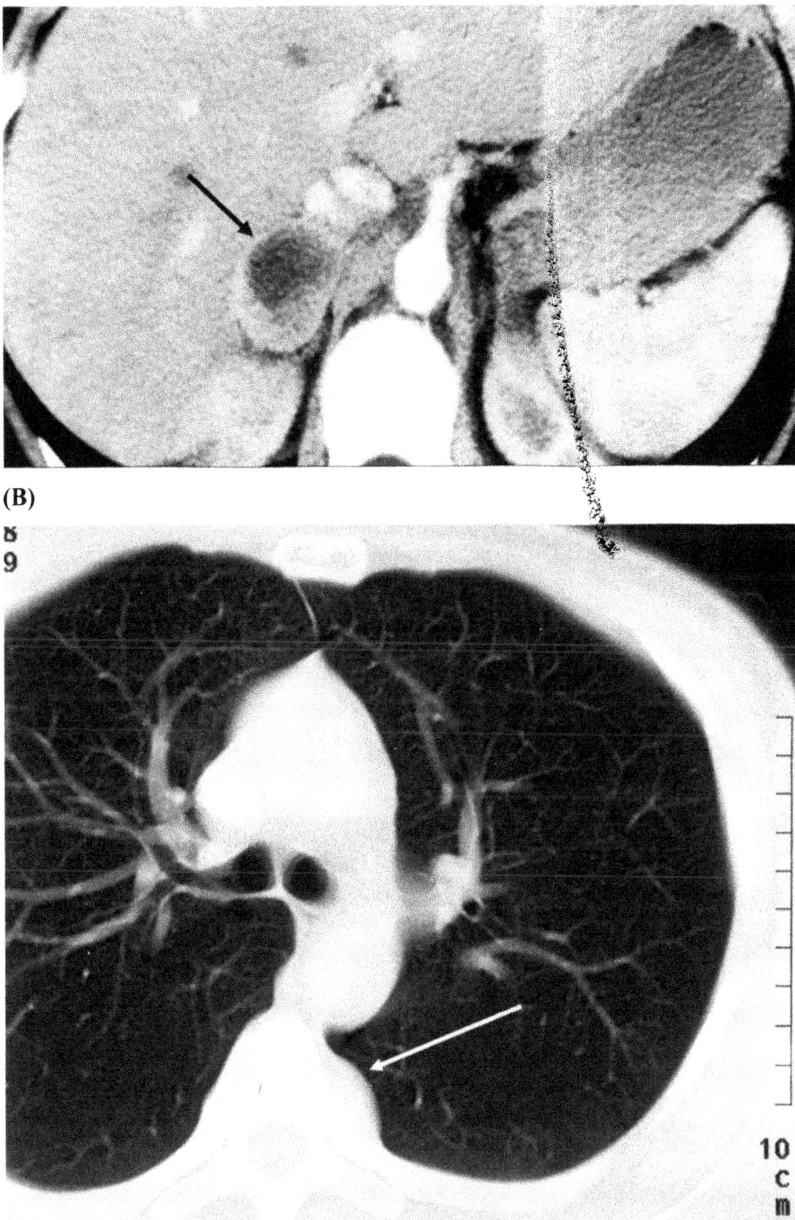

FIGURE 1. Paraganglioma syndrome in a 23-year-old women. This patient showed a mutation in the *SDHD* gene. **(A)** Right adrenal pheochromocytoma in CT (arrow), (**B**) and (**C**) thoracic paraganglioma (arrow) in CT (B) and MRI (C) and, (**D**) paraganglioma of the right glomus jugulare (arrow).

(C)

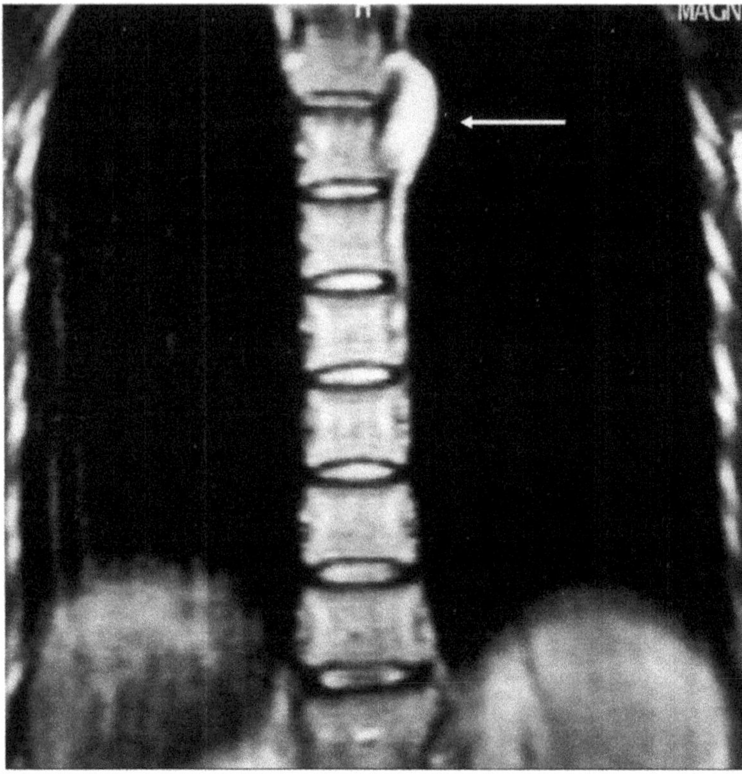

(D)

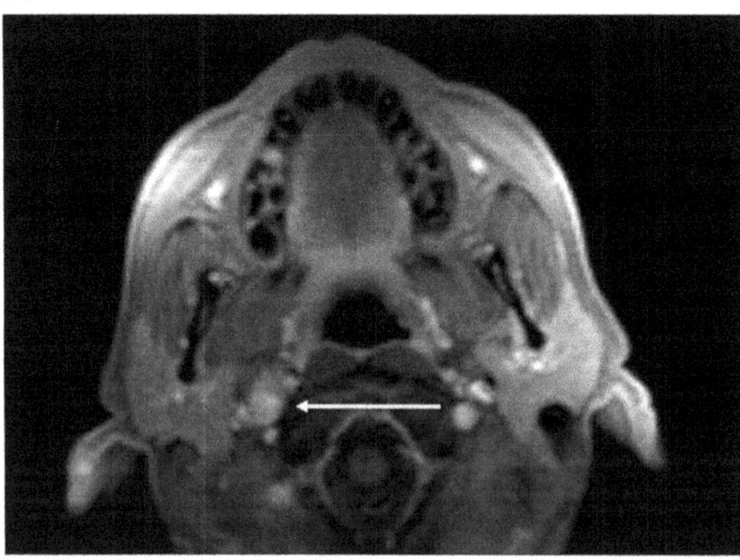

FIGURE 1. continued

TABLE 3. Malignant pheochromocytoma and paraganglioma associated with mutations of the *SDHB* gene (From Neumann *et al.* JAMA 2004[30])

Case	Sex	Location	Status 2004 or at death	Duration of disease (year)	SDHB mutation
1	f	Thoracic	Living 34 years	3	155 del C
2	m	Abdominal extra-adrenal[1]	Living 35 years	20	270 C/G
3	m	Neck	Living 45 years	11	271 G/A
4	m	Adrenal	Living 56 years	6	271 G/A
5	f	Abdominal extra-adrenal	Dead 45 years	32	300–4 del 5bp
6	f	Adrenal[2]	Dead 28 years	11	394 T/C
7	m	Abdominal extra-adrenal	Living 68 years	3	558–3 C/G
8	f	Adrenal[2]	Dead 36 years	2	847 del TCTC
9	m	Neck	Dead 64 years	32	859 G/A
10	m	Neck	Dead 64 years	2	859 G/A
11	m	Abdominal extra-adrenal	Living 66 years	6	899 + 1 GA

[1]Later associated with benign neck paraganglioma and thoracic pheochromocytoma.
[2]Multiple malignant tumors at this location.

PREDICTORS AND PREVALENCE OF A SYNDROME ASSOCIATED WITH MUTATIONS OF THE *SDHC* GENE

Mutations of the *SDHC* gene are rare in the literature at least prior to 2005 and restricted to manifestations with head and neck paragangliomas. We therefore sought to clinically characterize pheochromocytoma and PGL associated with *SDHC* mutations. In our publication in JAMA in 2005, we analyzed the *SDHC* gene in 371 unrelated pheochromocytoma patients who were not carriers of *VHL, RET, SDHB,* and *SDHD* mutations and had clinically no NF 1.[33] None of the pheochromocytoma patients had a germline *SDHC* mutation. This implies that pheochromocytoma presentations, in the absence of PGL, need not be offered *SDHC* testing. In the second part of this study, we analyzed 121 patients with head and neck paragangliomas (HNP) for mutations of the *SDHB, SDHC,* and *SDHD* genes. In this HNP series, mutations frequencies were 4% for *SDHC*, 7% for *SDHB*, and 17% for *SDHD*. Comparing 90 pheochromocytoma subjects without germline mutations to those carrying mutations of the genes *SDHB* ($n = 15$), *SDHC* ($n = 22$), or *SDHD* ($n = 42$) revealed more carotid body tumors in the *SDHC* group than in the sporadic HNP patients. Further, fewer instances of multiple tumors in *SDHC* mutation carriers than in *SDHD* mutation carriers, and no malignant tumors in *SDHC* mutation carriers compared to 6 out of 15 in patients with *SDHB* mutations were noted. There was a younger age at diagnosis in *SDHC* mutation carriers than in sporadic HNP patients (TABLE 4).

CONCLUSIONS

In summary, pheochromocytoma is a disorder in which over the last 22 years much progress has been achieved. Instrumental have been the inherited

TABLE 4. Comparison of major characteristics of head and neck paraganglioma (HNP) subgroup patients

Subgroup	*SDHC*	Sporadic	P (*SDHC* vs. spor.)	*SDHB*	P (*SDHC* vs. *SDHB*)	*SDHD*	P (*SDHC* vs. *SDHD*)	Comparison of all groups*
Patients with tumors (*n*)	22 (100%)	90 (100%)	-	15	-	42 (100%)	-	
Age at diagnosis (median, range)	46 (13–73)	53 (15–83)	0.03	39 (21–66)	0.56	36 (13–67)	0.04	<0.001
Carotid body tumors	13 (59%)	29 (32%)	0.03	10 (67%)	0.74	35 (83%)	0.07	<0.001
Jugular paragangliomas	6 (27%)	33 (37%)	0.46	2 (13%)	0.43	8 (19%)	0.53	0.10
Tympanic paragangliomas	2 (9%)	21 (23%)	0.24	0	0.50	4 (10%)	>0.99	0.04
Vagal paragangliomas	2 (9%)	3 (3%)	0.25	2 (13%)	>0.99	1 (2%)	0.27	0.16
Multiple tumors	2 (9%)	10 (11%)	0.30	4 (27%)	0.20	24 (57%)	<0.001	<0.001
Patients with malignant tumors	0 (0%)	0 (0%)	>0.99	6 (40%)	0.002	0 (0%)	>0.99	<0.001

^{n}denotes patients, not tumors.

*For this test as null hypothesis was assumed that there is no difference between the four groups for each parameter.

From Schiavi *et al.* 2005[33]

syndromes, such as MEN 2, VHL, and PGL. Such patients have benefited because of advances on clinical diagnostic means, molecular genetic diagnostic means, and endoscopic surgery.

ACKNOWLEDGMENTS

CE is a recipient of the Doris Duke Distinguished Clinical Scientist Award. HPHN is supported by grants from the Deutsche Krebshilfe (German Cancer Foundation) (70-3313-Ne 1) and the Deutsche Forschungsgemeinschaft (NE 571/5-2 to HPHN) (German Research Foundation), and the European Union (LSHC-CT-2005-518200).

REFERENCES

1. MAHER, E.R., L. ISELIUS, J.R. YATES, *et al.* 1991. Von Hippel-Lindau disease: a genetic study [see comment]. J. Med. Genet. **28:** 443–447.
2. NEUMANN, H.P. 1987. Basic criteria for clinical diagnosis and genetic counselling in von Hippel-Lindau syndrome. Vasa **16:** 220–226.
3. NEUMANN, H.P. & O.D. WIESTLER. 1991. Clustering of features of von Hippel-Lindau syndrome: evidence for a complex genetic locus [see comment]. Lancet **337:** 1052–1054.
4. GLAVAC, D., H.P. NEUMANN, C. WITTKE, *et al.* 1996. Mutations in the VHL tumor suppressor gene and associated lesions in families with von Hippel-Lindau disease from central Europe. Hum. Genet. **98:** 271–280.
5. NEUMANN, H.P., O.A. MULLER, B.A. PONDER, *et al.* 1989. Early diagnosis of multiple endocrine neoplasia type IIa. Klinische Wochenschrift **67:** 951–956.
6. NEUMANN, H.P., D.P. BERGER, G. SIGMUND, *et al.* 1993. Pheochromocytomas, multiple endocrine neoplasia type 2, and von Hippel-Lindau disease [see comment][erratum appears in N Engl J Med 1994 Dec 1;331(22):1535]. N. Engl. J. Med. **329:** 1531–1538.
7. EISENHOFER, G., J.W. LENDERS, W.M. LINEHAN, *et al.* 1999. Plasma normetanephrine and metanephrine for detecting pheochromocytoma in von Hippel-Lindau disease and multiple endocrine neoplasia type 2. N. Engl. J. Med. **340:** 1872–1879.
8. NEUMANN, H.P., B.U. BENDER, M. REINCKE, *et al.* 1999. Adrenal-sparing surgery for phaeochromocytoma [see comment]. Br. J. Surg. **86:** 94–97.
9. GAGNER, M., A. LACROIX & E. BOLTE. 1992. Laparoscopic adrenalectomy in Cushing's syndrome and pheochromocytoma. N. Engl. J. Med. **327:** 1033.
10. JANETSCHEK, G., G. FINKENSTEDT, R. GASSER, *et al.* 1998. Laparoscopic surgery for pheochromocytoma: adrenalectomy, partial resection, excision of paragangliomas. J. Urol. **160:** 330–334.
11. WALZ, M.K., K. PEITGEN, H.P. NEUMANN, *et al.* 2002. Endoscopic treatment of solitary, bilateral, multiple, and recurrent pheochromocytomas and paragangliomas. World J. Surg. **26:** 1005–1012.
12. WALZ, M.K., P.F. ALESINA, F.A. WENGER, *et al.* 2006. Laparoscopic and retroperitoneoscopic treatment of pheochromocytomas and retroperitoneal

paragangliomas—Results of 160 tumors in 126 patients. World J. Surg. **30:** 899–908.

13. HOEGERLE, S., E. NITZSCHE, C. ALTEHOEFER, *et al.* 2002. Pheochromocytomas: detection with 18F DOPA whole body PET–initial results. Radiology **222:** 507–512.
14. PACAK, K., G. EISENHOFER & D.S. GOLDSTEIN. 2004. Functional imaging of endocrine tumors: role of positron emission tomography. Endocr. Rev. **25:** 568–580.
15. HOEGERLE, S., N. GHANEM, C. ALTEHOEFER, *et al.* 2003. 18F-DOPA positron emission tomography for the detection of glomus tumours. Eur. J. of Nucl. Med. Mol. Imaging **30:** 689–694.
16. SEIZINGER, B.R., D.I. SMITH, M.R. FILLING-KATZ, *et al.* 1991. Genetic flanking markers refine diagnostic criteria and provide insights into the genetics of Von Hippel Lindau disease. Proc. Natl. Acad. Sci. USA **88:** 2864–2868.
17. LATIF, F., K. TORY, J. GNARRA, *et al.* 1993. Identification of the von Hippel-Lindau disease tumor suppressor gene [see comment]. Science **260:** 1317–1320.
18. BENDER, B.U., C. ALTEHOFER, A. JANUSZEWICZ, *et al.* 1997. Functioning thoracic paraganglioma: association with Von Hippel-Lindau syndrome. J. Clin. Endocrinol. Metab. **82:** 3356–3360.
19. MULLIGAN, L.M., J.B. KWOK, C.S. HEALEY, *et al.* 1993. Germ-line mutations of the RET proto-oncogene in multiple endocrine neoplasia type 2A. Nature **363:** 458–460.
20. MULLIGAN, L.M., C. ENG, C.S. HEALEY, *et al.* 1994. Specific mutations of the RET proto-oncogene are related to disease phenotype in MEN 2A and FMTC. Nat. Genet. **6:** 70–74.
21. ENG, C., D. CLAYTON, I. SCHUFFENECKER, *et al.* 1996. The relationship between specific RET proto-oncogene mutations and disease phenotype in multiple endocrine neoplasia type 2. International RET mutation consortium analysis. JAMA **276:** 1575–1579.
22. ENG, C. 1996. Seminars in medicine of the Beth Israel Hospital, Boston. The RET proto-oncogene in multiple endocrine neoplasia type 2 and Hirschsprung's disease. N. Engl. J. Med. **335:** 943–951.
23. ENG, C., H. HAMPEL & A. DE LA CHAPELLE. 2001. Genetic testing for cancer predisposition [erratum appears in Annu Rev Med 2002;53:xi]. Ann. Rev. Med. **52:** 371–400.
24. BAYSAL, B.E., R.E. FERRELL, J.E. WILLETT-BROZICK, *et al.* 2000. Mutations in SDHD, a mitochondrial complex II gene, in hereditary paraganglioma. Science **287:** 848–851.
25. ASTUTI, D., F. LATIF, A. DALLOL, *et al.* 2001. Gene mutations in the succinate dehydrogenase subunit SDHB cause susceptibility to familial pheochromocytoma and to familial paraganglioma [erratum appears in Am J Hum Genet 2002 Feb;70(2):565]. Am. J. Hum. Genet. **69:** 49–54.
26. NIEMANN, S. & U. MULLER. 2000. Mutations in SDHC cause autosomal dominant paraganglioma, type 3. Nat. Genet. **26:** 268–270.
27. GIMM, O., M. ARMANIOS, H. DZIEMA, *et al.* 2000. Somatic and occult germ-line mutations in SDHD, a mitochondrial complex II gene, in nonfamilial pheochromocytoma. Cancer Res. **60:** 6822–6825.
28. NEUMANN, H.P., B. BAUSCH, S.R. MCWHINNEY, *et al.* 2002. Germ-line mutations in nonsyndromic pheochromocytoma [see comment]. N. Engl. J. Med. **346:** 1459–1466.

29. ENG, C., M. KIURU, M.J. FERNANDEZ & L.A. AALTONEN. 2003. A role for mitochondrial enzymes in inherited neoplasia and beyond. Nat. Rev. Cancer **3:** 193–202.
30. NEUMANN, H.P., C. PAWLU, M. PECZKOWSKA, *et al.* 2004. Distinct clinical features of paraganglioma syndromes associated with SDHB and SDHD gene mutations [erratum appears in JAMA. 2004 Oct 13;292(14):1686]. JAMA **292:** 943–951.
31. GIMENEZ-ROQUEPLO, A.P., J. FAVIER, P. RUSTIN, *et al.* 2003. Mutations in the SDHB gene are associated with extra-adrenal and/or malignant phaeochromocytomas. Cancer Res. **63:** 5615–5621.
32. VANHARANTA, S., M. BUCHTA, S.R. MCWHINNEY, *et al.* 2004. Early-onset renal cell carcinoma as a novel extraparaganglial component of SDHB-associated heritable paraganglioma. Am. J. Hum. Genet. **74:** 153–159.
33. SCHIAVI, F., C.C. BOEDEKER, B. BAUSCH, *et al.* 2005. Predictors and prevalence of paraganglioma syndrome associated with mutations of the SDHC gene. JAMA **294:** 2057–2063.

Genetic Analyses of Apparently Sporadic Pheochromocytomas

The Rotterdam Experience

E. KORPERSHOEK,[a] F. H. VAN NEDERVEEN,[a] H. DANNENBERG,[a] B. J. PETRI,[a] P. KOMMINOTH,[b] A. PERREN,[b] J. W. LENDERS,[c] A. A. VERHOFSTAD,[c] W. W. DE HERDER,[a] R. R. DE KRIJGER,[a] AND W. N. M. DINJENS[a]

[a]*Department of Pathology, Josephine Nefkens Institute and Department of Internal Medicine, Erasmus MC - University Medical Center Rotterdam, Rotterdam, the Netherlands*

[b]*Department of Pathology, University Hospital Zürich, Switzerland*

[c]*Departments of Pathology and Internal Medicine, Radboud University Nijmegen Medical Center, Nijmegen, the Netherlands*

ABSTRACT: Pheochromocytomas (PCCs) are neuroendocrine tumors of chromaffin tissue that produce catecholamines. They are usually located in the adrenal medulla, although in about 10% the tumors arise from extra-adrenal chromaffin tissue. The majority of PCCs arise sporadically, but PCCs occur also in the context of hereditary cancer syndromes. Familial PCC is inherited as an autosomal dominant trait alone or as a component of the multiple endocrine neoplasia Type 2 (MEN2) syndrome (*RET* gene), Von Hippel–Lindau (VHL) disease (*VHL* gene), neurofibromatosis Type 1 (*NF1* gene), or familial pheochromocytoma–paraganglioma (PCC–PGL) syndrome (*SDHD/B* and *C* genes). It has been reported that 24% of apparently sporadic PCCs patients harbor germline mutations in these PCC-causing genes. We investigated the contribution of the inherited PCC-causing genes in a partly retrospectively and partly prospectively obtained series of 213 apparently sporadic PCCs. Mutation analysis was performed for *RET* (56 cases), *VHL* (136 cases), and *SDHD* (126 cases) and *SDHB* (47 cases). No germline *RET* mutations, six (4.4%) germline *VHL* mutations, two (1.5%) germline *SDHD* mutations, and one germline (1.6%) *SDHB* mutation were found. In total we found germline mutations in about 7.5% of the investigated apparently sporadic PCCs. Although 7.5% germline mutations in a series of apparently sporadic PCCs are far less than the more than 20% reported in the literature, the figure is significant enough to consider germline mutation testing for each patient with PCC.

Address for correspondence: Winand N. M. Dinjens, Department of Pathology, Josephine Nefkens Institute Room Be320a, Erasmus MC, University Medical Center Rotterdam, P.O. Box 1738, 3000DR Rotterdam, The Netherlands. Voice: +31-10-4087946; fax: 0031-10-4089487.
e-mail: w.dinjens@erasmusmc.nl

Ann. N.Y. Acad. Sci. 1073: 138–148 (2006).
doi: 10.1196/annals.1353.014

KEYWORDS: sporadic; germline; mutations; pheochromocytoma; *VHL; RET; SDHB; SDHD*

INTRODUCTION

Pheochromocytomas (PCCs) are usually benign tumors that arise from chromaffin cells of the adrenal medulla.[1] Autosomal dominant inherited cancer syndromes that may present with PCC include multiple endocrine neoplasia Type 2 (MEN2), Von Hippel–Lindau syndrome (VHL), and the pheochromocytoma–paraganglioma (PCC–PGL) syndrome.[1-3] There are three clinically distinct forms of the MEN2 syndrome: MEN2A, familial medullary thyroid carcinoma, and MEN2B. MEN2A is the most common subtype of MEN2, and almost 50% of patients develop PCCs. Most mutations associated with MEN2 are found in *RET* exons 10, 11, and 16. Approximately 85% of the germline RET mutations in MEN2 patients are missense mutations affecting codon 634. MEN2B makes up approximately 5% of the MEN2 patients, and has a more aggressive phenotype. Around half of the MEN2B patients develop PCCs.[4-7] Only three germline mutations are known to cause MEN2B (A883F in exon 15, M918T, and S922Y in exon 16).[6]

Patients with the VHL syndrome have predisposition to develop retinal and central nervous system hemangioblastomas, clear-cell renal-cell carcinomas, pheochromocytomas, pancreatic cysts and islet-cell tumors, cystadenomas of the epididymis, and endolymphatic-sac tumors.[8] Four phenotypic subclasses have been distinguished: VHL Type 1, Type 2a, Type 2b, and Type 2c, respectively. Only those with the Type 2 syndrome have a risk of developing PCC.[2,3,5,9]

Germline mutations in subunits of mitochondrial complex II, also known as succinate dehydrogenase (SDH), cause the PCC–PGL syndrome. The complex comprises four subunits, which are encoded by four different genes *SDHA* (5p15), *SDHB* (1p36), *SDHC* (1q23), and *SDHD* (11q23). Mutations associated with the PCC–PGL syndrome have only been demonstrated in *SDHB*, *SDHC*, and *SDHD*.[10] A large population-based study was performed by Neumann *et al.*, investigating the prevalence of *SDHB* and *SDHD* mutations in 334 unrelated patients with adrenal or extra-adrenal pheochromocytomas and 83 patients with head and neck paragangliomas.[11] They found that 12% of the patients had a mutation in either the *SDHB* or *SDHD* gene, with equal distribution between the two genes. *SDHC* mutations are extremely rare and have never been reported in PCC.[12,13] Germline mutations in *SDHA* cause Leigh syndrome,[14] but have never been discovered in patients with PGL or PCC.

When the family history of patients is negative for PCC or PGL, PCCs are termed "sporadic." However, this designation *sporadic*, based on clinical information, does not exclude the possibility of the presence of a germline mutation in one of the PCC susceptibility genes. Because patients with germline mutations in these genes need proper clinical treatment, and as patients harboring *SDHB* mutations have a higher risk for developing metastases[15,16] (van Nederveen *et al.* this issue), it is important to determine which mutations they carry. To investigate the prevalence of germline mutations in sporadic PCC, we have performed mutation analysis of *RET* exons 10, 11, and 16, and the entire coding sequence of *SDHB*, *SDHD,* and *VHL* in subgroups of a total of 213 cases of apparently sporadic PCC.

MATERIALS AND METHODS

Patients

Tissue specimens were retrieved from the archives of the Department of Pathology of the Erasmus MC (Rotterdam), the Radboud University Nijmegen Medical Center, and the University Hospital Zürich (Switzerland), following approval of the experimental design and protocols by the Medical Ethical Committee. Four unselected groups of sporadic PCC ($n = 213$ in total) were screened for mutations in either *RET*, *VHL*, *SDHB* or *SDHD*.

Tissue Preparation

Tumor DNA was isolated from paraffin-embedded tissue. Matching normal DNA was isolated from paraffin-embedded normal tissue of other organs removed at autopsy or from normal tissue within the tumor block. DNA isolation was performed by overnight incubation at 56°C in 180 μL Tris/HCl (pH8) and 20 μL proteinase K (20 mg/mL). After the incubation the samples were incubated at 100°C for 10 min.

Mutation Analysis

Published oligonucleotide primers and PCR conditions were used for mutation analysis of exons 10, 11, and 16 of the *RET* proto-oncogene in 56 PCC.[17,18] Single-strand conformation polymorphism (SSCP) analysis of 136 PCC patients was performed for *VHL* using primers and polymerase chain reaction (PCR) conditions previously reported.[19,20] *SDHD* mutation analysis of 126 PCCs was performed by SSCP and was previously reported by Dannenberg *et al.*[21] Both denaturating gradient gel electrophoresis (DGGE) and SSCP were used for mutation analysis of *SDHB* of 47 patients with PCCs. DGGE was previously described by Komminoth *et al.*[22] and the primers used are listed in TABLE 1.

TABLE 1. Primers used for mutation analysis of *SDHB*

Primer	Forward: 5′ → 3′	Reverse: 5′ → 3′	Product size (bp)	Method
SDHB 1	GAGCGACCTCGGGGTTAAG	GCTTTCCTGACTTTTCCCTC	157	SSCP
SDHB 2	cgcccgccgcgccccgcgcccggcccgccgcccccgcccg TTTTTCCTTTTTGTGAACTTT	AAGCATGTCCCTAAATCAAA	265	DGGE
SDHB 3	cgcccgccgcgccccgcgcccggcccgccgcccccgccc GGAACTTTACATAAATACCACTGGA	cgCTATCAGCTTTGGCCAGC	242	DGGE
SDHB 4	cgcccgccgcgccccgcgcccggcccgccgcccccgcccg aaataataaaTGATTCCGGATATGGGTGAG	cgtcccgcCCCCCATGCAAATAAAAACA	256	DGGE
SDHB 5	gcgcgTGATGATGGAATCTGATCCT	cgcccgccgcgccccgcgcccggcccgccgcccccgcccg aaataataaaCAGATTGAAACAATAAATA GGGA	261	DGGE
SDHB 6	cgcccgccgcgccccgcgcccggcccgccgcccccgcccg aaataataaaCCTCTCTTTTCTCCCCATAC	cgCAGCAATCTATTGTCCTCTTG	252	DGGE
SDHB 7	gcgcgAGCTAATCATCCCTGGTTTT	cgcccgccgcgccccgcgcccggcccgccgcccccgcccg aaataataaaTTGTGAGCACATGCTACTTC	270	DGGE
SDHB 8	cgcccgccgcgccccgcgcccggcccgccgcccccgcc cgGTGGGTTTTCCCTTTCAGTT	cgcccgccgcgccccgcgcccggcccgccgcccccgcccg GTGGGTTTTCCCTTTCAGTT	361	DGGE

DNA Sequencing

All samples demonstrating aberrant patterns were sequenced. PCR was performed in a final volume of 50 μL under identical conditions as the previous PCR, except that this mix contained 0.2 mM dNTPs instead of 0.02 mM dATPs and 0.8 μCi α^{32}P-dATP. The PCR products were purified using Nucleospin® Extract II (Macherey-Nagel, Düren, Germany) according to the manufacturer's instructions. The purification was followed by a sequence reaction using the BigDye® Terminator V3.1 cycle sequencing kit (Applied Biosystems, Foster City, CA). A total of 2 μL of Termination Ready Reaction mix, 2 μL of 5 × sequencing buffer, 1 μL forward or reverse primer (13.2 pM), and 14 μL of deionized water was added to 1 μL purified PCR product. The cycle sequencing program was performed for 25 cycles at 96°C for 10 sec, 50°C for 5 sec, and 4 min for 60°C. This was followed by a precipitation step, adding 13 μL deionized water, 3 μL 3M NaAc (pH 5.2), and 64 μL ethanol (100%) to the sequence reaction product and incubating overnight at room temperature before centrifuging for 20 min at 14,000 rpm. After washing the samples with 70% ethanol, and centrifuging them for 10 min at 14,000 rpm, the pellets were re-suspended in 20 μL formamide (Applied Biosystems, Warrington, UK). Products were analyzed on the ABI Prism 3100 genetic analyzer (Applied Biosystems).

RESULTS

RET Mutation Analysis

SSCP mutation analysis of *RET* exons 10, 11, and 16 was performed on 56 apparently sporadic PCCs. Four patients with benign PCCs and one with malignant PCC showed tumor-specific aberrant SSCP patterns. Sequence analysis revealed a C618Y mutation, an M918T mutation, and three C634R mutations, which were all absent in the normal DNA. One tumor with a C634R mutation was localized outside the adrenal gland, with regional lymph node metastases. The other tumors with *RET* mutations were all benign and located in the adrenal gland. Overall, 5 of 56 PCCs (9%) showed a somatic mutation in *RET* exons 10, 11, and 16, but no germline mutations were found.

VHL Mutation Analysis

Mutation analysis of the entire coding region of *VHL* was performed in 136 apparently sporadic PCCs, revealing 12 mutations. Somatic *VHL* mutations were found in 6 of 136 sporadic PCCs (4.4%), including 2 benign tumors (mutations: X > Cys+ 14AA (A854C) and Q164H) and 4 malignant PCCs (mutations: Q164H, R167W, G57E, L198P). Germline mutations were found

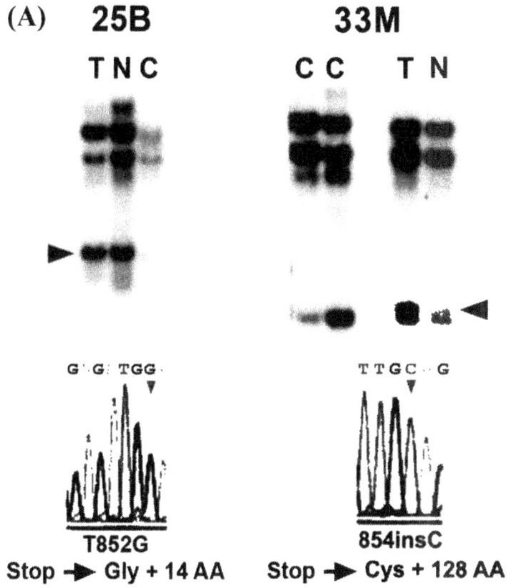

FIGURE 1. (**A**) *VHL,* SSCP, and sequence results of mutation T852G and insert 854insC (cDNA). *Arrowheads* point to aberrant patterns of tumor (T) and normal (N) DNA compared to a healthy control (C). (**B**) *Arrowheads* point to an aberrant SSCP pattern of a patient that harbored a L63P mutation (37) compared to a healthy control (C). (**C**) Sequence analysis, revealing the germline mutations causing I147T and G144Q amino acid substitutions on protein level. The *arrowheads* point to an aberrant sequence.* These pictures were modified with permission from Dannenberg *et al.* (**A**) and van der Harst *et al.* (**B** and **C**).

in 6 of 136 of the sporadic PCCs (4.4%), of which 1 was found in a malignant PCC (X > Cys+ 128AA [854insC]), whereas 5 were seen in benign PCC (mutations: X > Gly+ 14AA(T852G), P25L, L63P, I147T, G144Q) (FIG. 1).

SDHD Mutation Analysis

A total of 126 patients were tested for mutations in *SDHD*. Mutation analysis showed two germline mutations (1.6%) in exon 3 of *SDHD* (D92Y and L95P) (FIG. 2). D92Y was found in a patient with a benign adrenal PCC, who developed a second primary tumor (an extra-adrenal PCC) after 25 years. The patient carrying the L95P mutation was 25 years of age and had multiple extra-adrenal PCCs.

SDHB Mutation Analysis

DGGE and SSCP mutation analysis of 47 apparently sporadic PCCs revealed 2 mutations, a somatic S100F mutation (1.5%) in exon 4 and a germline

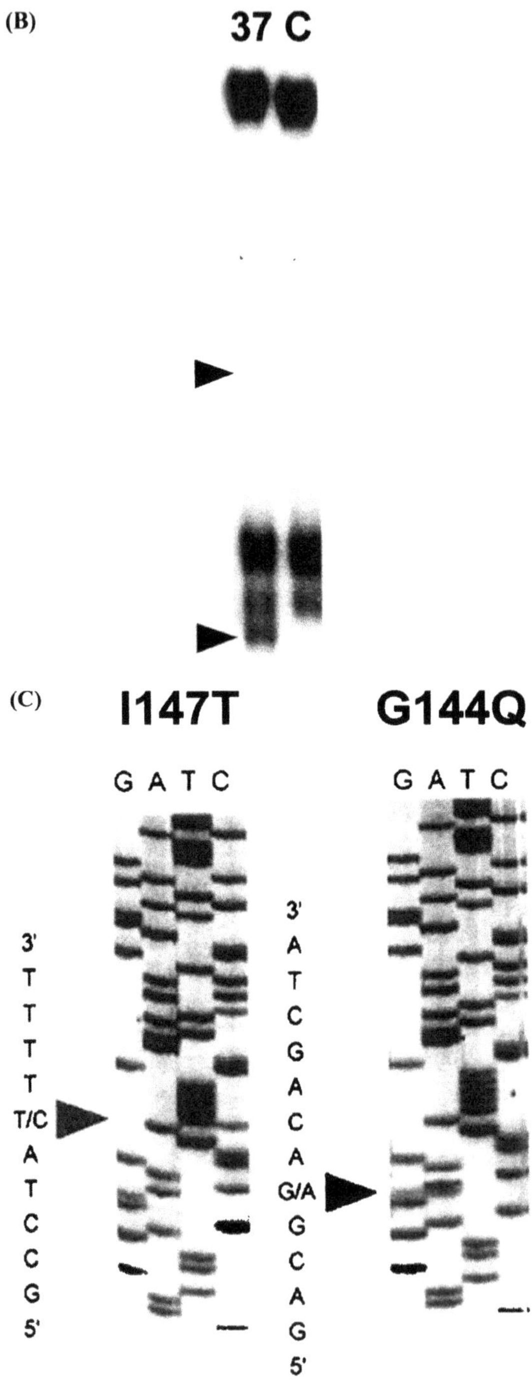

FIGURE 1 (*Continued*).

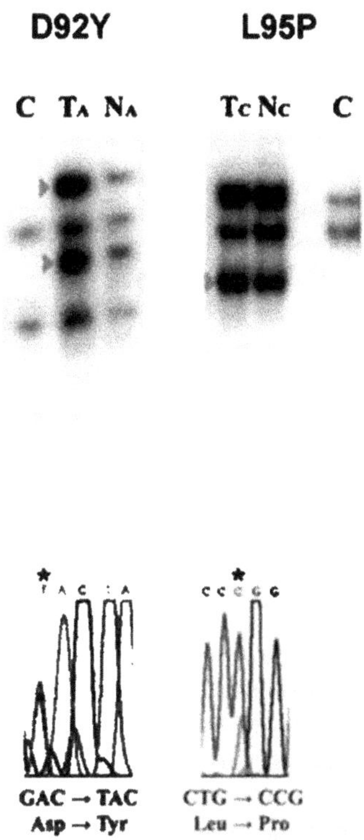

FIGURE 2. SSCP pattern of two patients baring a germline mutation in *SDHD*. Arrowheads point to an aberrant SSCP pattern of tumor (T_A) and normal (N_A) DNA of one patient baring a D92Y mutation, and tumor (T_C) and normal (N_C) DNA of another patient harboring the L95P mutation. The normal pattern is shown with a healthy control (C). "*" points to the changed sequence. This picture was adapted with permission from Dannenberg *et al.*[21]

mutation C243S (1.5%) in exon 7 (Results are not shown; these cases will be described in separate reports.). The former PCC was benign and extra-adrenal, localized within the urinary bladder, and was removed when the patient was at the age of 25 years. The germline C243S mutation was found in a metastatic lesion of a malignant PCC in a 63-year-old female.

DISCUSSION

In this study we have investigated 213 cases of apparently sporadic PCC for mutations in *RET* (exons 10, 11, and 16), *VHL*, *SDHD,* and *SDHB*. A total 7.5% of the apparently sporadic PCCs harbored germline mutations in the PCC susceptibility genes (0% *RET*, 4.4% *VHL*, 1.6% *SDHD,* and 1.5% *SDHB*) (TABLE 2).

TABLE 2. Germline mutations in patients with apparently sporadic PCC.

Number	Gender	Age (years)	Mal/ Ben	Location	Gene	Mutation cDNA	Mutation protein
10	F	38	B	A	VHL	C287T	P25L
37	M	26	B	A	VHL	T401C	L63P
19	F	58	B	A	VHL	T653C	I147T
48	F	39	B	A	VHL	G644A	G144Q
25B	F	49	B	A	VHL	T852G	X > Gly+ 14AA
33M	F	NK	M	A	VHL	854insC	X > Cys+ 128AA
F207	F	63	M	EA	SDHB	T861A	C243S
F188	F	27	B	A	SDHD	G285T	D92Y
F12	M	25	M	EA	SDHD	T295C	L95P

F = female; M = male; Mal = malignant; Ben = benign, A = adrenal; EA = extra-adrenal; NK = not known.

The somatic *RET* mutations found in the present study were the previously described C618Y, C634R, and M918T mutations.[6,18] In our study, no *RET* germline mutations were found. Gimenez-Roqueplo *et al.*[15] and Brauch *et al.*[23] did not find *RET* mutations either, but Cascon *et al.*[24] and Neumann *et al.*[25] published 5% and 5.7% germline *RET* mutations, respectively, in apparently sporadic PCC. However, the first patient with a germline *RET* mutation found by Cascon *et al.* also had C-cell hyperplasia, and the second patient had a positive family history.[24] So both cases had indication of possible syndrome-related disease. Furthermore, Neumann *et al.* revealed a positive family history for six of the patients with a germline *RET* mutation after final follow-up.[25] This would decrease the percentages germline mutations of truly sporadic PCC to 0% for Cascon *et al.* and 2.6% for Neumann *et al.*, which is more in concurrence with our results.

VHL mutations were the most abundant germline mutations discovered in our series, showing six germline mutations (4.4%), which have already been reported previously.[18,19] Brauch *et al.*[20] and Gimenez-Roqueplo *et al.*[23] reported 3.2% and 2.4% germline *VHL* mutations, respectively, which is in the same range as our data. In contrast, Neumann *et al.*[25] showed 11% *VHL* mutations in their 271 nonsyndromic PCC patients, which could be due to the presence of a "mutation belt" in the limited geographical area of that study.

SDHB mutation analysis in 47 PCCs revealed one germline mutation (1.5%). In addition, one somatic *SDHB* mutation in an extra-adrenal PCC was detected. The germline mutation frequency (1.5%) of our study is comparable with the 2.9% reported by Cascon *et al.*[24] and 4% of Neumann *et al.*[25] In contrast, Gimenez-Roqueplo *et al.* reported 9.5% *SDHB* mutations in a series of 84 patients with PCCs.[15] The difference in *SDHB* mutation frequencies in the study of Gimenez-Roqueplo *et al.*[15] compared to the other studies can again be explained by differences in the populations investigated.

Two (1.6%) germline *SDHD* mutations were found in our series of 126 apparently sporadic PCCs. This percentage is comparable to the published data.[15,24,25] Both mutations were previously described by Dannenberg *et al.*[21] and were seen in two patients with extra-adrenal PCC. The *SDHD* D92Y mutation is also known as a Dutch founder mutation in paragangliomas.[26]

In our study, the total percentage of germline mutations (7.5%) in *RET*, *VHL*, *SDHB*, and *SDHD* is comparable with several recent reports. Gimenez-Roqueplo *et al.* investigated 84 patients with apparently sporadic PCCs and found in total 11.9% germline mutations (0% *RET*, 2.4% *VHL*, 9.5% *SDHB*, and 0% *SDHD*).[15] In concurrence, Cascon *et al.* demonstrated 14.3% germline mutations in 35 patients (5.7% *RET*, 0% *VHL*, 2.9% *SDHB*, 5.7% *SDHD*).[24] In addition, Brauch *et al.*[23] investigated germline mutations in *RET* and *VHL* in sporadic PCCs and found only 2 of 62 (3.2%) patients with mutation in *VHL* and no *RET* mutations. However, mutation analysis was not performed for *SDHB* or *SDHD*, which could increase the percentage considerably. However, Neumann *et al.* detected germline mutations in 24% of patients with non-syndromic PCCs (*RET* (5%), *VHL* (11%), *SDHB* (4%), and *SDHD* (4%)).[25] Compared to Neumann *et al.*[25] the percentage of patients with a germline mutation reported in several studies, including ours, seems low. This could be due to differences in the studied populations in different geographical areas.

In conclusion, 7.5% of the 213 apparently sporadic PCCs investigated harbored germline mutations in *VHL*, *SDHB*, or *SDHD*. Although *RET* germline mutations were not found, we recommend germline genetic testing of all PCC susceptibility genes for newly diagnosed apparently sporadic PCCs.

REFERENCES

1. LENDERS, J.W. *et al.* 2005. Phaeochromocytoma. Lancet **366:** 665–675.
2. BRYANT, J. *et al.* 2003. Pheochromocytoma: the expanding genetic differential diagnosis. J. Natl. Cancer. Inst. **95:** 1196–1204.
3. MAHER, E.R. & C. ENG. 2002. The pressure rises: update on the genetics of phaeochromocytoma. Hum. Mol. Genet. **11:** 2347–2354.
4. ENG, C. 1996. Seminars in medicine of the Beth Israel Hospital, Boston. The RET proto-oncogene in multiple endocrine neoplasia type 2 and Hirschsprung's disease. N. Engl. J. Med. **335:** 943–951.
5. NEUMANN, H.P. *et al.* 2002. How many pathways to pheochromocytoma? Semin. Nephrol. **22:** 89–99.
6. PECZKOWSKA, M. & A. JANUSZEWICZ. 2005. Multiple endocrine neoplasia type 2. Fam. Cancer **4:** 25–36.
7. THAKKER, R.V. 2001. Multiple endocrine neoplasia. Horm Res. **56(Suppl 1)**: 67–72.
8. GIMM, O. 2005. Pheochromocytoma-associated syndromes: genes, proteins and functions of RET, VHL and SDHx. Fam. Cancer **4:** 17–23.
9. KIM, W.Y. & W.G. KAELIN. 2004. Role of VHL gene mutation in human cancer. J. Clin. Oncol. **22:** 4991–5004.
10. BAYSAL, B.E. 2003. On the association of succinate dehydrogenase mutations with hereditary paraganglioma. Trends Endocrinol. Metab. **14:** 453–459.

11. NEUMANN, H.P. *et al.* 2004. Distinct clinical features of paraganglioma syndromes associated with SDHB and SDHD gene mutations. JAMA **292:** 943–951.
12. MULLER, U., C. TROIDL & S. NIEMANN. 2005. SDHC mutations in hereditary paraganglioma/pheochromocytoma. Fam. Cancer **4:** 9–12.
13. BAYSAL, B.E. *et al.* 2004. An Alu-mediated partial SDHC deletion causes familial and sporadic paraganglioma. J. Med. Genet. **41:** 703–709.
14. BOURGERON, T. *et al.* 1995. Mutation of a nuclear succinate dehydrogenase gene results in mitochondrial respiratory chain deficiency. Nat. Genet. **11:** 144–149.
15. GIMENEZ-ROQUEPLO, A.P. *et al.* 2003. Mutations in the SDHB gene are associated with extra-adrenal and/or malignant phaeochromocytomas. Cancer Res. **63:** 5615–5621.
16. VAN NEDERVEEN, F.H. *et al.* 2006. The occurrence of SDHB gene mutations in pheochromocytomas. Ann. N. Y. Acad. Sci. This Volume.
17. KOMMINOTH, P. *et al.* 1995. Molecular diagnosis of multiple endocrine neoplasia (MEN) in paraffin-embedded specimens. Endocr. Pathol. **6:** 267–278.
18. VAN DER HARST, E. *et al.* 1998. Prognostic value of RET proto-oncogene point mutations in malignant and benign, sporadic phaeochromocytomas. Int. J. Cancer **79:** 537–540.
19. DANNENBERG, H. *et al.* 2003. Von Hippel-Lindau gene alterations in sporadic benign and malignant pheochromocytomas. Int. J. Cancer **105:** 190–195.
20. VAN DER HARST, E. *et al.* 1998. Germline mutations in the VHL gene in patients presenting with phaeochromocytomas. Int. J. Cancer **77:** 337–340.
21. DANNENBERG, H. *et al.* 2005. Clinical characteristics of pheochromocytoma patients with germline mutations in SDHD. J. Clin. Oncol. **23:** 1894–1901.
22. KOMMINOTH, P. *et al.* 1994. Detection of RET proto-oncogene point mutations in paraffin-embedded pheochromocytoma specimens by nonradioactive single-strand conformation polymorphism analysis and direct sequencing. Am. J. Pathol. **145:** 922–929.
23. BRAUCH, H. *et al.* 1997. Sporadic pheochromocytomas are rarely associated with germline mutations in the VHL tumor suppressor gene or the ret protooncogene. J. Clin. Endocrinol. Metab. **82:** 4101–4104.
24. CASCON, A. *et al.* 2004. Genetic and epigenetic profile of sporadic pheochromocytomas. J. Med. Genet. **41:** e30.
25. NEUMANN, H.P. *et al.* 2002. Germline mutations in nonsyndromic pheochromocytoma. N. Engl. J. Med. **346:** 1459–1466.
26. TASCHNER, P.E. *et al.* 2001. Nearly all hereditary paragangliomas in the Netherlands are caused by two founder mutations in the SDHD gene. Genes Chromosomes Cancer **31:** 274–281.

Familial Nonsyndromic Pheochromocytoma

GIUSEPPE OPOCHER,[a] FRANCESCA SCHIAVI,[a] MAURIZIO IACOBONE,[b] ANTONIO TONIATO,[a] SABINA SATTAROVA,[a] ZORAN ERLIC,[a] MADDALENA MARTELLA,[c] CATERINA MIAN,[a] ISABELLA MERANTE BOSCHIN,[a] LAURA ZAMBONIN,[a] PAOLA DE LAZZARI,[a] ALESSANDRA MURGIA,[c] MARIA ROSA PELIZZO,[a] GENNARO FAVIA,[b] AND FRANCO MANTERO[a]

[a]Department of Medical and Surgical Sciences, [b]Department of Pediatrics, and [c]Department of Gastroenterological Sciences, University Hospital of Padova, Padova, Italy

ABSTRACT: **Judging from recent data, heritable forms account for 30–40% of pheochromocytomas. The molecular basis for the familial pheochromocytoma has been largely elucidated and the role of germline mutation of the VHL, RET, SDHB, and SDHD genes has been established. However, on genotyping a group of 172 sporadic or familial pheochromocytomas, we characterized four unrelated probands with familial pheochromocytomas without any sequence variants of RET (exons 8, 10, 11, 13, 14, 15, and 16) or the entire coding sequence of VHL, SDHB, SDHC, SDHD, and EGLN3 (exon-intron boundaries included). The proband of family 1 is a man who had a bilateral pheochromocytoma at the age of 32 and a local recurrence at the age of 48 years. His brother died of malignant pheochromocytoma and his nephew died suddenly of an undiagnosed pheochromocytoma. The proband of family 2 is a female who had a 5-cm benign adrenal pheochromocytoma at the age of 34 years, while her cousin (maternal branch) had a monolateral pheochromocytoma at the age of 42 years. No other tumors had been reported in either family. The proband of family 3 is a female who had a bilateral pheochromocytoma at the age of 66 years. Her sister had a bilateral pheochromocytoma and breast cancer at the age of 54 years. Several other tumors were recorded in this family, including laryngeal cancer, leukemia, and a case of medullary thyroid carcinoma (MTC) in one brother. MTC was naturally ruled out in the proband and her sister. In family 4, the proband was a female who had a bilateral pheochromocytoma at the age of 46 years and a local recurrence a few years later, with liver metastases from the pheochromocytoma. Her brother had a monolateral benign pheochromocytoma. The proband also had a melanoma and bilateral renal cysts. This case revealed a VHL sequence**

Address for correspondence: Giuseppe Opocher, M.D., Endocrinology Unit, Department of Medical and Surgical Sciences University of Padova, Padova, Italy. Voice: +39 04982 13002; fax: +390 4982 13019.
e-mail: giuseppe.opocher@nipd.it

**Ann. N.Y. Acad. Sci. 1073: 149–155 (2006). © 2006 New York Academy of Sciences.
doi: 10.1196/annals.1353.015**

variant IVS2 + 43 A>G, which was also found in one other unrelated sporadic pheochromocytoma. VHL mRNA integrity is currently being evaluated. The proband had no cerebellar or spinal NMR findings or retinal alterations. In family 5, the proband was a female who had a right adrenal pheochromocytoma at the age of 50 years and a breast cancer at 49 years of age. Her mother had had a right adrenal pheochromocytoma at 61 years of age. Although other molecular mechanisms, such as particular variants in untranslated regions or partial gene deletions, cannot be ruled out, we think finding families with nonsyndromic pheochromocytoma without any RET, VHL, SDHB, SDHC, SDHD, or EGLN3 mutation may argue in favor of the presence of other pheochromocytoma susceptibility genes.

Keywords: familial pheochromocytoma; VHL gene; RET gene; succinate dehydrogenase; NF1 gene

INTRODUCTION

Our clinical and genetic understanding of pheochromocytoma and paraganglioma has been greatly enhanced in the last few years.[1,2] It has been demonstrated that the prevalence of hereditary pheochromocytomas is much higher than was once estimated (i.e., 30–40% instead of 10%) and that 10–24% of apparently sporadic forms also harbor a germline mutation in one of the pheochromocytoma susceptibility genes.[3] The discovery of the role of succinate dehydrogenase gene (SDHB, SDHD, and SDHC) mutations has also enabled the definition of pheochromocytoma/paraganglioma syndrome.[4]

Although some pheochromocytoma genes may still be unknown,[5] the role of the RET, VHL, SDHB, SDHD, and NF1 genes in the pathophysiology of pheochromocytoma is now well established.[6] Different phenotypes have also been better characterized[7] and the molecular basis for familial pheochromocytoma has been largely elucidated.

A new gene has recently been added to the long list of pheochromocytoma susceptibility genes: this is the EGLN3/PHD3 gene, which encodes for a prolyl hydroxylase. This protein may be one of the final steps in a common pathway that also involves VHL, RET, NF1, SDHB, and SDHD and controls neural crest-derived cell apoptosis.[8,9]

On genotyping a relatively large group of sporadic or familial pheochromocytomas, we characterized five unrelated probands with familial pheochromocytoma-only phenotypes, but without any sequence variant: the present article analyzes these cases.

MATERIAL AND METHODS

Patients with syndromic or nonsyndromic pheochromocytoma and neck or head paraganglioma were referred to our endocrine unit and included in the Padova Pheochromocytoma/Paraganglioma Register, which has accrued patients since 1996. The register comprises 172 index cases, classified as follows after extensive clinical and genetic evaluation: 32 cases syndromic to von Hippel–Lindau disease, 15 to type 2 A multiple endocrine neoplasia, 4 to type 1 neurofibromatosis, 16 cases syndromic to pheochromocytoma/paraganglioma syndrome, 91 cases of sporadic pheochromocytoma, and 19 of sporadic head and neck paraganglioma.

We characterized five index cases with nonsyndromic familial pheochromocytoma whose VHL, RET, SDHB, SDHD, and SHDC failed to reveal any mutation responsible for their disease: this particular group of patients forms the subject of the present investigation.

Molecular Analysis

All patients gave their written informed consent. Genomic DNA was isolated from peripheral blood using the Qiamp DNA blood Mini Kit according to the manufacturer's recommendations (Qiagen, GmbH, Hilden, Germany).

After specific polymerase chain reaction (PCR) amplification, germline DNA samples were tested as follows: mutation of the *VHL* gene was analyzed on the entire coding sequence and intron–exon boundaries by PCR–single-strand conformation polymorphism (PCR–SSCP) analysis, followed by direct sequencing of the amplicons; quantitative Southern blotting was also used to detect partial or complete gene deletions, as reported elsewhere.[10]

Mutation analysis of the RET, SDHB, SDHC, SDHD, and EGLN3 coding region and the intron–exon boundaries (exons 8, 10, 11,13, 14,15, of the RET gene, exons 1–8 of the SDHB gene, exons 1–6 of the SDHC gene, exons 1–4 of the SDHD gene, and exons 1–5 of the EGLN3 gene) was conducted as follows: primers for the amplification of the target sequences were based on published sequences for the RET, SDHB, SDHC, SDHD, and EGLN3 genes and designed using Primer Express™ Software v. 2.0 (Applied Biosystems, Foster City, CA, USA).

PCR amplification was performed in 20 μL of reaction mixture containing 1.5 mM $MgCl_2$, 0.2 mM dNTPs, 1 U AmpliTaq Gold (Applied Biosystems), and 0.5 μM of each forward and reverse primer. The amplification profile consisted of an initial denaturation step at 94°C for 5 min, followed by 35 cycles of denaturation at 94°C for 45 sec, annealing at 56–68°C for 45 sec, and extension at 72°C for 45 sec. A final extension step was carried out at 72°C for 7 min.

An aliquot of the PCR product was purified using ExoSAP-IT® (USB Corporation, Cleveland, OH, USA) at 37°C for 15 min and at 80°C for 15 min.

The purified amplicons were bidirectionally sequenced using the original primer pair and the Big-Dye Terminators v. 3.1 Cycle Sequencing Kit (Applied Biosystems) and analyzed on an ABI Prism 3100 DNA Analyzer (Applied Biosystems).

RESULTS

The proband of family 1 is a man who had a bilateral pheochromocytoma when 32 years of age and a local recurrence at the age of 48 years. His brother died of malignant pheochromocytoma and his nephew died suddenly of an undiagnosed pheochromocytoma.

Molecular analysis showed no VHL, RET, SDHD, SDHC sequence variants, but did reveal SDHB IVS1-111 G>A and IVS2 + 33 G>A sequence variants.

The proband of family 2 is a female who had a 5-cm benign adrenal pheochromocytoma at the age of 34 years, her cousin (maternal branch) had a monolateral pheochromocytoma at the age of 42 years . Molecular analysis showed no VHL, RET, SDHD, and SDHC sequence variants, while a SDHB IVS1-111 G>A sequence variant came to light.

No other tumors had been reported in families 1 or 2.

The proband of family 3 is a female who had a bilateral pheochromocytoma at the age of 66 years. Her sister had a bilateral pheochromocytoma and breast cancer at the age of 54 years. Several other tumors had been recorded in this family, including laryngeal cancer, leukemia, and also, in a brother, medullary thyroid carcinoma (MTC), which was naturally ruled out in the proband and her sister. Molecular analysis showed no VHL, SDHD, and SDHC sequence variants, but there were RET c.2712 C>G p.S904S and SDHB IVS1-111 G>A sequence variants.

In family 4, the proband was a female who had a bilateral pheochromocytoma at the age of 46 years that recurred locally with liver metastases a few years later. Her brother had a monolateral benign pheochromocytoma. The proband also had a melanoma and bilateral renal cysts. A VHL sequence variant IVS2 +43 A>G was found in this case and also in one other unrelated sporadic pheochromocytoma. Their VHL mRNA integrity is currently being assessed. The proband had no cerebellar or spinal NMR finding or retinal alterations. Molecular analysis showed the following sequence variants: VHL IVS2 +43 A>G, RET c.2071 G>A p.G691S, SDHD c.34 G>A p.G12S, IVS2-29 A>G, c.204 C>T p.S68S, and IVS3-32 T>C.

In family 5, the proband was a female who had a right adrenal pheochromocytoma at the age of 50 years and a breast cancer at 49 years. Her mother had had a right adrenal pheochromocytoma at 61 years. Molecular analysis showed no VHL, RET, SDHD, SDHB, or SDHC sequence variants.

EGLN3 gene point mutation was analyzed in all probands, revealing the following sequence variants: family 1: IVS4 + 66G>A (homozygous), family 2: IVS4 + 66G>A (homozygous), family 3: IVS4-20 delT (heterozygous), family 4: none, and family 5: IVS4-20 delT (homozygous).

DISCUSSION

Among 172 genotyped pheochromocytomas and paragangliomas, we isolated five unrelated probands with a positive family history but no clinical evidence of a syndromic form: we were unable to detect a genetic defect potentially linked to the hereditary nature of the disease in this group of subjects. This may mean that the spectrum of genetic defects in pheochromocytoma or paraganglioma should be expanded to include other, as yet unknown genes (unless a mutation of one of the six genes already identified as genetic causes of the syndrome escaped our notice in these five cases).

Early reports[11,12] showed that the majority of nonsyndromic familial pheochromocytoma index cases harbored a VHL gene mutation. Moreover, a pheochromocytoma-only subtype of VHL disease has been well characterized. So the most likely culprit is presumably VHL. In a review of 12 familial pheochromocytoma-only kindreds analyzed for susceptibility gene mutations, Astuti *et al.*,[13] recently demonstrated an SDHB or SDHD gene germline point mutation in only two cases. Therefore, 17% of non-VHL familial pheochromocytoma cases had SDH subunit mutation, showing that many familial pheochromocytoma-only kindreds may form a group with no currently known gene mutation—and our families probably belong to this group.

More recently,[14,15] it has been shown that complete or partial germline deletion of the SDHB gene may also be one of the genetic causes of pheochromocytoma/paraganglioma syndrome.

Direct sequencing of PCR-amplified fragments cannot detect large-size mutations, such as partial or complete deletions or gene rearrangements: this calls for quantitative Southern blot or real-time PCR fragment analyses. We performed such analyses on the VHL gene but were unfortunately still unable to detect any SDHB or SDHD large-size mutations. So the chances of some of our families having large-size SDHB/D mutations cannot be ruled out. This may be true of family 1, for instance, since two individuals had malignant pheochromocytoma. A high prevalence of SDHB mutations has been observed in malignant pheochromocytomas[16] and SDHB analysis is the first possibility to consider. The only sequence variants of SDHB that we detected in the proband of family 1, however, were localized in intron 1 and intron 2 (IVS1-111 G>A and IVS2 + 33 G>A): these two intronic variants were heterozygous and the only possible SDHB mutation would be a partial gene deletion not involving intron 1, exon 2, or intron 2, which we cannot detect at present.

Unlike the case in SDHB, we extensively analyzed the VHL gene, seeking partial or complete gene deletions too, although large-size VHL mutations have seldom been identified in pheochromocytoma. No VHL deletions were detected in any of our index cases, but the intronic sequence variant that we detected in family 4 (IVS2 + 43A>G) may have a role because we detected the same sequence variant in a case of sporadic pheochromocytoma. The presence of multiple renal cysts may also argue in favor of a VHL diagnosis. The index case has no other VHL lesions: the question remains unanswered until we have completed the VHL mRNA analysis now in progress.

Family 3 needs some specific comments too: the presence of a first-degree relative with medullary thyroid carcinoma strongly suggests a MEN 2 clinical diagnosis, but the two cases with bilateral adrenal pheochromocytoma had normal calcitonin, and FNAB of the thyroid nodules repeatedly excluded any medullary thyroid carcinoma. Of course, the RET gene was extensively analyzed but no mutation was found to justify the disease. Moreover, the particularly high prevalence of other types of cancer in this family may suggest a Li–Fraumeni-like syndrome, but no pheochromocytoma has been observed in this syndrome so far.[17]

In families 2 and 5, nothing worthy of note emerged from the genetic or clinical analyses so we think they are the best candidates to include in a familial non-syndromic pheochromocytoma group.

It has recently been suggested that all genetic lesions associated with paraganglioma/pheochromocytoma may have a single common pathway,[8,9] which reduces the likelihood of neural crest cell apoptosis. The key actor in this pathway is a protein initially identified as SM20, now known to be a 2-oxoglutarate-dependent prolyl hydroxylase named EglN3/PHD3.

Therefore, there is good reason to consider the EGLN3 gene as a new candidate for causing pheochromocytoma/paraganglioma, though no EGLN3 defects have been demonstrated in pheochromocytoma to date. The familial pheochromocytoma-only phenotype may be the ideal sample on which to test this hypothesis, but when we screened for point mutations of this gene, we found no sequence variants capable of changing this gene's activity in our probands.

Several studies indicating that chromosome loss is particularly frequent in pheochromocytoma may support the involvement of other candidate genes. We have found a particularly critical interval of 3.9 Mb, coming between 1p32.3 and 1p32.1, in the short arm of chromosome 1, which may be the site of one or more tumor suppressor loci involved in the genesis of pheochromocytoma.[5]

Very recently, Patricia Dahia[18] identified a large family in which pheochromocytoma transmission was consistent with a double recessive model. Two novel susceptibility loci were isolated at chromosome 2 and 16. Whether our families share the same molecular mechanism is under investigation.

In conclusion, we isolated a few cases of the familial pheochromocytoma-only phenotype without any significant genetic defects.

Although other molecular mechanisms, such as particular variants in untranslated regions and partial gene deletions, cannot be ruled out, we think that finding families with nonsyndromic pheochromocytoma without any RET, VHL, SDHB, SDHC, SDHD, or EGLN3 gene mutations may mean that other pheochromocytoma susceptibility genes exist.

ACKNOWLEDGMENTS

This study was supported by Grant 2004069534 from MIUR, Italy to G. Opocher.

REFERENCES

1. KOCH, C.A., K. PACAK & G.P. CHROUSOS. 2002. The molecular pathogenesis of hereditary and sporadic adrenocortical and adrenomedullary tumors. J. Clin. Endocrinol. Metab. **87:** 5367–5384.
2. BERTHERAT, J. & A.P. GIMENEZ-REQUEPLO. 2005. New insights in the genetics of adrenocortical tumors, pheochromocytomas and paragangliomas. Horm. Metab. Res. **37:** 384–390.
3. NEUMANN. H.P. *et al.* 2000. Germ-line mutations in nonsyndromic pheochromocytoma. N. Engl. J. Med. **346:** 1459–1466.
4. GIMM, O. *et al.* 2000. Somatic and occult germ-line mutations in SDHD, a mitochondrial complex II gene, in nonfamilial pheochromocytoma. Cancer Res. **60:** 6822–6825.
5. OPOCHER, G. *et al.* 2003. Fine analysis of the short arm of chromosome 1 in sporadic and familial pheochromocytoma. Clin. Endocrinol. (Oxf.) **59:** 707–715.
6. GIMM, O. *et al.* 2004. The genetic basis of pheochromocytoma. Front. Horm. Res. **31:** 45–60.
7. NEUMANN, H.P. *et al.* 2004. Distinct clinical features of paraganglioma syndromes associated with SDHB and SDHD gene mutations. JAMA **292:** 943–951.
8. MAXWELL, P.H. 2005 A common pathway for genetic events leading to pheochromocytoma. Cancer Cell. **8:** 91–93.
9. LEE, S. *et al.* 2005. Neuronal apoptosis linked to EglN3 prolyl hydroxylase and familial pheochromocytoma genes: developmental culling and cancer. Cancer Cell **8:** 155–167.
10. MURGIA, A. *et al.* 2000. Somatic mosaicism in von Hippel-Lindau disease. Hum. Mutat. **15:** 114.
11. CROSSEY, P.A. 1995. Molecular genetic diagnosis of Von Hippel-Lindau disease in familial pheochromocytoma. J. Med. Genet. **32:** 885–886.
12. WOODWARD, E.R. *et al.* 1997. Genetic predisposition to phaeochromocytoma analysis of candidate genes GDNF, RET and VHL. Hum. Mol. Genet. **6:** 1051–1056.
13. ASTUTI, D. *et al.* 2003. Genetic analysis of mitochondrial complex II subunits SDHD, SDHB and SDHC in paraganglioma and phaeochromocytoma susceptibility. Clin. Endocrinol. (Oxf.) **59:** 728–733.
14. CASCON, A. *et al.* 2005 Gross SDHB deletions in patients with paraganglioma detected by multiplex PCR: a possible hot spot? Genes Chromosomes Cancer 2005 Oct 28 [Epub ahead of print]; **45:** 213–219.
15. MCWHINNEY, S.R. *et al.* 2004. Large germline deletions of mitochondrial complex II subunits SDHB and SDHD in hereditary paraganglioma. J. Clin. Endocrinol. Metab. **89:** 5694–5699.
16. GIMENEZ-ROQUEPLO, A.P. *et al.* 2003. Mutations in the SDHB gene are associated with extra-adrenal and/or malignant phaeochromocytomas. Cancer Res. **63:** 5615–5621.
17. OLIVIER, M. *et al.* 2003. Li-Fraumeni and related syndromes: correlation between tumor type, family structure, and TP53 genotype. Cancer Res. **63:** 6643–6650.
18. DAHIA, P.L. *et al.* 2005. Novel pheochromocytoma susceptibility loci identified by integrative genomics. Cancer Res. **65:** 9651–9658.

Genetic Mutation Screening in an Italian Cohort of Nonsyndromic Pheochromocytoma/Paraganglioma Patients

M. CASTELLANO, L. MORI, M. GIACCHÈ, E. AGLIOZZO, R. TOSINI, A. PANAROTTO, C. CAPPELLI, P. MULATERO, D. CUMETTI, F. VEGLIO, AND E. AGABITI-ROSEI

Department of Internal Medicine, Laboratory of Molecular Medicine, University of Brescia and University of Turin, Italy

ABSTRACT: To assess the prevalence of genetic mutations in nonsyndromic pheochromocytoma/paraganglioma (PHEO/PGL) patients we have performed a systematic search for mutations in the succinate dehydrogenase (SDH) B, C, and D subunits, von Hippel–Lindau (VHL), and RET genes by direct bidirectional sequencing. Patients were selected from the medical records of hypertension centers. After exclusion of syndromic patients, 45 patients with familial (F+, $n = 3$) and sporadic (F−, $n = 42$) cases of isolated PHEO/PGL were considered. They included 35 patients with PHEO, 7 with PGL, and 3 with head/neck PGL (hnPGL). Three patients with PHEO (2F−, 1F+) presented VHL mutations (P86A, G93C, and R167W), six with PGL (4F−, 2F+) were positive for SDH or VHL mutations (SDHB R230G in two patients, SDHB S8F, R46Q, R90Q, and VHL P81L in one subject each), and one with hnPGL carried the SDHD 348–351delGACT mutation. We have also detected missense (SDHB S163P, SDHD H50R and G12S), synonymous (SDHB A6A, SDHD S68S), and intronic mutations that have been considered nonpathological polymorphic variants. No mutation was found in SDHC or RET genes. Our data indicate that germline mutations of VHL and SDH subunits are not infrequent in familial as well as in sporadic cases of nonsyndromic PHEO/PGL (overall, 12 of 45 probands, 22%). Accordingly, screening for such mutations seems to be justified. However, a more precise characterization of the functional relevance of any observed sequence variant and of other genetic and environmental determinants of neoplastic transformation is essential in order to plan appropriate protocols for family screening and follow-up.

KEYWORDS: pheochromocytoma; paraganglioma; genetics

Address for correspondence: Prof. M. Castellano, Dipartimento di Scienze Mediche e Chirurgiche, 2ˆMedicina Centro - Spedali Civili di Brescia, 25100 Brescia, Italy. Voice: +39 0303995251; fax +39 0303388147
e-mail: castella@med.unibs.it

**Ann. N.Y. Acad. Sci. 1073: 156–165 (2006). © 2006 New York Academy of Sciences.
doi: 10.1196/annals.1353.016**

INTRODUCTION

There is considerable variety in the definition of pheochromocytoma (PHEO) and paraganglioma (PGL). The common denominators are the embryological origin (a subset of neural crest–derived cells) and the histopathological appearance, whereas differential features derive from their anatomical location (adrenal medulla or paraganglia aligned to sympathetic or parasympathetic nervous system) and from the ability of producing catecholamine and various neuropeptides. The definition of PHEO should be reserved for catecholamine-producing tumors originating from the adrenal medulla, whereas the term of PGL is used for the extra-adrenal, usually catecholamine-producing tumors arising from sympathetic paraganglia located in the thorax-abdomen. The definition of head and neck PGL (hnPGL) is reserved for noncatecholamine-producing tumors originating from parasympathetic paraganglia (carotid body, glomus jugulotympanic). The overall incidence of these tumors is about 1 in 300,000.[1]

Clinical records suggest that approximately 10% of cases of PHEO/PGL and up to 50% of hnPGL occur in a familial setting.[2,3] There are four hereditary syndromes that are associated with PHEO/PGL: multiple endocrine neoplasia (MEN) Type 2A and 2B, neurofibromatosis (NF1) and von Hippel–Lindau syndrome (VHL); the genes involved are RET (OMIM 164761), NF1 (OMIM 162200), and VHL (OMIM 193300), respectively.

In addition, recent studies have shown that germline mutations in nuclear genes coding for the subunits B, D, and C of the mitochondrial succinate dehydrogenase complex II (SDH) are often associated with nonsyndromic, familial as well as apparently sporadic, PHEO/PGL. A growing body of data supports that the real prevalence of pathogenic germline mutations in these genes among patients presenting with nonsyndromic PHEO/PGL is probably much larger than supposed earlier on the basis of a positive family history for the disease.

We have therefore performed molecular screening in a sample of Italian patients referring to hypertension clinics for sporadic and familial nonsyndromic PHEO/PGL in order to evaluate the frequency of germline mutations in the genes coding for the VHL, RET, and SDH (B, C, and D) in this particular clinical setting.

PATIENTS AND METHODS

Patients

We have examined the medical records of patients referred to the hypertension centers of the University of Brescia and the University of Turin in the last 20 years and then selected those with PHEO/PGL. The diagnosis was supported by clinical, biochemical (plasma and/or urinary catecholamines, chromogranin A), and imaging data (computed tomography, magnetic resonance, ^{131}I-metaiodbenzylguanidine or In-111 Pentreotide scintigraphy, as needed). After exclusion of syndromic patients with MEN–2, von Hippel–Lindau, or neurofibromatosis features, only familial and sporadic cases of isolated PHEO/PGL were considered. Thus far, we have examined 45 probands, 35 with PHEO, 7 with PGL, and 3 with hnPGL. In this group of subjects there were three probands with a positive family history (1 PHEO, 1 PGL, and 1 hnPGL patient).

After obtaining an informed written consent, germline DNA was extracted from 10 mL of peripheral blood, using the DNA Isolation Kit for Mammalian Blood (Roche Diagnostic, Mannheim, Germany) according to the manufacturer's instructions.

Mutation Screening

DNA (200 ng) was amplified with intronic primers (TABLE 1) flanking the eight exons of SDHB, four exons of the SDHD,[4] six exons of SDHC, three exons of VHL[5] and exons 10, 11, 13, 14, 15, 16 of RET gene. Polymerase chain reaction (PCR) conditions were as follows: 5 min of denaturation at 94°C, then 38 cycles of denaturation (94°C), annealing (see TABLE 1 for temperature conditions), and polymerization (72°C) for 30 sec, respectively. PCR products were purified with Microcon 50 (Millipore, Billerica, MA) and sequenced using BigDye® Terminator v1.1 Sequencing Kit (Applied Biosystems, Foster City, CA). After a purification step performed with CentriSep Spin Columns (Princeton Separations, Adelphia, NJ), the products were analyzed on a 310 DNA Analyzer (Applied Biosystems).

RESULTS

No mutation in the examined RET gene exons was detected in our group of patients.

Each of the three patients (1 PGL, 1 PHEO, and 1 hnPGL) with a positive family history were carriers of genetic variants of potential pathogenic relevance. The patient presenting with familial PGL (Patient 5, see TABLE 2) had the mutation 688 C>G, corresponding to an arginine to glycine substitution (R230G) in exon 7 of the SDHB gene; Patient 8 (PHEO) presented the mutation 277G>T, G93C, in exon 1 of the VHL gene; and Patient 7 (hnPGL) presented the mutation 348–351delGACT in exon 4 of the SDHD gene.

Of the six patients with apparently sporadic PGL four were carriers of germinal sequence variants: one of them (Patient 2, 137G>A, R46Q, in exon 2 of SDHB) has been previously described in association with PHEO/PGL.[6] The remaining three variants (Patient 1, 23C>T, S8F, in exon 1 of SDHB; Patient 6, 688C>G, R230G, in exon 7 of SDHB; and Patient 10, 242C>T, P81L, in exon 1 of VHL) presented novel mutations to our knowledge.

TABLE 1. Set of primers and annealing temperature for PCR amplification of the different gene exons

		Temp (°C)
SDHB		
1F GGTCCTCAGTGGATGTAGGC	**1R** TCCTCCATCTCCCTGAGGCCTTG	61
2F TGGATATTGAATGCCTGCCT	**2R** GCCTTCCAAGGATGTGAAAA	63
3F ATTCCGAAGGTGACCTGAGA	**3R** CTCTATCAGCTTTGGCCAGC	63
4F CAGCAAGGAGGATCCAGAAG	**4R** ACAAATCCTGCCCTGAAAAA	63
5F CAGTGTCCAAGAAATGGGGT	**5R** TGAACGTTCCTCTCCAGAAT	63
6F GCACTGACCCCAAAGGTAAC	**6R** ATGGCAATGAAGGAAACCAG	63
7F CCAGAGCTTTGAGTTGAGCC	**7R** TGGTCCCTTTCCTTCTCAAA	63
8F AACCCCTATGGTTTTGAGGG	**8R** CTGCGGCAAGTAAAGGAACA	63
SDHD		
1F GTTGGTGGATGACCTTGAGC	**1R** TGAGTCCTCACTTCCATCCC	60
2F TCAGTCCTGTTAAAGGAGAGGTTC	**2R** CCTGCTAAAGGCATGACCA	55
3F AAAGATGTGTGTTTCTCACA	**3R** CAGCAAACAAACTGAGCAGACA	55
4F GTATAGTCTTCTAATTTCACT	**4R** CAATTCTTCAAAGTATGAAGT	55
SDHC		
1F CGTCACATGACACCCCCAAC	**1R** CTCCCAGTCCCACTGAA	60
2F AATCTATCCCTTCACCCCTA	**2R** ATCTCCAGACTTAGAAACTT	50
3F TCAAACGGTCATGGTTTTAT	**3R** CTCTGGCTCCAGAATCCTTC	55
4F ACTCTCTACTATGGTGTCAT	**4R** TGTGTAAAAACACATATACAT	50
5F AGCAGCTGTGACAAGCTACT	**5R** CTCCCTTCACAGAGAAAATG	55
6F CTGTTAATGTCCTATTTACT	**6R** CCAAGGAGATCTGAAAATACA	53
VHL		
1F TGGTCTGGATCGCGGAGGGA	**1R** GACCGTGCTATCGTCCCTGC	63
2F GTGGCTCTTTAACAACCTTTGC	**2R** ACTTACCACAACAACCTTATC	55
3F TTCCTTGTACTGAGACCCTAGT	**3R** TCCTGTATCTAGATCAAGACTC	55
RET		
10S GGAGGCTGAGTGGGCTACG	**10R** CTGGGAGGTGGTGGTGGTC	66,5
11S CTCTGGCGGTGCCAAGCCTC	**11R** GAAGGCAGCTGGGGAGGGCA	66,5
13S AACTTGGGCAAGGCGATGCA	**13R** AGAACAGGGCTGTATGGAGC	65
14S AAGACCCAAGCTGCCTGAC	**14R** GCTGGGTGCAGAGCCATAT	66
15S CCCCCGGCCCAGGTCTCAC	**15R** GCTCCACTAATCTTCGGTATCTTT	55
16S AGGGATAGGGCCTGGCCTTC	**16R** TAACCTCCACCCCAAGAGAG	55

In the two patients with sporadic hnPGL, genetic screening revealed one previously unreported mutation in Patient 3: a 269G>A transversion, leading to R90Q substitution, in exon 3 of SDHB.

The screening performed on 34 cases of apparently sporadic PHEO showed the presence of sequence variants in eight patients. Two of them were positive for mutations in the VHL gene: Patient 9, with 256C>G, P86A in exon 1 and Patient 11 with 561C>T, R167W in exon 3. Both mutations have been previously described in association with PHEO.[7,8] Patient 4 carried two distinct SDHB variants: a 18A>C transversion, A6A, in exon 1, known as genetic polymorphism[9] and a 487T>C, S163P, in exon 5; such missense mutation has been considered a polymorphic variant in a Spanish population,[10] but we have not found such variation in a series of 70 Italian controls (140 chromosomes).

TABLE 2. Clinical features of patients carrying sequence variants in SDHB, SDHD and VHL genes

Mutation type	Patient number	Clinical features tumor site	F	Malignancy	Age at first diagnosis	UC	Scintigraphy	Screened relatives/ carriers/ affected	Mutation reference
SDHB 23T>C S8F	1	Left para-adrenal PGL	–	–	28	–	MIBG +	3/2/0	New
SDHB 137G>A, R46Q	2	Right para-adrenal PGL	–	–	45	+	n.a.	5/0	6
SDHB 269G>A, R90Q	3	Bilateral tympanic and carotid hn-PGL	–	–	33	–	n.a.	3/0	New
SDHB 487T>C, S163P 18A>C A6A	4	Right adrenal PHEO	–	–	17	+	MIBG +	–	10, 9
SDHB 822C>G, R230G	5	Left juxta-adrenal interaortocaval multifocal PGL	+	+	9	+	MIBG-OCT +	16/6/1	New
	6	Right para-aortic PGL	–	–	28	+	MIBG +	29/16/2	
SDHD 348–351delGACT	7	Carotid glomous hn-PGL	+	Local invasivity	47	–	OCT +	–	30
VHL 277G>T G93C	8	Adrenal bilateral PHEO	+	–	31	+	n.a.	1/1/1	24
VHL 256C>G, P86A	9	Adrenal bilateral PHEO	–	–	9	+	MIBG +	0	7
VHL 242C>T, P81L	10	Left para-adrenal PGL	–	–	35	+	MIBG +	0	New
VHL 561C>T, R167W	11	Adrenal bilateral PHEO	–	–	28	+	MIBG +	0	8
SDHD 149A>G, H50R	12	Right adrenal PHEO	–	–	65	+	MIBG +	0	11
	13	PHEO	–	–	n.a.	+	n.a.	0	
SDHD 204C>T, S68S 34G>A, G12S	14	Left adrenal PHEO	–	–	54	+	n.a.	0	12
SDHB IVS1–111G>A	15	Right adrenal PHEO	–	–	45	+	MIBG +	0	4
SDHB IVS2 + 35G>A IVS4 + 60T>C	16	PHEO	–	–	40	+	n.a.	0	9

OCT = Octreoscan; UC = urinary catecholamine; n.a. = not available; F = familiarity; – = negative; + = positive; F = familial.

We have found additional known polymorphisms in five other patients with sporadic PHEO: two of them (Patients 12 and 13) presented the nonsynonymous 149A>G substitution, H50R, in exon 3 of SDHD[11] and Patient 14 was a carrier of two polymorphisms,[12] 34G>A, G12S and 204C>T, S68S in SDHD exon 1 and 3, respectively. Three additional intronic polymorphisms of the SDHB gene were found in Patient 15 (IVS1–111 G>A) and Patient 16 (IVS2 + 35 G>A and IVS4 + 60T>C).

We have further investigated the three missense mutations of SDHB gene (S8F, R90Q, and R230G), which have not been described before, in order to define their clinical relevance better. First, we have not found similar gene variants in a cohort of 70 healthy subjects. We have then considered whether the amino acids involved (S8, R90, R230) are conserved among different vertebrate and invertebrate species. As shown in FIGURE 1, positions S8 and S163 are conserved in different mammalian species (*Rattus norvegicus*, *Mus musculus*, *Pan troglodytes*, *Canis familiaris*), while positions R90 and R230 are identical both in mammalian and invertebrate species. We further evaluate loss of heterozygosis (LOH) in the available tumoral tissues; we were able to ex-

```
Homo sapiens         MAAVVALSLRRRLPATTLG--GACLQASRGAQTAAATAPRIKKFAIYRWDPDKAGDKPHM 58
Rattus norvegicus    MAAVVGVSLKRGFSATALGRVGLQFQACREAQTAAAAAPRIKTFAIYRWDPDKAGDKPRM
Mus Musculus         MAATVGVSLKRGFPAAVLGRVGLQFQACRGAQTAAAAAPRIKKFAIYRWDPDKTGDKPRM
Pan troglodytes      MAAVVALSLRRRLPATTLG--GACLQASRGAQTAAATAPRIKKFAIYRWDPDKAGDKPHM
Canis familiaris     MAAVVGVSLKRRFPAAALG--GACLQACRGAQTAAATAPRIKKFAIYRWDPDKTGDKPHM
Drosophila m.        LSRVGSLVARNQMRAISNG--TA--QLEQQAQPKEAQEPQIKKFEIYRWNPDNAGEKPYM
S.pombe                                                      LKTFEIYRWNPEKPEVKPKL
M.grisea                          PSAALR--KPAMVSVRSMASVGESESKMKTFQIYRWDPSQPSEKPRM
A.thaliana                     RLIPARWTSTGA—EAETKASSGGGRGSNLKTF  QIYRWNPDNPG-KPEL

Homo sapiens         QTYKVDLNKCGPMVLDALIKIKNEVDSTLTFRRSCREGICGSCAMNINGGNTLACTRRID 118
Rattus norvegicus    QTYKVDLNKCGPMVLDALIKIKNEIDSTLTFRRSCREGICGSCAMNINGGNTLACTRRID
Mus Musculus         QTYEVDLNKCGPMVLDALIKIKNEVDSTLTFRRSCREGICGSCAMNINGGNTLACTRRID
Pan troglodytes      QTYEVDLNKCGPMVLDALIKIKNEVDSTLTFRRSCREGICGSCAMNINGGNTLACTRRID
Canis familiaris     QTYEIDLNKCGPMVLDALIKIKNEIDSTLTFRRSCREGICGSCAMNINGGNTLACTRRID
Drosophila m.        QTYEVDLRECGPMVLDALIKIKNEMDPTLTFRRSCREGICGSCAMNIGGTNTLACISKID
S.pombe              QKYTVDLTKCGPMVLDALIKIKNEQDPTLTFRRSCREGICGSCAMNINGSNTLACICNIK
M.grisea             QTYTLDLNKTGPMVLDALVRIKNELDPTLTFRRSCREGICGSCAMNINGTNTLACLCRIP
A.thaliana           QNYQIDLKDCGPMVLDALIKIKNEMDPSLTFRRSCREGICGSCAMNIDGCNGLACLTKIQ

Homo sapiens         TNLNKVSKIYPLPHMYVIKDLVPDLSNFYAQYKSIEPYLKKKDESQE--GKQQYLQSIEERE 178
Rattus norvegicus    TDLGKVSKIYPLPHMYVIKDLVPDLSNFYAQYKSIEPYLKKKDESQE--GKQQYLQSIEDRE
Mus Musculus         TDLSKVSKIYPLPHMYVIKDLVPDLSNFYAQYKSIEPYLKKKDESQE--GKQQYLQSIEDRE
Pan troglodytes      TNLNKVS------------------SNFYAQYKSIEPYLKKKDESQE--GKQQYLQSIEERE
Canis familiaris     TNLSKVSKIYPLPHMYVIKDLVPDLSNFYAQYKSIEPYLKKKDESQE--GKQQYLQSIEDRE
Drosophila m.        INTSKSLKVYPLPHMYVVRDLVPDMNNFYEQYRNIQPWLQRKNEAGEKKGKAQYLQSVEDRS
S.pombe              KD-NKPTKIYPLPHCFIVKDLVPDLTYFYKQYKSIEPWLQNDNIPKD----KEFYQSRADRA
M.grisea             TEASSEVKIYPLPHTYVVKDLVPDLTHFYKQYRSIKPYLQRDEPAPDG---KEYRQSKEDRR
A.thaliana           DEASETT-ITPLPHMFVIKDLVVDMTNFYNQYKSIEPWLKRKTPASV--PAKEILQSKKDRA

Homo sapiens         KLDGLYECILCACCSTSCPSYWWNGDKYLGPAVLMQAYRWMIDSRDDFTEERLAKLQDPF 238
Rattus norvegicus    KLDGLYECILCACCSTSCPSYWWNGDKYLGPAVLMQAYRWMIDSRDEFTEERLAKLQDPF
Mus Musculus         KLDGLYECILCACCSTSCPSYWWNGDKYLGPAVLMQAYRWMIDSRDDFTEERLAKLQDPF
Pan troglodytes      KLDGLYECILCACCSTSCPSYWWNGDKYLGPAVLMQAYRWMIDSRDDFTEERLAKLQDPF
Canis familiaris     KLDGLYECILCACCSTSCPSYWWNGDKYLGPAVLMQAYRWMIDSRDDFTEERLAKLQDPF
Drosophila m.        KLDGLYECILCACCSTSCPSYWWNAEKYLGPAVLMQAYRWIIDSRDENSAERLNKLKDPF
S.pombe              KLDGLYECILCACCSTSCPSYWWNSEEYLGPAVLMQAYRWIIDSRDQATAKRLDVMQNSM
M.grisea             KLDGLYECILCACCSTSCPSYWWNSEEYLGPAILLQSYRWLADSRDQRKVERLALDNSM
A.thaliana           KLDGMYECILCACCSTSCPSYWWNPESYLGPAALLHANRWISDSRDEYTKERLEAIDDEF
```

FIGURE 1. Conservation of amino acid position S8, R90, S163, and R230 of SDHB protein among different species.

tract DNA from an abdominal, catecholamine-producing PGL from Patient 6 (R230G mutation) and amplify them with a set of primers surrounding microsatellites D1S199, D1S2644, D1S2697, and D1S507: the results (data not shown) confirmed somatic LOH. Finally we considered PHEO/PGL penetrance among relatives of probands carrying the same mutation. In particular, we have been able to examine two large kindreds from Patient 5 (familial PGL) and Patient 6 (sporadic PGL), both carriers of the R230G mutation in SDHB gene: among 22 carriers of such mutation found in the two kindreds, three more subjects were affected by PHEO/PGL.

DISCUSSION

In the present screening of an Italian sample of PHEO/PGL patients representative of the specialized hypertensive clinical setting, we have been able to find 17 sequence variants in genes potentially involved in PHEO/PGL pathogenesis. Of these, five (SDHB R46Q, SDHD 348-351 delGACT, VHL G93C, P86A, and R167W) have been previously described in association with PHEO/PGL, while three (SDHB S8F, R90Q, and R230G and VHL P81L) are novel mutations that presumably play a causative role. In addition, we have found eight known genetic polymorphisms. Accordingly, the overall prevalence of clinically significant mutations is 10 of 45 patients (22%), with relative contribution of 5 of 45 (11%), 4 of 45 (9%), and 1 of 45 (2%) for SDHB, VHL, and SDHD genes, respectively. If we limit our consideration to PHEO/PGLs presenting in a familial setting, the prevalence of pathogenically relevant mutations is 100% (3 of 3), but in sporadic forms the frequency of mutation is also very high, in substantial agreement with the literature, showing similar data in a large collection of patients with sporadic PHEO/PGL (TABLE 3).

In our sample no patient presented mutations of RET or SDHC genes. As a matter of fact, we preliminarily excluded PHEO/PGL occurring in syndromic form, and PHEO is almost never the first clinical manifestation of a MEN2 syndrome; on the other hand, only eight cases of SDHC-associated PGL have been reported thus far.

TABLE 3. Occult germline mutations in sporadic nonfamilial phaeochromocytomas

Gene	No. of patients	Subjects with mutations	Percent	Reference	Present data (%)
RET	712	22	3.1 (0–21.4)	16–26	0
VHL	586	41	7.0 (0–20)	18, 20, 23, 24–27	7.9
SDHB	536	39	7.3 (4.9–14.3)	25, 26, 28, 29	12.5
SDHD	561	27	4.8 (0–8)	25, 26, 28–30	0

It should also be noted that the prevalence of SDHD mutations is lower than previously reported, but this may be at least in part due to the small number of hnPGLs included in our samples, which are more frequently associated with SDHD mutations.

From these data and previous evidence from the literature, we may argue that the most cost-effective mutation screening strategy in the setting of hypertensive patients with nonsyndromic PHEO is probably the sequential analysis of VHL, SDHB, and SDHD, whereas in PGL the sequence should be SDHB, SDHD, VHL, and SDHC.

We have been able to perform an extended pedigree analysis only in two kindreds, both carrying the novel SDHB R230G mutation. Notably, only 5 of 22 mutation carriers had a diagnosis of PHE/PGL (two subjects in proband 6 family and three subjects in proband 5 family). None of the remaining 17 carriers, clinically asymptomatic, showed evidence of the disease on thorough biochemical and imaging investigation.

Although our mutation screening by direct bidirectional sequencing is very sensitive, we cannot exclude the occurrence of other mutations in intronic or, regulatory regions, large deletions of the entire gene,[13] or exon skipping promoted by Alu intronic sequence, as recently reported by various authors.[14,15] Southern blot or RNA analysis (RT-PCR or Northern blot) could give us more complete results.

In conclusion, the present findings in an Italian cohort of PHEO/PGL patients recruited through hypertension clinic facilities suggest that genetic screening for mutations of candidate genes (at least SDHB, VHL, and SDHD) is indicated not only in familial, but also in sporadic forms, given the relatively high prevalence of pathogenically relevant mutations. However, a more precise characterization of the functional relevance of any observed sequence variant and of other genetic and environmental determinants of neoplastic transformation is essential in order to plan appropriate protocols for family screening and follow-up.

ACKNOWLEDGMENTS

This work has been supported by research grants funded by the Italian MIUR, under PRIN No. 2004069534—002 and by the Fondazione della Communità Bresciana.

REFERENCES

1. Baysal, B.E. 2002. Hereditary paraganglioma targets diverse paraganglia. J. Med. Genet. **39**: 617–622.
2. Grufferman, S. *et al.* 1980. Familial carotid body tumors: case report and epidemiologic review. Cancer Rev. **46**: 2116–2122.

3. VAN DER MEY, A.G., P.D. MAASWINKEL-MOOY, C.J. CORNELISSE, *et al.* 1989. Genomic imprinting in hereditary glomus tumours: evidence for new genetic theory. Lancet **2:** 1291–1294.
4. BENN, D.E., M.S. CROXSON, K. TUCKER, *et al.* 2003. Novel succinate dehydrogenase subunit B (SDHB) mutations in familial phaeochromocytomas and paragangliomas, but an absence of somatic SDHB mutations in sporadic phaeochromocytomas. Oncogene **22**:1358–1364.
5. ASHIDA, S., H. OKUDA, M. CHIKAZAWA, *et al.* 2000. Detection of circulating cancer cells with von Hippel-Lindau gene mutation in peripheral blood of patients with renal cell carcinoma. Clin. Cancer. Res. **6:** 3817–3822.
6. GIMENEZ-ROQUEPLO, A.P., J. FAVIER, P. RUSTIN, *et al.* 2002. Functional consequences of a SDHB gene mutation in an apparently sporadic pheochromocytoma. J. Clin. Endocrinol. Metab. **87**: 4771–4774.
7. CHEN, F. *et al.* 1995. Germline mutations in the von Hippel-Lindau disease tumor suppressor gene: correlations with phenotype. Hum. Mutat. **5:** 66–75.
8. CROSSEY, P.A. *et al.* 1994. Identification of intragenic mutations in the von Hippel-Lindau disease tumour suppressor gene and correlation with disease phenotype. Hum. Mol. Genet. **3**: 1303–1308
9. CASCON, A., A. CEBRIAN, S. RUIZ-LLORENTE, *et al.* 2002. SDHB mutation analysis in familial and sporadic phaeochromocytoma identifies a novel mutation. J. Med. Genet. **39**: E64.
10. CASCON, A., S. RUIZ-LLORENTE, M.F. FRAGA, *et al.* 2004. Genetic and epigenetic profile of sporadic pheochromocytomas. J. Med. Genet. **41**: e30.
11. CASCON, A., S. RUIZ-LLORENTE, A. CEBRIAN, *et al.* 2003. G12S and H50R variations are polymorphisms in the SDHD gene. Genes Chromosomes Cancer **37**: 220–221.
12. KYTOLA, S., B. NORD, E.E. ELDER, *et al.* 2002. Alterations of the SDHD gene locus in midgut carcinoids, Merkel cell carcinomas, pheochromocytomas, and abdominal paragangliomas Genes Chromosomes Cancer **34**: 325–332.
13. MCWHINNEY, S.R., R.T. PILARSKI, S.R. FORRESTER & M.C. SCHNEIDER 2004. Large germline deletions of mitochondrial complex II subunits SDHB and SDHD in hereditary paraganglioma. J. Clin. Endocrinol. Metab. **89**: 5694–5699.
14. BAYSAL, B.E., J.E. WILLETT-BROZICK, P.A. FILHO, *et al.* 2004. An Alu-mediated partial SDHC deletion causes familial and sporadic paraganglioma. J. Med. Genet. **41**: 703–709.
15. BAYLEY, J.P., P. DEVILEE, & P.E. TASCHNER. 2005. The SDH mutation database: an online resource for succinate dehydrogenase sequence variants involved in pheochromocytoma, paraganglioma and mitochondrial complex II deficiency. BMC Med. Genet. **6:** 39.
16. ZEDENIUS, J. *et al.* 1994. Somatic and MEN 2A de novo mutations identified in the RET proto-oncogene by screening of sporadic MTC. Hum. Mol. Genet. **3:** 1259–1262.
17. BELDJORD, C. *et al.* 1995. The RET protooncogene in sporadic pheochromocytomas: frequent MEN 2-like mutations and new molecular defects. J. Clin. Endocrinol. Metab. **80**: 2063–2068.
18. ENG, C. *et al.* 1995. Mutations in the RET proto-oncogene and the von Hippel-Lindau disease tumour suppressor gene in sporadic and syndromic phaeochromocytomas. J. Med. Genet. **32**: 934–937.

19. LINDOR, N.M., R. HONCHEL, S. THIBODEAU, *et al.* 1995. Mutations in the RET protooncogene in sporadic pheochromocytomas. J. Clin. Endocrinol. Metab. **80**: 627–629.
20. HOFSTRA, R.M. *et al.* 1996. Extensive mutation scanning of RET in sporadic medullary thyroid carcinoma and of RET and VHL in sporadic pheochromocytoma reveals involvement of these genes in only a minority of cases. J. Clin. Endocrinol. Metab. **81**: 2881–2884.
21. TAKAYA, K. *et al.* 1996. The RET proto-oncogene in sporadic pheochromocytomas. Intern. Med. **35**: 449–452.
22. RODIEN, P., X. JEUNEMAITRE, C. DUMONT, *et al.* 1997. Genetic alterations of the RET proto-oncogene in familial and sporadic pheochromocytomas. Horm. Res. **47**: 263–268.
23. BRAUCH, H. 1997. Sporadic pheochromocytomas are rarely associated with germline mutations in the VHL tumor suppressor gene or the ret protooncogene. J. Clin. Endocrinol. Metab. **82**: 4101–4104.
24. NEUMANN, H.P. *et al.* 2002. Germ-line mutations in nonsyndromic pheochromocytoma. N. Engl. J. Med. **346**: 1459–1466.
25. BAUTERS, C. *et al.* 2003. Hereditary phaeochromocytomas and paragangliomas: a study of five susceptibility genes. J. Med. Genet. **40**: e75.
26. GIMENEZ-ROQUEPLO, A.P. 2003. Mutations in the SDHB gene are associated with extra-adrenal and/or malignant phaeochromocytomas. Cancer Res. **63**: 5615–5621.
27. VAN DER HARST, E. *et al.* 1998. Germline mutations in the VHL gene in patients presenting with phaeochromocytomas. Int. J. Cancer **77**: 337–340.
28. ASTUTI, D., N. HART-HOLDEN, F. LATIF, *et al.* 2003. Genetic analysis of mitochondrial complex II subunits SDHD, SDHB and SDHC in paraganglioma and phaeochromocytoma susceptibility. Clin. Endocrinol. (Oxf) **59**: 728–733.
29. NEUMANN, H.P. *et al.* 2004. Distinct clinical features of paraganglioma syndromes associated with SDHB and SDHD gene mutations. JAMA **25**: 943–951.
30. CASCON, A. *et al.* 2002. Identification of novel SDHD mutations in patients with phaeochromocytoma and/or paraganglioma. Eur. J. Hum. Genet. **10**: 457–461.

Frequent Genetic Changes in Childhood Pheochromocytomas

RONALD R. DE KRIJGER,[a] FRANCIEN H. VAN NEDERVEEN,[a] ESTHER KORPERSHOEK,[a] WOUTER W. DE HERDER,[b] SABINE M.P.F. DE MUINCK KEIZER-SCHRAMA,[c] AND WINAND N.M. DINJENS[a]

[a]*Department of Pathology, Josephine Nefkens Institute, Erasmus MC-University Medical Center, Rotterdam, the Netherlands*

[b]*Department of Internal Medicine, Erasmus MC-University Medical Center, Rotterdam, the Netherlands*

[c]*Department of Pediatrics, Subdivision Pediatric Endocrinology, Erasmus MC-Sophia, Rotterdam, the Netherlands*

ABSTRACT: **Pheochromocytomas (PCCs) are rare catecholamine-producing tumors of the adrenal gland which may also occur elsewhere in the abdomen and are then called paragangliomas. A proportion of PCCs occurs in hereditary cancer syndromes, including multiple endocrine neoplasia Type 2 (MEN2), caused by mutations in the *RET* proto-oncogene, von Hippel–Lindau (VHL) disease, caused by *VHL* gene abnormalities, and the pheochromocytoma–paraganglioma (PCC–PGL) syndrome, caused by mutations in SDHB and SDHD. Since a proportion of PCCs occurs in children we hypothesized that germline mutations in RET, VHL, succinate dehydrogenase subunit B (SDHB), and subunit D (SDHD) occur more frequently in the pediatric age range. From our single-institution collection of PCCs, we have selected 10 cases that occurred in individuals up to 18 years of age at diagnosis. In these, we have performed mutation analysis on normal and tumor tissues for exons 10, 11, and 16 of RET and for the entire coding sequence of VHL, SDHB, and SDHD. The 10 patients include 7 boys and 3 girls, with an average age of 15.5 years (range 9–18 years). Two patients had germline RET exon 11 mutations (C634R) and 1 patient had an R64P germline mutation in the VHL gene. In the remaining 7 patients there was one patient from a family fulfilling the clinical criteria for VHL disease. All tumors were benign (average follow-up: 12 years) and were located in the adrenal. From our findings we conclude that (a) a large proportion (40%) of pediatric PCC patients is diagnosed in the context of inherited cancer syndromes, and**

Address for correspondence: R.R. de Krijger, M.D. Ph.D., Department of Pathology, Josephine Nefkens Institute, Room Be222, Erasmus MC, P.O. Box 1738, 3000 DR Rotterdam, the Netherlands. Voice: +31-10-4087901; fax: +31-10-4089487.
e-mail: r.dekrijger@erasmusmc.nl

Ann. N.Y. Acad. Sci. 1073: 166–176 (2006).
doi: 10.1196/annals.1353.017

(b) candidate gene analysis appears to be indicated to detect germline mutations.

KEYWORDS: **pheochromocytoma; childhood; mutation analysis; genetics**

INTRODUCTION

Pheochromocytomas (PCCs) are catecholamine-producing tumors of chromaffin cells in the adrenal medulla which may also occur in extra-adrenal locations and are then called paragangliomas (PGLs). Such sympathetic PGLs should be distinguished from head and neck PGLs, which have a parasympathetic origin, do not usually produce catecholamines, and have a different genetic background.[1,2] PCCs were originally called "the 10% tumor" for the frequency of malignancy, familial occurrence, and the proportion of tumors presenting during childhood. However, several studies have challenged these percentages, and it is obvious now that the frequency of familial occurrence, that is, the proportion of PCC that is inherited, may be up to 25%.[3]

There are several heritable (endocrine) tumor syndromes, which all have an autosomal dominant mode of inheritance, that include PCC: von Hippel–Lindau disease (VHL), caused by abnormalities in the VHL tumor-suppressor gene; multiple endocrine neoplasia Type 2 (MEN2), caused by activating point mutations in the *RET* proto-oncogene; and the newly described PCC–PGL syndrome, caused by mutations in one of three genes encoding succinate dehydrogenase subunits (SDHB, SDHC, and SDHD). The incidence of VHL and MEN2 is approximately the same, 1 of 36,000, whereas this incidence is not yet known for the PCC–PGL syndrome.[4]

Until now, relatively little attention has been paid to PCC occurring during childhood and adolescence, with only a few studies describing larger series of patients, predominantly from a clinical point of view.[5–8] None of these studies has systematically studied molecular genetic abnormalities in the above-mentioned genes. Therefore, we have undertaken such an analysis in a single-institution-derived group of 10 patients under 18 years that presented with adrenal-based PCCs, covering the entire coding region of VHL, SDHB, and SDHD, and exons 10, 11, and 16 of RET.

MATERIALS AND METHODS

Patients

Tissue specimens were retrieved from the archives of the Department of Pathology of the Erasmus MC (Rotterdam), following approval of the experimental design and protocols by the Medical Ethical Committee. Ten PCCs were selected for mutation analysis for RET, VHL, SDHB, and SDHD, without knowing the patient or family history (for patient details see TABLE 1).

Tissue Preparation

Tumor DNA and matching normal DNA were isolated from paraffin-embedded tissue. DNA isolation was performed using Puregene (Gentra, Minneapolis, MN) according to the manufacturer's instructions.

Denaturating Gradient Gel Electrophoresis (DGGE)

Polymerase chain reaction (PCR) using genomic DNA as template was carried out in a 50-μL mixture of 1 × PCR buffer (Perkin Elmer Europe, Rotkreuz, Switzerland) containing 10 to 400 ng of template DNA, 200 μM of each intron-based primer (TABLE 1), and 1 μL Taq polymerase (Ampli Taq Gold, Perkin Elmer Europe). After a hot start of 7 min at 95°C, a "touch-down" procedure was used consisting of denaturation for 60 sec at 95°C, annealing for 60 sec at temperatures decreasing from 60 to 55°C during the first 11 cycles (with 0.5°C decremental steps in cycles 2 to 11), and ending with an extension step at 72°C for 60 sec. Ten cycles with an annealing temperature of 55°C and 15 cycles with an annealing temperature of 45°C followed with extension times of 90 sec. After a final extension for 10 min at 72°C, heteroduplex formation was induced by initial denaturation for 10 min at 98°C followed by incubations at 55°C for 30 min and 37°C for 30 min. For DGGE, 10 μL of the PCR product in 3 μL Ficoll-based loading buffer were loaded onto 10% polyacrylamide gels containing a urea-formamide gradient in 0. 5×Tris-acetate TAE-EDTA. The amplicons were electrophoresed at 60°C and 100 V for 16 h. DNA strands were visualized using silver staining as described previously.[9]

Single-Strand Conformation Polymorphism (SSCP) Analysis

PCR amplification of tumor DNA was performed with 10 to 100 ng DNA in a final volume of 15 μL containing 1.5 mM $MgCl_2$, 10 mM Tris-HCl, 50 mM KCl, 0.02 mM dATP, 0.2 mM dGTP, dTTP, and dCTP, 0.8 μCi α^{32}P-dATP (Amersham, Buckinghamshire, United Kingdom), 15 pmol of each forward and reverse primer (TABLE 2), and 3U Taq polymerase (Ampli Taq Gold, Perkin Elmer Europe). PCR was performed for 35 cycles of 95°C for 30 sec, 55°C for 45 sec, and 1 min at 72°C, followed by 1 cycle at 72°C for 10 min. PCR products were electrophoresed overnight at 8W on a nondenaturing gel, containing 8% polyacrylamide ([49:1] Fluka, Neu-Ulm, Germany) and 10% glycerol (v/v). After electrophoresis, the gel was dried and exposed to an X-ray film.

TABLE 1. Clinical details and results of mutation analysis in pediatric PCC patients

Patient	Age at operation (yr)	Sex	Side	Size (cm)	Weight (gram)	Follow up (yr)	Mutation in candidate genes	Syndrome
F18	17	M	right	6	60	20	None	
F30	14	M	right	3.2	20	15	None	
F31	15	M	right	8 × 4. 4 × 4	80	U	None	
F41	16	M	right	3	17	18	RET C634R	MEN2a
			left	3	15		RET C634R	MEN2a
F44	18	M	U	4 × 2.5	U	U	None[a]	
F68	9	M	left	4 × 2.8	U	U	None	
			right	1.7 × 1.3	U		None	
F80	18	F	left	3 × 2.5	U	12	RET C634R	MEN2a
			right	3 × 3	U		RET C634R	MEN2a
F95	13	F	left	7 × 3 × 1.5	U	10	None	U[c]
			right	5.5 × 5 × 2.5	U		None	
F107	17	M	right	2.5 × 1.5 × 1.5	U	7	None[b]	VHL[b]
F119	18	F	left	3	23	2	VHL R64P	VHL

NOTE: U = unknown; M = male; F = female; size has been indicated as greatest tumor diameter or alternatively in two or three dimensions, as recorded.

[a]In this patient an exom 5 TCT to CCT base change was found in SDHB, leading to an S163P amino acid change, which is presently considered as a polymorphism.

[b]This patient and his family fulfilled all clinical criteria for VHL disease, including clear-cell renal cell carcinoma and two hemangioblastomas in addition to the PCC in the index patient, but no VHL mutation was detected because of the inferior DNA quality of this sample.

[c]This patient presented with hemihypertrophy, multinodular adrenocartical hyperplasia, and fibroadenoma of the breast, in addition to bilateral PCC.

TABLE 2. Primers used for mutation analysis

	Forward	Reverse	Product size (bp)	Mutation analysis method
RET 10	5′-GCGCCCCAGGAGGCTGAGTG-3′	5′-cgcccgccgcgccccgcgcccgtcccgccgcc cccgcgTGGTGGTCCCGGCCGCC-3′	225	DGGE
RET 11	5′-CTCTGCGGTGCCAAGCCTCA-3′	5′-cgcccgccgcgccccgcgcccggcccgccgcccccgcccg GAGTAGCTGACCGGGAAGGC-3′	262	DGGE
RET 16	5′-cgcccgccgcgccccgcgcccggcccgccgcccccgcccga aataataaaAGGGATAGGGCCTGGGCTTC-3′	5′-ACCCCAAGAGAGCAACACCC-3′	224	DGGE
VHL 1a	5′-gcgcgcgAGCGCGTTCCATCCTCTAC-3′	5′-cgcccgccgcgccccgcgcccggcccgccgcccccgcccg AGGGCCGTACTCTTCGAC-3′	255	DGGE
VHL 1b	5′-gcgcgGCGGAGAACTGGGACGAG-3′	5′-cgcccgccgcgccccgcgcccggcccgccgcccccgcccg GCTTCAGACCGTGCTATCGT-3′	418	DGGE
VHL 2	5′-cgcccgccgcgccccgcgcccggcccgccgcccccgcccg aaataataaaCTTTAACAACCTTGCTT-3′	5′-cgtcccgcGTCTATCCTGTACTTACCAC-3′	266	DGGE
VHL 3	5′-gcgcgTTCCTTGTACTGAGACCCTAGT-3′	5′-cgcccgccgcgccccgcgcccggcccgccgcccccgcccg GCTTCAGACCGTGCTATCGT-3′	316	DGGE
SDHB 1	5′-GAGCGACCTCGGGGTTAAG-3′	5′-GCTTTCCTGACTTTTCCCTC-3′	157	SSCP
SDHB 2	5′-cgcccgccgcgccccgcgcccggcccgccgcccccgcccg AGCTGAGATGTGTGAACTTT-3′	5′-AAGCATGTCCCTAAATCAAA-3′	265	DGGE
SDHB 3	5′-cgcccgccgcgccccgcgcccggcccgccgcccccgccc GGAACTTTACATAAATACCACTGGA-3′	5′-cgCTATCAGCTTTGGCCAGC-3′	242	DGGE

(*Continued*.)

TABLE 2. *Continued*

	Forward	Reverse	Product size (bp)	Mutation analysis method
SDHB 4	5′-GATTCCGGATATGGGTGAG-3′5′cgcccgccg cgccccgcgcccggcccgccgcccccgcccgaaataa taaaT5′	5′-cgtcccgcCCCCCATGCAAATAAAAACA-3′	256	DGGE
SDHB 5	5′-gcgcgTGATGATGGAATCTGATCCT-3′	5′-cgcccgccgcgccccgcgcccggcccgccgcccccgcccgaaa taataaaCAGATTGAAACAATAAATAGGGA-3′	261	DGGE
SDHB 6	5′-cgcccgccgcgccccgcgcccggcccgccgcccccgccc gaaataataaaCCTCTCTTTTCTCCCCATAC-3′	5′-cgCAGCAATCTATTGTCCTCTTG-3′	252	DGGE
SDHB 7	5′-gcgcgAGCTAATCATCCCTGGTTTT-3′	5′-cgcccgccgcgccccgcgcccggcccgccgcccccgcccg aaataataaaTTGTGAGCACATGCTACTTC-3′	270	DGGE
SDHB 8	5′-cgcccgccgcgccccgcgcccggcccgccgcccccgcccg GTGGGTTTTCCCTTTCAGTT-3′	5′-cgcccgccgcgccccgcgcccggcccgccgcccccgccc gGTGGGTTTTCCCTTTCAGTT-3′	361	DGGE
SDHD 1	5′-cgcccgccgcgccccgcgcccggcccgccgcccccgcccg GTGGGTTTTCGACCTTGAGCCCTCA GGAACG-3′	5′-cgcccgccgcgccccgcgcccggcccgccgcccccgc ccgaaataataaaT5′-gcgcgTCAGGGTGGGA AGACCCCT-3′	153	DGGE
SDHD 2	5′-GATCATCCTAATGACTCTTTCC-3′	5′-AGCAGCAGCGATGGAGAGAA-3′	168	SSCP
SDHD 3	5′-ATCTGGTCCTTTTTG-3′	5′-cgcccgccgcgccccgcgcccggcccgccgcccccgcccg CTTTTATGA5′-gcgcgCAACTATATTTGGA ATTGCTATAC-3′	245	DGGE
SDHD 4	5′-GATTTTTTCTTTTTCT-3′	5′-cgcccgccgcgccccgcgcccggcccgccgcccccgcccg TGATGTTAT5′-gcgcgCAATTCTTCAAAGT ATGAAGTCA-3′	269	DGGE

DNA Sequencing

All samples demonstrating aberrant patterns were sequenced. PCR was performed in a final volume of 50 μL under identical conditions as the previous PCR, except that this mix contained 0.2 mM dNTPs instead of 0.02 mM dATPs and 0.8 μCi α^{32}P-dATP. The PCR products were purified using Nucleospin® Extract II (Macherey-Nagel, Düren, Germany) according to the manufacturer's instructions. The purification was followed by a sequence reaction using the BigDye® Terminator V3.1 cycle sequencing kit (Applied Biosystems, Foster City, CA). Two microliters of Termination Ready Reaction mix, 2 μL of 5 × Sequencing buffer, 1 μL forward or reverse primer (13.2 pM), and 14 μL of deionized water was added to 1 μL purified PCR product. The cycle sequencing program was performed for 25 cycles of 96°C for 10 sec, 50°C for 5 sec, and 4 min for 60°C. This was followed by a precipitation step, adding 13 μL deionized water, 3 μL 3M NaAc (pH 5.2), and 64 μL ethanol (100%) to the sequence reaction product and incubating overnight at room temperature before centrifuging 20 min at 14,000 rpm. After washing the samples with ethanol 70%, centrifuging them 10 min at 14,000 rpm, the pellets were resuspended in 20 μL formamide (Applied Biosystems, Warrington, UK). Products were analyzed on the ABI Prism 3100 genetic analyzer (Applied Biosystems).

RESULTS

Patients and Tissues

All patient characteristics have been summarized in TABLE 1. In our series of 10 patients, representing 6.4% of all cases of PCC in our institution over a 17-year period, 70% were in boys, 40% of patients presented with bilateral tumors, and 40% had mutations in RET or VHL (see below) or fulfilled the clinical criteria for VHL, leading to a diagnosis of MEN2A or VHL disease in two patients each. In contrast, there were neither extra-adrenal tumors nor tumors with malignant behavior, after an average follow-up of 12 years, in this group of patients.

Mutation Analysis

The results from the mutation analysis of RET exons 10, 11, and 16, as well as the entire coding region of VHL (3 exons), SDHB (8 exons), and SDHD (4 exons) are summarized in TABLE 1 as well. In three of these we found a germline RET or VHL mutation present in both normal and tumor DNA of these patients. In one patient the family history convincingly indicated the presence of VHL disease, although this could not be confirmed in the normal and PCC tumor tissue of this patient on account of the inferior DNA quality. Furthermore, one patient showed an S163P alteration in the SDHB gene, which was interpreted as a polymorphism, based on findings in the literature and our own investigations (data not shown). Although all tumors that were available for this study ($n = 14$) yielded sufficient DNA for analysis, 35% of amplicons tested did not give an analyzable result.

The result of the SSCP analysis of VHL exon 1 of patient F119 and the sequence result of the alteration in exon 5 of SDHB in patient F44 are shown in FIGURES 1A and 1B, respectively.

DISCUSSION

In this study we have shown that in a small series of childhood PCCs up to 40% of patients have familial disease as evidenced by the presence of germline mutations in RET and VHL. This finding indicates that routine molecular analysis and a thorough family history are essential in patients presenting with PCC under the age of 18.

The clinical findings of our patient series are generally in good agreement with the larger series of childhood PCC patients that have been published.[5–8] There is a male predominance, with 60–75% of patients being boys, compatible with a figure of 70% in this study. Secondly, childhood PCCs are frequently bilateral, ranging from 25% to 55% in the literature, in agreement with our finding of 40% bilateral tumors. There is less concordance on extra-adrenal occurrence, with one study in agreement with our results, reporting no extra-adrenal PCC, whereas there are two studies that found 8% and 18% of such localization. Finally, the issue of malignancy in childhood PCC is difficult to assess in the various published studies, as it is not always entirely clear what criteria for malignancy have been applied. In our opinion, only PCCs with histologically proven metastases can be classified as malignant, although an exception could be made for cases where elevated catecholamine levels persist after primary tumor resection and are supported by a positive metaiodobenzylguanidyl scan in an area of the body where chromaffin cells do not normally occur. Applying the above criteria, we did not find any malignant case, after an average follow-up of 12 years. Although there are recent attempts to develop histological criteria that might indicate malignancy, these studies await further confirmation.[10,11]

There are only few case studies that have reported on mutation analysis of RET, VHL, or the SDH genes in childhood PCC.[12,13] In one, an MEN2A family was identified when a father presented with a PCC first, and 18 years later his son had a medullary thyroid carcinoma (MTC).[12] In the other study, a *de novo* VHL germline mutation was unexpectedly discovered in an incidentally found adrenal PCC in a 10-year-old boy.[13] In the present study, we report two MEN2A patients, both with a C634R mutation in RET exon 11, and both presenting

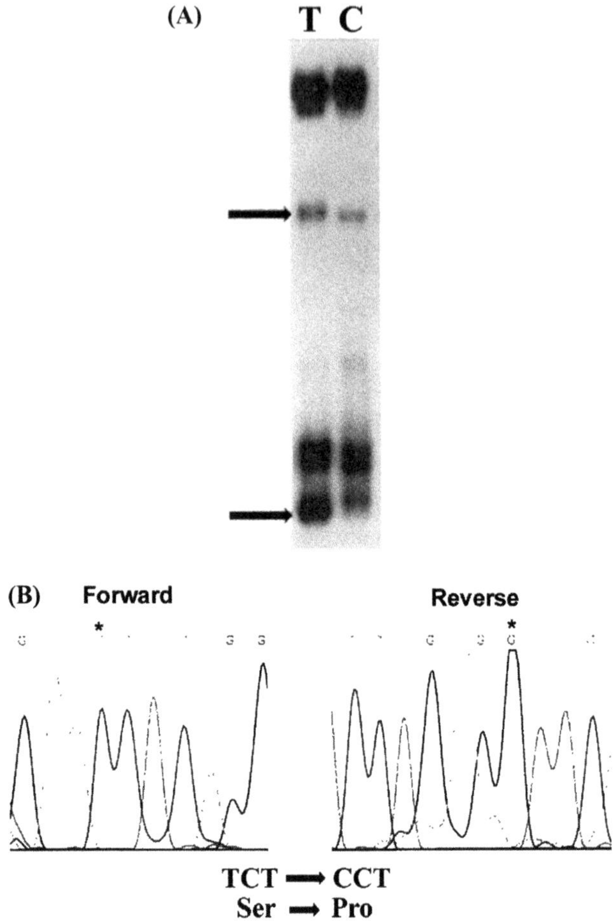

FIGURE 1. (**A**) Single strand conformational polymorphism analysis, showing comparison of the banding pattern of VHL exon 1 between tumor (T) and control (C) sample in patient F119. Clearly, the tumor sample shows the presence of two aberrant bands (*arrows*). Upon sequence analysis, a mutation in codon 64 was detected, leading to an amino acid change from arginine to proline. (**B**) Forward (*left*) and reverse (*right*) sequence analysis results from SDHB exon 5 in patient F44, showing a TCT to CCT change, indicated by an *asterisk*, leading to an amino acid change from serine to proline. Because this change occured at equal frequency in normal individuals and PCC patients, this alteration is regarded as a polymorphism, and not as a tumor-related mutation.

with bilateral PCCs. Although all tests were performed without knowledge of the clinical patient history, it was revealed after genetic analysis that both patients came from MEN2A families that had already been recognized. It is interesting to note that the particular mutation in these patients has been associated with a more aggressive phenotype of MTC, although such prognostic information is lacking for PCC behavior.[14] Further, we found one patient with an exon 1 VHL mutation, who also came from a known VHL family. One other patient also came from a family with a clinical history that was compatible with VHL, presenting with two hemangioblastomas and a clear-cell renal cell carcinoma in addition to the PCC. Because of the relatively inferior DNA quality, however, we could not obtain a result for all VHL exons tested in this patient, which may have led to our failure to detect a VHL mutation. Alternatively, there may have been other *VHL* gene abnormalities, such as a large deletion, which we may have missed with our technique, although VHL patients with PCCs usually have missense mutations. Finally, there was one patient in whom we found a missense alteration in exon 5 of SDHB. Although this alteration represents an amino acid change in this codon, the same change is found in 2.3% of a control population in the literature, which is comparable to the frequency that we have found in a series of 150 PCCs in our laboratory (unpublished data), favoring the idea that this change should be considered a polymorphism.[15] Apart from these patients with known tumor syndromes, there was one girl who presented with metachronous bilateral PCCs at the ages of 13 and 17 years, who also had several other benign tumors or tumor-like conditions, including multinodular adrenocortical hyperplasia, a fibroadenoma of the breast, as well as hemihypertrophy. This patient has been extensively discussed in a separate case report, to which the reader is referred.[16]

In conclusion, mutation analysis of the most relevant candidate genes presently available, including VHL, RET, SDHB, and SDHD, reveals a mutation frequency of 40% in a small series of childhood PCCs, which strongly favors mutation screening in each childhood PCC patient in a prospective fashion. The presence of other tumors or congenital abnormalities in such patients should be registered as well, to facilitate investigations into other disease-causing genes.

REFERENCES

1. Dannenberg, H. *et al.* 2000. Losses of chromosomes 1p and 3q are early genetic events in the development of sporadic pheochromocytomas. Am. J. Pathol. **157:** 353–359.
2. Dannenberg, H. *et al.* 2001. Differential loss of chromosome 11q in familial and sporadic parasympathetic paragangliomas detected by comparative genomic hybridization. Am. J. Pathol. **158:** 1937–1942.
3. Neumann, H.P.H. *et al.* 2002. Germ-line mutations in nonsyndromic pheochromocytoma. N. Engl. J. Med. **346:** 1459–1466.
4. Bryant, J. *et al.* 2003. Pheochromocytoma: the expanding genetic differential diagnosis. J. Natl. Cancer Inst. **95:** 1196–1204.
5. Révillon, Y. *et al.* 1992. Pheochromocytoma in children: 15 cases. J. Pediatr. Surg. **27:** 910–911.

6. PEREL, Y. *et al.* 1997. Pheochromocytoma and paraganglioma in children: a report of 24 cases of the French Society of Pediatric Oncology. Pediatr. Hematol. Oncol. **14:** 413–422.
7. CIFTCI, A.O. *et al.* 2001. Pheochromocytoma in children. J. Pediatr. Surg. **36:** 447–452.
8. BELTSEVICH, D.G. *et al.* 2004. Pheochromocytoma surgery: epidemiologic peculiarities in children. World J. Surg. **28:** 592–596.
9. KOMMINOTH, P. *et al.* 1994. Detection of RET proto-oncogene point mutations in paraffin-embedded pheochromocytoma specimens by nonradioactive single-strand conformation polymorphism analysis and direct sequencing. Am. J. Pathol. **145:** 922–929.
10. THOMPSON, L.D. 2002. Pheochromocytoma of the Adrenal gland Scaled Score (PASS) to separate benign from malignant neoplasms: a clinicopathologic and immunophenotypic study of 100 cases. Am. J. Surg. Pathol. **26:** 551–566.
11. KIMURA, N. *et al.* 2005. Histological grading of adrenal and extra-adrenal pheochromocytomas and relationship to prognosis: a clinicopathological analysis of 116 adrenal pheochromocytomas and 30 extra-adrenal sympathetic paragangliomas including 38 malignant tumors. Endocr. Pathol. **16:** 23–32.
12. BECK, O. *et al.* 2004. Pheochromocytoma in childhood: implications for further diagnostic procedures. Acta Paediatr. **93:** 1630–1634.
13. POZO, J. *et al.* 2005. Sporadic pheochromocytoma in childhood: clinical and molecular variability. J. Pediatr. Endocrinol. Metab. **18:** 527–532.
14. SZINNAI, G. *et al.* 2003. Review of multiple endocrine neoplasia type 2A in children: therapeutic results of early thyroidectomy and prognostic value of codon analysis. Pediatrics. **111:** E132–E139.
15. CASCON, A. *et al.* 2004. Genetic and epigenetic profile of sporadic pheochromocytomas. J. Med. Genet. **41:** e30.
16. VAN DEN AKKER, E.L.T. *et al.* 2002. Congenital hemihypertrophy and pheochromocytoma, not a coincidental combination? Eur. J. Pediatr. **161:** 157–160.

The Occurrence of SDHB Gene Mutations in Pheochromocytoma

FRANCIEN H. VAN NEDERVEEN, WINAND N. M. DINJENS, ESTHER KORPERSHOEK, AND RONALD R. DE KRIJGER

Department of Pathology, Josephine Nefkens Institute, Erasmus MC—University Medical Center Rotterdam, Rotterdam, the Netherlands

ABSTRACT: Pheochromocytomas (PCCs) are rare tumors arising from neural crest–derived chromaffin cells. The majority of these tumors are located in the adrenals and gives rise to catecholamine overproduction. In at least 10% of the cases the tumors are located outside the adrenal gland, in extra-adrenal sites like the bladder and the organ of Zuckerkandl. Recent investigations have found mutations in succinate dehydrogenase subunit B (SDHB), the gene coding for subunit B of the respiratory chain complex II. Mutations in the SDHB gene, with additional loss of the wild-type allele, result in loss of function of respiratory complex II and appear to correlate with extra-adrenal location of PCCs. Also, a link has been established between malignant behavior and inactivating mutations of SDHB. In this article we review the published SDHB gene mutations, as well as the location and behavior of the resulting PCCs.

KEYWORDS: pheochromocytoma (PCC); succinate dehydrogenase subunit B (SDHB); genetics; extra-adrenal; malignancy

INTRODUCTION

Pheochromocytomas (PCCs) are rare catecholamine-producing tumors located in the adrenal medulla, but they occur elsewhere in the abdomen in approximately 10% of cases, including the organ of Zuckerkandl, the bladder, and the prostate. Recent research has indicated that approximately 20–25% of PCCs are hereditary and caused by mutations in one of four genes that are responsible for three heritable (endocrine) tumor syndromes, including multiple endocrine neoplasia type 2 (MEN2), von Hippel–Lindau disease (VHL), and the pheochromocytoma–paraganglioma (PCC–PGL) syndrome.[1] The latter syndrome is caused by mutations in one of three genes encoding subunits of the mitochondrial respiratory chain complex II, succinate dehydrogenase subunits B, C, and D (SDHB, SDHC, and SDHD).

Address for correspondence: F. H. van Nederveen, M.D., Erasmus MC—University Medical Center Rotterdam, Josephine Nefkens Institute, Room Be 232, P. O. Box 1738, 3000 DR, Rotterdam, the Netherlands. Voice: +31-10-408-7901; fax: +31-10-408-9478.
e-mail: f.vannederveen@erasmusmc.nl

Ann. N.Y. Acad. Sci. 1073: 177–182 (2006). © 2006 New York Academy of Sciences.
doi: 10.1196/annals.1353.018

SDHD was the first of these genes to be discovered, and is located on 11q23, corresponding to the putative PGL1 region. Large series of apparently sporadic PCCs have been screened for mutations in the SDHD gene, which were found at low frequency.[2,3] The majority of patients that harbored an SDHD mutation were diagnosed with head and neck PGL.[3–5] A recent publication, however, reports the occurrence of PCC in 20% of patients harboring a mutation in SDHD or having a positive family history for head and neck PGL.[6] With respect to SDHC, located on 1q21, to date only few gene mutations have been found, with no convincing evidence of other tumors than head and neck PGL. In contrast, SDHB germline mutations were found in several PCCs, including apparently sporadic tumors. SDHB is located in the putative PGL4 region, and is mapped to 1p36. A correlation between SDHB mutations and both extra-adrenal location and malignant behavior has been described in the literature.[7–9] In this article we review the presently published SDHB mutations in PCC in relation to the location and clinical behavior of these tumors.

SDHB FUNCTION

The mitochondrial complex II, which is responsible for electron transport in the respiratory chain, is composed of four subunits. In addition, this complex plays an important role in the Krebs cycle. SDHB is one of the four subunits of the complex, and together with the A subunit forms the catalytic domain, whereas the C and D subunits are the integral membrane proteins. In the catalytic domain the B subunit is an iron sulfur protein, and the A subunit is a flavoprotein.

Recently, a link has been established between the hypoxic phenotype of VHL-related tumors, which include PCC, and the PCCs resulting from SDHB and SDHD mutations, all showing decreased oxidoreductase activity, through comparison of RNA expression profiles of these tumor groups. It was suggested that in all VHL- or SDH-related PCCs, hypoxia-inducible factor 1α (HIF1α) plays a central role in a cascade of events that ultimately lead to reduced SDHB protein expression.[10]

SDHB GENE MUTATIONS IN PCC

So far, no somatic SDHB mutations and only a single somatic SDHD mutation have been described.[11] For this paper, we have analyzed the literature for germline SDHB mutations in families and in patients with apparently sporadic PCCs. Apparently patients with sporadic disease are those with a negative family history for PCC and/or PGL at any location. Patients with familial disease are defined as those with a PCC and at least one other family member with a PCC and/or a PGL at any location. These data have been summarized in

TABLE 1. SDHB gene mutations in familial PCC

Exon/Intron	Mutation	Location[a]	Malignancy	Reference	Number of families
Exon 2	K40E	EA	No	12	1
Exon 2	R46X	EA	No	13	1
Exon 2	R46Q	A	No	13	1
Exon 2	88 del C	Unknown	Yes	13	1
Exon 2	R64Q	A	No	13	1
Exon 2	L65H[b]	EA	Yes	13	1
Intron	Inv2 + 3 G/C[b]	EA	Yes	13	1
Exon 3	R90X	EA	Yes	13, 14	4
		EA	Unknown		
		EA	Unknown		
		A	Unknown		
Exon 4	H132P	EA	Yes	8	1
Exon 5	INVS4-1G>A	EA	No	13	1
Exon 6	P197R	EA	No	14, 3	2
Exon 6	R242H	EA	Yes	15	
Intron	inv 4-1G>A	EA	No	13	1
	1kb deletion 5′	EA	No	16	1

[a]A = adrenal; EA = extra-adrenal.
[b]Same patient.

TABLES 1 and 2, respectively. When available the tumor location and the clinical behavior are indicated. A total of 16 families has been described, comprising 36 individuals carrying an SDHB germline mutation.[3,8,12–16] In these families, 14 different mutations or other genetic abnormalities have been found in the SDHB gene, without evidence for a mutation hotspot. Because most studies performed so far are case reports, and no population-based analysis has been done, the frequency of familial SDHB mutations in the general population remains unclear. In addition, a total number of 527 patients with apparently sporadic PCC has been investigated.[1,3,7,9,10,14] In these, 34 individuals with a germline SDHB mutation were found, representing 6.5% of all apparently sporadic PCCs. Again, no mutation hotspot regions in the SDHB gene were noted.

SDHB GENE MUTATIONS AND MALIGNANT BEHAVIOR

In general, the frequency of malignant behavior in PCC is 10%. It would be expected that in the group of 34 sporadic and 16 familial cases of PCC (see TABLES 1 and 2), all carrying germline SDHB mutations, approximately 5 tumors would be malignant, if allowing for sufficient follow-up. However, according to the published data, at least 6 familial and 12 sporadic PCC were malignant, leading to an overall frequency of 36%, which is more than threefold higher than expected. It should be added at this point that the follow-up period has not been specified in all studies, which could potentially lead to an even

TABLE 2. SDHB gene mutations in apparently sporadic PCC

Exon	Mutation	Location[a]	Malignancy	Reference	Families
Exon 1	155 del C	EA	Yes	9	1
Exon 2	R27X	EA	Unknown	1	1
Exon 2	A29-Q30 insertion	EA	Unknown	1	1
Exon 2	A43P	EA	Yes	7	1
Exon 2	R46G	EA	Yes	1, 7	3
		A	No		
		A	No		
Exon 2	R46Q	A	Yes	7, 9	3
		EA+A	Unknown		
		A	Yes		
Exon 2	G53R	A	Unknown	9	1
Exon 2	300-4 del CCTCA	A	Yes	9	1
Exon 2	L65P	EA+A	Unknown	9	1
Exon 3	L87S	A	Yes	9	3
		EA	Unknown		
		EA	Unknown		
Exon 4	C101Y	EA	Unknown	1	2
Exon 4	I127N	A	Unknown	3	1
Exon 5	inv 4-3C>G	Unknown	Unknown	10	1
Exon 5	558-3 C/G	EA	Yes	9	1
Exon 6	C192R	EA	Unknown	1	1
Exon 6	C196Y	EA	Unknown	1	1
Exon 6	S198R	Unknown	Unknown	10	1
Exon 6	D221X	A	Unknown	3	1
Exon 6	R230C	Unknown	Unknown	10	1
Exon 6	725 del C	A	No	14, 7	2
		EA	Unknown		
Exon 6	754-55 del TG	EA	Yes	7	2
		EA	Yes		
Exon 7	847-49 del TCTC	EA	No	1, 9	2
		A	Yes		
Exon 7	F230 C	A	Yes	7	1
Exon 7	R242H	EA	Yes	1,9	1
Exon 7	C249X	EA	Unknown	1	1

[a]A = adrenal; EA = extra-adrenal.

higher frequency of malignancy. This is also true for the fact that in 18 cases of sporadic PCC the clinical behavior has been reported as unknown.[1,3,7,9,10,14] Taken together, the joint data clearly support the notion that SDHB mutations are related to malignant behavior.

SDHB GENE MUTATIONS AND EXTRA-ADRENAL LOCATION

As for the frequency of malignancy, the frequency of extra-adrenal occurrence of PCC has been reported as 10%. Again, this would mean that 5 of the

52 published cases would involve an extra-adrenal tumor. However, 13 familial and 20 sporadic PCCs were located outside the adrenal glands, yielding a frequency of 66%, which is more than sixfold higher than expected.[1,3,7–9,12–16] There were one familial and three sporadic cases of PCC in which the tumor location was unknown, leaving 3 familial and 11 sporadic PCCs with an adrenal location. This clearly indicates a correlation between extra-adrenal location of PCC and the presence of SDHB gene mutations.

CONCLUSION

In view of an aggregate mutation frequency of 25% in the four candidate genes for PCC, we recommend genetic testing of each PCC for RET, VHL, SDHD, and SDHB. In case of a malignant or extra-adrenal PCC, with or without a positive family history, SDHB mutation analysis would appear to be the first choice. Furthermore, finding germline SDHB mutations has important implications for index patients and their family members, as SDHB-related PCCs are often extra-adrenal and malignant.

REFERENCES

1. NEUMANN, H.P.H. *et al.* 2002. Germ-line mutations in nonsyndromic pheochromocytomas. N. Engl. J. Med. **19:** 1459–1466.
2. DANNENBERG, H. *et al.* 2005. Clinical characteristics of pheochromocytoma patients with germline mutations in SDHD. J. Clin. Oncol. **23:** 1894–1901.
3. ASTUTI, D. *et al.* 2003. Genetic analysis of mitochondrial complex II subunits SDHD, SDHB and SDHC in paraganglioma and phaeochromocytoma susceptibility. Clin. Endocrinol. **59:** 728–733.
4. BAYSAL, B.E. *et al.* 2002. Prevalence of SDHB, SDHC, and SDHD germline mutations in clinic patients with head and neck paragangliomas. J. Med. Genet. **39:** 178–183.
5. DANNENBERG, H. *et al.* 2002. Frequent germ-line succinate dehydrogenase subunit D gene mutations in patients with apparently sporadic parasympathetic paraganglioma. Clin. Cancer Res. **8:** 2061–2066.
6. VAN HOUTUM, W.H. *et al.* 2005. Increased prevalence of catecholamine excess and phaeochromocytomas in a well-defined Dutch population with SDHD-linked head and neck paragangliomas. Eur. J. Endocrinol. **152:** 87–94.
7. GIMENEZ-ROQUEPLO, A. *et al.* 2003. Mutations in the SDHB gene are associated with extra-adrenal and/or malignant pheochromocytomas. Cancer Res. **63:** 5615–5621.
8. MAIER-WOELFLE, M. *et al.* 2004. A novel succinate dehydrogenase subunit B gene mutation, H132P, causes familial malignant sympathetic extraadrenal paragangliomas. J. Clin. Endocrinol. Metab. **89:** 362–367.
9. NEUMANN, H.P. *et al.* 2004. Distinct clinical features of paraganglioma syndromes associated with SDHB and SDHD gene mutations. JAMA **292:** 943–951.
10. DAHIA, P.L. *et al.* 2005. A HIF1 alpha regulatory loop links hypoxia and mitochondrial signals in pheochromocytomas. PLoS Genet. Epub July 25.

11. GIMM, O. *et al.* 2000. Somatic and occult germ-line mutations in SDHD, a mitochondrial complex II gene, in nonfamilial pheochromocytoma. Cancer Res. **60:** 6822–6825.
12. MCDONNELL, C.M. *et al.* 2004. K40E: a novel succinate dehydrogenase (SDH)B mutation causing familial pheochromocytoma and paraganglioma. Clin. Endocrinol. **61:** 510–514.
13. BENN, D.E. *et al.* 2003. Novel succinate dehydrogenase subunit B (SDHB) mutations in familial phaeochromocytomas and paragangliomas, but an absence of somatic SDHB mutations in sporadic phaeochromocytomas. Oncogene **22:** 1358–1364.
14. ASTUTI, D. *et al.* 2001. Gene mutations in the succinate dehydrogenase subunit SDHB cause susceptibilty to familial pheochromocytoma and familial paraganglioma. Am. J. Hum. Genet. **69:** 49–54.
15. YOUNG, A.L. *et al.* 2002. Familial malignant cathecholamine-secreting paraganglioa with prolonged survival associated with mutation in the succinate dehydrogenase B gene. J. Clin. Endocrinol. Metab. **87:** 4101–4105.
16. MCWHINNEY, S.R. *et al.* 2004. Large germline deletions of mitochondrial complex II subunits SDHB and SDHD in hereditary paraganglioma. J. Clin. Endocrinol. Metab. **89:** 5694–5699.

SDH Mutations in Patients Affected by Paraganglioma Syndromes

A Personal Experience

M. MANNELLI,[a] L. SIMI,[b] T. ERCOLINO,[a] M.S. GAGLIANÒ,[a] L. BECHERINI,[a] S. VINCI,[b] R. SESTINI,[c] F. GENSINI,[c] P. PINZANI,[b] M. MASCALCHI,[d] L. GUERRINI,[d] C. PRATESI,[e] G. NESI,[f] F. TORTI,[g] F. CIPOLLINI,[h] G.P. BERNINI,[i] AND M. GENUARDI[c]

[a]Section of Endocrinology, [b]Clinical Biochemistry, [c]Medical Genetic, and [d]Radiology, Department of Clinical Physiopathology, [e]Section of Vascular Surgery, Department of Clinical and Surgical Critical Care, and [f]Department of Human Pathology and Oncology, University of Florence Medical School, Florence, Italy
[g]ICP Istituti Clinici di Perfezionamento, Padiglione Alfieri, Milan, Italy
[h]Internal Medicine 2, Pistoia Hospital, Pistoia, Italy
[i]Department of Internal Medicine, University of Pisa, Pisa, Italy

ABSTRACT: Mutations in genes encoding mitochondrial succinate dehydrogenase (SDH) are frequently involved in the development of neural crest-derived (NCD) tumors, such as pheochromocytomas (PHEOs) or paragangliomas (PGLs). In this study we report the results of sequencing analysis in leukocyte DNA of patients affected by PHEO/PGL who turned out to be SDH mutation carriers. A nonsense germline heterozygous mutation (Q109X) was found in the exon 4 of the SDHD gene in the index cases of six unrelated families affected by PHEO/PGL. Haplotype analysis showed the presence of a founder effect. Affected patients showed high clinical variability, ranging from monolateral to bilateral glomus tumors, variably associated or not with PGLs or PHEOs. A novel missense SDHD variant, T112I, was also found in one of our families. A new missense G106D mutation, involving a highly conserved amino acid, was found in two sisters affected by bilateral glomus tumors. A P81L mutation associated with abdominal and head and neck PGL was detected in three families. A G12S variant of the SDHD gene was found in one patient affected by a PHEO. The finding of this variant in 3 of 100 control subjects suggests that it is a polymorphism and not a mutation. A novel IVS2-1G>T variant was found at intron 2 of SDHD gene in one patient affected by a glomus tumor. All the tumors associated with SDHD

Address for correspondence: Prof. M. Mannelli, Endocrinology Section, Department of Clinical Physiopathology, University of Florence, Viale Pieraccini 6 50139, Florence, Italy. Voice: ++39-055-4271428; fax: ++39-055-4271413.
e-mail: m.mannelli@dfc.unifi.it

Ann. N.Y. Acad. Sci. 1073: 183–189 (2006). © 2006 New York Academy of Sciences.
doi: 10.1196/annals.1353.019

mutations were benign. Conversely, the only mutation we found in SDHB gene (IVS3 + 1G>A) was associated with a malignant PHEO.

Keywords: succinate dehydrogenase; founder effect; neural crest–derived tumors

INTRODUCTION

Succinate dehydrogenase (SDH) is the major component of the mitochondrial complex II of the respiratory chain, and consists of four nuclear-encoded polypeptides: the flavoprotein (SDHA), the iron sulfur protein (SDHB), and the two integral membrane proteins, SDHC and SDHD. The mitochondrial complex II is involved in both the tricarboxylic acid cycle and the aerobic respiratory chain, where it performs the oxidation of succinate and is responsible for the electron transport from FADH to CoQ.

In several recent studies it has been shown that germline mutations of SDHD, SDHC, and SDHB genes are responsible for hereditary paraganglioma syndromes named PGL-1, PGL-3, and PGL-4, respectively. SDHD is reported to be the most commonly mutated gene in multiple and benign head and neck paragangliomas (PGLs), while SDHB seems to be frequently associated with malignant and abdominal tumors.[1–5]

In this article we report on the SDH mutations found at genetic analysis in a series of patients affected by pheochromocytomas (PHEOs) or PGLs.

PATIENTS AND MATERIALS

Fifty-three patients affected by single, multiple, or recurrent PHEOs or PGLs, with or without a positive family history, were systematically evaluated for the presence of germline mutations in the susceptibility genes VHL, RET, SDHB, SDHC, and SDHD.

Each patient gave written informed consent for genetic analysis. Genomic DNA was extracted from leukocytes using a commercial kit and following manufacturer's instructions (NucleoSpin Blood L, Macherey-Nagel, Duren, Germany). DNA sequencing analysis was performed by using Big Dye Terminator chemistry and electropherograms were obtained by using ABIPrism 310 Genetic Analyser (Applied Biosystems, Foster City, CA). Amplification of SDHB, SDHD, and SDHC exons was performed using specific primers as previously reported.[6]

Tumor specimens were obtained at surgery and immediately frozen in liquid nitrogen. Microdissection of frozen tissue sections was performed using PALM laser microbeam system (PALM Microlaser Technologies AG, Bernried, Germany) that allows isolation of single cells or groups of cells. Microdissected cells were isolated from sections stained with hematoxylin and eosin mounted onto a polyethylene membrane slide and catapulted into the lid of a 0.5-mL reaction tube using the laser pressure catapulting technique of the instrument. For the DNA isolation, tubes were incubated overnight at 37°C with 20 mL of proteinase K digestion buffer (20 mmol/L Tris pH 8.0, 2 mmol/L EDTA, 0.5% Igepal CA-630 (Sigma, Milano, Italy), and 20 mg/mL proteinase K), and then inactivated at 95°C for 10 min. Lysate was directly used for subsequent polymerase chain reaction (PCR) and sequencing analysis to assess loss of heterozygosity (LOH).

Simple tandem repeat polymorphisms used for SDHD haplotype analysis have been described previously.[2] Genotypes in our samples were established for markers D11S5017, D11S5015, D11S5019, D11S5030, and D11S1347. All markers were amplified using fluorescently labeled primers under standard PCR conditions and amplicons submitted to ABI Prism 310 GeneScan analysis.

RESULTS

Genetic analysis assessed the presence of two VHL, one SDHB, and six different SDHD variants, while no mutations were found in RET and SDHC genes.

All the SDH variants found in our experience are listed in TABLE 1. All the tumors associated with SDHD mutations were benign, while the SDHB-mutated PHEO reported a malignant result.

The most frequent SDHD mutation was constituted by a C to T substitution in exon 4 leading to a stop codon (Q109X). This mutation was found in six index cases of six apparently unrelated families. Haplotype analysis spanning a region of 304 bp did not show any evidence of a recombination event and demonstrated the presence of a founder effect. These data have been reported in detail in a recent article.[6]

TABLE 1. SDHB and SDHD mutations found in the present study and some of their principal characteristics

Gene	Name	Type	Region	Conserved Domain	Phenotype	Reference
SDHB	IVS3+1G>A	Splicing site	Intron 3	–	Pheo	Undescribed
SDHD	Q109X	Nonsense mutation	Exon 4	High	PGL-Pheo	2, 6
	T112L	Rare variant	Exon 4	Low	None/Pheo	Undescribed
	G106D	Missense mutation	Exon 4	Very high	PGL	Undescribed
	P81L	Missense mutation	Exon 3	High	Pheo/PGL	2, 7–11
	G12S	Polymorphism	Exon 1	Very low	Pheo	3, 10, 12–15
	IVS2-1G>T	Splicing site	Intron 2	–	PGL	16

So far, 44 of 83 heterozygote carriers were identified (21 females and 23 males).

Affected patients and family members who accepted to participate underwent measurement of urinary metanephrines and plasma chromogranin A as well as extensive radiologic examinations (NMR of the neck, thorax, and abdomen and scintigraphy with ^{123}I-metaiodobenylguanidine and/or ^{111}In-pentetreotide to investigate the presence of neural crest–derived (NCD) tumors. Eighteen affected patients were identified (8 males and 10 females) and 51 tumors documented, 4 PHEOs and 47 PGL. The majority of PGLs were in the head–neck region ($n = 37$), followed by abdominal ($n = 8$) and thoracic PGLs ($n = 2$). Secreting tumors were revealed in six patients—three affected by PHEO (one bilateral), two by abdominal PGL and one by thoracic PGL. Plasma chromogranin A was elevated in 71% of patients. Patients with only head–neck PGLs did not show elevated levels of urinary metanephrines. The mean age of clinical presentation was 39 years (range 14–69 years). Penetrance was 33% to 83% at 30 and 60 years, respectively. Affected patients showed high clinical variability in the age of onset, in the type of clinical presentation, and in the number, localization, and secreting properties of the tumors. In one of these families we also identified a novel missense SDHD variant (T112I) that segregated independently from the Q109X mutation. The T112I variation was not detected in 100 control subjects and in the six mutated members of our family it was not associated with any clinical manifestations, while the same mutation has been found in one unrelated patient affected by PHEO (Opocher and Schiavi, personal data). As the affected patient shows the same haplotype, this variant is probably to be considered a low-penetrance mutation. Sequencing performed on DNA extracted from tumoral cells isolated by laser capture–microdissection techniques demonstrated loss of maternal wild-type allele. Microsatellite analysis is still to be done in order to define the extension of allelic loss.

The P81L mutation was found in three index cases. Overall four NCD tumors were revealed: one glomus tumor, one thoracic PGL, one abdominal PGL, and one PHEO; the last two were secreting tumors. A 30-year-old man who inherited this germline mutation from the father is still unaffected by NCD tumors. This mutation has been previously reported in several studies.[2,7–11] Whether this mutation is recurrent or due to a founder effect is still controversial. In our experience, haplotype analysis revealed different results from those previously described.

A new missense mutation in exon 4 (G106D) has been found in two sisters affected by bilateral glomus tumors. This mutation was not found in 100 control samples. Moreover, glycine at codon 106 is conserved in all the species available in the GenBank database (see TABLE 2), suggesting the importance of this residue for conformational and/or enzymatic function of SDHD protein.

The G12S variant was found in one patient with a secreting PHEO. This variant has been previously reported and it is still unclear whether it represents

TABLE 2. Degree of interspecies amino acid conservation at loci where SDHD mutations have been found in exon 4

Genus and species	Amino acid position								Length
	106	107	108	109	110	111	112	113	
Bos taurus	G	I	G	Q	V	V	T	D	158 aa
Mus musculus	G	L	G	Q	V	V	T	D	159 aa
Rattus norvegicus	G	I	G	Q	V	V	T	D	158 aa
Xenopus tropicalis	G	L	G	Q	V	V	T	D	152 aa
Danio rerio	G	L	G	Q	V	V	T	D	158 aa
Branchiostoma belcheri	G	F	E	Q	I	L	T	D	154 aa
Drosophila melanogaster	G	V	E	A	M	V	V	D	182 aa
Drosophila pseudosomas	G	V	E	A	M	V	V	D	182 aa
Caernorhabditis elegans	G	I	H	G	V	V	Y	D	145 aa
Neurospora crassa	G	F	G	N	I	I	V	D	166 aa
Aspergillus	G	S	Q	A	S	I	I	D	171 aa

a polymorphism or a mutation.[3,10,12–15] In our experience, analysis performed in 100 control samples has revealed the presence of the same variant in three healthy subjects confirming that it is a polymorphism.

The IVS-1G>T mutation was found in a patient affected by a glomus tumor. This mutation involves a splice site and functional analysis defining its role in the transcription has already been reported by other authors.[16]

An intronic mutation (IVS3 + 1G>A) involving a splice site at intron 3 of SDHB gene was found in one patient affected with a malignant PHEO. The extent to which this mutation affects gene function is at present under investigation.

CONCLUSIONS

In this study 15 of 53 patients (28.3%) affected with NCD tumors, with or without a family history of PHEO/PGL, were found to be a carrier of germline mutation in one of the susceptibility genes.

In our series, the most frequent variant was found in the SDHD gene. Among these six variants, three were found in exon 4 in the amino acid region (ranging from 106th to 112th position), one in exon 3, one in exon 1, and one intronic. All the tumors detected in SDHD mutation carriers had a benign manifestation and were found in patients deriving the mutation from the father, thus confirming the apparent maternal imprinting.

Clinical variability was a constant feature of PGL1, even in families affected by the same founder mutation.

The single SDHB mutation was associated with a malignant PHEO, thus confirming the widely reported association between SDHB mutations and malignancy.

Our study confirms the importance of genetic analysis in the clinical management of patients affected by NCD tumors.

ACKNOWLEDGMENTS

This work was partly supported by grants from MIUR (Ministero dell'Istruzione, dell'Universitá e della Ricerca) (prot. 2004069534) and the Department of Clinical Pathophysiology, University of Florence.

REFERENCES

1. BAYSAL, B.E. 2002. Hereditary paraganglioma targets diverse paraganglia. J. Med. Genet. **39:** 617–622.
2. BAYSAL, B.E. *et al.* 2002. Prevalence of SDHB, SDHC, and SDHD germline mutations in clinic patients with head and neck paragangliomas. J. Med. Genet. **39:** 178–183.
3. GIMENEZ-ROQUEPLO, A.P. *et al.* 2003. Mutations in the SDHB gene are associated with extra-adrenal and/or malignant phaeochromocytomas. Cancer Res. **63:** 5615–5621.
4. BENN, D.E. *et al.* 2003. Novel succinate dehydrogenase subunit B (SDHB) mutations in familial phaeochromocytomas and paragangliomas, but an absence of somatic SDHB mutations in sporadic phaeochromocytomas. Oncogene **22:** 1358–1364.
5. NEUMANN, H.P. *et al.* AND THE EUROPEAN AMERICAN PARAGANGLIOMA STUDY GROUP. 2004. Distinct clinical features of paraganglioma syndromes associated with SDHB and SDHD gene mutations. JAMA **292:** 943–951 [Erratum in JAMA **292:** 1686].
6. SIMI, L. *et al.* 2005. Phenotype variability of neural crest derived tumours in six Italian families segregating the same founder SDHD mutation Q109X. J. Med. Genet. **42:** e52.
7. MHATRE, A.N. *et al.* 2004. SDHB, SDHC, and SDHD mutation screen in sporadic and familial head and neck paragangliomas. Clin. Genet. **66:** 461–466.
8. ASTUTI, D. *et al.* 2003. Genetic analysis of mitochondrial complex II subunits SDHD, SDHB and SDHC in paraganglioma and phaeochromocytoma susceptibility. Clin. Endocrinol. **59:** 728–733.
9. MILUNSKY, J.M. *et al.* 2001. Novel mutations and the emergence of a common mutation in the SDHD gene causing familial paraganglioma. Am. J. Med. Genet. **100:** 311–314.
10. GIMM, O. *et al.* 2000. Somatic and occult germ-line mutations in SDHD, a mitochondrial complex II gene, in nonfamilial PHEOchromocytoma. Cancer Res. **60:** 6822–6825.
11. BAYSAL, B.E. 2000. Mutations in SDHD, a mitochondrial complex II gene, in hereditary paraganglioma. Science **287:** 848–851.
12. LEUBE, B. *et al.* 2004. SDHD mutation analysis in seven German patients with sporadic carotid body paraganglioma: one novel mutation, no Dutch founder mutation and further evidence that G12S is a polymorphism. Clin. Genet. **65:** 61–63.

13. CASCON, A. *et al.* 2003. G12S and H50R variations are polymorphisms in the SDHD gene. Genes Chromosomes Cancer **37:** 220–221.
14. PERREN, A. *et al.* 2002. Absence of somatic SDHD mutations in sporadic neuroendocrine tumors and detection of two germline variants in paraganglioma patients. Oncogene **21:** 7605–7608.
15. KYTOLA, S. *et al.* 2002. Alterations of the SDHD gene locus in midgut carcinoids, Merkel cell carcinomas, PHEOchromocytomas, and abdominal paragangliomas. Genes Chromosomes Cancer **34:** 325–332.
16. RENARD, L. *et al.* 2003. A novel mutation in the SDHD gene in a family with inherited paragangliomas—implications of genetic diagnosis for follow up and treatment. Head Neck **25:** 146–151.

Paraganglioma Syndrome

SDHB, SDHC, and SDHD Mutations in Head and Neck Paragangliomas

FRANCESCA SCHIAVI,[a] THEODOROS SAVVOUKIDIS,[a] FRANCO TRABALZINI,[b] FRANCO GREGO,[c] MICHELE PIAZZA,[c] PIETRO AMISTÀ,[d] SERENA DEMATTÈ,[e] ANTONELLA DEL PIANO,[e] MARIA ENRICA CECCHINI,[e] ZORAN ERLIC,[a] PAOLA DE LAZZARI,[a] FRANCO MANTERO,[a] AND GIUSEPPE OPOCHER[a]

[a]*Department of Endocrinology, Padova University Hospital, Padova, Italy*

[b]*Department of Oto-Surgery, Padova University Hospital, Padova, Italy*

[c]*Department of Vascular Surgery, Padova University Hospital, Padova, Italy*

[d]*Department of Neuroradiology, Padova University Hospital, Padova, Italy*

[e]*S.Chiara Hospital, Trento, Italy*

ABSTRACT: Paraganglioma syndrome includes head and neck paraganglioma and pheochromocytoma, and is classified according to the three susceptibility genes involved, SDHB, SDHC, and SDHD. This study assessed the prevalence of germline mutations in SDHB, SDHC, and SDHD genes in a consecutive population admitted to Padova Hospital consisting of 20 patients with head and neck paraganglioma (HNP). Mutations were identified in the three genes in four affected individuals, three sporadic cases and one with family history of HNP. The novel SDHB p.R242C mutation was identified in a sporadic monolateral carotid body tumor. The SDHC p.Q147X mutation, the first to be described in Italy, was detected in a sporadic monolateral jugulotympanic paraganglioma. The SDHD p.Y114C mutation was identified in two unrelated patients, one familial case of bilateral carotid body tumor and one multiple paraganglioma. SDHB, SDHC, and SDHD molecular screening is important in all HNPs, with or without primary indicators of paraganglioma syndrome, to orient mutation-driven clinical screening for additional HNPs and pheochromocytoma.

KEYWORDS: head and neck paraganglioma; SDHB; SDHC; SDHD

Address for correspondence: Francesca Schiavi, Ph.D., Unità di Endocrinologia, Dipartimento Scienze Mediche e Chirurgiche, Università di Padova, Italy. Voice: 0039 049 8213018; fax: 0039 049 657391.

e-mail: francesca.schiavi@unipd.it

Ann. N.Y. Acad. Sci. 1073: 190–197 (2006). © 2006 New York Academy of Sciences.
doi: 10.1196/annals.1353.020

INTRODUCTION

Head and neck paragangliomas (HNPs) are highly vascularized benign tumors deriving from neuroectodermal cells. They are commonly located in the carotid bifurcation, the jugular foramen, the vagal nerve, and the middle ear. HNPs are generally hormonally silent and often asymptomatic. From 10% to 50% of HNPs are inherited.[1,2]

So far, four loci—PGL 1 (SDHD gene), PGL 2, PGL 3 (SDHC gene), and PGL 4 (SDHB gene)—have been identified in hereditary paraganglioma,[3–6] while investigations are under way on the gene responsible for PGL 2.[7]

The SDHB, SDHC, and SDHD genes encode three subunits of the mitochondrial complex II (succinate dehydrogenase), a heterotetrameric complex involved in the Krebs cycle and the aerobic electron-transport chain.

Transmission is autosomal dominant with incomplete penetrance. Maternal transmission of the SDHD gene does not cause tumor on account of maternal imprinting.[8]

HNPs can be part of the paraganglioma syndrome, with (SDHD, SDHB mutations) or without (SDHC mutations) associated pheochromocytoma.

The aim of this study was to review the cases of HNP referred to the Padova Hospital, in the oto-surgery, vascular surgery or endocrinology departments, in the last 10 years, and to assess the prevalence of SDHB, SDHC, and SDHD germline mutations.

MATERIAL AND METHODS

Patient and Clinical Data Collection

We retrospectively reviewed the clinical records of 20 patients with HNP admitted to the Endocrinology (1 patient), Oto-Surgery (11), and Vascular Surgery Units (8) of the Padova University Hospital from January 1996 to August 2005.

These patients were reviewed at the outpatients' clinic of the Endocrinology Unit, where their personal and family history was collected. All patients gave their informed consent.

DNA Isolation and DNA Sequencing

Genomic DNA was isolated from peripheral blood using the Qiamp DNA blood Mini Kit according to the manufacturer's recommendations (Qiagen, GmbH, Hilden, Germany).

We analyzed the SDHB, SDHC, and SDHD coding region and the intron–exon boundaries (eight exons of the SDHB gene, six exons of the SDHC gene, and four exons of the SDHD gene).

Primers for amplifying the target sequences were based on published sequences for the SDHB, SDHC, and SDHD genes (NM_003000, NM_003001, and NM_003002, respectively) and were designed using Primer Express™ Software v. 2.0 (Applied Biosystems, Foster City, CA, USA).

Polymerase chain reaction (PCR) amplification was done in 20 μL reaction mixture containing 1.5 mM $MgCl_2$, 0.2 mM dNTPs, 1U AmpliTaq Gold (Applied Biosystems), 0.5 μM of each forward and reverse primer. The amplification profile consisted of an initial denaturation step at 94°C for 5 min, followed by 35 cycles of denaturation at 94°C for 45 sec, annealing at 56–68°C for 45 sec, and extension at 72°C for 45 sec. A final extension step was carried out at 72°C for 7 min.

An aliquot of the PCR product was purified using ExoI/Shrimp alkaline phosphatase treatment (USB, Cleveland, OH, USA) at 37°C for 15 min and 80°C for 15 min.

The purified amplicons were bidirectionally sequenced using the original primer pair and Big-Dye Terminators v. 3.1 Cycle Sequencing Kit (Applied Biosystems) and analyzed on an ABI Prism 3100 DNA Analyzer (Applied Biosystems).

RESULTS

Clinical Findings

In all, 24 HNP patients were admitted to Padova University Hospital in the last 10 years; we reviewed 20 of them.

All 20 patients, 4 men and 16 women, were referred as having sporadic forms, but accurate collection of their personal and family history showed that one was a familial case.

Among these patients, there were 7 (35%) carotid body tumors, 10 (50%) jugulotympanic paragangliomas, 1 (5%) paraganglioma in the proximity of the vagal nerve, 1 (5%) bilateral carotid body tumor, and 1 (5%) multiple paraganglioma, bilateral carotid body tumor, and jugulotympanic paraganglioma (TABLE 1).

So far, none of the HNPs included in this study have shown signs of malignancy.

Fourteen patients (70%) were symptomatic: the most common presenting symptom was pulsatile tinnitus, occurring in 43% of cases, followed by hearing loss (33%).

Thirteen patients (65%) had a small mass (less than 3 cm).

Local recurrences were identified by magnetic resonance imaging (MRI) in three patients (two sporadic cases and one familial).

Mutational Analysis

Genetic screening of the SDHB, SDHC, and SDHD genes in the 20 affected individuals identified a 724C-T transition in exon 7 of the SDHB gene resulting in an arg242 to cys (p.R242C) substitution, a 439C-T transition in exon 6 of the SDHC gene resulting in a glu147 to term (p.Q147X) substitution, and a 341G-C transversion in exon 4 of the SDHD gene resulting in a tyr114 to cys (p.Y114C) substitution.

These SDHB, SDHC, or SDHD mutations prompted the diagnosis of paraganglioma syndrome.

Clinical Characteristics of Patients Harboring SDHB-C-D Mutations

Patient 1 exhibited a missense mutation, c.724C>T p.R242C in exon 7 of the SDHB gene. This mutation has never been described before, but a different mutation affecting the same amino acid (c.725G>A p.R242H) was described in a man and his son, both with metastatic catecholamine-secreting paragangliomas.[9]

Patient 1 was 51 years old and was first referred to our hospital in 1995 for acute pain in the right eye associated with a right neck mass suggestive of a 3.5-cm carotid body tumor. During the surgical resection of the mass, he had a hypertensive episode with a diastolic pressure higher than 150 mm Hg. Histology revealed a benign paraganglioma. The complete clinical characterization of the proband and the molecular investigation of his relatives are in progress.

Patient 2 exhibited a nonsense mutation c.439C>T p.Q147X in exon 6 of the SDHC gene. This was the first time said mutation was described.[10]

This 50-year-old patient was first referred to our hospital in 2003 complaining of vertigo and right-sided hearing loss, associated with a right-sided 7 × 5 × 4.5 cm tympanic paraganglioma. He was normotensive with normal chromogranin A and negative abdominal and chest CT scans. His mother (73 years old) was also found to carry the mutation, associated with a left-sided 2-cm carotid body tumor. His brother (47 years old) and sister (36 years old) were found to carry the mutation, but their neck and skull base MRI revealed no lesions.

Patients 3 and 4 exhibited a missense mutation c.341G>C p.Y114C in exon 4 of the SDHD gene, a mutation first identified in affected members of a German family with hereditary paragangliomas.[11]

Patient 3, 64 years old, was referred to our hospital in 1996 with chronic headache and migraine associated with bilateral carotid body tumors, removed surgically. Follow-up MRI of the neck in 2001 showed no relapses. One brother carried the same SDHD mutation. His clinical screening is in progress.

Patient 4, 37 years old, had suffered progressive hearing loss since she was 15 years old. A jugulotympanic paraganglioma had been removed surgically in 1983, and in 1991 a recurrent tumor had also been resected; a left carotid body tumor was found in the same year. In 1996, a second recurrence of the jugulotympanic paraganglioma was identified and treated surgically. In 2003, a computed tomography scan revealed a right carotid body tumor. Clinically, the patient had a right-sided neck mass, left-deviated tongue, right-deviated rima

TABLE 1. Major characteristics of HNP patients in this study

Characteristics	Patient 1 SDHB c.724C>T p.R242C	Patient 2 SDHC c.439C>T p.Q147X	Patient 3 SDHD c.341G>C p.Y114C	Patient 4 SDHD c.341G>C p.Y114C	Sporadic Cases ($n = 16$)
Age at diagnosis year or median (range) (yr)	41	33	55	15	55 (20–71)
Tumor site (no.)					
Carotid body	1		2	2	6
Jugular-tympanic		1		1	9
Vagal					1
Multiple tumors	0	0	1	1	0
Malignant tumors	0	0	0	0	0

oris, and motor impairment of the scalene muscle block. The asymptomatic brother had the same mutation. Clinical screening is in progress.

DISCUSSION

HNPs are rare, generally benign, highly vascularized, slow-growing tumors of the paraganglia. Most HNPs are sporadic, but they can also be familial in proportions varying from 9.5% to 50%, depending on the population analyzed.[12]

Germline mutations in the SDHB, SDHC, and SDHD genes have been found not only in the majority of familial HNPs, but also in sporadic cases. In individuals with SDHB and SDHD mutations, HNP can be associated with pheochromocytoma, as part of the paraganglioma syndrome.

This study assessed the prevalence of germline mutations in SDHB, SDHC, and SDHD genes in a consecutive population of 20 patients with HNP admitted to Padova Hospital.

Mutations were identified in one of the three genes in four affected individuals, three sporadic cases and one with a family history of HNP. The prevalence of SDHB, SDHC, and SDHD mutations was 5% (1/20 cases), 5% (1/20 cases), and 10% (2/20 cases), respectively.

These figures differ slightly from the prevalence of SDHB, SDHC, and SDHD mutations reported in other studies, but are similar to the prevalences recorded in the only population-based registry (TABLE 2).

Mutation carriers had a normal catecholamine excretion and no evidence of pheochromocytoma so far.

In this series of patients, the frequency of head paraganglioma is higher than reported elsewhere in the literature: this may be because our oto-surgery team is particularly qualified for tympanic tumor surgery (most of the patients came from northeast Italy, but a few were from central Italy). In this study,

TABLE 2. Prevalence of SDHB, SDHC, and SDHD mutation in this study and in four different series of HNP cases

	Cases (No.)	SDHB Mutation % (No.)	SDHC Mutation % (No.)	SDHD Mutation % (No.)
This study	20	5 (1)	5 (1)	10 (2)
Schiavi, F. *et al.*, 2005[10,a]	121	6.6 (8)	4.1 (5)	16.5 (20)
Mhatre, A.N. *et al.*, 2004[18]	17	5.9 (1)	0 (0)	5.9 (1)
Badenhop, R.F. *et al.*, 2003[19]	34	8.8 (3)	0 (0)	32.4 (11)
Baysal, B.E. *et al.*, 2002[12]	47	6.4 (3)	0 (0)	14.9 (7)

[a]Cases from the population-based International HNP Registry.

11 individuals were initially referred to the Oto-Surgery unit, 8 to Vascular Surgery, and 1 to Endocrinology.

Both the one familial case and the one bilateral sporadic case carried the same SDHD mutation. These two patients came from the same geographic area in northern Italy (Valsugana, Trentino), but were unrelated. Anecdotal reports have suggested a high incidence of HNP in this particular part of northern Italy, and isolating two unrelated probands sharing the same SDHD mutation and the same country of origin may suggest a founder effect. A detailed study of HNP patients coming from this country is in progress.

SDHD founder effects have been described in the Netherlands (D92Y and L139P)[13] and the United States (P81L),[14] one has also been identified in Tuscany, Italy (Q109X),[15] and probably another two in Spain (c.337-340 delGATC and W43X).[16]

The low malignancy, incomplete penetrance, and absence of disease when the mutation is inherited from the mother probably help SDHD mutation to spread and this may help to explain the large number of SDHD founder effects detected so far for this rare disease.

A positive family history, early onset, and the presence of multiple tumors have been suggested as primary indicators of paraganglioma syndrome.

In the current report, only two of the four mutation carriers had these features, while the other two patients were sporadic and monolateral cases developing in the fourth decade. In the latter two patients, HNP was only classified as part of the syndrome after molecular screening of their SDHB, SDHC, and SDHD genes. There may be several reasons for this: incomplete penetrance and genomic imprinting may result, in the case of the SDHD gene, in a negative family history. The clinical diagnosis may also be reached several years after the onset of the HNP, which is hormonally silent, frequently asymptomatic, slow growing, often presenting late as a space-occupying mass.

Molecular screening is therefore necessary in cases of apparently sporadic HNP, even without any primary indicators of the paraganglioma syndrome.

Identifying a germline mutation in the SDHB, SDHC, or SDHD genes enables the diagnosis of paraganglioma syndrome.

Detecting a particular mutation may help to predict the tumor's behavior because paraganglioma syndrome differs in its clinical characteristics of penetrance and expression, depending on the mutated gene involved (this has been established in a relatively small number of subjects).

In SDHB mutation carriers, HNP is found in 31% of cases, adrenal pheochromocytoma in 28%, extra-adrenal pheochromocytoma in 59%, multifocal tumors in 28%, and malignant tumors in 34%.[17]

In SDHD mutation carriers, HNP is found in 79% of cases, adrenal pheochromocytoma in 53%, extra-adrenal pheochromocytoma in 39%, and multifocal tumors in 74%, while there are no malignant tumors.[17]

In SDHC mutation carriers, HNP occurs in 100% of cases, but there are no adrenal or extra-adrenal pheochromocytomas, or malignant tumors.[10]

A mutation-driven clinical screening for additional HNPs and pheochromocytoma may be advisable in such patients.

Molecular diagnosis may also affect prevention and clinical outcome. Since large tumors may be hazardous to nearby nerves and vessels, early diagnosis may facilitate the surgical removal of the paragangliomas, reducing their local invasiveness and the risk of recurrence.

In conclusion, in a cohort of 20 patients consecutively referred with sporadic HNP, we identified four carriers of a mutation in one of the paraganglioma syndrome susceptibility genes, resulting in a 25% prevalence of heritable forms. One patient with an SDHD mutation was only identified as a familial case after careful consideration of the family history, while two carriers of mutations (affecting SDHB and SHDC) had no primary evidence of syndromic HNP, being affected by sporadic, monolateral HNP of apparent onset in the fourth decade.

SDHB, SDHC, and SDHD molecular screening enables the detection of potentially heritable cases with a diagnosis of paraganglioma syndrome and should be recommended in cases of sporadic HNP too.

ACKNOWLEDGMENTS

This study was supported by Grant 2004069534 from MIUR, Italy to G. Opocher.

REFERENCES

1. GRUFFERMAN, S. *et al.* 1980. Familial carotid body tumors: case report and epidemiologic review. Cancer **46:** 2116–2122.
2. VAN DER MEY A.G. *et al.* 1989. Genomic imprinting in hereditary glomus tumours: evidence for new genetic theory. Lancet **2:** 1291–1294.

3. BAYSAL, B.E. *et al.* Fine mapping of an imprinted gene for familial nonchromaffin paragangliomas, on chromosome 11q23. Am. J. Hum. Genet. **60:** 121–132.
4. BAYSAL, B.E. *et al.* 2000. Mutations in SDHD, a mitochondrial complex II gene, in hereditary paraganglioma. Science **287:** 848–851.
5. ASTUTI, D. *et al.* 2001. Gene mutations in the succinate dehydrogenase subunit SDHB cause susceptibility to familial pheochromocytoma and to familial paraganglioma. Am. J. Hum. Genet. **69:** 49–54.
6. NIEMANN, S. & U. MULLER. 2000. Mutations in SDHC cause autosomal dominant paraganglioma, type 3. Nat. Genet. **26:** 268–270.
7. MARIMAN E.C.M. *et al.* 1993. Analysis of a second family with hereditary nonchromaffin paragangliomas locates the underlying gene at the proximal region of chromosome 11q. Hum. Genet. **91:** 357–361.
8. BAYSAL, B.E. 2004. Genomic imprinting and environment in hereditary paraganglioma. Am. J. Med. Genet. C. Semin. Med. Genet. **129:** 85–90.
9. YOUNG, A.L. *et al.* 2002. Familial malignant catecholamine-secreting paraganglioma with prolonged survival associated with mutation in the succinate dehydrogenase B gene. J. Clin. Endocrinol. Metab. **87:** 4101–4105.
10. SCHIAVI, F. *et al.* 2005. Predictors and prevalence of paraganglioma syndrome associated with mutations of the SDHC gene. JAMA **294:** 2057–2063.
11. MILUNSKY, J.M. *et al.* 2001. Novel mutations and the emergence of a common mutation in the SDHD gene causing familial paraganglioma. Am. J. Med. Genet. **100:** 311–314.
12. BAYSAL, B.E. 2002. Hereditary paraganglioma targets diverse paraganglia. J. Med. Genet. **39:** 617–622.
13. TASCHNER, P.E. *et al.* 2001. Nearly all hereditary paragangliomas in the Netherlands are caused by two founder mutations in the SDHD gene. Genes Chromosomes Cancer **31:** 274–281.
14. BAYSAL, B.E. 2002. Prevalence of SDHB, SDHC, and SDHD germline mutations in clinic patients with head and neck paragangliomas. J. Med. Genet. **39:** 178–183.
15. SIMI, L. *et al.* 2005. Phenotypc variability of neural crest derived tumours in six Italian families segregating the same founder SDHD mutation Q109X. J. Med. Genet. **42:** e52.
16. VELASCO, A. *et al.* 2005. Mutation analysis of the SDHD gene in four kindreds with familial paraganglioma: description of one novel germline mutation. Diagn. Mol. Pathol. **14:** 109–114.
17. NEUMANN, H.P. *et al.* 2004. Distinct clinical features of paraganglioma syndromes associated with SDHB and SDHD gene mutations. JAMA **292:** 943–951.
18. MHATRE, A.N. 2004. SDHB, SDHC, and SDHD mutation screen in sporadic and familial head and neck paragangliomas. Clin. Genet. **66:** 461–466.
19. BADENHOP, R.F. *et al.* 2004. The prevalence of SDHB, SDHC, and SDHD mutations in patients with head and neck paraganglioma and association of mutations with clinical features. J. Med. Genet. **41:** e99.

Germline Mutation of von Hippel–Lindau (VHL) Gene 695 G>A (R161Q) in a Patient with a Peculiar Phenotype with Type 2C VHL Syndrome

LIBERO SANTARPIA,[a] DANIELA LAPA,[a]
AND SALVATORE BENVENGA[a,b,c]

[a]*Sezione di Endocrinologia del Dipartimento Clinico Sperimentale di Medicina e Farmacologia Policlinico Universitario, Messina, Italy*

[b]*Programma Infradipartimentale di Endocrinologia Molecolare Clinica Università di Messina, A.O.U. Policlinico G. Martino, Messina, Italy*

[c]*Master di Endocrinologia dell'Infanzia, dell'Adolescenza e della Donna, Università di Messina, Messina, Italy*

ABSTRACT: Von Hippel–Lindau (VHL) disease is an autosomal dominant familial neoplastic disorder with an estimated birth incidence of approximately 1:36000 live. VHL has intrafamilial variability expression and it is characterized by the predisposition to develop hemangioblastomas of the central nervous system and retina, pheochromocytomas, clear-cell renal carcinoma, adenomas, and carcinomas of the pancreas, paragangliomas, renal and pancreatic cysts, papillary cystadenomas of the epididymis and, rarely, cystadenomas of the endolymphatic sac tumor and broad ligament. We describe a Sicilian girl with type 2C VHL who showed the apparently *de novo* mutation R161Q in association with an extra-axial supratentorial frontal meningioma, which can be included as a characteristic sign in VHL.

KEYWORDS: mutation detection; VHL gene; tumor suppressor gene; genotype–phenotype; meningioma

INTRODUCTION

Von Hippel–Lindau (VHL; MIM 193300) disease is an autosomal-dominant familial cancer syndrome predisposing to retinal and central nervous system hemangioblastomas, pheochromocytomas, and renal and pancreatic tumors.

Address for correspondence: Salvatore Benvenga, M.D., Programma di Endocrinologia Molecolare Clinica, Azienda Policlinico Universitario, Padiglione H, 4 piano Via Consolare Valeria, 1 Messina, I-98125, Italy. Voice: +39-090-221-3517; fax: +39-090-221-3518.
e-mail: s.benvenga@me.nettuno.it

**Ann. N.Y. Acad. Sci. 1073: 198–202 (2006). © 2006 New York Academy of Sciences.
doi: 10.1196/annals.1353.021**

Clinically, VHL can be subdivided into type 1 or type 2 based on the absence or presence of pheochromocytomas. The occurrence of renal cell carcinoma allows a further distinction between type 2A (low risk) and type 2B (high risk).[1–3] The presence of pheochromocytomas without the other classical features of VHL constitutes type 2C. These clinical types correlate with the type of the VHL gene mutations: type 1 families frequently harbor *VHL* deletions or truncation mutations, while type 2 families almost invariably harbor *VHL* missense mutation.[1,3,4] VHL is a pleiotropic tumor suppressor gene that is widely expressed in both fetal and adult tissues,[5,6] including tissues that are unaffected by VHL.[7,8]

The VHL gene product, pVHL, forms a multiprotein complex that contains elongin B, elongin C, Cul-2, and Rbx1, and negatively regulates hypoxia-inducible mRNAs including VEGF mRNA (vascular endothelial growth factor).[9–11] pVHL regulates cell cycle exit and extracellular matrix formation.[12,13]

Many germline mutations have been found in VHL-affected individuals,[3,4,14,15] as well as somatic mutations in sporadic tumors.[16–20]

We have analyzed the VHL gene in a von Hippel–Lindau family in whom the proband had bilateral pheochromocytomas, and multiple paragangliomas. This patient had a relatively common VHL gene mutation 695 G>A (R161Q), but also a peculiar phenotype characterized by the presence of an extra-axial right-sided supratentorial frontal meningioma (16 mm in diameter).

Meningioma has been rarely reported in association with VHL.

MATERIALS AND METHODS

A 26-year-old woman with VHL was referred to us with a two-step development of bilateral pheochromocytomas, and subsequent appearance of multiple paragangliomas. VHL begun at 11 years of age as a unilateral pheochromocytoma. Another pheochromocytoma also developed in the contralateral adrenal gland 13 years later as did two concurrent paragangliomas of the abdominal aorta and urinary bladder. Bilateral pheochromocytomas and paragangliomas were surgically removed. During the follow-up of this patient, a meningioma was detected by magnetic resonance imaging. The 51-year-old father, 48-year-old mother, 22-year-old sister, and 19-year-old brother were asymptomatic. Informed consent for genetic testing was obtained from each individual.

Genomic DNA was extracted by conventional methods from peripheral blood lymphocytes. The entire coding sequence of the gene was polymerase chain reaction (PRC) amplified with 35-cycle reactions and with the use of primers previously described.[3] The amplification products were subjected to denaturing high-performance liquid chromatography (DHPLC) analysis. PCR products showing different DHPLC peaks compared to normal controls were subjected to direct sequencing (ABI Prism 310, Applied Bio System, Bosten City, CA).

RESULTS AND DISCUSSION

In DHPLC analysis, only exon 3 of the proband's genomic DNA showed a heterozygous peak. Indeed, subsequent sequence analysis showed a missense mutation: G>A substitution at cDNA nucleotide 695, corresponding to a predicted R161Q change in the VHL gene product. This kind of mutation is consistent with the type 2C phenotype of our patient (see INTRODUCTION). This mutation has been reported frequently in VHL patients.[1,14] However, this mutation has never been described in association with meningioma, a tumor that has rarely been reported to be associated with VHL.[21–26] Only for the type 2B patient described by Kanno *et al.*[21] is the VHL gene mutation known. Interestingly enough, this was another missense mutation (Leu158Val), which is localized in a codon very close to the codon mutated in our patient.

Plasma and urine catecholamines (including metanephrines) were repeatedly normal in the proband's relatives. Of these relatives, only the father's genomic DNA showed a small, but reproducibly so, heterozygous peak. This heterozygosity, corresponding to 695 G>A, was confirmed by direct sequencing of the exon 3. The lower than 50:50 ratio between the wild-type G and the mutated A peak was consistent with mosaicism. This hypothesis will be tested in further detail in upcoming studies on DNA isolated from a number of somatic cells such as buccal cells, hair roots, and skin fibroblasts. Asymptomatic mosaic carriers have been described in various disorders and have been demonstrated to be the cause of many cases of recurrence and late-onset disease.[27,28]

We conclude that missense mutation causing amino acid replacement in a pVHL region that includes residues 158 and 161 might result in the formation of VHL-associated meningiomas. In addition, apparently asymptomatic carriers of VHL may exist because of somatic mosaicism.

REFERENCES

1. CHEN, F., T. KISHIDA, M. YAO, *et al.* 1995. Germline mutations in the von Hippel-Lindau disease tumor suppressor gene: correlations with phenotype. Hum. Mutat. **5:** 66–75.
2. CHEN, F., L. SLIFE, T. KISHIDA, *et al.* 1996. Genotype-phenotype correlation in von Hippel–Lindau disease: identification of a mutation associated with VHL type 2A. J. Med. Genet. **33:** 716–717.
3. CROSSEY, P.A., F.M. RICHARDS, K. FOSTER, *et al.* 1994. Identification of intragenic mutations in the von Hippel–Lindau disease tumour suppressor gene and correlation with disease phenotype. Hum. Mol. Genet. **3:** 1303–1308.
4. ZBAR, B., T. KISHIDA, F. CHEN, *et al.* 1996. Germline mutations in the Von Hippel–Lindau disease (VHL) gene in families from North America, Europe, and Japan. Hum. Mutat. **8:** 348–357.
5. KAELIN, W.G. JR & E.R. MAHER. 1998. The VHL tumour-suppressor gene paradigm. Trends Genet. **14:** 423–426.

6. OHH, M. & W.G. KAELIN, JR. 1999. The von Hippel–Lindau tumour suppressor protein: new perspectives. Mol. Med .Today **5:** 257–263.
7. LATIF, F., K. TORY, J. GNARRA, *et al.* 1993. Identification of the von Hippel–Lindau disease tumor suppressor gene. Science **260:** 1317–1320.
8. RICHARDS, F.M., P.N. SCHOFIELD, S. FLEMING, *et al.* 1996. Expression of the von Hippel–Lindau disease tumour suppressor gene during human embryogenesis. Hum. Mol. Genet. **5:** 639–644.
9. ILIOPOULOS, O., C. JIANG, A.P. LEVY, *et al.* 1996. Negative regulation of hypoxia-inducible genes by the von Hippel–Lindau protein. Proc. Natl. Acad. Sci. USA **93:** 10595–10599.
10. SIEMEISTER, G., K. WEINDEL, K. MOHRS, *et al.* 1996. Reversion of deregulated expression of vascular endothelial growth factor in human renal carcinoma cells by the von Hippel–Lindau protein. Cancer. Res. **56:** 2299–2301.
11. STEBBINS, C.E., W.G. KAELIN, JR. & N.P. PAVLETICH. 1999. Structure of the VHL-ElonginC-ElonginB complex: implications for VHL tumor-suppressor function. Science **284:** 255–461.
12. OHH, M., R.L. YAUCH, K.M. LONERGAN, *et al.* 1998. The von Hippel–Lindau tumor suppressor protein is required for proper assembly of an extracellular fibronectin matrix. Mol. Cell. **1:** 959–968.
13. PAUSE, A., S. LEE, R.A. WORRELL, *et al.* 1997. The von Hippel–Lindau tumour suppressor gene product forms a stable complex with human CUL-2, a member of the Cdc53 family of proteins. Proc. Natl. Acad. Sci. USA **93:** 1770–1775.
14. GLAVAC, D., H.P. NEUMAN, C. WITTKE, *et al.* 1996. Mutations in the VHL tumor suppressor gene and associated lesions in families with von Hippel–Lindau disease from central Europe. Hum. Genet. **99:** 271–280.
15. STOLLE, C., G. GLENN, B. ZBAR, *et al.* 1998. Improved detection of germline mutations in the von Hippel–Lindau disease tumor suppressor gene. Hum. Mutat. **12:** 417–423.
16. ENG, C., P.A. CROSSEY, L.M. MULLIGAN, *et al.* 1995. Mutations in the RET proto-oncogene and the von Hippel–Lindau disease tumour suppressor gene in sporadic and syndromic phaeochromocytomas. J. Clin. Genet. **32:** 934–937.
17. GNARRA, J.R., K. TORY, Y. WENG, *et al.* 1994. Mutations of the VHL tumor suppressor gene in renal carcinoma. Nat. Genet. **7:** 85–90.
18. KANNO, H., K. KONDO, S. ITO, *et al.* 1994. Somatic mutations of the von Hippel–Lindau tumor suppressor gene in sporadic central nervous system hemangioblastomas. Cancer Res. **54:** 4845–4847.
19. NEUMANN, H.P., B. BAUSCH, S.R. MCWHINNEY, *et al.* 2002. Freiburg-Warsaw-Columbus Pheochromocytoma Study Group: germ-line mutations in nonsyndromic pheochromocytoma. N. Engl. J. Med. **346:** 1459–1466.
20. KONDO, K., M. YAO, M. YOSHIDA, *et al.* 2002. Comprehensive mutational analysis of the VHL gene in sporadic renal cell carcinoma: relationship to clinicopathological parameters. Genes Chromosomes Cancer. **34:** 58–68.
21. KANNO, H., I. YAMAMOTO, M. YOSHIDA, *et al.* 2003. Meningioma showing VHL gene inactivation in a patient with von Hippel–Lindau disease. Neurology **60:** 1197–1199.
22. MELMON, K.L. & S.W. ROSEN. 1964. Lindau's disease: review of the literature and study of a large kindred. Am. J. Med. **36:** 595–617.
23. HULL, M.T., K.A. WARFEL, J. MULLER, *et al.* 1979. Familial islet cell tumors in Von Hippel-Lindau's disease. Cancer. **44:** 1523–1526.

24. NEUMANN, H.P., E. DINKEL, H. BRAMBS, *et al.* 1991. Pancreatic lesions in the von Hippel–Lindau syndrome. Gastroenterology **101:** 465–471.
25. SALAZAR, F.G. & J.M. LAMIELL. 1980. Early identification of retinal angiomas in a large kindred von Hippel–Lindau disease. Am. J. Ophthalmol. **89:** 540–545.
26. GOVERNALE, L.S., A.O. VORTMEYER, Z. ZHUANG, *et al.* 2001. Fibrous meningioma in a patient with von Hippel–Lindau disease: a genetic analysis. J. Neurosurg. **95:** 1045–1049
27. COLMAN, S.D., S.A. RASMUSSEN, V.T. HO, *et al.* 1996. Somatic mosaicism in a patient with neurofibromatosis type 1. Am. J. Hum. Genet. **58:** 484–490.
28. ZLOTOGORA, J. 1998. Germ line mosaicism. Hum. Genet. **102:** 381–386.

Von Hippel–Lindau Gene Mutation in Non-Syndromic Familial Pheochromocytomas

AN-LI TONG,[a] ZHENG-PEI ZENG,[a] HAN-ZHONG LI,[b] DI YANG,[c] LIN LU,[a] MING LI,[a] YA-RU ZHOU,[a] JING ZHANG,[a] SHI CHEN,[a] AND WEI LIANG[a]

[a]*Department of Endocrinology, Peking Union Medical College Hospital, Chinese Academy of Medical Sciences and Peking Union Medical College, 100730 Beijing, China*

[b]*Department of Urology, Peking Union Medical College Hospital, Chinese Academy of Medical Sciences and Peking Union Medical College, 100730 Beijing, China*

[c]*Department of Pathology, Peking Union Medical College Hospital, Chinese Academy of Medical Sciences and Peking Union Medical College, 100730 Beijing, China*

ABSTRACT: **Approximately 50% of patients with non-syndromic familial pheochromocytomas had germline von Hippel–Lindau (VHL) gene mutations, but no reports on the subject were available in China. A total of five unrelated Chinese families with non-syndromic familial pheochromocytomas were screened for VHL gene mutation by polymerase chain reaction (PCR) and subsequent direct sequencing. Missense germline mutations of VHL gene were detected in four of the five families. Arg161Gln (695G-A) mutation was found in two families, and the other two families had Leu163Phe (700C-T) and Arg167Trp (712C-T) mutation, respectively. In conclusion, VHL gene may have frequent mutation in Chinese patients with non-syndromic familial pheochromocytomas.**

KEYWORDS: **non-syndromic familial pheochromocytomas; von Hippel–Lindau gene; mutation**

INTRODUCTION

Most pheochromocytomas are sporadic, and approximately 10–15% of the pheochromocytoma patients have been believed to be of hereditary origin.

Address for correspondence: Dr. Zheng-Pei Zeng, M.D., Department of Endocrinology, Peking Union Medical College Hospital, 100730 Beijing, China. Voice: 86-10-65295071; fax: 86-10-65230460.
e-mail: zengzhengpei@yahoo.com.cn

Ann. N.Y. Acad. Sci. 1073: 203–207 (2006).
doi: 10.1196/annals.1353.022

Hereditary familial pheochromocytomas may be one of the manifestations of some hereditary syndromes, such as multiple endocrine neoplasia type 2A (MEN 2A) or type 2B (MEN 2B), von Hippel–Lindau (VHL) disease, and type 1 neurofibromatosis (NF1), which are associated with the mutations of RET gene, VHL gene, and NF1 gene, respectively. A group of familial non-syndromic pheochromocytomas has also been characterized. Recently, germline mutations of the genes for succinate dehydrogenase subunit D (SDHD) and succinate dehydrogenase subunit B (SDHB) were found in families with isolated paraganglioma and/or pheochromocytomas.[1] Molecular genetic studies revealed that approximately 50% of patients with apparent familial non-syndromic pheochromocytomas might have germline VHL gene mutations. These patients may be the members of VHL type 2C family, who have no other symptoms of VHL but pheochromocytomas only.[2,3] Up to now, there is no report about gene mutation in patients with familial non-syndromic pheochromocytomas in Chinese patients. The purpose of this research is to study the mutation of VHL gene in Chinese patients with non-syndromic familial pheochromocytomas.

MATERIALS AND METHODS

Patients

A total of five unrelated Chinese families with non-syndromic familial pheochromocytomas involving 11 patients (including 5 males and 6 females) were studied for VHL gene mutation (FIG. 1). Eight of the 11 patients had bilateral pheochromocytomas, and three had unilateral pheochromocytoma. The patients and their familial members had no clinical manifestation of hereditary syndromes, including MEN 2A, MEN 2B, VHL disease, and NF1. The laboratory and image examinations also excluded the presence of the above-mentioned hereditary syndromes.

Mutation Identification

Genomic DNA was extracted from peripheral blood leukocytes by using DNAzol (GIBCO/BRL, Rockville, MD). Subsequent polymerase chain reaction (PCR) amplifications of the three exon regions were performed in 50 μL of mixture containing 200 μM dNTP, 2 μM of each primer flanking the exons analyzed, 100–200 ng of genomic DNA, and 2 U Taq Polymerase (dNTP and Taq Polymerase were purchased from TaKaRa, Japan). PCR conditions of the three reactions were similar, which consisted of 30 cycles of 60 s at 95°C, 60 s at 62°C, and 90 s at 72°C, followed by a 7-min final extension at 72°C. The primers used in the amplification

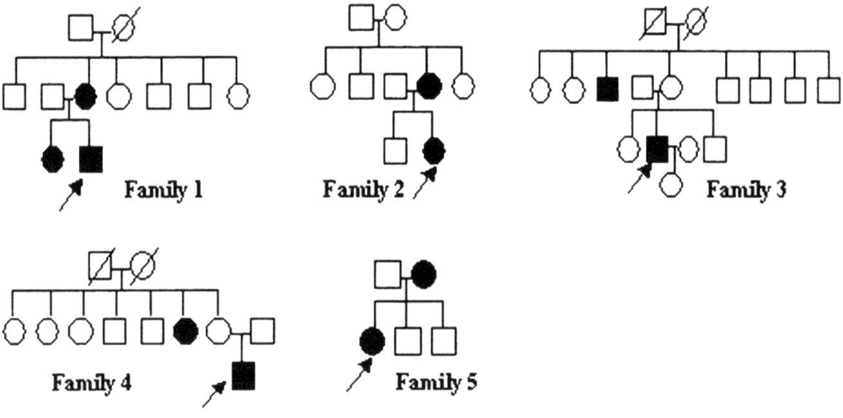

FIGURE 1. Five families with non-syndromic familial pheochromocytoma.

were[4]: exon 1: forward, 5′-TGGTCTGGATCGCGGAGGGAAT-3′, and reverse, 5′-GCTGGGTCGGGCCTAAGCGCCGGGCCCGT-3′; exon 2: forward 5′-GTGGCTCTTTAACAACCTTTGC-3′, and reverse, 5′-CCTGTACTTAC CACAACAACCTTATC-3′; and for exon 3 : forward 5′-TTCCTTGTACTGA GACCCTAGT-3′, and reverse, 5′-AGCTGAGATGAAACAGTGTAAGT-3′. The PCR products were purified, and bidirectionally sequenced with an ABI 3730XL DNA sequencer (AME Bioscience, Toroed, Norway).

RESULTS

Missense germline mutations of the VHL gene were detected in four of the five families. All of the gene mutations took place in exon 3. Missense VHL gene mutation Arg161Gln (695G-A) was found in two families, and the other two families had Leu163Phe (700C-T) and Arg167Trp (712C-T) mutations, respectively (FIG. 2). Except for the proband with 700C-T gene mutation, whose relatives were not available for the study, the genetic studies were completed in the patients of the other families, and the same mutations were detected in the patients of the same families.

DISCUSSION

The VHL syndrome is an autosomal dominant neoplasia caused by germline deletions or mutations in the tumor-suppressor VHL gene. The mutations can lead to the development of tumors and cysts, including retinal and craniospinal hemangioblastomas, renal cell carcinoma (RCC) or cysts, pancreatic tumors or cysts, pheochromocytomas, and endolymphatic sac tumors, etc. Clinically,

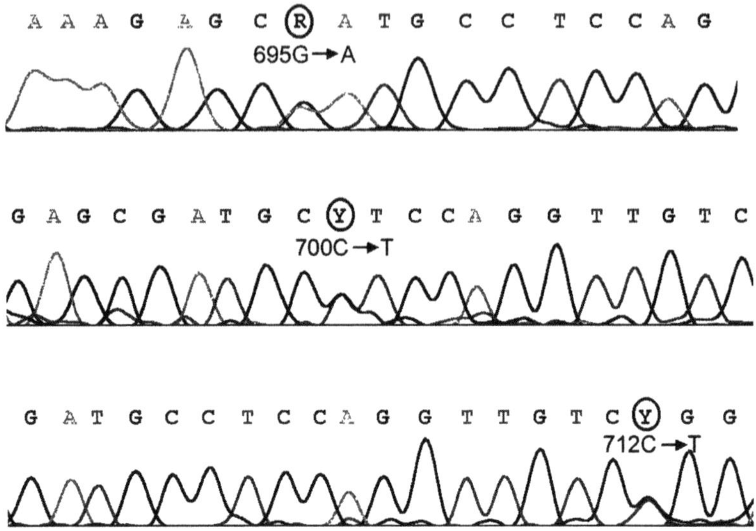

FIGURE 2. The three mutation locus of VHL gene.

VHL disease falls into four subtypes, depending on the presence of pheochromocytoma or RCC. Type 1 has no pheochromocytoma and type 2 has the presence of both hemangioblastoma and pheochromocytomas, either with relatively low incidence (type 2A) or high incidence (type 2B) of RCC and pancreatic tumors. VHL2C is characterized by a pheochromocytoma-only phenotype.[5,6]

More than 300 germline mutations have been identified in familial VHL disease, and most germline VHL mutations occurred in 1–2 families.[5,7] Mutations in the VHL gene are restricted to an area between nucleotide 375 (codon 55) and nucleotide 820 (codon 202). There are close correlations between genotype and phenotype. Deletions and protein-truncating mutations predominate in type 1 families, whereas 96% of type 2 families had missense mutations.[8,9]

However, there was no report about the mutation detection of VHL gene in pheochromocytoma patients in China. In our study, four of the five families with non-syndromic familial pheochromocytoma had missense mutations of VHL gene, and three distinct intragenic germline mutations were detected. It is well known that a hotspot for VHL germline mutations is readily visible at the beginning of exon 3, or more specifically at nucleotides 712/713 (in codon 167).[8] All the three gene mutations in our series were at the start of exon 3, and one was at codon 167. Missense mutations at codon 167 are associated with a much higher risk of pheochromocytoma,[2] and 43% of type 2 families had missense mutations at codon 167.[9]

Arg161Gln (695G-A) mutation was detected in two families in our study. This mutation had been reported in a Spanish patient, who also had non-syndromic familial pheochromocytoma.[10] In addition, an alteration, Leu163Phe (700C-T), which had not been reported before, was detected in one of our patients. Further study has to be conducted to prove the association between the mutation and the disease.

VHL gene may have frequent mutations in Chinese patients with non-syndromic familial pheochromocytomas. The patients with VHL gene mutation are probably of VHL type 2C. The patients with non-syndromic familial pheochromocytomas should be examined for the change of VHL gene, and the genetic tests are of importance in the early detection of asymptomatic pheochromocytoma and in the screening of other members in VHL families.

REFERENCES

1. BRYANT, J. *et al.* 2003. Pheochromocytoma: the expanding genetic differential diagnosis. J. Natl. Cancer Inst. **95:** 1196–1204.
2. RICHARDS, F.M. *et al.* 1998. Molecular genetic analysis of von Hippel-Lindau disease. J. Intern. Med. **243:** 527–533.
3. HES, F.J. *et al.* 2003. Pheochromocytoma in von Hippel-Lindau disease. J. Clin. Endocrinol. Metab. **88:** 969–974.
4. GUO, H.F. *et al.* 2004. Somatic mutations of VHL gene and HIF-1α expression in primary renal clear cell carcinomas. Chin. J. Surg. **42:** 196–200.
5. SIMS, K.B. 2001. Von Hippel-Lindau disease: gene to bedside. Curr. Opin. Neurol. **14:** 695–703.
6. LONSER, R.R. *et al.* 2003. von Hippel-Lindau disease. Lancet **361:** 2059–2067.
7. ZBAR, B. *et al.* 1996. Germline mutations in the Von Hippel-Lindau disease (VHL) gene in families from North America, Europe, and Japan. Hum. Mutat. **8:** 348–357.
8. HES, F.J. *et al.* 2001. Molecular genetic aspects of von Hippel-Lindau (VHL) disease and criteria for DNA analysis in subjects at risk. Neth. J. Med. **59:** 235–243.
9. FRIEDRICH, C.A. 2001. Genotype-phenotype correlation in von Hippel-Lindau syndrome. Hum. Mol. Genet. **10:** 763–767.
10. RUIZ-LLORENTE, S. *et al.* 2004. Genetic characterization and structural analysis of VHL Spanish families to define genotype-phenotype correlations. Hum. Mutat. **23:** 160–169.

Transcription Association of *VHL* and *SDH* Mutations Link Hypoxia and Oxidoreductase Signals in Pheochromocytomas

PATRICIA L.M. DAHIA FOR THE FAMILIAL PHEOCHROMOCYTOMA CONSORTIUM

Departments of Medicine and Cellular & Structural Biology, San Antonio Cancer Institute, University of Texas Health Science Center, San Antonio, Texas, USA

ABSTRACT: Pheochromocytomas and paragangliomas are neural-crest–derived tumors that arise from mutations in *RET, VHL, NF1,* and in the genes-encoding succinate dehydrogenase (SDH) subunits B (*SDHB*), C (*SDHC*), and D (*SDHD*). Despite their genetic diversity, these tumors cannot be clearly distinguished on the basis of their primary mutation. We recently identified two major transcriptional programs embedded within familial and sporadic pheochromocytomas and paragangliomas using global expression profiling. This review will summarize the major results of these studies and discuss their implications. The transcription data revealed that: (a) tumors with mutations in *VHL, SDHB,* and *SDHD* genes share a transcription signature of hypoxia, angiogenesis, and oxidoreductase imbalance; (b) SDHB protein is suppressed in tumors with mutations in *SDHB and SDHD*, and also in a subset of tumors with *VHL* mutations; and (c) HIF1α is involved in the SDHB downregulation observed in these tumors. These results are consistent with the existence of a close interconnection between the *VHL* and *SDH* pathways mediated predominantly by hypoxia and oxidoreductase signals. It further suggests that low SDHB levels indicative of impaired mitochondrial complex II function may be a shared element of these pheochromocytomas. SDHB may thus constitute a marker for tumors with abnormal hypoxic profile.

KEYWORDS: hypoxia; hypoxia-inducible factor (HIF); hypoxia-inducible factor subunit; microarray; multiple endocrine neoplasia Type 2 (MEN 2); mutation; neurofibromatosis Type 1 (NF1); oxidoreductase; oxidative stress; paraganglioma; pathway intersection; pheochromocytoma; prolyl hydroxylase; RET; intracellular signaling; succinate dehydrogenase (SDH); succinate dehydrogenase subunit B (SDHB); succinate dehydrogenase subunit C (SDHC); succinate dehydrogenase subunit D (SDHD); transcription profiling; von Hippel–Lindau (VHL)

Address for correspondence: Patricia Dahia, Departments of Medicine and Cellular & Structural Biology, University of Texas Health Science Center, 7703 Floyd Curl Drive, Room No. 5053-R3, MC 7880, San Antonio-TX 8229-3900, USA. Voice: 210-567-4866; fax: 210-567-1956.
e-mail: dahia@uthscsa.edu

**Ann. N.Y. Acad. Sci. 1073: 208–220 (2006). © 2006 New York Academy of Sciences.
doi: 10.1196/annals.1353.023**

Pheochromocytomas and paragangliomas are catecholamine-secreting tumors derived from chromaffin cells of neural crest origin located in the adrenal medulla and extra-adrenal sympathetic paraganglia, respectively.[1] These tumors can arise as a result of mutations in *RET*, *VHL*, *NF1,* and in subunits *B, C,* or *D* of the succinate dehydrogenase (*SDH*) genes, which underlie multiple endocrine neoplasia Type 2 (MEN2), von Hippel–Lindau (VHL), neurofibromatosis Type 1 (NF1), and familial paraganglioma syndromes Type 4 (PGL4), 3 (PGL3), and 1 (PGL1), respectively.[2] Currently, fewer than 30% of sporadic pheochromocytomas can be attributed to mutations within the genes related to these hereditary syndromes.[2–4] A question that remains unanswered is how these distinct genetic lesions lead to a similar tumor phenotype.

To establish whether the disruption of various genetic signals that predispose to pheochromocytoma interacts to determine tumor development, we generated global expression signatures of a large group of hereditary and sporadic primary pheochromocytomas and paragangliomas.[5] We found that tumors with *VHL* and *SDHB* or *D* mutations form a single cluster (Cluster 1), which is distinct from "Cluster 2" pheochromocytomas: those with mutations in *RET, NF1,* and novel familial pheochromocytoma variants without a known primary genetic defect (named familial pheochromocytoma [FP])[5,6] (TABLE 1). In this series, sporadic pheochromocytomas were distributed between the two major clusters. This transcription-based partition was shown to have high predictive value by cross-validation/permutation methods. Importantly, independent validation was obtained by the identification of novel mutations in genes belonging to the predicted cluster in a number of samples that had not been previously screened. Hence, novel *VHL* or *SDHB* mutations were detected in tumors that aligned with Cluster 1, while *RET* or *FP*-type deletions were identified in tumors that segregated with Cluster 2.[5,6] The robust predictive value of this two-cluster structure provided an underlying framework for characterization of the interaction between tumors with mutations in independent genes. A pathway-enrichment method, gene-set enrichment analysis (GSEA), was thus applied to the data to delineate the underlying biological programs embedded in each of these clusters.[5,7]

HYPOXIA, ANGIOGENESIS, AND SUPPRESSED OXIDOREDUCTASE SIGNATURES ARE PROMINENT FEATURES OF TUMORS WITH *VHL, SDHB,* AND *SDHD* MUTATIONS

Increased hypoxic signals have been previously associated with *VHL* mutations, as a result of VHL's role in regulating the HIF-mediated hypoxia response.[8,9] Under normoxic conditions VHL, the substrate recognition component of an E3 ligase complex, promotes ubiquitination of hydroxylated forms of HIF1α, which will ultimately undergo degradation by the 26S proteasome.[10,11]

TABLE 1. The pheochromocytoma transcriptome

Cluster	Hereditary pheochromocytoma syndrome (susceptibility gene)	Significantly represented pathways	Representative differentially expressed genes
1	VHL/*VHL*	Hypoxia	IGFBP3
			VEGF
	PGL4/*SDHB*	Angiogenesis	Proline 4-hydroxylase
			Stanniocalcin 1 and 2
		Oxidoreductase	Lactate dehydrogenase
			Hexokinase
	Sporadic tumors (Type 1)	Electron transport chain	Lysyl oxidase
		Krebs Cycle	Thrombospondin 2
		Adhesion	Collagen type V, XIV
		Proteasome degradation	Laminin
			Notch 3
			Thioredoxin
			Aldo-keto reductase 1, C1, C2
			Glutaryl-Coenzyme A dehydrogenase
			Glutaredoxin 2
			Thioltransferase
2	MEN 2/*RET*	Protein synthesis and translation	Glutamate receptor
	NF1/*NF1*		Adrenergicα2a receptor
		Kinase signaling	PHOX2a
	FP/unknown		PNMT
			Monoamine oxidase B
	Sporadic tumors ("type 2")	Neurodevelopment	RET tyrosine kinase
		Endocytosis	PI3-kinase-p85α subunit
		Adrenergic metabolism	MAPK 13
			src-family-associated phosphoprotein2
			IGF 1 receptor

VHL: von Hippel-Lindau; SDHB: succinate dehydrogenase subunit B; SDHD: succinate dehydrogenase subunit D; MEN 2: multiple endocrine neoplasia, NFI: neurofibromatosis type 1; FP: familial pheochromocytoma (novel hereditary variant).

VHL mutations prevent VHL binding to hydroxylated HIF1α, which results in increased HIF1α availability. HIF1α is able to translocate to the nucleus, where it dimerizes with HIF1β and binds to hypoxia-response elements (HREs) within the regulatory region of target genes.[12,13]

Hydroxylation of HIF1α is carried out by three oxygen-dependent prolyl hydroxylases (PHD), PHD1, PHD2, and PHD3, and requires 2-oxoglutarate, Fe(II), and ascorbate for this activity.[14–18] The end products of PHD activity, in addition to hydroxylated HIF, are succinate and CO_2. Under hypoxic conditions, PHD activity is suppressed and HIF exerts its downstream effects.[18] HIF activates a well-recognized set of genes involved in a variety of physiological processes, including angiogenesis, proliferation, cell survival and death, glucose transport, and glycolysis.[19] Several of these genes, including vascular endothelial growth factor (VEGF), hexokinase, lactate dehydrogenase, thrombospondin, and others, were highly expressed in *VHL* mutant compared with pheochromocytomas with *RET* or *NF1* mutations (TABLE 1).

A hypoxic-angiogenic signature was also notable amongst *SDH* (both *SDHB* and *SDHD*) mutant pheochromocytomas, indicating that these tumors similarly activate hypoxic signals.[5] This is in agreement with recent reports describing a HIF-mediated mechanism to explain the pathogenesis of *SDH*-related tumors.[20,21] These studies suggest that inhibition of PHD activity is the central defect that ultimately results in increased HIF availability in *SDH* loss-of-function.[22] Accumulation of succinate resulting from SDH dysfunction blocks the activity of PHD by a "product inhibition" effect[20] Low PHD activity in turn leads to increased HIF availability. In support for this theory, increased levels of succinate have been recently reported in primary pheochromocytomas and paragangliomas.[23,24] Inhibition of PHD activity was also recently shown to be at the center of the mechanism for increased HIF levels detected in tumors with loss-of-function of the *fumarate hydratase* (FH) gene.[25] FH, like SDH, is a component of the Krebs cycle, which has been associated with predisposition to renal carcinoma, and leiomyomas of the skin and uterus.[26] The shared metabolic functions of both enzymes and their role in cancer predisposition syndromes represent the strongest evidence yet for linking the hypoxia pathway with energy metabolism signaling.

An alternative (and not mutually exclusive) concept has also been suggested to explain the increased levels of HIF observed as a result of disrupted PHD activity. This model is based on the findings that increased production of reactive oxygen species (ROS) also diminishes activity of PHDs.[27] Through a yet unknown mechanism, ROS-mediated suppression of PHD activity leads to enhanced HIF availability. The finding of elevated ROS in an SDHC-null *C. elegans* model[28] and in a fibroblast cell line expressing a loss-of-function *SDHC* mutation[29] is in agreement with a "ROS theory" to explain SDH-mediated HIF activation, but has yet to be characterized in human pheochromocytomas or paragangliomas.

In addition to the hypoxia profile described above, a clear oxidoreductase component was identified in the transcription signature of *VHL*- and *SDH*-mutated tumors.[5] This pattern was predominantly defined by a coordinated suppression of redox-related genes, such as flavin reductase, glutaredoxin, aldo-keto reductase, glutaryl dehydrogenase, etc. While abnormal transcription of genes involved in the oxidative response might be expected in view of the oxidoreductase role of SDH, disrupted redox function has not been previously described in *VHL* mutations. As a result of our investigation of markers of the oxidoreductase imbalance displayed by this group of pheochromocytomas

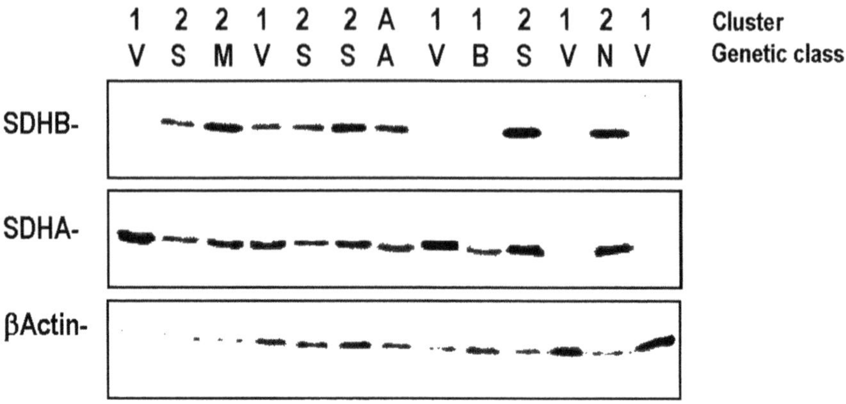

FIGURE 1. Low expression of SDHB is a general feature of cluster 1 tumors. (A) Expression of SDHB and SDHA protein in pheochromocytomas of various distinct genetic origins. SDHB expression segregates with transcription cluster distribution (1 or 2, as in TABLE 1). Western blot analysis of SDHB of whole cell lysates from primary tumors was performed as described in Dahia *et al.*[5] Genetic classes are defined as follows: MEN2 (M), NF1 (N), sporadic (S), VHL (V), SDHB (B), SDHD (D) tumors, normal adrenal medulla (A). β-Actin was used as a loading control.

we found consistently low expression of SDHB, but not SDHA, in protein lysates from tumors with mutations in *SDHB,* possibly as a result of instability caused by a mutant SDHB protein. However, the finding of equally suppressed levels of SDHB in pheochromocytomas with mutations in *SDHD* and the majority of *VHL*-mutated tumors, as well as in sporadic pheochromocytomas that belonged to Cluster 1 was surprising (FIG. 1). In contrast, tumors with *RET* and *NF1* mutations, components of Cluster 2, showed SDHB levels comparable to those of normal adrenal medulla (FIG. 1). Thus the reduction in SDHB protein expression appears to be representative of the underlying general oxidoreductase deficit displayed by pheochromocytomas in this group. It will be important to determine which other components of the oxidative response are similarly affected in these tumors.

Taken together with results from previous studies demonstrating loss of complex II function in tumors carrying *SDHB* and *SDHD* mutations,[3,30] the suppressed levels of SDHB in mutant tumors observed in this series of pheochromocytomas suggest that decreased SDHB expression may function as a marker for disrupted SDH/complex II activity. In addition, low SDHB levels in three of five VHL tumors and in sporadic pheochromocytomas that belonged to transcriptional Cluster 1 might indicate that not only tumors with mutations of *SDH* subunits, but some pheochromocytomas defective in *VHL* function and possibly other related pathways that affect sporadic tumors in this group, may also have a mitochondrial complex II dysfunction. As mentioned above, despite a clear segregation of SDHB expression with cluster distribution of the various subtypes of pheochromocytomas, we did not observe a similar

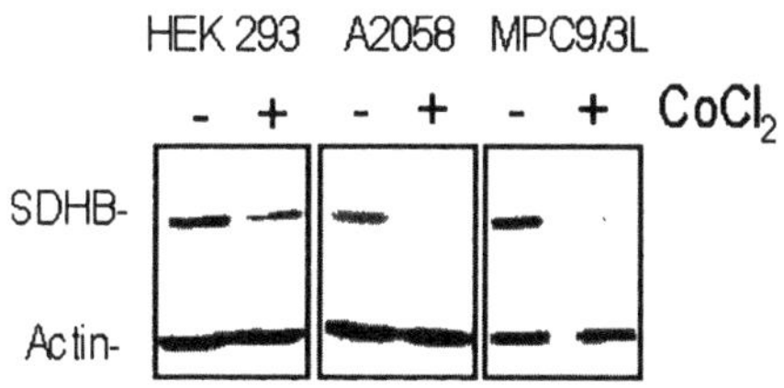

FIGURE 2. Hypoxic-like stimulus reduces SDHB levels. Cell lines of distinct tissue and embryonic origins, including embryonic kidney HEK293, melanoma A2058, and mouse pheochromocytoma MPC9/3L cell lines show consistent reduction of SDHB protein levels after exposure to the hypoxic mimetic agent, cobalt chloride ($CoCl_2$). Furthermore, transient expression in HEK293 cells of a HIF1α double mutant (P402A/P564A) that is resistant to VHL-mediated degradation has a similar effect on SDHB expression.[5] Conversely, A2058 cell lines where HIF1α expression was blocked by stable expression of a HIF1α short hairspin RNA (shHIF1α) do not show changes in SDHB after exposure to $CoCl_2$, in contrast to similarly treated cells that express a control shGFP RNA.

correspondence with SDHA expression. The reason for the lack of suppression of SDHA in Cluster 1 tumors is unclear and might reflect increased stability of this subunit despite the mitochondrial complex II dysfunction, or the presence of a highly homologous SDHA isoform that has been described to be co-expressed in chromaffin tissue and might be indistinguishably detected by our current methods.[24,31]

HIF1α IS INVOLVED IN THE SDHB DOWNREGULATION OF VHL TUMORS

Because HIF plays a central role in the hypoxic profile of VHL dysfunction, and, as indicated by these initial data, also of *SDH*-null tumors, we hypothesized that HIF might be implicated in the downregulation of SDHB. In agreement with this hypothesis, we first found that a variety of cell lines, both of chromaffin and nonchromaffin origin, responded to a hypoxic mimetic agent, cobalt chloride ($CoCl_2$), with reduction of SDHB protein levels (FIG. 2). In addition, overexpression of a nondegradable form of HIF1α, mutated at the prolyl residues that are targeted for PHD hydroxylation (HIF1αP402A/P564A), resulted in reduction of SDHB protein levels in HEK293 cells, which have an intact hypoxia signaling machinery.[5] Conversely, suppression of HIF1α by chronic expression of a HIF1α short-hairpin-RNA (shRNA), but not by control shRNA, in neural-crest-derived cell lines prevented downregulation of SDHB mediated by $CoCl_2$.[5] These results are consistent with a role for HIF1α in contributing to the decreased SDHB protein levels.

The precise mechanism for HIF's effects on SDHB remains unclear. The SDHB promoter lacks canonical hypoxia-responsive elements (HRE) typical of HIF1α target genes.[32] However, recent evidence indicates that HIF may

TABLE 2. Significant pathways in VHL- and SDH- related pheochromocytomas revealed by transcription profiling in addition to hypoxia-angiogenesis and oxidoreductase

Pathway/ontology	*P* value
Cell–cell signaling	0.04
Cell cycle	0.04
Chromatin	0.04
Agglutinin	0.03
Extracellular matrix component	0.007
Microtubule-associated complex	0.004
Nuclear cytoplasmic transport	0.002

affect expression of a variety of genes without the requirement for an HRE promoter site.[33–35] Studies examining whether this response is mediated by a transcriptional or posttranscriptional event are currently under way. At any rate, our preliminary results are consistent with a model whereby HIF1α activation reduces complex II function through SDHB downregulation (FIG. 3). Disrupted complex II would lead to reduced PHD activity either through ROS or elevated succinate levels. Low activity of PHD would enhance HIF1α availability with consequent activation of downstream targets, thus completing the feedback loop.

ADDITIONAL PATHWAYS MAY BE IMPLICATED IN THE TUMORIGENIC PROCESS RELATED TO LOSS OF SDH AND VHL FUNCTION

Despite the clear hypoxia/defective redox signature observed in *VHL*- and *SDH*-related tumors, other pathways were also found to be significantly enriched in the transcription profiling of these tumors (TABLE 2).[5] This suggests that the tumorigenic process defined by these mutations involves concurrent disruptions of multiple signals.

Although HIF operates as a central element in the VHL pathway, its role as the primary tumorigenic trigger in the lack of VHL function has been highly debatable.[36–40] In particular, *VHL* mutations that occur in Type 2C disease, which is characterized by familial occurrence of pheochromocytoma without other manifestations typical of the von Hippel–Lindau syndrome, suggest the existence of HIF-independent functions of VHL.[41,42] Furthermore, dysfunction of extracellular matrix formation has been identified independently from HIF in genetic studies of the *VHL* ortholog in *C. elegans*.[43] In support for additional pathways activated by dysfunctional VHL, a recent study has indicated that defective apoptosis of chromaffin precursor cells triggered by HIF-independent signals might be a common event in multiple pheochromocytoma syndromes.[44] Further clues on additional functions of VHL and SDH might be obtained by examining the coordinate regulation of genes with common

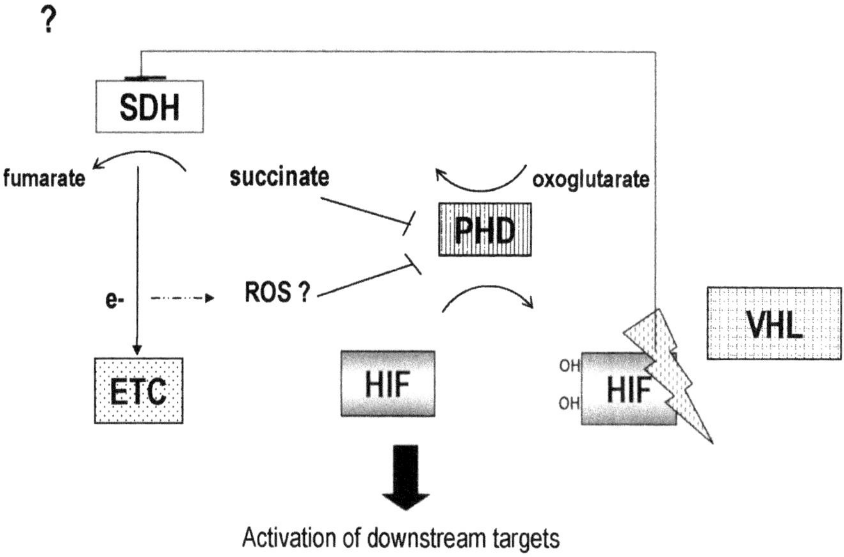

FIGURE 3. Diagram showing the interaction of the VHL, SDH, and HIF pathways. Mutations in *VHL* and *SDH* genes increase HIF1α availability due to reduced proteasome-mediated degradation of HIF or to reduced activity of prolyl hydroxylase (PHD), respectively. PHD hydroxylates HIF (HIF-OH) and makes it a target for VHL recognition and degradation by the proteasome pathway (*lightning-shaped arrow*). The dual function of SDH at the Krebs cycle and electron transport chain (ETC) may, when disrupted, contribute to reduce PHD activity. Elevated succinate levels that result from loss of the Krebs cycle function reduce PHD activity by a product inhibition effect. Mutations in *SDH* may also affect PHD function by a putative increase in generation of reactive oxygen species (ROS). Reduced PHD activity leads to stabilization of HIF1α. Furthermore, HIF1α can down-regulate SDHB, which may lead to instability of complex II, and consequently, reduced PHD activity. The mechanisms of HIF's suppression of SDHB are still unknown. Increased HIF1α activity results in transcription of downstream targets, including angiogenic factors.

transcription factor binding sites within specific tumor classes with mutations in *VHL, SDHB,* and *SDHD.*

TRANSLATIONAL POTENTIAL OF THE TRANSCRIPTION PROFILING: SDHB AS A MARKER TO DISTINGUISH SUBTYPES OF PHEOCHROMOCYTOMAS

Identification of markers of pheochromocytoma subgroups can have an impact on diagnosis and may be a useful tool for follow-up and surveillance of discrete tumor subtypes.[45] We used the information obtained from the expression profiling analysis to verify the value of SDHB immunostaining to distinguish pheochromocytomas belonging to Cluster 1 (*VHL, SDHB,* and

SDHD mutants) from tumors represented by Cluster 2 (MEN 2- and NF1-related pheochromocytomas). The majority of tumors with mutations in *SDHB* and *SDHD* (80% and 67%, respectively) and also, though to a lesser extent, *VHL*-mutant pheochromocytomas (40%) showed almost undetectable SDHB staining, while all tumors with *RET* and *NF1* mutations tested had very high expression levels of SDHB, determined both by intensity and percentage of stained tumor cells (P. Dahia and V. Nose, unpublished results).[5] In contrast, SDHA expression had an opposing staining pattern in these tumors. This is similar to results from a study of head and neck paragangliomas with *SDHB* or *SDHD* mutations.[46] Our pilot results suggest that the SDHB and SDHA immunostaining pattern may function as markers for distinguishing Cluster 1 from Cluster 2 pheochromocytomas. Expanded series will be required to validate this initial finding.

In summary, our findings provide a link between pheochromocytomas with mutations in distinct genes, *VHL, SDHB,* and *SDHD*, which share a common effect on the hypoxia response, and also suggest that mitochondrial complex II inhibition may contribute to enhance HIF1α signals. It is tempting to speculate that mitochondrial complex II inhibition may contribute to the development of a broader group of tumors with an increased hypoxic response. Importantly, since hypoxic signals are found in a variety of cancers, and have been suggested to define a more severe prognosis for these tumors,[47,48] the current findings may have broad implications for a variety of malignancies. Identification of the underlying molecular mechanisms for the link between hypoxia and energy signals may offer opportunities to explore future therapeutic targets in tumors with prominent hypoxic profile. Along these lines, the use of enhancers of PHD activity as a means to reverse increased HIF1α levels may constitute a promising new avenue for future testing in *SDH*- and *VHL*-null models.[49]

APPENDIX

Familial Pheochromocytoma Consortium (FP Consortium) members and their affiliations follow:

Gail Adler, Brigham and Women's Hospital, Boston, MA 02115; Seth M. Arum, Boston Medical Center, Boston, MA; Marta Barontini, Center of Endocrinology Investigations CEDIE, Buenos Aires, Argentina; Diana E. Benn, Royal North Shore Hospital and Kolling Institute of Medical Research, University of Sydney, Australia; Ana Valéria B. de Castro, Universidade Estadual Paulista, Botucatu, SP, Brazil; Robert Dluhy, Brigham and Women's Hospital, Boston, MA, Judy Garber, Department of Population Sciences, Dana-Farber Cancer Institute, Harvard Medical School, Boston, MA; John Godine, Massachusetts General Hospital, Diabetes Center, Boston, MA; Ashley Grossman, St. Bartholomew's Hospital, London, UK; Shirin Haddady, Division of Endocrinology, University of Massachusetts Memorial

Medical Center, Worcester, MA, Shannon Heitritter, Brigham and Women's Hospital, Boston, MA, Richard Hodin, Department of Surgery, Massachusetts General Hospital, Boston, MA; Márta Korbonits, St. Bartholomew's Hospital, London, UK; Deborah J. Marsh, Royal North Shore Hospital and Kolling Institute of Medical Research, University of Sydney, Australia; Francis Moore, Jr, Brigham and Women's Hospital, Boston, MA, Célia Nogueira, Universidade Estadual Paulista, Botucatu, SP, Brazil; Vania Nosé, Department of Pathology, Brigham and Women's Hospital, Boston, MA; I. Tolgay Ocal, Yale University, New Haven, CT; Pascal Pigny, Regional University Hospital, CHRU, Lille, France; James A. Powers, Tufts New England Medical Center, Boston, MA; Bruce G. Robinson, Royal North Shore Hospital and Kolling Institute of Medical Research, University of Sydney, Australia; Marie Rosales, Division of Endocrinology, University of Massachusetts Memorial Medical Center, Worcester, MA; Gabriela Sanso, Center of Endocrinology Investigations CEDIE, Buenos Aires, Argentina; Sandro Santagata, Department of Pathology, Brigham and Women's Hospital, Boston, MA; Kathy Schneider, Department of Population Sciences, Dana-Farber Cancer Institute, Harvard Medical School, Boston, MA; Julie Ann Sosa, Yale University, New Haven, CT; Charles D. Stiles, Dana-Farber Cancer Institute, Harvard Medical School, Boston, MA; Arthur S. Tischler, Tufts New England Medical Center, Boston, MA; Sérgio P. A. Toledo, University of São Paulo, School of Medicine, São Paulo SP, Brazil.

ACKNOWLEDGMENTS

Patricia Dahia is a recipient of a South Texas Health Research Center (STHRC) Junior Faculty Award and a UTHSCSA Executive Research Committee (ERC) New Investigator Award.

REFERENCES

1. MANGER, W.M. & R.W. GIFFORD. 2002. Pheochromocytoma. J. Clin. Hypertens. (Greenwich) **4:** 62–72.
2. BRYANT, J. *et al.* 2003. Pheochromocytoma: the expanding genetic differential diagnosis. J. Natl. Cancer. Inst. **95:** 1196–1204.
3. GIMENEZ-ROQUEPLO, A.P. *et al.* 2003. Mutations in the SDHB gene are associated with extra-adrenal and/or malignant phaeochromocytomas. Cancer Res. **63:** 5615–5621.
4. NEUMANN, H.P. *et al.* 2002. Germ-line mutations in nonsyndromic pheochromocytoma. N. Engl. J. Med. **346:** 1459–1466.
5. DAHIA, P.L.M. *et al.* 2005. A HIF1α regulatory loop links hypoxia and mitochondrial signals in pheochromocytomas. PLoS Genet. **1:** e8.
6. DAHIA, P.L.M. *et al.* 2005. Novel pheochromocytoma susceptibility loci identified by integrative genomics. Cancer Res. **65:** 9651–9658.

7. SUBRAMANIAN, A. *et al.* 2005. From the cover: gene set enrichment analysis: a knowledge-based approach for interpreting genome-wide expression profiles. Proc. Natl. Acad. Sci. USA **102:** 15545–15550.
8. WYKOFF, C.C. *et al.* 2001. The HIF pathway: implications for patterns of gene expression in cancer. Novartis Found. Symp. **240:** 212–225; discussion 225-231.
9. EISENHOFER, G. *et al.* 2004. Distinct gene expression profiles in norepinephrine and epinephrine producing hereditary and sporadic pheochromocytomas: activation of hypoxia-driven angiogenic pathways in von Hippel-Lindau syndrome. Endocr. Relat. Cancer **11:** 897–911.
10. KAELIN, W.G. JR. 2003. The von Hippel-Lindau gene, kidney cancer, and oxygen sensing. J. Am. Soc. Nephrol. **14:** 2703–2711.
11. KAELIN, W.G. JR. 2002. How oxygen makes its presence felt. Genes Dev. **16:** 1441–1445.
12. SEMENZA, G.L. 2004. Hydroxylation of HIF-1: oxygen sensing at the molecular level. Physiology (Bethesda). **19:** 176–182.
13. SEMENZA, G.L. 2002. HIF-1 and tumor progression: pathophysiology and therapeutics. Trends Mol. Med. **8:** S62–S67.
14. IVAN, M. *et al.* 2001. HIFα targeted for VHL-mediated destruction by proline hydroxylation: implications for O_2 sensing. Science **292:** 464–468.
15. JAAKKOLA, P. *et al.* 2001. Targeting of HIFα to the von Hippel-Lindau ubiquitylation complex by O_2-regulated prolyl hydroxylation. Science **292:** 468–472.
16. APPELHOFF, R.J. *et al.* 2004. Differential function of the prolyl hydroxylases PHD1, PHD2, and PHD3 in the regulation of hypoxia-inducible factor. J. Biol. Chem. **279:** 38458–38465.
17. MAXWELL, P.H. & P.J. RATCLIFFE. 2002. Oxygen sensors and angiogenesis. Semin. Cell Dev. Biol. **13:** 29–37.
18. EPSTEIN, A.C. *et al.* 2001. *C. elegans* EGL-9 and mammalian homologs define a family of dioxygenases that regulate HIF by prolyl hydroxylation. Cell **107:** 43–54.
19. SEMENZA, G.L. 2002. Involvement of hypoxia-inducible factor 1 in human cancer. Intern. Med. **41:** 79–83.
20. SELAK, M.A. *et al.* 2005. Succinate links TCA cycle dysfunction to oncogenesis by inhibiting HIFα prolyl hydroxylase. Cancer Cell **7:** 77–85.
21. GIMENEZ-ROQUEPLO, A.P. *et al.* 2002. Functional consequences of a SDHB gene mutation in an apparently sporadic pheochromocytoma. J. Clin. Endocrinol. Metab. **87:** 4771–4774.
22. GOTTLIEB, E. & I.P. TOMLINSON. 2005. Mitochondrial tumour suppressors: a genetic and biochemical update. Nat. Rev. Cancer **5:** 857–866.
23. POLLARD, P.J. *et al.* 2005. Accumulation of Krebs cycle intermediates and overexpression of HIF1α in tumours which result from germline FH and SDH mutations. Hum. Mol. Genet. **14:** 2231–2239.
24. BRIERE, J.J. *et al.* 2005. Mitochondrial succinate is instrumental for HIF1α nuclear translocation in SDHA-mutant fibroblasts under normoxic conditions. Hum. Mol. Genet. **14:** 3263–3269.
25. ISAACS, J.S. *et al.* 2005. HIF overexpression correlates with biallelic loss of fumarate hydratase in renal cancer: novel role of fumarate in regulation of HIF stability. Cancer Cell **8:** 143–153.
26. TOMLINSON, I.P. *et al.* 2002. Germline mutations in FH predispose to dominantly inherited uterine fibroids, skin leiomyomata and papillary renal cell cancer. Nat. Genet. **30:** 406–410.

27. GERALD, D. *et al.* 2004. JunD reduces tumor angiogenesis by protecting cells from oxidative stress. Cell **118:** 781–794.
28. ISHII, N. *et al.* 1998. A mutation in succinate dehydrogenase cytochrome B causes oxidative stress and ageing in nematodes. Nature **394:** 694–697.
29. ISHII, T. *et al.* 2005. A mutation in the SDHC gene of complex II increases oxidative stress, resulting in apoptosis and tumorigenesis. Cancer Res. **65:** 203–209.
30. GIMENEZ-ROQUEPLO, A.P. *et al.* 2001. The R22X mutation of the SDHD gene in hereditary paraganglioma abolishes the enzymatic activity of complex II in the mitochondrial respiratory chain and activates the hypoxia pathway. Am. J. Hum. Genet. **69:** 1186–1197.
31. TOMITSUKA, E. *et al.* 2003. Direct evidence for expression of type II flavoprotein subunit in human complex II (succinate-ubiquinone reductase). Biochem. Biophys. Res. Commun. **311:** 774–779.
32. AU, H.C. & I.E. SCHEFFLER. 1998. Promoter analysis of the human succinate dehydrogenase iron-protein gene—both nuclear respiratory factors NRF-1 and NRF-2 are required. Eur. J. Biochem. **251:** 164–174.
33. GUSTAFSSON, M.V. *et al.* 2005. Hypoxia requires notch signaling to maintain the undifferentiated cell state. Dev. Cell. **9:** 617–628.
34. KOSHIJI, M. *et al.* 2005. HIF-1α induces genetic instability by transcriptionally downregulating MutSalpha expression. Mol. Cell. **17:** 793–803.
35. KOSHIJI, M. *et al.* 2004. HIF-1α induces cell cycle arrest by functionally counteracting Myc. EMBO J. **23:** 1949–1956.
36. WYKOFF, C.C. *et al.* 2004. Gene array of VHL mutation and hypoxia shows novel hypoxia-induced genes and that cyclin D1 is a VHL target gene. Br. J. Cancer **90:** 1235–1243.
37. MACK, F.A. *et al.* 2003. Loss of pVHL is sufficient to cause HIF dysregulation in primary cells but does not promote tumor growth. Cancer Cell **3:** 75–88.
38. KONDO, K. *et al.* 2003. Inhibition of HIF2α is sufficient to suppress pVHL-defective tumor growth. PLoS Biol. **1:** E83.
39. KIM, W. & W.G. KAELIN JR. 2003. The von Hippel-Lindau tumor suppressor protein: new insights into oxygen sensing and cancer. Curr. Opin. Genet. Dev. **13:** 55–60.
40. RAVAL, R.R. *et al.* 2005. Contrasting properties of hypoxia-inducible factor 1 (HIF-1) and HIF-2 in von Hippel-Lindau-associated renal cell carcinoma. Mol. Cell. Biol. **25:** 5675–5686.
41. CLIFFORD, S.C. *et al.* 2001. Contrasting effects on HIF-1α regulation by disease-causing pVHL mutations correlate with patterns of tumourigenesis in von Hippel-Lindau disease. Hum. Mol. Genet. **10:** 1029–1038.
42. HOFFMAN, M.A. *et al.* 2001. von Hippel-Lindau protein mutants linked to type 2C VHL disease preserve the ability to downregulate HIF. Hum. Mol. Genet. **10:** 1019–1027.
43. BISHOP, T. *et al.* 2004. Genetic analysis of pathways regulated by the von Hippel-Lindau tumor suppressor in *Caenorhabditis elegans*. PLoS Biol. **2:** e289.
44. LEE, S. *et al.* 2005. Neuronal apoptosis linked to EglN3 prolyl hydroxylase and familial pheochromocytoma genes: developmental culling and cancer. Cancer Cell **8:** 155–167.
45. EISENHOFER, G. *et al.* 2004. Malignant pheochromocytoma: current status and initiatives for future progress. Endocr. Relat. Cancer **11:** 423–436.
46. DOUWES DEKKER, P.B. *et al.* 2003. SDHD mutations in head and neck paragangliomas result in destabilization of complex II in the mitochondrial respiratory

chain with loss of enzymatic activity and abnormal mitochondrial morphology. J. Pathol. **201:** 480–486.

47. Birner, P. *et al.* 2000. Overexpression of hypoxia-inducible factor 1α is a marker for an unfavorable prognosis in early-stage invasive cervical cancer. Cancer Res. **60:** 4693–4696.
48. Aebersold, D.M. *et al.* 2001. Expression of hypoxia-inducible factor-1α: a novel predictive and prognostic parameter in the radiotherapy of oropharyngeal cancer. Cancer Res. **61:** 2911–2916.
49. Temes, E. *et al.* 2005. Activation of HIF-prolyl hydroxylases by R59949, an inhibitor of the diacylglycerol kinase. J. Biol. Chem. **280:** 24238–24244.

A Phenotypic Perspective on Mammalian Oxygen Sensor Candidates

BORA E. BAYSAL

Department of Obstetrics, Gynecology and Reproductive Sciences, University of Pittsburgh School of Medicine, Pittsburgh, Pennsylvania, USA

ABSTRACT: Chronic hypoxic stimulation in mammals can induce several phenotypic changes, such as polycythemia, pulmonary vascular changes, pulmonary hypertension, and carotid body (CB) enlargement. These phenotypic alterations provide a tool to test whether an oxygen sensor candidate is involved in an organism's response to environmental hypoxia. Here I evaluate the phenotypic evidence for several commonly considered oxygen sensor candidates. Germline mutations in NADPH oxidase, mitochondrial complexes I, III, IV, and heme oxygenase 2 genes cause different phenotypic consequences, suggesting distinct physiological roles rather than oxygen sensing. Germline mutations in *VHL* and HIF1 prolyl hydroxylase 2 genes cause polycythemia consistent with their role in oxygen homeostasis. However, it is unclear whether environmental variations affecting oxygen availability modify their phenotype, as would be expected from a defect in an oxygen sensor. Succinate dehydrogenase (SDH); mitochondrial complex II) germline mutations cause CB paragangliomas and there is evidence that the severity and the population genetics of paragangliomas may be influenced by altitude. Thus, from a phenotypic perspective, succinate dehydrogenase (SDH) appears to be a well-supported oxygen sensor candidate. It is suggested that a universal oxygen sensor candidate must be supported by evidence from multiple layers of biological complexity.

KEYWORDS: hereditary paraganglioma; *SDHD* gene; mitochondrim; reductionist approach

INTRODUCTION

Oxygen is critical for life in mammals. Homeostatic mechanisms that compensate for oxygen deprivation are well recognized and reviewed extensively.[1,2] At the organismic level, hypoxia is sensed within seconds by the carotid body

Address for correspondence: Bora E. Baysal, M.D., Ph.D., Department of Obstetrics, Gynecology and Reproductive Sciences, University of Pittsburgh School of Medicine, Magee-Women's Research Institute-Room 424, 204 Craft Avenue, Pittsburgh, PA, 15213. Voice: 412-641-6093; fax: 412-641-6156.
e-mail: baysalb@mwri.magee.edu

Ann. N.Y. Acad. Sci. 1073: 221–233 (2006). © 2006 New York Academy of Sciences.
doi: 10.1196/annals.1353.024

(CB), a small highly vascular organ located at the bifurcation of the common carotid artery, to stimulate the cardiorespiratory system and increase the ventilation and heart rates.[3] Chronic hypoxia leads to longer-term adaptive changes through transcriptional activation of many genes critical for survival under hypoxia. For example, erythropoietin (Epo), which is synthesized primarily by kidney upon hypoxic challenge, increases erythrocyte production by the bone marrow to compensate for the reduced oxygen delivery to the peripheral tissues. The transcriptional response to chronic hypoxia is thought to be primarily regulated by hypoxia-inducible factor (HIF), a heterodimer protein composed of an oxygen-regulated alpha subunit and a constitutively active beta subunit.[4]

Chronic hypoxic exposure, as occurs in mammals dwelling in high altitudes or in certain medical conditions, such as cyanotic heart and chronic lung diseases, induces certain phenotypic changes, such as polycythemia secondary to Epo stimulation,[5] pulmonary vascular changes, pulmonary hypertension[6] and ensuing right heart failure,[7] and CB enlargement and paragangliomas.[8] It is possible that additional and currently less-recognized phenotypic features may also be associated with chronic hypoxic exposure. The presence of these phenotypes without an obvious hypoxic condition may suggest inborn defects in oxygen homeostasis. The more specific a phenotype for chronic hypoxia, the more pathognomonic it will be to suspect an underlying condition associated with hypoxic stimulation. For example, polycythemia secondary to Epo stimulation and CB paragangliomas are highly specific indicators of chronic hypoxic stimulation because their incidence, especially of the head and neck paragangliomas ($\sim$1 in 1,000,000), is rather low.[9] In contrast, right heart failure and pulmonary hypertension are common medical conditions with great etiologic diversity.

Although homeostatic mechanisms against hypoxia suggest the presence of oxygen-sensing mechanisms in mammals, the molecular identity of a universal mammalian oxygen sensor has not been confirmed. Over the years several molecules have been proposed as oxygen sensors and multiple oxygen-sensing mechanisms have been suggested.[10] Oxygen sensor candidates were often proposed on the basis of at least these two observations: first, the candidate molecule interacts with molecular oxygen, and second *in vitro* structural or functional perturbations in the candidate sensor disrupt regulation of certain known hypoxia-induced pathways. Because these observations were made on experimental and molecular systems, I would like to refer to this methodology to select an oxygen sensor candidate as the molecular-reductionist approach.

An alternative, but much less emphasized, approach to identify an oxygen sensor involves elucidation of the genetic bases of rare cases and families with chronic hypoxic phenotypes in the absence of any hypoxic challenge. This approach can be referred to as the phenotypic-genetic approach. The phenotypic-genetic perspective to identify an oxygen sensor is based on a simple rationale. The quantitative reduction either in the molecular oxygen levels or in the proteins that sense them through physical interaction must have the same phenotypic consequences. If a molecule is involved in the sensation of environmental oxygen levels, then its reduced levels caused by loss of function mutations should mimic hypoxia and recapitulate the phenotypic characteristics seen among subjects challenged by chronic hypoxia.

Ideally, if either the molecular-reductionist or the phenotypic-genetic approach correctly identifies an oxygen sensor, the other method should provide confirmatory evidence. In other terms, a candidate oxygen sensor molecule identified by the molecular-reductionist approach should create a hypoxic phenotype when it is mutated. Similarly, the protein product of a gene identified by the phenotypic-genetic approach should interact with molecular oxygen, and its alterations *in vitro* should disrupt regulation of oxygen-sensing pathways. Here, I will briefly examine evidence for several oxygen sensor candidates: two oxygen sensor candidates suggested by the phenotypic-genetic approach and then four candidates identified by the molecular-reductionist approaches.

OXYGEN SENSOR CANDIDATES OF THE PHENOTYPIC-GENETIC APPROACH

Chuvash Polycythemia

Polycythemias refer to an abnormal increase in circulating red blood cell numbers. Primary polycythemias are caused by abnormalities in red cell precursors, whereas secondary polycythemias are caused by increased Epo levels.[11] Chuvash polycythemia (CP) is caused by a homozygous missense founder mutation (598C>T) in the *VHL* gene. The *VHL* is the gene mutated in the Von Hippel–Lindau syndrome, which in characterized by cerebellar and retinal hemangiomas, clear-cell renal cell carcinomas, and pheochromocytomas. The *VHL* protein product (pVHL) is involved in the degradation of hydroxylated HIF1-α subunits during normoxia. In normoxia, the HIF1-α subunit is hydroxylated at prolyl and asparaginyl residues by a class of oxygen-, ascorbate-, Fe^{2+}-dependent hydroxylases. In hypoxia, HIF1-α subunits are not hydroxylated and escape the degradation pathway. The accumulation of HIF1-α subunits triggers the formation of transcriptionally active HIF1 dimer.[12]

CP is phenotypically similar to the polycythemias with high Epo levels that develop upon chronic hypoxic exposure, as occurs in congenital heart and chronic lung disorders and in certain hemoglobin abnormalities with high oxygen affinity. Therefore, the genetic defect in CP mimics a chronic hypoxic phenotype and confirms the role for pVHL suggested by the molecular evidence in the oxygen homeostasis.[13] CP is endemic to the Chuvash population in Russia, although the same mutation was also detected in other polycythemia cases. Interestingly, the same founder mutation was also discovered in distant regions, such as in southern Italy.[14] Environmental factors and population history involved in the dissemination of this founder mutation in such geographically distant populations are unknown. It has been speculated that this mutation may have conferred a selective advantage in phenotypically normal heterozygous carriers against iron-deficiency anemia, which may be predisposed by certain environmental or dietary factors.[14] The CP founder mutation provides a unique opportunity to shed further light on the pVHL's biological role.

Hereditary Paraganglioma

Hereditary paraganglioma (PGL) is characterized by the development of highly vascularized tumors of the paraganglionic system and is caused by germline heterozygous mutations in the *SDHB, SDHC,* and *SDHD* subunit genes of succinate dehydrogenase (SDH).[9] SDH oxidizes succinate to fumarate in Krebs cycle and also functions as mitochondrial complex II by directly transferring the electrons extracted from succinate to ubiquinone. The CB and other head and neck paragangliomas develop frequently among SDH mutation carriers, especially those with *SDHD* mutations. Because CB paragangliomas also develop in mammals dwelling at high altitudes, SDH is a candidate complex involved in oxygen sensing and signaling.[15]

The precise role of SDH in the oxygen-sensing pathway is unknown. Global gene expression analysis of PGL tumors strongly confirms the disruption of oxygen-sensing pathways.[16] Selak *et al.*[17] showed that experimental down-regulation of SDH leads to hypoxic pathway induction and proposed that the impact of SDH mutations on oxygen sensing is attributable to the accumulation of succinate, which inhibits HIF1 hydroxylases. However, it is unknown what would make succinate particularly important for the *in vivo* regulation of HIF1 hydroxylases, because other organic molecules, including fumarate,[18] oxaloacetate, and pyruvate,[19] seem to regulate HIF1 hydroxylase enzymatic activities. We previously analyzed genotype–phenotype–altitude interactions in subjects carrying *SDHD* mutations and the population genetics of *SDHD* founder mutations and suggested that increased altitudes increase severity of paraganglioma tumors.[20] Indeed, altitude seems to correlate well with the population genetic characteristics of PGL tumors. The higher the altitude, the lower the frequency of *SDHD* mutations in the etiology of PGL tumors.[21] This is thought to be a consequence of the elimination of *SDHD* mutations in populations residing at higher altitudes. In contrast, the *SDHD* mutations in populations residing in lower altitudes, such as the Netherlands, may increase in frequency. The influence of altitude on the PGL phenotype suggests that SDH activity may be directly regulated by molecular oxygen (see discussion below), although no biochemical evidence exists yet to support this prediction.

OXYGEN SENSOR CANDIDATES OF THE MOLECULAR-REDUCTIONIST APPROACH

NADPH Oxidase

Several models of O_2 sensing include the involvement of redox-dependent reactions and implicate reactive oxygen species (ROS) in the signaling process.[10] NADPH oxidase is a key enzyme in neutrophils, where it is involved in the bactericidal production of ROS. NADPH oxidase uses NADPH as the electron donor and reduces oxygen to superoxide. Identification of NADPH oxidase-like enzymes in non-neutrophil cells suggested that NADPH oxidase-derived ROS could play a role in oxygen-sensitive processes, including hypoxic pulmonary vasoconstriction (HPV), CB chemoreceptor activation, and Epo gene expression.[22] In general, it has been suggested that hypoxia depresses ROS levels generated by NADPH oxidase in O_2-sensitive cells. These suggestions were derived primarily from experiments using (*a*) pharmacologic inhibitors of NADPH oxidase, such as iodonium compounds diphenyleneiodonium (DPI) or iodonium diphenyl (ID); (*b*) chemicals, such as hydrogen peroxide (H_2O_2) that alter the redox status of cells; and (*c*) data demonstrating widespread expression of NADPH subunit genes.

NADPH oxidase is a multisubunit enzyme consisting of a flavocytochrome, which is a heterodimer. The smaller or α subunit is approximately 22 kDa (p22-phox), while the larger β subunit is approximately 91 kDa (gp91-phox). Upon activation of NADPH, three other polypeptides of 67 kDa (p67-phox), 47 kDa (p47-phox), and 40 kDa (p40-phox) join the complex. Activity of the complex also involves at least two G proteins, Rap1A and p21rac2. These proteins alternate between binding GDP (inactive state) and GTP (active state).

Germline mutations in four of the five subunits of NADPH oxidase cause chronic granulomatous disease (CGD). CGD is a primary immunodeficiency disorder of the innate immune system.[23] The mutations result in an absence or very low level of enzymatic activity that leads to a defective production of microbicidal superoxides, such as hydrogen peroxide and hydroxyl radical, and impairs killing of potential pathogens. Consequently, CGD patients sometimes suffer fatal recurrent bacterial and fungal infections. More than half of all CGD cases are caused by mutations in the X-linked *CYBB* gene that encodes the gp91-phox subunit.

Experiments testing the integrity of oxygen-sensing pathways on transgenic mice lacking the gp91 subunit of NADPH oxidase have generated conflicting results. While some studies suggested disruption of oxygen sensing in transgenic mouse,[24] others found preservation of oxygen-sensing mechanisms in Epo-producing cells, pulmonary vascular cells, and in the CB.[25–27]

The phenotypic characteristics of the genetic impairment of NADPH oxidase subunits in humans suggest a physiological role to provide natural barriers in the respiratory tract and lymph nodes against bacteria and fungi, rather than oxygen homeostasis. To support the hypothesis that NADPH oxidase has a role in oxygen sensing at the organism level, it is essential to demonstrate that chronic hypoxic exposure increases risk of such infections in normal subjects.

Mitochondrial Oxidative Phosphorylation Complexes

Mitochondria have received much attention in regulating responses to hypoxia. Respiratory stimulation effects of many poisons are linked to their inhibitory effects on oxidative phosphorylation (OXPHOS) complexes in mitochondria. OXPHOS is composed of five multimeric complexes. Complexes I–IV make up the electron transport chain (ETC), whereas complex V is the ATP synthase. Dietary carbohydrate and fat are oxidized to common reducing elements NADH + H^+ and $FADH_2$, which transfer their electrons to mitochondrial complex I (NADH + H^+-ubiquinone oxidoreductase) and complex II (succinate-ubiquinone oxidoreductase), respectively. The sequential transfer of electrons from the reducing elements to ubiquione (coenzyme Q) through complex I/II, then to cytochrome *c* through complex III (ubiquinole-cytochrome C oxidoreductase), and then to molecular oxygen through complex IV (cytochrome *c*:oxygen oxidoreductase; cytochrome oxidase) is accompanied by proton pumping, which generates an electrochemical potential energy that is used by complex V to synthesize ATP.[28]

The role of mitochondria in oxygen sensing has been debated on the basis of conflicting results obtained in *in vitro* models. For example, each of the four OXPHOS complexes were claimed to be critical in CB's oxygen sensing.[29] These experiments often employed drug inhibitors of OXPHOS complexes, such as rotenone, myxothiazol, antimycin A, cyanide, and mitochondria-depleted cell lines to study alterations in either stabilization of HIF1-α and/or in ion channel activities causing hypoxic chemotransduction in oxygen-sensitive cells.[29,30] More recently, inhibition of OXPHOS complex activities by means of small interfering RNA (siRNA) was employed to study the role of mitochondria in oxygen sensing.[31] Some studies supported an important role for mitochondria while others questioned it.[32] Studies emphasizing the role of mitochondria in oxygen sensing have not converged on specific OXPHOS complexes or on specific mechanisms to explain the sensing process.[31–33] As a result, consensus remains elusive for answers to several important questions, such as: (1) which OXPHOS complex(es) senses the reduced oxygen concentrations; (2) what conformational/enzymatic changes the sensor acquires during hypoxia; (3) whether ROS or another secondary messenger is involved in activating the hypoxic pathways; and (4) if ROS is involved, whether its levels decrease or increase during hypoxic signaling.

Subunits for all OXPHOS complexes, with the exception of complex II, are encoded by both nuclear and mitochondrial genomes. All subunits of complex II are encoded by the nuclear genome. Complex I is composed of approximately

42 subunits. Complex II, III, IV, and V are composed of 4, 11, 13, and 16 subunits, respectively. It is surprising that although mitochondria have been frequently implicated as an oxygen sensor organelle in *in vitro* experiments using mitochondrial inhibitors, confirmatory evidence in transgenic mouse models carrying mutations in OXPHOS complex subunits have been rarely sought. Piruat *et al.*[34] tested the integrity of oxygen sensing by the CB in a transgenic mouse model carrying heterozygous gene deletion in the *SDHD* subunit of complex II. They found that the heterozygous mouse did not develop paragangliomas and that CB showed persistent hypersensitivity to hypoxia but retained hypoxia responsiveness. Unfortunately, embryonic lethality of the homozygous null mouse and the failure to recapitulate the CB paragangliomas prevented a more definitive assessment of the role of complex II in CB's oxygen sensing.

The phenotype in inherited OXPHOS defects in humans is very complex and diverse.[35] Mutations in OXPHOS complex subunit genes were associated with Leber optic atrophy, Leigh syndrome, syndromic encephalopathy, leukodystrophy, myoclonic epilepsy, pediatric hypotonia, vomiting, strabismus, and central nervous system atrophy. The underlying pathophysiology may involve impairment of ATP production, oxidative stress, or uncontrolled apoptosis. It is unknown whether any of these phenotypes are associated with defective oxygen sensing.[28] Specifically, there is no evidence that the subunit mutations in complex I, complex III, and complex IV lead to hypoxia-related phenotypes, such as polycythemia and CB paraganglioma that would suggest involvement of these complexes in oxygen-sensing pathways. Thus far, the only established genetic link between OXPHOS complexes and oxygen-sensing pathways has come from PGLs that are caused by mutations in mitochondrial complex II subunits SDHB, SDHC, and SDHD.

In summary, the germline mutations in the subunits of OXPHOS complexes that are considered as oxygen sensors in experimental models do not appear to provide much supportive evidence for their involvement in oxygen homeostasis at the organism level.

HIF1-α Hydroxylases

Whereas mitochondria and NADPH oxidases were considered as oxygen sensor candidates, partly because of their role in redox-dependent events and ROS production, a newer group of candidates emerged by studying the regulation of HIF1-α. HIF1-α is bound by pVHL tumor suppressor protein and targeted for proteasomal destruction upon hydroxylation at proline and asparagine residues under normoxic conditions. When oxygen concentrations fall, HIF1-α is stabilized. It has been demonstrated that inhibition of HIF1-α hydroxylation under hypoxic conditions prevents its degradation and leads to its stabilization as a transcription factor. Because the enzymes that hydroxylate HIF1-α, referred to as HPH1/PHD1/EGLN1,

HPH2/PHD2/EGLN2, HPH3/PHD3/EGLN3, and FIH, use molecular oxygen as well as Fe^{2+} and 2-oxoglutarate (2-OG, α-ketoglutarate) in a concentration-dependent manner, they were suggested as cellular oxygen sensors.[36,37]

Although HIF1 hydroxylases were shown to be sensitive to changes in oxygen concentrations *in vitro*, increasing numbers of observations implicate other proteins and molecules affecting their activities as well. For example, in addition to the substrates oxygen, Fe^{2+} and 2-OG, HIF1 hydroxylase enzymatic activities could be altered by ROS, nitric oxide (NO), and Krebs cycle intermediates, such as succinate and fumarate, as well as other molecules of intermediary metabolism. Furthermore, HIF1 hydroxylase activities could be subject to further regulation by other oxygen-regulated proteins, such as HIF, Siah1 and 2.[38] The complexity level involved in the regulation of HIF hydroxylase and their multiplicity makes it difficult to appreciate whether the HIF hydroxylases are regulated *in vivo* directly by molecular oxygen during hypoxia, as expected from an oxygen sensor, or whether other cellular and metabolic alterations induced by hypoxia have temporally more proximate roles in their inhibition.

There is a limited amount of information on the phenotypic consequences of mutations in genes encoding the HPH/EGLN/PHD family of HIF1 hydroxylases. Transgenic animal models with inactivated HPH/PHD/EGLN genes have yet to be reported. A small family with three affected individuals (father and two children) with erythrocytosis has been very recently identified carrying a heterozygous mutation in the HPH2/PHD2/EGLN2 gene.[39] However, in contrast to Chuvash polycythemia, where the affected individuals carrying homozygous *VHL* 598 C>T mutation have ~tenfold increase in serum Epo levels compared to normal controls,[11] the two polycythemic subjects with HPH2 mutations had Epo levels close to the lower boundary of the normal range. The description of this polycythemic family carrying a PHD2 heterozygous mutation is important because it supports the *in vitro* data defining a critical role for HIF1 hydroxylases in the regulation of erythropoiesis and provides a phenotypic tool to test their presumed roles as oxygen sensors. For example, it is important to know whether the phenotype recapitulates the secondary erythrocytosis seen in secondary hypoxia and whether environmental oxygen pressures could modify the phenotype.

Hemoxygenase-2

Hemoxygenase (HO) is a membrane-bound enzyme that catabolizes heme to CO, biliverdin, and iron using oxygen and NADPH as the electron donor. Most heme is derived from the degradation of erythrocytes. Type 1 isoform of HO (HO-1) can be induced by the administration of heme. The other isoform, HO-2 is constitutively expressed in most cells, most abundantly in neurons, testicular Leydig cells and spermatocytes. HO-1 and HO-2 are monomeric peptides encoded by distinct genes in the genome.[40]

Expression of HO may provide protection against oxidation as both biluribin and biliverdin are known to be potent antioxidants. HO-2 may function by sequestering and inactivating free radicals, such as ROS and NO. In addition, HO-2 may counter the effects of oxidants by regulating the levels of heme and synthesis of NO synthase (NOS). Because HO-1 is expressed at very low levels, except in spleen, HO-2 activity may be the primary defense enzyme inactivating the free radicals.

Recently, Williams *et al.*[41] showed that hemoxygenase-2 is part of the oxygen-sensitive BK channel complex in the CB and increases its channel activity in normoxia. The channel activity is reduced during hypoxia in excised membrane patches. The channel activity was also reduced by the knockdown of HO-2 expression, but rescued by CO, a product of HO-2. Thus CB cells demonstrated HO-2-dependent hypoxic BK channel inhibition, which suggested that HO-2 is an oxygen sensor that controls channel activity during oxygen deprivation.

Mouse knockout models for both HO-1 and HO-2 are available. Targeted disruption suggested a role for HO-1 in cytoprotection through augmentation of iron efflux and enhancing cell viability.[42] Similarly, HO-2 knockout animals were sensitized to oxidative injury in the lung, presumably as a result of blockage in the turnover of lung iron.[43] Subsequent studies in knockout animals also supported a role for HO-2 in the regulation of oxidative injury in cortical neurons and astrocytes.[44] A recent study found that mice lacking HO-2 showed an attenuated hypoxic ventilatory response and, as a result, hypoxemia and right heart hypertrophy.[45] Although the weakening of the hypoxic ventilatory response in the HO-2 knockout mouse might seem to support a role in the oxygen-sensing pathway, the hypoxia-induced increased ventilation rate, which is mediated by the CB, did not show a significant difference between the wild-type and the HO-2 null mouse.[45] Thus, it is unclear whether the diminished overall hypoxic ventilatory response in the mouse is caused by a defect in the oxygen sensor apparatus *per se*, or is a consequence of the oxidative injury in lung, which may secondarily decrease the tidal volume and lead to an overall decrease in ventilation capacity upon hypoxic exposure.

Online Mendelian Inheritance in Man (OMIM) does not contain any human genetic cases carrying a germline mutation in the HO-2 gene. However, Yachie *et al.*[46] described a 26-month-old patient deficient in the HO-1 gene product as a result of homozygous germline mutations. The subject showed growth retardation, anemia, iron deposition, and vulnerability to stressful injury similar to those observed in the corresponding knockout mice.

DISCUSSION

I have briefly reviewed data on several commonly considered oxygen sensor candidates: four are suggested by the molecular-reductionist approach and two are suggested by the phenotypic-genetic approach. I explored whether the candidates identified by one approach have the support of data from the other approach. The phenotypic features of the mutations in the three candidates of the molecular-reductionist approach, namely NADPH oxidase, mitochondrial respiratory chain complexes I, III, and IV, and the CB oxygen sensor candidate heme oxygenase-2, do not appear to recapitulate the specific phenotypic characteristics of chronic hypoxic exposure, but instead suggest other physiological roles for the mutated genes. Although it is possible that currently unknown genetic models of these oxygen sensor candidates may provide more supportive data for oxygen sensing in the future. The phenotypic data for HIF1 hydroxylases are still too sketchy to reach a conclusion. In contrast, the two candidates of the phenotypic-genetic approach, namely pVHL and SDH, have had consistent support from molecular data regarding their role in oxygen-sensing pathways. From a methodological perspective, these findings suggest that the predictive power of models might be higher when they are formed on the basis of observations at the phenotypic level. Stated differently, the molecular-reductionist approach may not have high predictive power to identify which molecule is truly relevant to oxygen sensing at the organism level. Perhaps this is not surprising because almost 60 reactions in which molecular oxygen directly participates have been uncovered.[47] Although disruption of some of these reactions *in vitro* may alter oxygen homeostasis, this may not necessarily indicate their involvement in oxygen-sensing at the organism level.

An analogy might be helpful to show how *in vitro* perturbations of certain gene products, which are not involved in oxygen sensing, can still disrupt oxygen homeostasis. Suppose that there is a room with a fuel-based heating system and suppose that the internal temperature is kept at 20°C in winter with the help of a heat sensor. If the room temperature goes down (hypoxia), it is the sensor that first detects it and sends a signal to a transducer, which then turns on the fuel-burning furnace (e.g., HIF1 transcriptional machinery) to bring back the room temperature. One can imagine many ways other than the dysfunction of the sensor that this whole heating system can be made to fail. For example, the fuel delivery could be stopped, the signaling wire from the sensor could be disconnected, the furnace could fail, the room's walls can collapse, etc. Furthermore, if some of the nonsensor components are defective (mutations) or frozen (extreme nonphysiological hypoxia), the heating system may malfunction either by not working at all or by constitutively working to overheat the house irrespective of the outside temperature. Hence a complete system malfunction would make it difficult to identify whether the problem is in the sensor or in the other components of the system. Perhaps one could suspect a problem specifically in the sensor if the system stabilizes the room temperature at 10°C or 30°C, instead of 20°C. Then the furnace would turn off when the outside temperature reaches above 10°C (hypoactive hypoxic response) or 30°C (hyperactive hypoxic response), instead of 20°C (normal hypoxic response). Thus in contrast to nonsensor defects, which are likely to make the system completely unresponsive to the environment, the system should retain its capacity to interact with the environment with the sensor defects, although at an abnormal homeostatic threshold. It is hoped that this analogy may help to convey the rationale behind the suggestion that the phenotypes caused by certain defects in an oxygen sensor should demonstrate evidence of an aberrant interaction threshold with the environment, as suggested by the interaction of *SDHD* mutations with altitude.

In conclusion, by contrasting the molecular and phenotypic data, I have attempted to highlight a problem inherent in the molecular-reductionist approaches to identify a universal oxygen sensor and emphasized the essentiality of confirmation at the phenotypic level. I have argued that complex homeostatic systems possessing sensors could be broken down by defects in many of its components, which themselves do not function as sensors. Thus, it is conceivable that some of the experimental approaches that show disruption of oxygen homeostasis may have targeted such nonsensor components of the mammalian oxygen-sensing system. The phenotypic confirmation of a universal oxygen sensor candidate will also help to advance our understanding of how aberrations in oxygen-sensing have in impact on our health and disease.

ACKNOWLEDGMENTS

I thank Susan Felsenfeld for her valuable stylistic suggestions. The author's work is supported by NIH Grant 1R01CA112364–01.

REFERENCES

1. Bunn, H.F. & R.O. Poyton. 1996. Oxygen sensing and molecular adaptation to hypoxia. Physiol. Rev. **76:** 839–885.
2. Weir, E.K. *et al.* 2005. Acute oxygen-sensing mechanisms. N. Engl. J. Med. **353:** 2042–2055.
3. Gonzalez, C. *et al.* 1994. Carotid body chemoreceptors: from natural stimuli to sensory discharges. Physiol. Rev. **74:** 829–898.
4. Semenza, G.L. 2001. Hypoxia-inducible factor 1: oxygen homeostasis and disease pathophysiology. Trends Mol. Med. **7:** 345–350.
5. Bernardi, L. *et al.* 2003. Ventilation, autonomic function, sleep and erythropoietin: chronic mountain sickness of Andean natives. Adv. Exp. Med. Biol. **543:** 161–175.
6. Howell, K. *et al.* 2004. Structural basis of hypoxic pulmonary hypertension: the modifying effect of chronic hypercapnia. Exp. Physiol. **89:** 66–72.
7. Maggiorini, M. 2003. Cardio-pulmonary interactions at high altitude: pulmonary hypertension as a common denominator. Adv. Exp. Med. Biol. **543:** 177–189.
8. Arias-Stella, J. & J. Valcarcel. 1976. Chief cell hyperplasia in the human carotid body at high altitudes: physiologic and pathologic significance. Hum. Pathol. **7:** 361–373.

9. BAYSAL, B.E. 2002. Hereditary paraganglioma targets diverse paraganglia. J. Med. Genet. **39:** 617–622.
10. ACKER, T. & H. ACKER. 2004. Cellular oxygen sensing need in CNS function: physiological and pathological implications. J. Exp. Biol. **207:** 3171–3188.
11. GORDEUK, V.R., D.W. STOCKTON & J. T. PRCHAL. 2005. Congenital polycythemias/erythrocytoses. Haematologica **90:** 109–116.
12. SAFRAN, M. & W.G. KAELIN JR., 2003. HIF hydroxylation and the mammalian oxygen-sensing pathway. J. Clin. Invest. **111:** 779–783.
13. ANG, S.O. *et al.* 2002. Disruption of oxygen homeostasis underlies congenital Chuvash polycythemia. Nat. Genet. **32:** 614–621.
14. PERROTTA, S. *et al.* 2006. Von Hippel-Lindau-dependent polycythemia is endemic on the island of Ischia: identification of a novel cluster. Blood **107:** 514–519.
15. BAYSAL, B.E. *et al.* 2000. Mutations in SDHD, a mitochondrial complex II gene, in hereditary paraganglioma. Science **287:** 848–851.
16. DAHIA, P.L. *et al.* 2005. A HIF1alpha regulatory loop links hypoxia and mitochondrial signals in pheochromocytomas. PLoS. Genet. **1:** 72–80.
17. SELAK, M.A. *et al.* 2005. Succinate links TCA cycle dysfunction to oncogenesis by inhibiting HIF-alpha prolyl hydroxylase. Cancer Cell **7:** 77–85.
18. ISAACS, J.S. *et al.* 2005. HIF overexpression correlates with biallelic loss of fumarate hydratase in renal cancer: novel role of fumarate in regulation of HIF stability. Cancer Cell. **8:** 143–153.
19. LU, H. *et al.* 2005. Reversible inactivation of HIF-1 prolyl hydroxylases allows cell metabolism to control basal HIF-1. J. Biol. Chem. **280:** 41928–41939.
20. ASTROM, K. *et al.* 2003. Altitude is a phenotypic modifier in hereditary paraganglioma type 1: evidence for an oxygen-sensing defect. Hum. Genet. **113:** 228–237.
21. BAYSAL, B.E. 2004. Genomic imprinting and environment in hereditary paraganglioma. Am. J. Med. Genet. C. Semin. Med. Genet. **129:** 85–90.
22. JONES, R.D., J.T. HANCOCK & A.H. MORICE. 2000. NADPH oxidase: a universal oxygen sensor? Free Radic. Biol. Med. **29:** 416–424.
23. HEYWORTH, P.G., A.R. CROSS & J.T. CURNUTTE. 2003. Chronic granulomatous disease. Curr. Opin. Immunol. **15:** 578–584.
24. FU, X.W. *et al.* 2000. NADPH oxidase is an O2 sensor in airway chemoreceptors: evidence from K+ current modulation in wild-type and oxidase-deficient mice. Proc. Natl. Acad. Sci. USA **97:** 4374–4379.
25. THOMPSON, R.J. *et al.* 2002. Developmental regulation of O(2) sensing in neonatal adrenal chromaffin cells from wild-type and NADPH-oxidase-deficient mice. Pflugers Arch. **444:** 539–548.
26. SANDERS, K.A. *et al.* 2002. Role of components of the phagocytic NADPH oxidase in oxygen sensing. J. Appl. Physiol. **93:** 1357–1364.
27. ARCHER, S.L. *et al.* 1999. O2 sensing is preserved in mice lacking the gp91 phox subunit of NADPH oxidase. Proc. Natl. Acad. Sci. USA **96:** 7944–7949.
28. WALLACE, D.C. 1999. Mitochondrial diseases in man and mouse. Science **283:** 1482–1488.
29. DONNELLY, D.F. & J.L. CARROLL. 2005. Mitochondrial function and carotid body transduction. High Alt. Med. Biol. **6:** 121–132.
30. WYATT, C.N. & K.J. BUCKLER. 2004. The effect of mitochondrial inhibitors on membrane currents in isolated neonatal rat carotid body type I cells. J. Physiol. **556:** 175–191.

31. GUZY, R.D. *et al.* 2005. Mitochondrial complex III is required for hypoxia-induced ROS production and cellular oxygen sensing. Cell. Metab. **1:** 401–408.
32. WENGER, R.H. 2006. Mitochondria: oxygen sinks rather than sensors? Med. Hypotheses **66:** 380–383.
33. MANSFIELD, K.D. *et al.* 2005. Mitochondrial dysfunction resulting from loss of cytochrome c impairs cellular oxygen sensing and hypoxic HIF-alpha activation. Cell. Metab. **1:** 393–399.
34. PIRUAT, J.I. *et al.* 2004. The mitochondrial SDHD gene is required for early embryogenesis, and its partial deficiency results in persistent carotid body glomus cell activation with full responsiveness to hypoxia. Mol. Cell. Biol. **24:** 10933–10940.
35. SHOFFNER, J.M. 2001. Oxidative phosphorylation diseases. *In* The Metabolic & Molecular Basis of Inherited Disease 8th ed., chap. 104. C.R. Scriver, A.L. Beaudet, W.S. Sly & D. Valle, Eds.: 2367–2423. McGraw-Hill, New York, NY.
36. IVAN, M. *et al.* 2001. HIFalpha targeted for VHL-mediated destruction by proline hydroxylation: implications for O2 sensing. Science **292:** 464–468.
37. JAAKKOLA, P. *et al.* 2001. Targeting of HIF-alpha to the von Hippel-Lindau ubiquitylation complex by O2-regulated prolyl hydroxylation. Science **292:** 468–472.
38. KAELIN, W.G. 2005. Proline hydroxylation and gene expression. Annu. Rev. Biochem. **74:** 115–128.
39. PERCY, M.J. *et al.* 2006. A family with erythrocytosis establishes a role for prolyl hydroxylase domain protein 2 in oxygen homeostasis. Proc. Natl. Acad. Sci. USA **103:** 654–659.
40. MAINES, M.D. & P.E. GIBBS. 2005. 30 some years of heme oxygenase: from a "molecular wrecking ball" to a "mesmerizing" trigger of cellular events. Biochem. Biophys. Res. Commun. **338:** 568–577.
41. WILLIAMS, S.E. *et al.* 2004. Hemoxygenase-2 is an oxygen sensor for a calcium-sensitive potassium channel. Science **306:** 2093–2097.
42. POSS, K.D. & S. TONEGAWA. 1997. Reduced stress defense in heme oxygenase 1-deficient cells. Proc. Natl. Acad. Sci. USA **94:** 10925–10930.
43. DENNERY, P.A. *et al.* 1998. Oxygen toxicity and iron accumulation in the lungs of mice lacking heme oxygenase-2. J. Clin. Invest. **101:** 1001–1011.
44. REGAN, R.F., J. CHEN & L. BENVENISTI-ZAROM. 2004. Heme oxygenase-2 gene deletion attenuates oxidative stress in neurons exposed to extracellular hemin. BMC Neurosci. **5:** 34.
45. ADACHI, T. *et al.* 2004. Hypoxemia and blunted hypoxic ventilatory responses in mice lacking heme oxygenase-2. Biochem. Biophys. Res. Commun. **320:** 514–522.
46. YACHIE, A. *et al.* 1999. Oxidative stress causes enhanced endothelial cell injury in human heme oxygenase-1 deficiency. J. Clin. Invest. **103:** 129–135.
47. VANDERKOOI, J.M., M. ERECINSKA & I. A. SILVER. 1991. Oxygen in mammalian tissue: methods of measurement and affinities of various reactions. Am. J. Physiol. **260:** C1131–C1150.

Molecular Implications of RET Mutations for Pheochromocytoma Risk in Multiple Endocrine Neoplasia 2

TARANJIT S. GUJRAL AND LOIS M. MULLIGAN

Division of Cancer Biology and Genetics, Cancer Research Institute, Queen's University, Kingston, Ontario, K7L 3N6 Canada

ABSTRACT: **Multiple endocrine neoplasia Type 2 (MEN 2) is an inherited cancer syndrome characterized by medullary thyroid carcinoma (MTC). The disease has three subtypes, which are distinguished by the presence of additional phenotypes. In particular, pheochromocytoma occurs in approximately 50% of patients with the MEN 2A or MEN 2B subtypes, but is not found in patients with the milder disease subtype, familial MTC (FMTC). All subtypes of MEN 2 are caused by activating mutations of the RET (REarranged in Transfection) proto-oncogene. RET encodes a transmembrane receptor tyrosine kinase, required for development of neuroendocrine cell types and the kidneys. All MEN 2 subtypes are associated with single amino acid substitution mutations that are found in either the extracellular domain or in the kinase domain of RET. There are strong genotype–phenotype correlations in MEN 2 between patient phenotype and the specific residue that is mutated. MEN 2A is primarily associated with substitutions at five extracellular cysteine residues, while 95% of MEN 2B is associated with a single methionine to threonine mutation in the kinase domain (M918T). In FMTC, RET mutations are more broadly distributed, with both extracellular cysteines and intracellular sites implicated. In all cases, MEN 2-RET mutations result in constitutive activation of the receptor, although the mechanism and relative functional effects of the mutations vary. Recent advances in functional characterization and development of molecular models of RET and of various MEN 2-RET mutants are helping us understand tissue-specific differences in oncogenic potential conferred by the different RET mutations. Here, we discuss and compare several well-characterized mutations of the extracellular and kinase domains, which have quite varied functional implications.**

KEYWORDS: **RET; MEN 2; pheochromocytoma; genotype–phenotype**

Address for correspondence: Dr. Lois M. Mulligan, Department of Pathology and Molecular Medicine, Cancer Research Institute, Botterell Hall Room 329, Queen's University, Kingston, ON, Canada K7L 3N6. Voice: 1-613-533-6000 X 77475; fax: 1-613-533-6830.
e-mail: mulligal@post.queensu.ca

Ann. N.Y. Acad. Sci. 1073: 234–240 (2006). © **2006 New York Academy of Sciences.**
doi: 10.1196/annals.1353.025

Multiple endocrine neoplasia, Type 2 (MEN 2), is an inherited cancer syndrome characterized by medullary thyroid carcinoma (MTC), a tumor of the thyroid C cells. The disease has three subtypes, based on the combination of clinical manifestations. The most common disease subtype, MEN 2A, represents more than 85% of all disease cases. MEN 2A is characterized by MTC and, in addition, is associated with pheochromocytoma (PC) in about 50% of cases, and parathyroid hyperplasia or adenoma (HPT) in 15–30% of cases. MEN 2B, which represents approximately 5% of all MEN 2 diagnoses, is the most aggressive and earliest-onset disease subtype. It is also characterized by MTC and PC, but not HPT, and is further associated with a number of developmental anomalies including decreased upper/lower body ratio, marfanoid habitus, skeletal deformations, mucosal neuromas, ganglioneuromatosis of the intestinal tract, and myelinated corneal nerves (reviewed in Ref. 1). The final MEN 2 subtype, familial MTC (FMTC), has the mildest phenotype, having MTC as its only disease feature.

All subtypes of MEN 2 are caused by germline mutations of the RET (*RE*arranged in *T*ransfection) proto-oncogene. *RET* encodes a receptor tyrosine kinase required for the development of neural crest–derived cell types, the kidney, and spermatogonia.[2,3] Under normal conditions, activation of *RET* is induced by interaction of *RET* with a complex comprising a soluble ligand member of the glial cell line–derived neurotrophic factor (GDNF) family, and a co-receptor of the GDNF family receptor alpha proteins.[4] In MEN 2, oncogenic point mutations of RET, leading to single amino acid substitutions in the extracellular or tyrosine kinase domains, result in aberrant activation of the receptor and induction of downstream signals.[4] These gain-of-function mutations have been found in fewer than two dozen codons to date, and the majority of MEN 2 cases are accounted for by mutation at one of only 12 *RET* codons (FIG. 1).[5] Further, strong genotype–phenotype correlations between specific *RET* mutations and the associated patient disease phenotypes have been recognized.[6,7] The MEN 2A phenotype is primarily associated with mutations of cysteine residues in the extracellular domain of *RET*, which result in ligand-independent dimerization and activation of the receptor. MEN 2B is caused by a small group of mutations in the tyrosine kinase domain, with more than 95% of the disease attributable to a methionine-to-threonine substitution of residue 918 (M918T). FMTC is associated with the most diverse spectrum of mutations, including mutations of both extracellular and kinase domain residues.

As we might predict, the association of disease subtype with specific *RET* mutations reflects differences in the risk of specific tumors in individuals with those mutations. For example, substitutions of cysteine residue 634, in the extracellular domain of *RET*, occur in about 85% of MEN 2A cases and, as a corollary, this substitution is a strong predictor of risk for both PC and HPT.[6,8–11] Other mutations within the same region, such as substitutions of cysteine codons 609 or 611, are only rarely associated with PC, although they

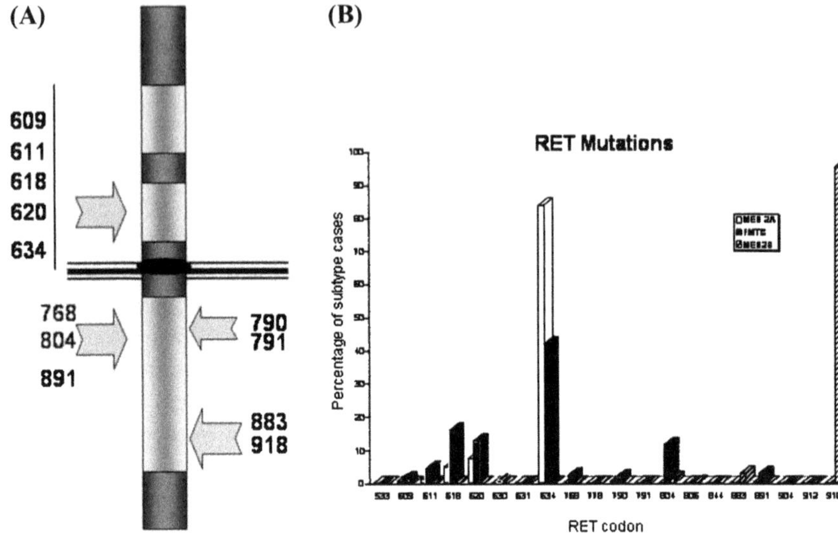

FIGURE 1. Distribution of RET mutations. (**A**) Schematic diagram of the RET receptor showing the codons most frequently mutated in MEN 2. (**B**) Distribution of RET mutations for MEN 2A, MEN 2B, and FMTC. Data are taken from published reports and, as a consequence, rarer mutations, which are disproportionately reported, are overrepresented in this summary.

can confer significant risk of MTC or its precursor C-cell hyperplasia.[6,8,11] A possible explanation of these findings is that there are differences in the oncogenicity of different *RET* mutations, which correlate with the penetrance of MEN 2 disease phenotypes. Although each of these mutant *RET* isoforms is associated with the occurrence of MTC *in vivo, in vitro* assays have suggested that codon 634 mutations are the most oncogenic, while mutations of other cysteine residues in the extracellular domain (609, 611, 618, 620) have lower transforming ability.[12,13] These variations in oncogenicity have been suggested to arise from differences in the ability of mutant RET proteins to mature and localize to the cell surface (e.g., FIG. 2).[12,13] Relatively fewer mature receptors containing mutations of codons 609, 611, 618, or 620 are translocated to the cell surface as compared to normal RET proteins or to receptors mutated at codon 634. As a result, although these mutants of RET are all able to form dimers and autophosphorylate in the absence of ligand, there is a reduced number of receptors available on the cell surface to form dimers and initiate unregulated signals (FIG. 2).

The prevalence of individual MEN 2 disease phenotypes, such as PC and HPT, correlates well with the relative oncogenicity of different extracellular domain RET mutants, suggesting a functional mechanism that may underlie this genotype–phenotype correlation. Taken together, these data have suggested

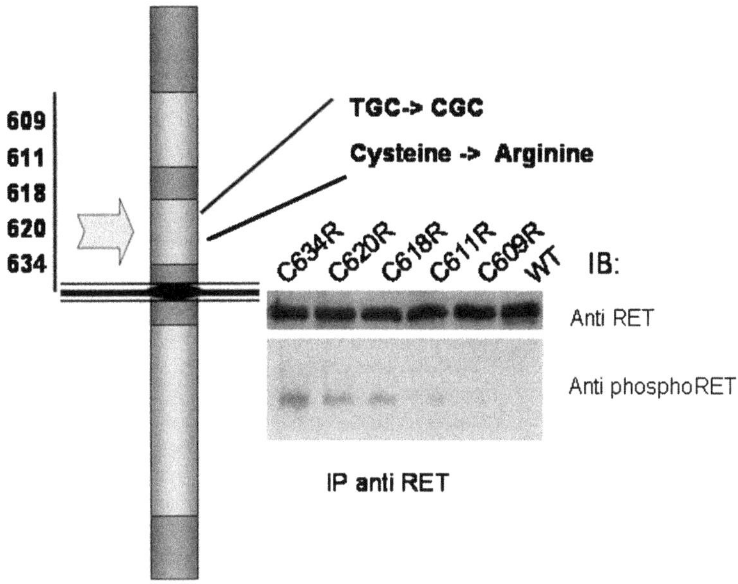

FIGURE 2. Functional effects of RET mutations of extracellular cysteine residues. Amino acid substitutions in the extracellular domain of RET primarily affect one of five cysteine residues (left). While these mutant receptors are generally expressed in normal levels (upper right), dimerization and activation of the receptors, in the absence of ligand varies, as indicated by autophosphorylation (lower right).

that there are tissue-specific sensitivities to the effects of aberrant RET activation.[6,14] The association of C-cell disease with all RET mutations predicts that these cells are most sensitive to RET activation, and that any of the oncogenic RET mutations is transforming in this cell type. Conversely, the lower penetrance of both PC and of HPT suggests that adrenal chromaffin cells and the parathyroid may either require a more highly oncogenic protein to confer RET's transforming ability, or are at relatively lower risk of a transforming event in the presence of less oncogenic proteins. Thus, although all MEN 2A-type mutations confer a risk of PC and HPT, and examples exist of co-occurrence of these phenotypes with mutations of the most codons, overall, some mutations confer upon the individual much lower risks of PC or HPT.

Similar correlations of *RET* mutation genotype and variation in associated phenotype are found in the *RET* mutations of the tyrosine kinase domain (FIG. 1). The pathognomonic MEN 2B mutation, M918T, and the rare and relatively benign FMTC mutation Y791F, both lie within the RET kinase domain. Tyrosine 791 lies within the N-terminal lobe of the kinase, where a mutation to phenylalanine (Y791F) may alter local spatial interactions, resulting in conformational changes and partial activation.[15] The M918T mutation lies within the catalytic core of the RET kinase and has been predicted either to induce

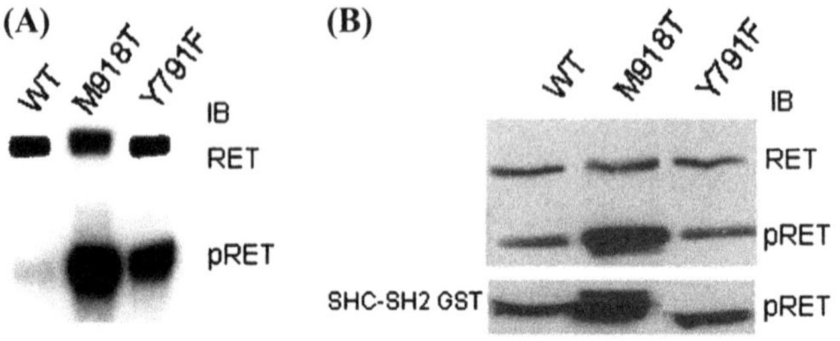

FIGURE 3. RET mutants of the intracellular domain have different functional implications. (**A**) RET phosphorylation in the absence of ligand. RET receptors with either the M918T or Y791F mutation are highly phosphorylated even without stimulation, while the wild-type receptor (WT) has very little autophosphorylation. (**B**) RET phosphorylation and substrate binding after ligand stimulation. After GDNF treatment, WT and Y791F RET forms have similar levels of autophosphorylation, and binding to a purified GST-SHC-SH2 domain protein. However, M918T RET is significantly more phosphorylated and binds more SHC-SH2 domain.

a conformational change in the kinase catalytic core, activating RET without dimerization, or to alter the substrate specificity of RET, making it more similar to that of cytoplasmic tyrosine kinases, such as SRC, or both.[16–18] FIGURE 3A shows that, *in vitro*, both RET-Y791F and RET-M918T mutant forms are dramatically activated and autophosphorylated in the absence of any ligand stimulation. However, while ligand stimulation increases phosphorylation of both wild-type RET, as expected, and RET-M918T, the level of phosphorylation of RET-Y791F is not increased further by ligand addition (FIG. 3B). Interestingly, the relative level of autophosphorylation, and of binding to known RET substrates (e.g., SHC), is very similar for ligand-activated wild-type RET and the RET-Y791F mutant, irrespective of ligand activation (FIG. 3). RET-M918T is more highly phosphorylated and binds more SHC than either of the above receptors, and both binding and phosphorylation are further increased in the presence of ligand. Together, these data suggest that the M918T and Y791F mutations differ in the way they affect the ability of RET receptors to become activated. In M918T mutants, RET retains the ability to respond to ligand-mediated activation, while the Y791F mutant can no longer be further stimulated in this way. These data suggest that, while RET-Y791F is more active than a wild-type RET receptor, and hence has transforming potential, this is relatively modest in comparison to the much more transforming RET-M918T mutant that can be stimulated by both normal and mutation-associated mechanisms. Relative risk of disease phenotypes similarly correlates with RET mutant activity, with approximately 50% of MEN 2B cases having PC while instances of Y791F-associated PC are extremely rare.[11,19]

The association of MEN 2 disease phenotype and RET mutation genotype has been recognized for some time. Functional analyses are now beginning to dissect the underlying mechanisms of these disease associations. Our data, and that of others, suggest that the correlation of specific MEN 2 disease phenotypes, such as PC or HPT, with specific RET mutations may provide a clinical representation of relative transforming activity of different RET mutations. However, although this variation can be observed for several classes of mutations affecting different RET receptor domains, the mechanisms by which the range of transforming potential is conferred is different and in fact unique for the specific RET mutations observed and most particularly the domains in which they lie.

REFERENCES

1. BRAUCKHOFF, M. *et al.* 2004. Multiple endocrine neoplasia 2B syndrome due to codon 918 mutation: clinical manifestation and course in early and late onset disease. World J. Surg. **28:** 1305–1311.
2. SCHUCHARDT, A. *et al.* 1994. Defects in the kidney and enteric nervous system of mice lacking the tyrosine kinase receptor Ret. Nature **367:** 380–383.
3. MENG, X. *et al.* 2000. Regulation of cell fate decision of undifferentiated spermatogonia by GDNF. Science **287:** 1489–1493.
4. ARIGHI, E., M.G. BORRELLO & H. SARIOLA. 2005. RET tyrosine kinase signaling in development and cancer. Cytokine Growth Factor Rev. **16:** 441–467.
5. MARX, S.J. 2005. Molecular genetics of multiple endocrine neoplasia types 1 and 2. Nat. Rev. Cancer **5:** 367–375.
6. MULLIGAN, L.M. *et al.* 1994. Specific mutations of the *RET* proto-oncogene are related to disease phenotype in MEN 2A and FMTC. Nat. Genet. **6:** 70–74.
7. SCHUFFENECKER, I. *et al.* 1994. *RET* proto-oncogene mutations in French MEN 2A and FMTC families. Hum. Mol. Genet. **3:** 1939–1943.
8. SCHUFFENECKER, I. *et al.* 1998. Risk and penetrance of primary hyperparathyroidism in multiple endocrine neoplasia type 2A families with mutations at codon 634 of the RET proto-oncogene. Groupe D'etude des Tumeurs a Calcitonine. J. Clin. Endocrinol. Metab. **83:** 487–491.
9. ENG, C. *et al.* 1996. The relationship between specific *RET* proto-oncogene mutations and disease phenotype in multiple endocrine neoplasia type 2: International *RET* Mutation Consortium. JAMA **276:** 1575–1579.
10. MULLIGAN, L.M. *et al.* 1995. Genotype-phenotype correlation in multiple endocrine neoplasia type 2: report of the International *RET* Mutation Consortium. J. Intern. Med. **238:** 343–346.
11. YIP, L. *et al.* 2003. Multiple endocrine neoplasia type 2: evaluation of the genotype-phenotype relationship. Arch. Surg. **138:** 409–416.
12. CHAPPUIS-FLAMENT, S. *et al.* 1998. Dual effect on the RET receptor of MEN 2 mutations affecting specific extracytoplasmic cysteines. Oncogene **17:** 2851–2861.
13. PELET, A. *et al.* 1998. Various mechanisms cause RET-mediated signaling defects in Hirschsprung's disease. J. Clin. Invest. **101:** 1415–1423.
14. TAKAHASHI, M. *et al.* 1999. Co-segregation of MEN2 and Hirschsprung's disease: the same mutation of RET with both gain and loss-of-function? Hum. Mutat. **13:** 331–336.

15. PLAZA-MENACHO, I. *et al.* 2005. RET-familial medullary thyroid carcinoma mutants Y791F and S891A activate a Src/JAK/STAT3 pathway, independent of glial cell line-derived neurotrophic factor. Cancer Res. **65:** 1729–1737.
16. SONGYANG, Z. *et al.* 1995. Catalytic specificity of protein-tyrosine kinases is critical for selective signalling. Nature **373:** 536–539.
17. SANTORO, M. *et al.* 1995. Activation of *RET* as a dominant transforming gene by germline mutations of MEN2A and MEN2B. Science **267:** 381–383.
18. GUJRAL, T.S. *et al.* Molecular mechanisms of RET receptor-mediated oncogenesis in multiple endocrine neoplasia 2B. Nat. Genet. Under review.
19. BERNDT, I. *et al.* 1998. A new hot spot for mutations in the ret proto-oncogene causing familial medullary thyroid carcinoma and multiple endocrine neoplasia type 2A. J. Clin. Endocrinol. Metab. **83:** 770–774.

Transcriptional Regulation of Phenylethanolamine *N*-Methyltransferase in Pheochromocytomas from Patients with von Hippel–Lindau Syndrome and Multiple Endocrine Neoplasia Type 2

THANH-TRUC HUYNH,[a] KAREL PACAK,[b] DONA L. WONG,[c] W. MARSTON LINEHAN,[d] DAVID S. GOLDSTEIN,[a] ABDEL G. ELKAHLOUN,[e] PETER J. MUNSON,[f] AND GRAEME EISENHOFER[a]

[a]*Clinical Neurocardiology Section, National Institute of Neurological Disorders and Stroke, National Institutes of Health, Bethesda, Maryland 20892, USA*

[b]*Reproductive Biology and Medicine Branch, National Institute of Child Health and Human Development, National Institutes of Health, Bethesda, Maryland 20892, USA*

[c]*Department of Psychiatry, Harvard Medical School and Laboratory of Molecular and Developmental Neurobiology, McLean Hospital, Belmont, Massachusetts 02478, USA*

[d]*Urologic Oncology Branch National Cancer Institute, National Institutes of Health, Bethesda, Maryland 20892, USA*

[e]*Genome Technology Branch, National Human Genome Research Institute, National Institutes of Health, Bethesda, Maryland 20892, USA*

[f]*Mathematical and Statistical Computing Laboratory, Center for Information Technology, National Institutes of Health, Bethesda, Maryland 20892, USA*

ABSTRACT: Pheochromocytomas in multiple endocrine neoplasia type 2 (MEN-2) express phenylethanolamine *N*-methyltransferase (PNMT), the enzyme that catalyzes conversion of norepinephrine to epinephrine, whereas those in von Hippel–Lindau (VHL) syndrome do not. Consequently, pheochromocytomas in MEN-2 produce epinephrine, whereas those in VHL syndrome produce mainly norepinephrine. This study examined whether transcription factors known to regulate expression of PNMT explain the different tumor phenotypes in these syndromes.

Address for correspondence: Graeme Eisenhofer, Ph.D., Building 10, Room 6N252, National Institutes of Health, 10 Center Drive, MSC-1620, Bethesda, MD 20892-1620. Voice: 301-496-8925; fax: 301-402-0180.
e-mail: ge@box-g.nih.gov

Ann. N.Y. Acad. Sci. 1073: 241–252 (2006).
doi: 10.1196/annals.1353.026

Quantitative polymerase chain reaction (PCR) and Western blotting were used to assess levels of mRNA and protein for the glucocorticoid receptor, early growth response 1 (Egr-1), the Sp1 transcription factor (Sp1), and MYC-associated zinc finger protein (MAZ) in 6 MEN-2 and 13 VHL tumors. Results were cross-checked with data obtained using microarray gene expression profiling in a further set of 10 MEN-2 and 12 VHL tumors. Pheochromocytomas in MEN-2 and VHL syndrome did not differ in expression of the glucocorticoid receptor, Egr-1, Sp1, or MAZ as assessed by quantitative PCR and Western blotting. Microarray data also indicated no relevant differences in expression of the glucocorticoid receptor, Egr-1, MAZ, and the AP2 transcription factor. Thus, our results do not support a role for the above transcription factors in determining differences in expression of PNMT in pheochromocytomas from patients with VHL syndrome and MEN-2. Microarray analysis, however, did indicate differences in expression of genes involved in neural crest cell lineage and chromaffin cell development, consistent with differential survival of PNMT-expressing cells in the two syndromes.

Keywords: pheochromocytoma; transcription factors; phenylethanolamine N-methyltransferase; catecholamines; microarray

INTRODUCTION

Pheochromocytomas are rare neuroendocrine tumors arising from chromaffin cells and characterized by excessive production of catecholamines. Pheochromocytomas in patients with multiple endocrine neoplasia type 2 (MEN-2) and von Hippel–Lindau (VHL) syndrome have distinctly different gene expression profiles, patterns of catecholamine production, and clinical presentations.[1–3] Pheochromocytomas in MEN-2 patients express phenylethanolamine N-methyltransferase (PNMT), the enzyme that converts norepinephrine to epinephrine, whereas VHL tumors do not express PNMT. Consequently, pheochromocytomas in MEN-2 produce norepinephrine and epinephrine, and are characterized by an adrenergic biochemical phenotype, whereas those in VHL syndrome produce only norepinephrine and are characterized by a noradrenergic phenotype.

The glucocorticoid dependence of adrenal medullary expression of PNMT, originally described by Wurtman and Axelrod,[4] is mediated by binding to nuclear glucocorticoid receptors and subsequent activation of the glucocorticoid response element in the promotor region of the PNMT gene.[5] Numerous other transcription factors, including early growth response 1 (Egr-1),[6] the Sp1 transcription factor (Sp1),[7] the MYC-associated zinc finger protein (MAZ),[8] and the AP2 transcription factor[9] are now also identified as participating in the regulation of PNMT gene expression.

On the basis of the above findings, we hypothesized that differences in catecholamine phenotypes in pheochromocytomas from patients with MEN-2 and

VHL syndrome might be on account of differences in expression of transcription factors known to regulate PNMT. We therefore used quantitative polymerase chain reaction (PCR) and Western blotting to assess levels of mRNA and protein for the glucocorticoid receptor, Egr-1, Sp1, and MAZ in pheochromocytomas from patients with MEN-2 and VHL syndrome. Differences in gene expression were further examined using our cDNA and oligonucleotide microarray gene expression databases.

MATERIALS AND METHODS

Patients

The study population included 31 patients with pheochromocytoma, 13 on account of MEN-2 and 18 on account of VHL syndrome. The diagnosis of MEN-2 or VHL syndrome was confirmed by identification of germline mutations of the *RET* proto-oncogene or the *VHL* tumor-suppressor gene. Blood and tumor tissue samples were obtained under studies approved by the appropriate institutional review boards, with informed consent obtained from all patients.

Collection of Tissue and Blood Samples

Samples of tumor tissue were obtained within 90 min of surgical removal of pheochromocytomas. Dimensions of tumors were recorded, and small samples (50–400 mg) were dissected away, placed on dry ice, and then stored at −80°C. Blood samples were obtained from patients using an intravenous catheter inserted into a forearm vein, with patients supine for at least 20 min before blood collection. Blood samples were transferred into tubes containing heparin as anticoagulant and immediately placed on ice until centrifuged (4°C) to separate the plasma. Plasma was stored at −80°C until assayed.

Tissue and Plasma Catecholamines

Tissue and plasma concentrations of catecholamines (norepinephrine, epinephrine, and dopamine) were quantified by liquid chromatography with electrochemical detection.[10] Samples of tumor tissue were weighed frozen and homogenized in 5–10 volumes of 0.4-M perchloric acid containing 0.5-mM EDTA. Homogenates were centrifuged and supernatants collected for catecholamine determinations. Plasma concentrations of metanephrines (normetanephrine and metanephrine) were determined using a different liquid chromatography procedure after extraction onto solid-phase ion exchange columns.[11]

Quantitative PCR

RNA was extracted from frozen samples of pheochromocytoma tissue after homogenization in TRIzol reagent (Invitrogen, Carlsbad, CA) followed by RNeasy Maxi (Qiagen, Valencia, CA) according to the manufacturer's recommendations. Total RNA (2 μg) was reversibly transcribed to cDNA using random hexamers. Real-time quantitative PCR (TaqMan PCR), using a 7000 Sequence Detector (Applied Biosystems, Foster City, CA), was used for quantification of mRNA for the glucocorticoid receptor, Egr-1, Sp1, and MAZ. The primers and TaqMan probes were designed from the human glucocorticoid receptor, Egr-1, Sp1, and MAZ gene sequences using the Primer Express program from Applied Biosystems (TABLE 1).

Expression of mRNA for the glucocorticoid receptor, Egr-1, Sp1, and MAZ was normalized for differences in total RNA using 18S ribosomal RNA (Human 18S rRNA Pre-Developed TaqMan Assay Reagents, Applied Biosystems). PCR amplifications of 18S rRNA and the glucocorticoid receptor, Egr-1, Sp1, and MAZ were carried out in the same tubes. Reaction tubes contained 20 ng cDNA product as template, 1 × TaqMan Universal PCR Master Mix, 0.9 μmol/L for each of the forward and reverse primers for the glucocorticoid receptor, Egr-1, Sp1, and MAZ, 0.2 μmol/L for TaqMan probes for the glucocorticoid receptor, Egr-1, Sp1, and MAZ, and 1 × human 18S rRNA primers and probe, all to a final volume of 50 μL with H_20. PCR involved 40 cycles at the following temperature parameters: 15 s at 95°C and 1 min at 60°C. Input RNA amounts were calculated manually using the comparative Ct method for the target genes and 18S rRNA.

Western Blot Analysis

Nuclear proteins were prepared according to the procedure of Andrews and Faller.[12] Samples of pheochromocytoma tissue (approximately 15 mg)

TABLE 1. Oligonucleotide primers and probes used in PCR

Primers	Oligonucleotide sequence
Egr-1	
Forward	5′-TTT GCC AGG AGC GAT GAA C
Reverse	5′- TTT GTC TGC TTT CTT GTC CTT CTG
TaqMan	5′ (FAM)- CAA GAG GCA TAC CAA GAT CCA CTT GCG-(TAMRA)
Sp1	
Forward	5′-TGG CAC AGT CAC TGT GAA TGC
Reverse	5′- GTA CCC AAT GCA CTG AGG TTA ATG
TaqMan	5′ (FAM)- CTC TCC TCC ATG CCA GGC CTC CA-(TAMRA)
MAZ	
Forward	5′-CCA TGC CTG CGA GAT GTG T
Reverse	5′- TCC GAG TGC GAC AGC TTG T
TaqMan	5′ (FAM)- CGC GAC GTC TAC CAC CTG AAC CGA-(TAMRA)

were homogenized using a Dounce homogenizer in 0.5 mL of 10 mmol/L HEPES-KOH buffer (pH 7.9) containing 1.5 mmol/L $MgCl_2$, 10 mmol/L KCl, 0.5 mmol/L dithiothreitol, and 0.2 mmol/L phenylmethylsulfonyl fluoride together with protease inhibitors and incubated on ice for 10 min. Nuclear fractions pellets were collected by centrifugation at 17, 000 *g* for 10 s (4°C). The pellets were lysed in 0.1 mL of 20 mM HEPES-KOH (pH 7.9) buffer containing 25% glycerol, 420 mM NaCl, 1.5 mM $MgCl_2$, 0.2 mM EDTA, 0.5 mM DTT, and 0.2 mM PMSF together with protease inhibitors and incubated on ice for 20 min. Supernatant nuclear fractions were collected by centrifugation at 17,000 *g* for 2 min (4°C) and stored at −80°C.

Nuclear proteins (20 μg) were electrophoresed on a 10% SDS-polyacrylamide and transferred onto polyvinylidene fluoride (PVDF) membranes (Millipore, Bedford, MA). Membranes were incubated in blocking buffer (50 mM Tris, pH 7.4, 0.9% NaCl, 0.05% Tween-20, and 10% dry milk) overnight at 4°C. Membranes were then washed three times for 10 min each with Tris buffer saline (50 mM Tris, pH 7.4, 0.9% NaCl) containing 0.05% Tween-20, and then incubated with either rabbit anti-Egr-1 polyclonal antibody (1:1000, Santa Cruz Biotechnology, Santa Cruz, CA) or rabbit anti-Sp1 polyclonal antibody (1:1000, Santa Cruz Biotechnology) or mouse anti-MAZ monoclonal antibody (1:400, kind gift from Dr. Kenneth Marcu, Stony Brook, New York) or glucocorticoid receptor antibody for 1 h at room temperature. Membranes were then washed again three times for 10 min each with Tris buffer saline containing 0.05% Tween-20 and incubated for 1 h with horseradish peroxidase conjugated anti-rabbit IgG or anti-mouse IgG, respectively at 1:2000. Membranes were again washed three times for 10 min each with Tris buffer saline containing 0.05% Tween-20. Proteins were visualized using an enhanced chemiluminescence method (SuperSignal West Pico Chemiluminescent kit, Pierce, Rockford, IL).

Microarray Databases

Gene expression databases were generated from cDNA and oligonucleotide microarrays of tumor samples from patients with MEN-2 and VHL syndrome as described elsewhere.[2,13] Databases were explored for differences in expression of transcription factors known to be involved in regulation of PNMT as well as other genes associated with neural crest cell lineage development and chromaffin cell differentiation.

Statistical Analysis

Differences in tissue and plasma catecholamines and expression of transcription factors and the glucocorticoid receptor were examined using the Student's *t*-test. A *P* value 0.05 was considered significant.

TABLE 2. Concentrations of catecholamines in tumor tissue and of catecholamines and metanephrines in plasma

	VHL (n = 18)	MEN-2 (n = 13)
Tumor catecholamines		
Norepinephrine (μmol/g)	15.0 ± 2.7	32.0 ± 8.1*
Epinephrine (μmol/g)	0.3 ± 0.1	27.8 ± 6.9**
Plasma catecholamines		
Norepinephrine (nmol/L)	5.8 ± 1.1	4.8 ± 1.3
Epinephrine (nmol/L)	0.1 ± 0.0	1.0 ± 0.3**
Plasma metanephrines		
Normetanephrine (nmol/L)	2.4 ± 0.4	5.6 ± 1.9
Metanephrine (nmol/L)	0.2 ± 0.0	3.5 ± 1.7**

All values are means ± SEM.
*$P < 0.05$, **$P < 0.001$.

RESULTS

Tumor and Plasma Catecholamines

Norepinephrine accounted for 98% of the total catecholamine contents in pheochromocytomas from VHL patients, whereas in MEN-2 patients, norepinephrine accounted for only 53% and epinephrine 47% of total tumor catecholamine contents (TABLE 2). Pheochromocytoma tissue concentrations of epinephrine were 93-fold higher ($P < 0.001$) in tumors from MEN-2 patients than in those from VHL patients, while norepinephrine concentrations in MEN-2 tumors were twofold higher ($P < 0.04$) than in VHL tumors. Plasma concentrations of epinephrine were ninefold higher ($P < 0.001$) and those of metanephrine 18-fold higher ($P < 0.001$) in MEN-2 patients than in VHL patients.

Quantitative PCR and Western Blot Analyses

Expression of glucocorticoid receptor (alpha and beta) protein tended to be lower in VHL than MEN-2 tumors, while mRNA expression tended to the opposite direction (FIG. 1A). These differences, however, did not reach significance. Similarly, quantitative PCR and Western blot analyses indicated no consistent differences in expression of Egr-1, Sp1, and MAZ mRNA or protein between pheochromocytomas in MEN-2 and VHL syndrome (FIG. 1B, C, and D).

Microarray Databases

Both cDNA and oligonucleotide microarray analyses indicated higher ($P <$ 0.0001) levels of expression of PNMT in MEN-2 tumors than in VHL tumors.

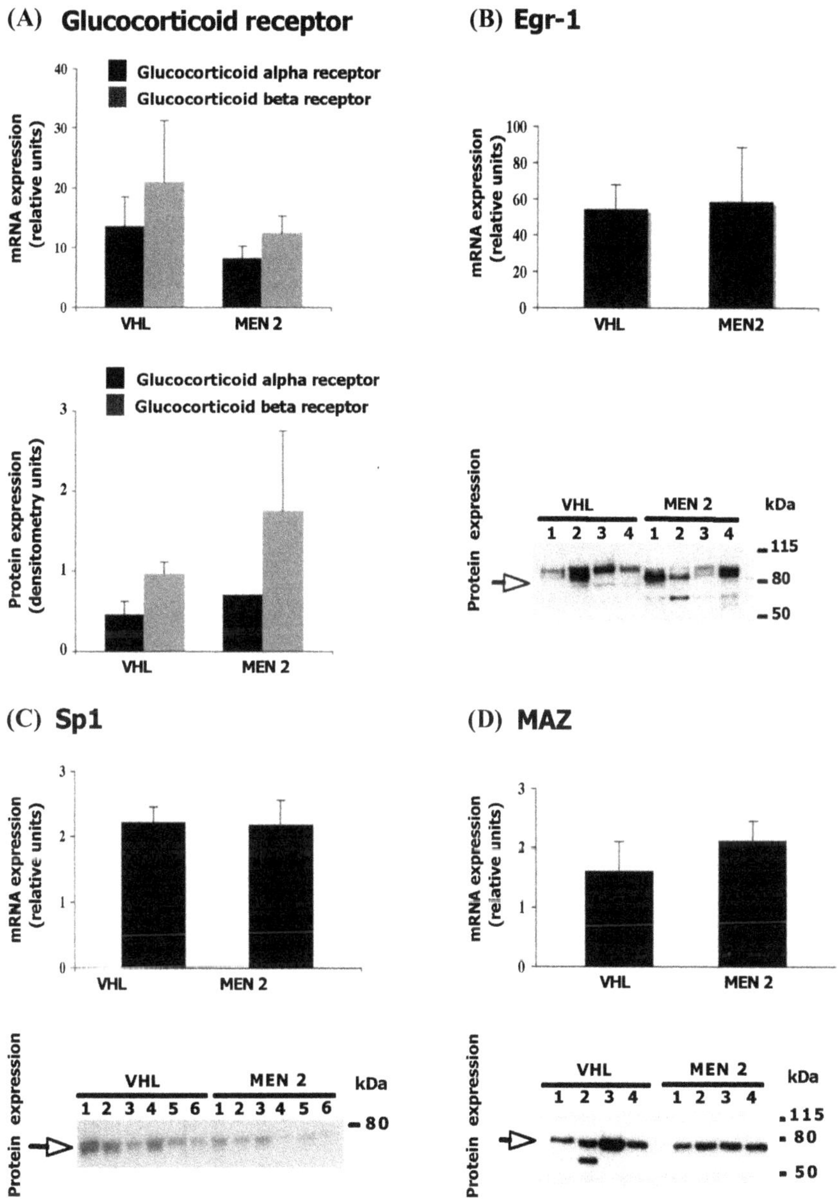

FIGURE 1. Expression of the glucocorticoid receptor, Egr-1, Sp1, and MAZ mRNA and protein in pheochromocytomas from patients with MEN-2 and VHL syndrome. Expression of mRNA was determined by TaqMan PCR, with expression shown relative to that of 18S ribosomal mRNA, as described in the "Methods" section. Expression of glucocorticoid receptor protein in Western blots was determined by densitometry using NIH image 1.62 software. Levels of expression of Egr-1, Sp1, and MAZ protein are shown in the Western blot images.

TABLE 3. Selection of differentially expressed genes from microarray expression profiles

	Gene symbols	*P* value
VHL > MEN-2		
Endothelial PAS domain 1	EPAS1, HIF 2α	<0.0001*
RE1-silencing transcription factor	REST	<0.0004*
Insulin-like growth factor 2 (somatomedin A)	IGF2	<0.0001
Glial cell-derived neurotrophic factor	GDNF	<0.0004
GDNF receptor alpha 1	GFRalpha1	<0.0003
neuregulin 1	NRG1, GGF	<0.0002
neuritin 1	NRN	<0.0003
MEN-2 > VHL		
Ret proto-oncogene	RET	<0.0001
Neural cell adhesion molecule 1	NCAM1	<0.0001
Neural cell adhesion molecule 2	NCAM2	<0.001
Astrotactin	ASTN	<0.001
Achaete-scute complex-like 1	ASCL1, MASH1	<0.0001
Bone morphogenetic protein 8b	BMP8B, OP2	<0.0001

*P value from cDNA array database (all other P-values from oligonucleotide array database).

Consistent with the quantitative PCR results, there were no differences in expression of the glucocorticoid receptor, Egr-1, and MAZ by either of the microarray analyses. Expression of alpha, beta, and gamma isoforms of the AP2 transcription factor also showed no relevant differences consistent with higher expression of PNMT in MEN-2 than VHL tumors. However, microarray analyses indicated differences in expression of other genes involved in neural crest cell lineage and chromaffin cell development that might contribute to different noradrenergic and adrenergic catecholamine phenotypes of pheochromocytomas (TABLE 3).

DISCUSSION

Our study revealed no consistent differences in expression, at both mRNA and protein levels, of the glucocorticoid receptor, Egr-1, Sp1, and MAZ in pheochromocytomas from patients with MEN-2 and VHL syndrome. Microarray analyses also indicated no relevant difference in expression of the AP2 transcription factor. Differences in synthesis of epinephrine in pheochromocytomas from patients with MEN-2 and VHL syndrome are therefore unlikely to be on account of any continuing influence of these transcription factors in regulating expression of PNMT. As shown elsewhere,[14] the adrenergic phenotype of adrenal pheochromocytomas can be maintained after spread of tumor cells to sites distant from adrenal sites of steroid production. This observation is consistent with the view that expression of PNMT does not depend on continuing high local concentrations of glucocorticoids.

The above interpretation does not exclude the possibility that glucocorticoids and related transcription factors may be transiently involved in influencing expression of PNMT during differentiation of neural crest cells, either before or during development into tumor cells. Other levels of regulation that our methods did not identify, such as differences in posttranslational phosphorylation of those transcription factors, also remain possible.

Our findings in hereditary pheochromocytomas contrast with previous findings by others of greater expression of Egr-1 in sporadic adenergic than noradrenergic tumors.[15] Epinephrine production and the adrenergic phenotype in hereditary tumors may therefore reflect different mechanisms than in sporadic tumors.

Pheochromocytomas in MEN-2 and VHL syndrome have been suggested to develop from different populations of noradrenergic and adrenergic chromaffin cells.[2] However, while distinct populations of adrenergic and noradrenergic chromaffin cells are present in the adrenals of many mammalian species, almost all chromaffin cells in the adult human adrenal medulla express PNMT.[16] This observation suggests that development of adrenal pheochromocytomas producing almost exclusively norepinephrine, such as in VHL syndrome, might reflect dedifferentiation, with loss of expression of PNMT and other aspects of the adrenergic phenotype.

Findings by Lee *et al.*[17] now suggest an alternative explanation to the above for the development of pheochromocytomas with distinct mutation-dependent phenotypes. That study indicated that familial pheochromocytomas may be explained by a single pathway linking mutations in several disease-causing genes (i.e., *RET, VHL, NF1, SDHB,* and *SDHD*) to failure of apoptosis after withdrawal of growth factors during chromaffin cell development.

How would a single pathway lead to divergent phenotypes in different hereditary forms of pheochromocytoma? We speculate that there are different susceptibilities of the pathway to effects of mutations of specific genes at different stages of neural crest development and differentiation. According to this notion, pheochromocytomas in VHL syndrome would develop from neural crest progenitors before differentiation into PNMT-expressing and epinephrine-producing adrenal chromaffin cells, whereas epinephrine-producing tumors in MEN-2 would develop on account of susceptibility of fully differentiated PNMT-expressing chromaffin cells to the effects of activating *RET* mutations.

Preliminary support for the above view comes from our microarray data indicating differential expression in MEN-2 versus VHL tumors of a number of genes involved in the differentiation of neural crest progenitor cells. Endothelial PAS domain protein 1 (EPAS1), also known as hypoxia inducible factor 2α, is expressed in greater abundance in VHL and sporadic noradrenergic tumors than in MEN-2 and sporadic adrenergic tumors.[2] Apart from functions in endothelial cell hypoxia-induced signaling pathways, EPAS1 is also expressed in embryonic norepinephrine-producing sympathetic nerves and chromaffin cells, where it regulates the expression of tyrosine hydroxylase, the rate limiting enzyme in catecholamine synthesis.[18,19] In such cells, impaired degradation of EPAS1, on account of defective VHL protein, might lead to failure of apoptosis at a critical period, with subsequent development of norepinephrine-producing chromaffin cell tumors

Other genes involved in neural crest cell lineage development indicated by expression profiling to be more highly expressed in VHL than MEN-2 tumors included the RE1-silencing transcription factor, insulin-like growth factor 2 (IGF2), glial cell-derived neurotrophic factor (GDNF), and GDNF receptor alpha 1. The RE1-silencing transcription factor, a repressor that silences transcription of neuron-specific genes in non-neuronal cells, has been implicated to regulate PNMT expression in chromaffin cells.[20] IGF2 is expressed in particularly high amounts in pheochromocytomas,[21,22] and acting through the IGF-I receptor substantially decreases catecholamine synthesis.[23] GDNF and other neurotrophin family members acting through a variety receptors (e.g., RET and GDNF receptor alpha 1) are important for the differentiation of neural crest cells, promoting survival of tyrosine hydroxylase positive cells,[24] and in chromaffin cells, a change from an endocrine to a neuronal morphology.[25]

Genes involved in neural crest cell lineage development indicated by expression profiling to be more highly expressed in MEN-2 than VHL tumors included the expected RET proto-oncogene, neural cell adhesion molecules 1 and 2, and achaete-scute homolog-1 (MASH1). The neural cell adhesion molecules have been previously implicated in the differentiation and morphological arrangement of PNMT-positive adrenergic and PNMT-negative noradrenergic cells of the developing adrenal medulla.[26,27] Furthermore, findings in transgenic mice lacking MASH1, show that this transcription factor is essential for the correct phenotypic differentiation of adrenal chromaffin cells.[28] In particular, chromaffin cells lacking MASH1 do not express catecholamine-synthesizing enzymes, including PNMT.

In summary, the present findings indicate that maintenance of PNMT expression and epinephrine production in pheochromocytomas from MEN-2 patients, and lack of PNMT in tumors from VHL patients, are unlikely to reflect influences of any continuing difference in expression of transcription factors known to regulate the PNMT gene (i.e., glucocorticoid receptor, Egr-1, Sp-1, MAZ, and AP2). Our microarray results lead to the alternative hypothesis that the differing catecholamine phenotypes in VHL and MEN-2 tumors reflect origins from developmentally distinct chromaffin cell progenitors, with presence or absence of PNMT maintained independently of the above transcription factors.

ACKNOWLEDGMENTS

We gratefully acknowledge the gift of MAZ rabbit antibody from Kenneth B. Marcu, State University of New York at Stony Brook, Stony Brook, USA.

This research was supported by the Intramural Research Program of the NIH, National Institute of Neurological Disorders and Stroke, National Cancer Institute, National Institute of Child Health and Human Development, National Human Genome Research Institute, and Center for Information Technology.

REFERENCES

1. EISENHOFER, G. *et al.* 2001. Pheochromocytomas in von Hippel-Lindau syndrome and multiple endocrine neoplasia type 2 display distinct biochemical and clinical phenotypes. J. Clin. Endocrinol. Metab. **86:** 1999–2008.
2. EISENHOFER, G. *et al.* 2004. Distinct gene expression profiles in norepinephrine- and epinephrine-producing hereditary and sporadic pheochromocytomas: activation of hypoxia-driven angiogenic pathways in von Hippel-Lindau syndrome. Endocr. Rel. Cancer **11:** 897–911.
3. HUYNH, T.-T. *et al.* 2005. Different expression of catecholamine transporters in phaeochromocytomas from patients with von Hippel-Lindau syndrome and multiple endocrine neoplasia type 2. Eur. J. Endocrinol. **153:** 551–563.
4. WURTMAN, R.J. & J. AXELROD. 1966. Control of enzymatic synthesis of adrenaline in the adrenal medulla by adrenal cortical steroids. J. Biol. Chem. **241:** 2301–2305.
5. TAI, T.C. *et al.* 2002. Glucocorticoid responsiveness of the rat phenylethanolamine N-methyltransferase gene. Mol. Pharmacol. **61:** 1885–1892.
6. EBERT, S.N. *et al.* 1994. Egr-1 activation of rat adrenal phenylethanolamine N-methyltransferase gene. J. Biol. Chem. **269:** 20885–20898.
7. EBERT, S.N. & D.L. WONG. 1995. Differential activation of the rat phenylethanolamine N-methyltransferase gene by Sp1 and Egr-1. J. Biol. Chem. **270:** 17299–17305.
8. HER, S. *et al.* 1999. Phenylethanolamine N-methyltransferase gene expression. Sp1 and MAZ potential for tissue specific expression. J. Biol. Chem. **274:** 8698–8707.
9. WONG, D.L. *et al.* 1998. Phenylethanolamine N-methyltransferase gene expression. Synergistic activation by Egr-1, AP-2 and the glucocorticoid receptor. Mol. Brain Res. **61:** 154–161.
10. EISENHOFER, G. *et al.* 1986. Simultaneous liquid-chromatographic determination of 3,4-dihydroxyphenylglycol, catecholamines, and 3,4-dihydroxyphenylalanine in plasma, and their responses to inhibition of monoamine oxidase. Clin. Chem. **32:** 2030–2033.
11. LENDERS, J.W. *et al.* 1993. Determination of metanephrines in plasma by liquid chromatography with electrochemical detection. Clin. Chem. **39:** 97–103.
12. ANDREWS, N.C. & D.V. FALLER. 1991. A rapid micropreparation technique for extraction of DNA-binding proteins from limiting numbers of mammalian cells. Nucleic Acids Res. **19:** 2499.
13. BROUWERS, F.M. *et al.* 2006. Gene expression profiling of pheochromocytomas. Ann. N.Y. Acad. Sci. In press.
14. EISENHOFER, G. *et al.* 2005. Pheochromocytoma catecholamine phenotypes and prediction of tumor size and location by use of plasma free metanephrines. Clin. Chem. **51:** 735–744.

15. Isobe, K. *et al.* 2000. Enhanced expression of mRNA coding for the adrenaline-synthesizing enzyme phenylethanolamine-N-methyl transferase in adrenaline-secreting pheochromocytomas. J. Urol. **163:** 357–362.
16. Cleary, S. *et al.* 2005. Expression of the noradrenaline transporter and phenylethanolamine N-methyltransferase in normal human adrenal gland and phaeochromocytoma. Cell Tissue Res. **27:** 448–453.
17. Lee, S. *et al.* 2005. Neuronal apoptosis linked to EglN3 prolyl hydroxylase and familial pheochromocytoma genes: developmental culling and cancer. Cancer Cell **8:** 155–167.
18. Tian, H. *et al.* 1998. The hypoxia-responsive transcription factor EPAS1 is essential for catecholamine homeostasis and protection against heart failure during embryonic development. Genes Dev. **12:** 3320–3324.
19. Favier, J. *et al.* 1999. Cloning and expression pattern of EPAS1 in the chicken embryo. Colocalization with tyrosine hydroxylase. FEBS Lett. **462:** 19–24.
20. Evinger, M.J. 1998. Determinants of phenylethanolamine-N-methyltransferase expression. Adv. Pharmacol. **42:** 73–76.
21. Haselbacher, G.K. *et al.* 1987. Insulin-like growth factor II in human adrenal pheochromocytomas and Wilms tumors: expression at the mRNA and protein level. Proc. Natl. Acad. Sci. USA **84:** 1104–1106.
22. Suzuki, T. *et al.* 1989. IGF-II-like immunoreactivity in human tissues, neuroendocrine tumors, and PC12 cells. Diabetes Res. Clin. Pract. **7**(Suppl I)**:** S21–S27.
23. Bach, L.A. & K.S. Leeding. 2002. Insulin-like growth factors decrease catecholamine content in PC12 rat pheochromocytoma cells. Horm Metab. Res. **34:** 487–491.
24. Maxwell, G.D. *et al.* 1996. Glial cell line-derived neurotrophic factor promotes the development of adrenergic neurons in mouse neural crest cultures. Proc. Natl. Acad. Sci. USA **93:** 13274–13279.
25. Forander, P., C. Broberger & I. Stromberg. 2001. Glial-cell-line-derived neurotrophic factor induces nerve fibre formation in primary cultures of adrenal chromaffin cells. Cell Tissue Res. **305:** 43–51.
26. Leon, C. *et al.* 1992. Expression of cell adhesion molecules and catecholamine synthesizing enzymes in the developing rat adrenal gland. Brain Res. Dev. Brain Res. **70:** 109–121.
27. Leon, C. *et al.* 1992. L1 Cell adhesion molecule is expressed by noradrenergic but not adrenergic chromaffin cells: a possible major role for L1 in adrenal medullary design. Eur. J. Neurosci. **4:** 201–209.
28. Huber, K. *et al.* 2002. Development of chromaffin cells depends on MASH1 function. Development **129:** 4729–4738.

Expression of mRNAs for Succinate Dehydrogenase Subunits and Related Genes in Pheochromocytoma

KAZUMASA ISOBE,[a] SUMIKO NISSATO,[a] ICHIRO TATSUNO,[b] TORU YASHIRO,[c] KAZUHIRO TAKEKOSHI,[a] AND YASUSHI KAWAKAMI[a]

[a]*Department of Clinical Pathology, Institute of Clinical Medicine, University of Tsukuba, 1-1-1 Tennnoudai, Tsukuba, Ibaraki 305-8575, Japan*

[b]*Department of Clinical Cell Biology, Graduate School of Medicine, Chiba University, 1-8-1 Inohana, Tyuou-ku, Chiba, Chiba 260-8655, Japan*

[c]*Department of Surgery, Institute of Clinical Medicine, University of Tsukuba, 1-1-1 Tennnoudai, Tsukuba, Ibaraki 305-8575, Japan*

ABSTRACT: **Mutations in the genes encoding succinate dehydrogenase (SDH) have been associated with susceptibility to pheochromocytoma. However, few reports have examined the level of SDH mRNAs expression. In this study, we examined the level of expression of mRNAs encoding SDHB, SDHC, and SDHD in pheochromocytoma, pheochromocytoma subgroups, and normal adrenal gland, and compared the expression of these genes to the level of expression of related genes in the same tissues. The mean relative level of expression of SDHB, SDHC, SDHD and VHL mRNA was 28.7 ± 6.2%, 16.6 ± 4.8%, 214 ± 47.5% and 25.9 ± 8.2%, respectively, in pheochromocytoma tissues compared to normal adrenal gland. Furthermore, the mean relative level of the *RET* proto-oncogene mRNA was 707 ± 149% in pheochromocytoma compared to normal adrenal gland. The level of expression of the SDH genes was highly correlated in each individual sample ($P < 0.0001$). The level of expression of the SDH mRNAs correlated with the level of VHL mRNA ($P < 0.0001$), but not with the level of RET mRNA. The level of SDH mRNAs expression also correlated with the expression of phenylethanolamine N-methyl transferase (PNMT), an adrenaline synthesizing enzyme ($P < 0.01$), which may explain the correlation between SDH expression and adrenaline content ($P < 0.05$). The level of SDH mRNAs expression correlated strongly with the expression of VEGF mRNA ($P < 0.0001$). In multiple endocrine neoplasia (MEN) 2a, the expression of the SDH genes and VHL mRNA was significantly higher than that observed in adrenal or extra-adrenal pheochromocytoma. The expression of the corticotropin-releasing hormone (CRH) mRNA was**

Address for correspondence: Kazumasa Isobe, Department of Clinical Pathology, Institute of Clinical Medicine, University of Tsukuba, 1-1-1 Tennnoudai, Tsukuba, Ibaraki 305-8575, Japan. Voice and fax: +81-29-853-3054.
e-mail: k-isobe@md.tsukuba.ac.jp

**Ann. N.Y. Acad. Sci. 1073: 253–262 (2006). © 2006 New York Academy of Sciences.
doi: 10.1196/annals.1353.027**

significantly higher in extra-adrenal pheochromocytoma than in adrenal pheochromocytoma or MEN2a. Thus, tumor-specific gene expression exists in pheochromocytoma, which may explain the characteristics of the tumor.

KEYWORDS: **SDHB; SDHC; SDHD; RET; VHL; mRNA expression**

INTRODUCTION

Pheochromocytomas are catecholamine-producing tumors arising most often from the adrenal medulla. Extra-adrenal pheochromocytomas are also called paragangliomas. Approximately 80% of pheochromocytomas are of a sporadic nature. However, familiality has been observed when the following diseases are either underlying or coexisting: multiple endocrine neoplasia (MEN) type 2a/b, von Hippel–Lindau syndrome (VHL), and neurofibromatosis type 1.

Certain genes are overexpressed in tumor cells, such as those encoding hormone-synthesizing enzymes. We have reported that the expression of mRNAs encoding catecholamine-synthesizing enzymes is increased in pheochromocytoma.[1,2] However, the mechanisms responsible for this increase have not yet been established. Evaluation of tumor DNA has identified germline mutations in the genes coding for subunits of mitochondrial complex II succinate dehydrogenase (SDH), which plays an important role in oxidative phosphorylation and the Krebs cycle.[3] Hereditary paraganglioma type 1 is characterized by vascularization and slow growth. The SDHD gene has been identified as a susceptibility gene for paraganglioma type 1, whereas mutations in the SDHC and SDHB genes have been linked to paraganglioma type 3 and 4, respectively.[4] In addition, several studies have linked loss of heterozygosity of wild-type SDHD and SDHB alleles to the development of paragangliomas and pheochromocytomas, suggesting that these genes function as tumor, suppressors.

The Ret gene encodes a transmembrane tyrosine kinase receptor, and is believed to be a proto-oncogene. RET activation normally occurs via binding to any of the ligands: glial cell line–derived neurotrophic factor (GDNF), neutrin, persephin, and artemin. RET mRNA overexpression is frequently found in pheochromocytomas.[5] Moreover, 50% of sporadic pheochromocytomas exhibit high levels of tyrosine phosphorylation of the ret protein and an increase in the level of the GDNF ligand.[6]

The VHL gene encodes for two proteins, the smaller pVHL19, which results from internal translation initiation from an in-frame ATG at codon 54 to produce a 160-amino acid protein, and the larger 213-amino acid pVHL30. pVHL has been shown to influence several processes, including cell cycle control, mRNA stability, and regulation of hypoxia-inducible gene expression. In contrast to RET, pVHL is considered to be a tumor suppressor and

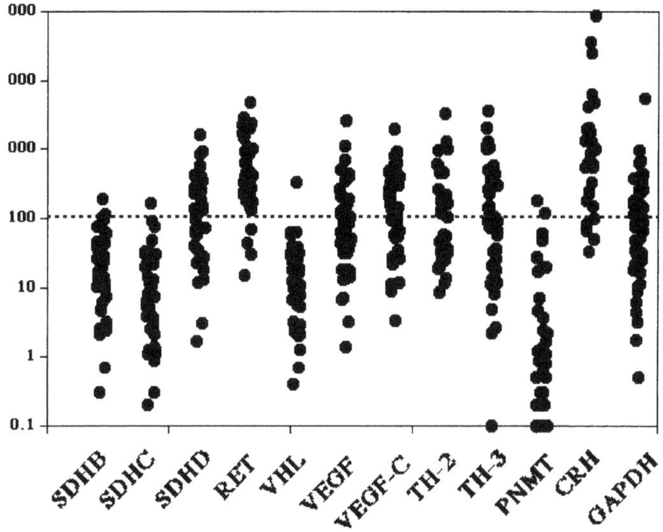

FIGURE 1. Relative level of expression mRNAs encoding SDHB, SDHC, SDHD, RET, VHL, VEGF, VEGF-C, TH exon2, TH exon3, PNMT, CRH, and GAPDH in pheochromocytoma tissues compared to normal adrenal gland.

most VHL-associated pheochromocytomas show loss of heterozygosity of this gene.

In this study, we report the expression of the mRNAs encoding SDH subunits, RET, and VHL in 44 clinical samples of pheochromocytoma. Furthermore, we compared the expression of the mRNAs encoding SDH subunits, RET, and VHL in pheochromocytoma subgroups (adrenal, extra-adrenal pheochromocytoma, and MEN2a). We also examined the correlation between the level of these genes' expression with the cellular content of epinephrine and norepinephrine and the level of mRNA encoding hormone-synthesizing enzymes and vascular factors.

MATERIALS AND METHODS

Tissue Samples

Pheochromocytoma tissues were obtained from patients at the time of excision. Informed consent for the experimental use of the samples was obtained from all donors. Each of these specimens was frozen immediately after surgical resection and was stored at −80°C until use. A total of 44 clinical samples of pheochromocytomas were analyzed in this study. Total human RNA from the adrenal gland and brain was purchased from Clontech (Palo Alto, CA, USA).

TABLE 1. Characteristics of 44 pheochromocytomas

Case	Age	Sex	Size (mm)	Weight (g)	*SDHB* (%)	*SDHC* (%)	*SDHD* (%)	*RET* (%)	*VHL* (%)	*TERT*	A (ng/mg)	Malignancy	Diagnosis	Complication
1	51	M	ϕ20		6.2	32.1	553.3	0.0	11.3	11	194	+	para	
2	61	F	125×100×110	700			558.4	193.4		6	166	+	pheo	
3	27	M		193	0.0	0.0	0.0	0.0	0.0	140	5	+	pheo	
4	15	M	50×40×35	39	4.9	2.6	34.2	42.6	12.4	0	3	+	pheo	
5	76	M	ϕ40		0.0	0.0	0.0	0.0	0.0	0		+	pheo	
6	36	F	30×30×20				236.8	2853.9		0	28204	–	pheo	
7	49	M	30×36×40	49	34.1	14.6	264.5	938.5	24.2	0	15735	–	para	
8	70	M	50×40×30							0	13160	–	pheo	diabetes[d] Hashimoto disease
9	37	F	70×40×30		193.3	169.7	1597.4	1044.1	331.5	0	10844	–	MEN2a[a]	thyroid medullary carcinoma
10	67	F	52×35×20	24	14.6	2.9	180.1	314.8	34.8	0	10805	–	pheo	essential hypertension
11	61	F	50×35×40	30	44.9	32.3	422.5	2245.9	61.5	0	8228	–	pheo	diabetes
12	68	M	38×24×12	9.7	28.0	13.1	152.8	4707.8	19.0		7746	–	pheo[b]	diabetes[c]
13	55	M	40×22	18.5	104.1	92.8	854.6	233.2	62.9	3	7666	–	pheo	
14	52	M	55×30×25	25	23.8	3.7	248.9	451.2	5.6		7581	–	pheo	diabetes[c]
15	58	M	55×45×30	34	117.2	75.7	921.4	2320.8	31.5		7282	–	pheo	diabetes
16	47	M			19.6	10.6	173.0	852.5	25.7	0	5772	–	para	diabetes[d]
17	28	M	35×53×40	50	10.3	3.9	94.8	631.6	17.8	0	3620	–	pheo	
18		M			11.9	2.3	134.3	148.1	2.0		3600	–	pheo	diabetes
19	51	M	50×50×60		13.7	4.4	70.2	650.4	12.2	0	2378	–	pheo	diabetes
20	55	F	55×40×40		2.8	0.9	13.0	170.7	1.3		2338	–	pheo	
21	40	F			0.3	0.2	1.7	181.9	0.4	0	1972	–	pheo	
22	33	F	36×40×25	16	2.1	1.1	61.9	1629.7	7.2	0	1809	–	pheo	
23	53	F	ϕ24	1.8	97.2	47.3	406.9	2034.8	37.6	0	1738	–	pheo	
24	23	F	28×30×25	17	75.6	30.2	234.1	1452.9	28.9	0	1653	–	pheo	
25	33	M	45×25×35		10.5	5.4	40.5	221.7	6.7	29	1417	–	pheo	
26	30	F	40×50×60	80	17.1	6.4	61.3	240.0	40.0	0	1228	–	pheo	diabetes
27	36	F	23×18×11	10	7.6	1.4	73.6	277.0	7.7		1067	–	pheo	diabetes[b]

Continued

TABLE 1. *Continued*

Case	Age	Sex	Size (mm)	Weight (g)	*SDHB* (%)	*SDHC* (%)	*SDHD* (%)	*RET* (%)	*VHL* (%)	*TERT*	A (ng/mg)	Malignancy	Diagnosis	Complication
28	41	M	40×30×25	18	12.7	5.1	58.2	458.5	10.3	0	1026	–	pheo	hyperlipidemia
29	50	F	75×50×45	120	26.5	19.4	272.9	1661.3	57.7	7	922	–	pheo	
30	49	M	110×75×35	643	14.4	8.0	109.7	400.8	9.9	0	863	–	pheo	
31	58	M	26×43×58	57	38.7	21.9	140.2	328.3	31.3	11	797	–	pheo	diabetes
32	30	M	75×60×38		28.9	12.0	78.8	607.3	33.8	0	689	–	pheo	diabetes, hyperlipidemia
33	62	F	50×55×60		4.7	1.3	11.7	0.0	2.3	0	506	–	pheo	
34	67	M	33×25×28	18	2.3	1.1	23.0	14.8	3.3	0	167	–	pheo	diabetes
35	24	M	75×65×25	58	2.6	1.3	34.3	0.0	2.6	0	135	–	pheo	
36	59	M	150×100×40		3.2	1.3	27.3	1003.9	5.5		132	–	pheo	
37	48	M	55×50×30		26.5	10.0	596.3	505.1	26.0	0	102	–	para	von Recklinghausen disease
38	58	M	33×32×26	35	0.7	0.3	3.2	69.1	0.7		61	–	pheo	diabetes
39	26	M	50×30×25	18	63.2	21.9	356.7	228.3	16.5		12	–	pheo	
40	72	M	ϕ35	53	0.0	0.0	0.0	0.0	0.0	0	0	–	pheo	
41	25	M	70×55×35	26	9.8	2.1	22.3	30.2	2.1		0	–	pheo	chronic renal failure
42	44	M	75×50×20		2.5	1.1	27.8	415.6	3.0			–	pheo	diabetes
43	36	F	60×48×40	50	44.1	7.5	17.7	131.0	10.7			–	pheo	
44	35	F	60×40×30		61.1	30.0	74.0	0.0	62.8			–	MEN2a[a]	
ad.gl.					100.0	100.0	100.0	100.0	100.0					
brain					203.3	57.5	74.0	85.3	11.4					

Abbreviations: *SDH* = succinate dehydrogenase; *VHL* = von Hippel–Lindau disease; *TERT* = telomerase transcriptase; A = adrenaline pheo = pheochromocytoma; MENIIa = multiple endocrine neoplasm a; para = paraganglioma.

[a]*RET* mutation 634 TGC→TGT = [b]*SDHD* mutation c.111 G→A.

[c]Has DM in family.

[c]Improved dramatically after surgery.

TABLE 2. Pearson correlation matrix showing correlation coefficients between age, *SDHB*, *SDHC*, *SDHD*, *RET*, *VHL*, *VEGF*, *VEGF*-C, *nNOS*, *TH* exon2,3, *PNMT*, *PACAP*, *POMC*, *CRH* mRNA expressions and A, NA contents in pheochromocytoma tissues

	Age	*SDHB*	*SDHC*	*SDHD*	*RET*	*VHL*	*VEGF*	*VEGF-C*	*nNOS*	*TH* exon2	*TH* exon3	*PNMT*	*PACAP*	*POMC*	*CRH*	A	NA
Age																	
SDHB	0.019																
SDHC	0.049	0.944‡															
SDHD	0.105	0.891‡	0.943‡														
RET	0.272	0.326	0.221	0.221													
VHL	−0.044	0.790‡	0.870‡	0.806‡	0.155												
VEGF	0.012	0.642‡	0.695‡	0.658‡	−0.003	0.470†											
VEGF-C	0.139	0.583‡	0.600‡	0.600‡	0.079	0.363*	0.933‡										
nNOS	−0.070	0.615‡	0.719‡	0.663‡	0.126	0.914‡	0.304	0.155									
TH exon2	0.163	0.411*	0.235	0.204	0.466†	0.041	0.046	0.150	−0.041								
TH exon3	0.039	0.119	0.034	0.022	0.448*	0.043	−0.081	0.051	0.024	0.413*							
PNMT	0.204	0.707‡	0.714‡	0.729‡	0.394*	0.455†	0.419*	0.393*	0.319	0.228	0.115						
PACAP	0.225	0.549†	0.520†	0.575‡	0.322	0.200	0.331	0.355*	0.085	0.301	0.191	0.940‡					
POMC	0.057	−0.030	−0.009	0.007	0.168	0.083	0.003	−0.021	0.382*	0.098	0.314	−0.067	0.013				
CRH	0.087	0.011	0.061	0.315	−0.052	−0.007	0.140	0.208	−0.042	0.041	−0.121	−0.013	0.033	−0.037			
A	0.317	0.446*	0.437*	0.470†	0.381*	0.430*	0.237	0.266	0.272	0.096	0.279	0.507†	0.392*	−0.105	−0.138		
NA	0.092	−0.013	−0.104	−0.039	0.167	0.018	−0.126	0.030	0.140	0.259	0.385*	−0.132	−0.029	0.633‡	−0.005	0.183	

Abbreviations: *SDH* = succinate dehydrogenase; *VHL* = von Hippel–Lindau; *VEGF* = vascular endothelial growth factor; *nNOS* = neural NO-synthase; *TH* = tyrosine hydroxylase; *PNMT* = phenylethanolamine N-methyltransferase; *PACAP* = pituitary adenylate cyclase-activating polypeptide; *POMC* = proopiomelanocortin; *CRH* = corticotropin-releasing hormone; A = adrenaline; NA = noradrenaline.

* < 0.05.

† < 0.01.

‡ < 0.001.

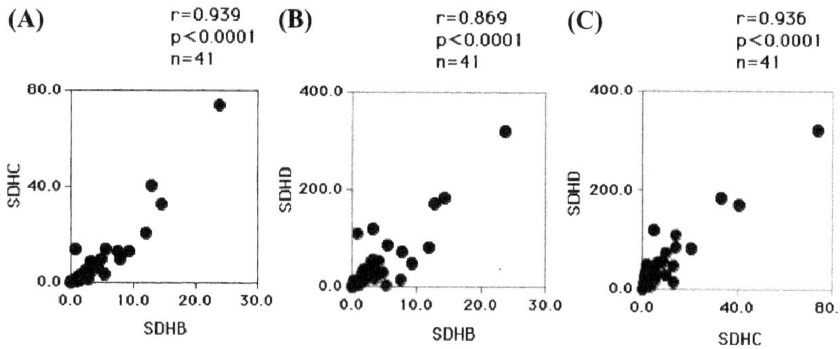

FIGURE 2. Real-time PCR analysis comparing the expression of SDHB, SDHC, and SDHD mRNA. Correlations are shown between SDHB and SDHC (**A**), SDHB and SDHD (**B**), SDHB and SDHD (**C**) in pheochromocytoma tissues.

Real-Time PCR

The PCR reaction mixture was prepared using a Taqman PCR master reagent kit (PE Applied Biosystems, CA) according to the manufacturer's instructions. The thermal cycling protocol was 2 min at 50°C and 10 min at 95°C, followed by 40 cycles of 95°C for 15s and 60°C for 1 min. Thermal cycling, fluorescence detection, and data analysis were performed on the ABI PRISM 7700 Sequence Detector using the software provided with the instrument. For GAPDH detection, we used TaqMan GAPDH Detection Reagents (PE Applied Biosystems).

Determination of Catecholamine Concentrations

Tissue concentrations of catecholamines (epinephrine, norepinephrine, and dopamine) were determined using a catecholamine autoanalyzer (H8030,

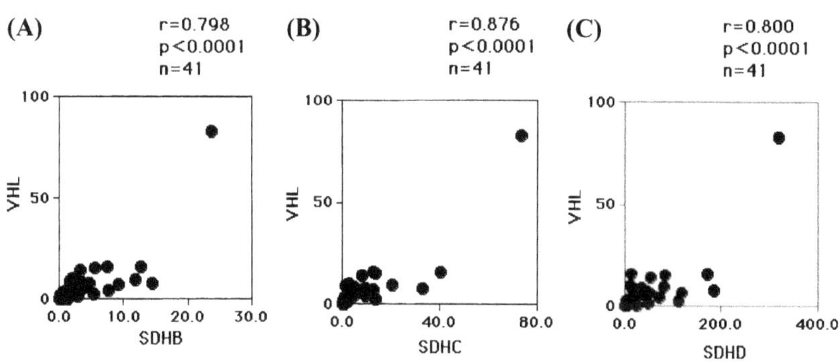

FIGURE 3. Real-time PCR analysis comparing the expression of SDHB, SDHC, SDHD, and VHL mRNA. Correlations are shown between SDHB and VHL (**A**), SDHC and VHL (**B**), and SDHD and VHL (**C**) in pheochromocytoma tissues.

TOSOH, Tokyo) with built-in high-performance liquid chromatography and spectrofluorometer.

Statistical Analysis

All data are expressed as the mean ± SE. The Pearson correlation was used to examine relationships between variables. Significance was indicated by a P value less than .05. Statistical significance between adrenal pheochromocytoma, extra-adrenal pheochromocytoma, and MEN2a was determined by Tukey-Kramer test, with the significance level at $P < 0.05$. All statistical analyses were performed using Statview version 5.0 for Macintosh.

RESULTS AND DISCUSSION

Patient's characteristics and data are provided in TABLE 1.

The mean relative expression of the mRNAs encoding SDHB, SDHC, SDHD and VHL in the samples of pheochromocytoma compared to their expression in a sample of normal adtrenal gland were 28.7 ± 6.2%, 16.6 ± 4.8%, 215 ± 47.5%, and 25.9 ± 8.2%, respectively. However, the mean relative expression of the mRNA encoding the RET proto-oncogene was 707 ± 149% in the samples of pheochromocytoma versus normal adrenal tissues. Thus, there was reduced expression of genes previously suggested to function as tumor suppressors (with the exception of SDHD), whereas the expression of the Ret proto-oncogene was increased in pheochromocytoma relative to normal adrenal tissues. In samples of MEN2a, in which mutations in ret increase ret signaling, the expression of the SDH genes and VHL was significantly higher than that in sporadic pheochromocytomas, suggesting that ret signaling may affect the expression of these genes, although there was no difference in the level of RET mRNA expression in these cells.

FIGURE 1 also shows the relative expression of a set of related genes in these tumors. Expression of these genes was variable. The expression of phenylethanolamine N-methyl transferase (PNMT) and corticotropin-releasing hormone (CRH) mRNA was found to be lower and higher in pheochromocytomas, respectively, than that observed in normal adrenal gland. Takaya *et al.*[7] have also reported that RET is overexpressed in a majority of cases of sporadic pheochromocytoma and suggested that this high level of expression may be relevant to the development or growth of pheochromocytoma.

TABLE 2 shows a correlation matrix between the patients' age, the level of expression of SDHB, SDHC, SDHD, RET, VHL, vascular endothelial growth factor (VEGF), VEGF-C, neuronal NO synthase (nNOS), tyrosine hydroxylase (TH) exon 2, TH exon 3, PNMT, pituitary adenylate cyclase–activating polypeptide (PACAP), proopiomelanocortin (POMC), CRH and epinephrine, norepinephrine, and dopamine contents in pheochromocytoma

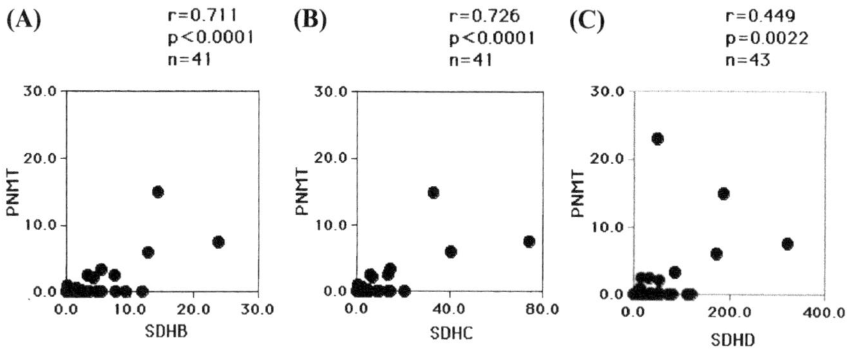

FIGURE 4. Real-time PCR analysis comparing the expression of SDHB, SDHC, SDHD, and PNMT mRNA. Correlations are shown between SDHB and PNMT (**A**), SDHC and PNMT (**B**), and SDHD and PNMT (**C**) in pheochromocytoma tissues.

tissues. The expression of the CRH mRNA was significantly higher in extra-adrenal pheochromocytoma than that in adrenal pheochromocyoma or MEN2a.

The individual SDH genes were expressed at similar relative ratios in the samples of pheochromocytoma we examined, suggesting that expression of these genes is coordinately controlled in pheochromocytoma ($P < 0.0001$, FIG. 2). The level of expression of SDH mRNAs was also correlated with the expression of VHL mRNA ($P < 0.0001$, FIG. 3), but not with the expression of RET mRNA. Both SDH and VHL have been reported to act as oxygen sensors, and their expression may be coordinately regulated.

The level of expression of SDH mRNAs correlated with PNMT mRNA expression ($P < 0.01$, FIG. 4), which may explain the correlation of the former with adrenaline content ($P < 0.05$). The expression of SDH mRNAs correlated

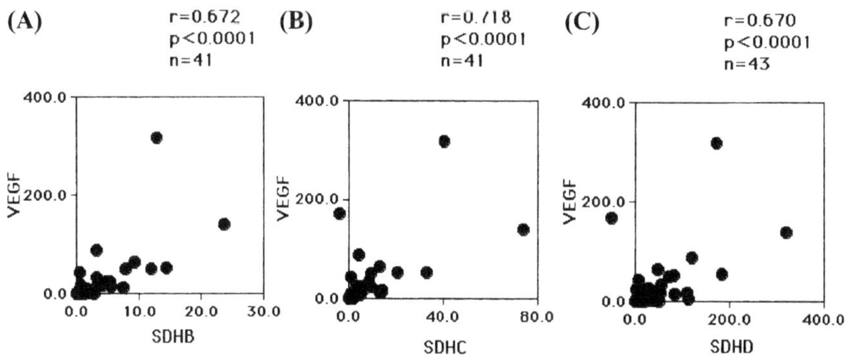

FIGURE 5. Real-time PCR analysis comparing the expression of SDHB, SDHC, SDHD, and VEGF mRNA. Correlations are shown between SDHB and VEGF (**A**), SDHC and VEGF (**B**), SDHD and VEGF (**C**) in pheochromocytoma tissues.

with the expression of VEGF mRNA ($P < 0.0001$, FIG. 5). The level of VEGF mRNA expression has been reported to be significantly higher in paragangliomas carrying a mutation in the SDHD gene than in sporadic pheochromocytoma.[8] Hypoxia in pheochromocytoma cells may induce the both SDHs and VEGF mRNA.

Thus, tumor-specific mRNA expressions exist in pheochromocytoma, and the level of expression of SDH genes, RET, VHL, VEGF, TH, PNMT, CRH mRNA we examined differs significantly in samples of pheochromocytomas. These differences in expression may explain variations in presenting signs and symptoms in these tumors and may also provide useful information about the tumor, such as its adrenal or extra-adrenal location, and the underlying mutation in suspected hereditary cases.

ACKNOWLEDGMENTS

This study was supported in part by a Grant from the Ministry of Education 15590927.

REFERENCES

1. ISOBE, K., T. NAKAI, N. YUKIMASA, *et al.* 1998. Expression of mRNA coding for four catecholamine-synthesizing enzymes in human adrenal pheochromocytomas. Eur. J. Endocrinol. **138:** 383–387.
2. ISOBE, K., T. NAKAI, T. YASHIRO, *et al.* 2000. Enhanced expression of mRNA coding for the adrenaline-synthesizing enzyme phenylethanolamine-N-methyltransferase in adrenaline-secreting pheochromocytomas. J. Urol. **163:** 357–362.
3. BAYSAL, B.E. 2002. Hereditary paraganglioma targets diverse paraganglia. J. Med. Genet. **39:** 617–622.
4. ASTROM, K., J.E. COHEN, J.E. WILLETT-BROZICK, *et al.* 2003. Altitude is a phenotypic modifier in hereditary paraganglioma type 1: evidence for an oxygen-sensing defect. Hum. Genet. **113:** 228–237.
5. EDSTROM, E., T. FRISK, F. FARNEBO, *et al.* 2000. Expression analysis of RET and the GDNF/GFRa-1 and NTN/GFRa-2 ligand complexes in pheochromocytomas and paragangliomas. Int. J. Mol. Med. **6:** 469–474.
6. HIR, H.L., L.G. COLUCCI-D'AMATO, N. CHARLET-BERGUERAND, *et al.* High levels of tyrosine phosphorylated proto-ret in sporadic pheochromocytomas. Cancer Res. **60:** 1365–1370.
7. TAKAYA, K., T. YOSHIMASA, H. ARAI, *et al.* 1996. Expression of the RET proto-oncogene in normal human tissues, pheochromocytomas, and other tumors of neural crest origin. J. Mol. Med. **74:** 617–621.
8. GIMENEZ-ROQUEPLO, A.P., J. FAVIER, P. RUSTIN, *et al.* 2001. The R22X mutation of the SDHD gene in hereditary paraganglioma abolishes the enzymatic activity of complex II in the mitochondrial respiratory chain and activates the hypoxia pathway. Am. J. Hum. Genet. **69:** 1186–1197.

The Norepinephrine Transporter and Pheochromocytoma

SUSANNAH CLEARY[a,b] AND JACQUELINE K. PHILLIPS[a]

[a]*Division of Health Sciences, Murdoch University, Perth, Western Australia, 6150, Australia*

[b]*National Institute of Neurological Disorders and Stoke, National Institutes of Health, Bethesda, Maryland, 20892, USA*

ABSTRACT: **Pheochromocytomas are rare neuroendocrine tumors of chromaffin cell origin that synthesize and secrete excess quantities of catecholamines and other vasoactive peptides. Pheochromocytomas also express the norepinephrine transporter (NET), a molecule that is used clinically as a means of incorporating radiolabelled substrates such as ^{131}I-MIBG (iodo-metaiodobenzylguanidine) into pheochromocytoma tumor cells. This allows the diagnostic localization of these tumors and, more recently, ^{131}I-MIBG has been used in trials in the treatment of pheochromocytoma, potentially giving rise to NET as a therapeutic target. However, because of varying levels or activities of the transporter, the ability of ^{131}I-MIBG to be consistently incorporated into tumor cells is limited, and therefore various strategies to increase NET functional activity are being investigated, including the use of traditional chemotherapeutic agents such as cisplatin or doxorubicin. Other aspects of NET discussed in this short review include the regulation of the transporter and how novel protein–protein interactions between NET and structures such as syntaxin 1A may hold the key to innovative ways to increase the therapeutic value of ^{131}I-MIBG.**

KEYWORDS: **norepinephrine transporter; PC12 cells; uptake assay; cisplatin**

INTRODUCTION

The norepinephrine transporter (NET) is a member of the solute carrier family 6 (SCL6) gene family of Na^+/Cl^--sensitive neurotransmitter transporters, which play a crucial role in the active termination and regulation of extracellular monoamine levels following their release from neuronal or endocrine stores. NET is characteristically expressed in noradrenergic neurons

Address for correspondence: Jacqueline Phillips, Division of Health Sciences, Murdoch University, South Street, MURDOCH, 6150, Perth, Western Australia, Australia. Voice: +61-8-9360-2257; fax: +61-8-9310-4144.
e-mail: j.k.phillips@murdoch.edu.au

Ann. N.Y. Acad. Sci. 1073: 263–269 (2006). © 2006 New York Academy of Sciences.
doi: 10.1196/annals.1353.029

of the brainstem and sympathetic nerves of the periphery, in addition to other nonneuronal sites including the lungs[1] and the placenta.[2] NET expression is also prominent in chromaffin cells of the adrenal gland,[3–6] and also in the neoplastic derivatives of chromaffin cells, pheochromocytomas.[7,8] In addition to its role as a target for psychostimulants such as cocaine, and several antidepressants, NET also plays a key role in imaging and treatment modalities using agents such as ^{131}iodo-metaiodobenzylguanidine (^{131}I-MIBG)[9–11] and ^{18}F-fluorodopamine (^{18}F-FDA).[12,13] For this reason, NET represents an area of interest for those who study pheochromocytomas and other tumors of neural crest lineage including neuroblastoma.

NET: A "Molecular Gateway" for Strategies in Pheochromocytoma Treatment

^{131}I- and ^{123}I-labelled MIBG is an imaging agent that provides excellent specificity (95–100%) but somewhat diminished sensitivity (56–90%)[13,14] for diagnostic localization of pheochromocytoma, presumably due in part to differences in the functional activity or expression levels of the transporter. ^{131}I-MIBG may also serve as a therapeutic tool for tumors of neural crest origin, with a number of reports suggesting that partial or occasionally complete eradication of malignant pheochromocytoma may be achieved through the use of this therapy.[15–17] Similar results have also been reported in the treatment of metastatic carcinoid.[18] The use of ^{131}I-MIBG therapy may be augmented by combinational therapy, where other treatments are used in concert with ^{131}I-MIBG in order to enhance delivery of this substrate into tumor cells. Central to this premise is the use of agents with a specific effect on NET expression, including the ability to increase transcription of NET, or more importantly, to increase the cell-surface activity of existing or newly synthesized transporter molecules.

A number of reports in neuroblastoma, both *in vitro* and *in vivo*, have suggested that pretreatment with traditional chemotherapeutic agents, including doxorubicin and cisplatin, may improve the effectiveness of ^{131}I-MIBG as a treatment modality,[19–21] and that this may be due to increased transcription of the transporter itself.[19] However, unpublished data from our laboratory suggests that there are intrinsic differences between the pheochromocytoma and neuroblastoma cell lines, as pretreatment of the rat pheochromocytoma PC12 cell line with cisplatin does not increase the functional activity of the transporter (FIG. 1). With the exception of data demonstrating that prolonged exposure to ketamine causes upregulation NET in cultured bovine chromaffin cells,[22] to date, very few studies have shown treatments that work to increase NET activity in either pheochromocytoma-derived cell lines or other cell types expressing the transporter.[23–26] Interestingly however, recent data with the topoisomerase I inhibitor topotecan on neuroblastoma cell lines has suggested that this drug may improve accumulation of ^{131}I-MIBG.[27] Although no studies using this

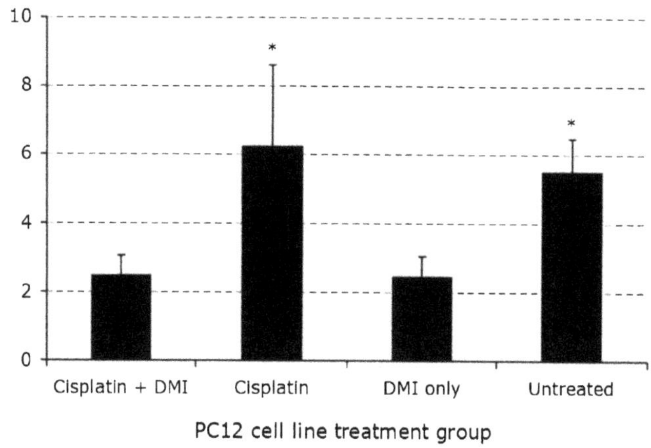

FIGURE 1. NET functional activity in response to cisplatin pretreatment. American Type Culture Centre (ATCC) PC12 cells were incubated for 24 h with cisplatin (10^{-6}M) prior to assessment of NET functional activity, as determined by the uptake of tritiated norepinephrine ([^{3}H]NE) in the absence and presence of desipramine (DMI 10 μM; a specific inhibitor of NET; $n = 8$; for detailed methodology see Ref. 32). Although treatment with DMI significantly reduced the uptake of [^{3}H]NE, pretreatment of the cells with cisplatin did not alter NET functional activity in PC12 cells relative to untreated controls. Statistical analysis was performed with SPSS software using OneWay ANOVA and Tukeys HSD PostHoc with significance set at 0.05.

drug have been conducted either *in vivo*, or in pheochromocytoma cell lines or tumor grafts, this may represent a promising lead for therapeutic use of ^{131}I-MIBG.

Manipulation Through Regulation

The widely accepted paradigm of the NET as a "plasma membrane" transporter contrasts with studies demonstrating that in chromaffin cells, NET is largely expressed within the cytoplasm.[5,6,8] Furthermore, the transporter has been found to associate with secretory granules.[4,8] Cell fractionation studies in PC12 cells indicate that the majority of NET is expressed in fractions containing norepinephrine vesicles, suggesting an association between the transporter and secretory granules and/or large, dense core vesicles. This predominant intracellular localization of NET appears surprising given the role of the transporter for reuptake of norepinephrine. However, numerous findings support the notion of a dynamic process in which transporter molecules are recycled to and from the cell surface. This trafficking ability may be mediated by either direct or indirect phosphorylation of the transporter molecule, a concept supported by both the presence of putative phosphorylation sites on the genes encoding transporters, and also via experimental data in which application of phosphorylating agents (e.g., phorbol esters) leads to transporter trafficking (for a comprehensive review see Ref. 28). Alternatively, it has also been hypothesized that an association between NET and secretory vesicles may be important in the intracellular trafficking of the transporter,[4] supporting other lines of evidence which argue that phosphorylation does not occur by direct interactions with the transporter, but rather at nonconsensus sites and via indirect mechanisms. Sequestered neurotransmitter can also be rereleased. This process involves the fusion of secretory vesicles with the plasma membrane and is facilitated by interactions between vesicular components including vesicular SNAREs (soluble N-ethymaleimide-sensitive attachment factor attachment protein receptor) and the plasma membrane.[4] Findings by Sung *et al.* have demonstrated a direct interaction between NET and the SNARE protein, syntaxin 1A, a protein involved in vesicle trafficking and docking. Their study suggested that PKC activation alters cell-surface NET/syntaxin 1A interactions, diminishing NET activity,[29] thus supporting the idea that transporter trafficking occurs by novel protein–protein interactions, rather than activation of the transporter directly.

Pheochromocytomas arise either as sporadically occurring tumors or as part of hereditary syndromes such as multiple endocrine neoplasia Type 2 (MEN2) and the von Hippel–Lindau (VHL) syndrome. In a study assessing the differences in NET expression between hereditary pheochromocytoma groups, we have recently shown that both NET mRNA and protein levels are greater in MEN2 than in VHL tumors.[7] Whether such differences in syntaxin 1A and/or the expression of other SNARE proteins also exists between hereditary tumors, and these correlate with, or play a role in the differences in NET expression, remains to be determined. Thorough understanding of monoamine transporter biology including aspects of transporter regulation and trafficking, and emerging concepts including protein–protein interactions such as the syntaxin 1A and NET interactions, may inspire innovative therapeutic strategies and classes of drugs capable of enhancing NET activity, thus further broadening the scope of ^{131}I-MIBG efficacy in a clinical setting.

NET and Cellular Phenotype

Pheochromocytomas from MEN2 patients are characterized by their ability to produce significant quantities of the catecholamine epinephrine, and are described as possessing an "adrenergic" phenotype. In contrast, tumors arising from VHL mutations produce negligible amounts of epinephrine, nor do they contain the enzyme responsible for the synthesis of epinephrine: phenylethanolamine N-methyltransferase (PNMT), and are thus termed "noradrenergic."[30,31] The observation of significantly greater levels of NET expression in adrenergic versus noradrenergic tumors may prompt speculation that such differences are associated with the preferential expression of NET in epinephrine-producing cells. This notion is supplemented by our findings that NET is expressed exclusively in adrenergic chromaffin cells of the rat[5] and human.[8] However, when examining both adrenergic and noradrenergic sporadic pheochromocytomas, we determined that expression of NET is found in both PNMT-negative and PNMT-positive chromaffin cells. Taken together, these data support the view that for tumors occurring independently of familial syndromes, NET expression cannot be predicted on the basis of cellular (or tumor) biochemical phenotype. Our study also noted that pheochromocytomas are capable of possessing a range of levels of NET immunoreactivity, but again this was not related to either tumor or cellular phenotype.

CONCLUSION

A greater understanding of the regulation and expression profile of NET will help enhance the use of agents that rely on its activity for diagnostic and treatment modalities not only for pheochromocytomas of both sporadic and familial origin, but also for other tumors such as neuroblastoma and carcinoids. Novel protein–protein interactions between NET and structures such as syntaxin 1A may hold the key to innovative ways to increase the therapeutic value of ^{131}I-MIBG.

REFERENCES

1. BRYAN-LLUKA, L.J., N.N. WESTWOOD & S.R. O'DONNELL. 1992. Vascular uptake of catecholamines in perfused lungs of the rat occurs by the same process as Uptake1 in noradrenergic neurones. Naunyn Schmiedeberg's Arch. Pharmacol. **345:** 319–326.
2. RAMAMOORTHY, S., P.D. PRASAD, P. KULANTHAIVEL, *et al.* 1993. Expression of a cocaine-sensitive norepinephrine transporter in the human placental syncytiotrophoblast. Biochemistry **32:** 1346–1353.
3. CUBELLS, J.F., K.S. KIM, H. BAKER, *et al.* 1995. Differential in vivo regulation of mRNA encoding the norepinephrine transporter and tyrosine hydroxylase in rat adrenal medulla and locus ceruleus. J. Neurochem. **65:** 502–509.
4. KIPPENBERGER, A.G., D.J. PALMER, A.M. COMER, *et al.* 1999. Localization of the noradrenaline transporter in rat adrenal medulla and PC12 cells: evidence for its association with secretory granules in PC12 cells. J. Neurochem. **73:** 1024–1032.
5. PHILLIPS, J.K., R. DUBEY, E. SESIASHVILVI, *et al.* 2001. Differential expression of the noradrenaline transporter in adrenergic chromaffin cells, ganglion cells and nerve fibres of the rat adrenal medulla. J. Chem. Neuroanat. **21:** 95–104.
6. SCHROETER, S., S. APPARSUNDARAM, R.G. WILEY, *et al.* 2000. Immunolocalization of the cocaine- and antidepressant-sensitive l-norepinephrine transporter. J. Comp. Neurol. **420:** 211–232.
7. HUYNH, T.T., K. PACAK, F.M. BROUWERS, *et al.* 2005. Different expression of catecholamine transporters in phaeochromocytomas from patients with von Hippel-Lindau syndrome and multiple endocrine neoplasia type 2. Eur. J. Endocrinol. **153:** 551–563.

8. CLEARY, S., F.M. BROUWERS, G. EISENHOFER, *et al.* 2005. Expression of the noradrenaline transporter and phenylethanolamine N-methyltransferase in normal human adrenal gland and phaeochromocytoma. Cell Tissue Res. **July**: 1–11.
9. MAUREA, S., A. CUOCOLO, J.C. REYNOLDS, *et al.* 1993. Iodine-131-metaiodobenzylguanidine scintigraphy in preoperative and postoperative evaluation of paragangliomas: comparison with CT and MRI. J. Nucl. Med. **34:** 173–179.
10. SHAPIRO, B., J.C. SISSON, B.L. SHULKIN, *et al.* 1995. The current status of metaiodobenzylguanidine and related agents for the diagnosis of neuro-endocrine tumors. Q. J. Nucl. Med. **39:** 3–8.
11. SISSON, J.C. & B.L. SHULKIN. 1999. Nuclear medicine imaging of pheochromocytoma and neuroblastoma. Q. J. Nucl. Med. **43:** 217–223.
12. PACAK, K., G. EISENHOFER, J.A. CARRASQUILLO, *et al.* 2001. 6-[18F]fluorodopamine positron emission tomographic (PET) scanning for diagnostic localization of pheochromocytoma. Hypertension **38:** 6–8.
13. ILIAS, I., J. YU, J.A. CARRASQUILLO, *et al.* 2003. Superiority of 6-[18F]-fluorodopamine positron emission tomography versus [131I]-metaiodobenzylguanidine scintigraphy in the localization of metastatic pheochromocytoma. J. Clin. Endocrinol. Metab. **88:** 4083–4087.
14. PACAK, K., W.M. LINEHAN, G. EISENHOFER, *et al.* 2001. Recent advances in genetics, diagnosis, localization, and treatment of pheochromocytoma. Ann. Int. Med. **134:** 315–329.
15. LOH, K.C., P.A. FITZGERALD, K.K. MATTHAY, *et al.* 1997. The treatment of malignant pheochromocytoma with iodine-131 metaiodobenzylguanidine (^{131}I-MIBG): a comprehensive review of 116 reported patients. J. Endocrinol. Invest. **20:** 648–658.
16. ROSE, B., K.K. MATTHAY, D. PRICE, *et al.* 2003. High-dose ^{131}I-metaiodobenzylguanidine therapy for 12 patients with malignant pheochromocytoma. Cancer **98:** 239–248.
17. SAFFORD, S.D., R.E. COLEMAN, J.P. GOCKERMAN, *et al.* 2003. Iodine-131 metaiodobenzylguanidine is an effective treatment for malignant pheochromocytoma and paraganglioma. Surgery **134:** 956–962.
18. SAFFORD, S.D., R.E. COLEMAN, J.P. GOCKERMAN, *et al.* 2004. Iodine-131 metaiodobenzylguanidine treatment for metastatic carcinoid: results in 98 patients. Cancer **101:** 1987–1993.
19. ARMOUR, A., S.H. CUNNINGHAM, M.N. GAZE, *et al.* 1997. The effect of cisplatin pretreatment on the accumulation of MIBG by neuroblastoma cells in vitro. Br. J. Cancer **75:** 470–476.
20. MASTRANGELO, R., A. TORNESELLO, R. RICCARDI, *et al.* 1995. A new approach in the treatment of stage IV neuroblastoma using a combination of [^{131}I]metaiodobenzylguanidine (MIBG) and cisplatin. Eur. J. Cancer **31A:** 606–611.
21. MECO, D., A. LASORELLA, A. RICCARDI, *et al.* 1999. Influence of cisplatin and doxorubicin on ^{125}I-meta-iodobenzylguanidine uptake in human neuroblastoma cell lines. Eur. J. Cancer **35:** 1227–1234.
22. HARA, K., K. MINAMI, S. UENO, *et al.* 2002. Up-regulation of noradrenaline transporter in response to prolonged exposure to ketamine. Naunyn Schmiedebergs Arch. Pharmacol. **365:** 406–412.
23. IKEDA, T., S. KITAYAMA, K. MORITA, *et al.* 2001. Nerve growth factor downregulates the expression of norepinephrine transporter in rat pheochromocytoma (PC12) cells. Brain Res. Mol. Brain. Res. **86:** 90–100.

24. ORDWAY, G.A., W. JIA, J. LI, *et al.* 2005. Norepinephrine transporter function and desipramine: residual drug effects versus short-term regulation. J. Neurosci. Methods **143:** 217–225.
25. ZHU, M.Y. & G.A. ORDWAY. 1997. Down-regulation of norepinephrine transporters on PC12 cells by transporter inhibitors. J. Neurochem. **68:** 134–141.
26. ZHU, M.Y., S. SHAMBURGER, J. LI, *et al.* 2000. Regulation of the human norepinephrine transporter by cocaine and amphetamine. J. Pharmacol. Exp. Ther. **295:** 951–959.
27. MCCLUSKEY, A.G., M. BOYD, M.N. GAZE, *et al.* 2005. [(131)I]MIBG and topotecan: A rationale for combination therapy for neuroblastoma. Cancer Lett. **228:** 221–227.
28. ZAHNISER, N.R. & S. DOOLEN. 2001. Chronic and acute regulation of Na+/Cl−-dependent neurotransmitter transporters: drugs, substrates, presynaptic receptors, and signaling systems. Pharmacol. Ther. **92:** 21–55.
29. SUNG, U., S. APPARSUNDARAM, A. GALLI, *et al.* 2003. A regulated interaction of syntaxin 1A with the antidepressant-sensitive norepinephrine transporter establishes catecholamine clearance capacity. J. Neurosci. **23:** 1697–1709.
30. EISENHOFER, G., J.W. LENDERS, W.M. LINEHAN, *et al.* 1999. Plasma normetanephrine and metanephrine for detecting pheochromocytoma in von Hippel-Lindau disease and multiple endocrine neoplasia type 2. N. Engl. J. Med. **340:** 1872–1979.
31. EISENHOFER, G., M.M. WALTHER, T.T. HUYNH, *et al.* 2001. Pheochromocytomas in von Hippel-Lindau syndrome and multiple endocrine neoplasia type 2 display distinct biochemical and clinical phenotypes. J. Clin. Endocrinol. Metab. **86:** 1999–2008.
32. DIXON, D.N., R.A. LOXLEY, A. BARRON, *et al.* 2005. Comparative studies of PC12 and mouse pheochromocytoma-derived rodent cell lines as models for the study of neuroendocrine systems. In Vitro Cell Dev. Biol. Anim. **41:** 197–206.

Expression and Effect of Adrenomedullin in Pheochromocytoma

ZHENG-PEI ZENG,[a] DONG-MEI LIU,[a] HAN-ZHONG LI,[b] XIN-RONG FAN,[b] GUO-QIANG LIU,[a] WEI-GANG YAN,[a] AN-LI TONG,[a] AND XIN ZHENG[a]

[a]*Department of Endocrinology, Peking Union Medical College Hospital, Chinese Academy of Medical Sciences & Peking Union Medical College, Beijing 100730, China*

[b]*Department of Urology, Peking Union Medical College Hospital, Chinese Academy of Medical Sciences & Peking Union Medical College, Beijing 100730, China*

ABSTRACT: This study investigates the expression of human adrenomedullin (ADM) and its receptor–receptor activity modifying protein 2/calcitonin receptor-like receptor (RAMP2/CRLR) mRNA in pheochromocytoma by reverse transcriptase polymerase chain reaction (RT-PCR) and its effect on the proliferation of pheochromocytoma cells by MTT. The mRNA expression of ADM and its receptor RAMP2/CRLR was present in normal adrenal medulla and pheochromocytoma tissues. The mRNA expression of ADM, RAMP2, and CRLR is markedly higher in pheochromocytomas than in normal medulla. ADM inhibits the proliferation of human pheochromocytoma cells and exerts a possible autocrine or paracrine effect in the adrenal.

KEYWORDS: adrenomedullin; expression; proliferation; adrenomedullin receptor; pheochromocytoma

INTRODUCTION

Adrenomedullin (ADM) is a potent vasodilator peptide that was isolated from human pheochromocytoma in 1993.[1] It has been shown to be widely distributed in a variety of tissues and cells that are abundant in the adrenal medulla and pheochromocytoma. But the effect of ADM on the pathogenesis of pheochromocytoma was not identified. The influence of ADM on the proliferation of pheochromocytoma cells is unknown. McLatchie *et al.* reported that the calcitonin receptor-like receptor (CRLR) would function either as a calcitonin gene-related peptide (CGRP) receptor or as an ADM receptor,[2]

Address for correspondence: Zheng-Pei Zeng, M.D., Department of Endocrinology, Peking Union Medical College Hospital, Beijing 100730, China. Voice: 86-10-65295071; fax: 86-10-65230460. e-mail: zengzhengpei@yahoo.com.cn

Ann. N.Y. Acad. Sci. 1073: 270–276 (2006).
doi: 10.1196/annals.1353.030

depending on the expression of receptor activity–modifying proteins (RAMPs). RAMP2/CRLR serves as an ADM receptor.[3,4] To date there has been no report about whether ADM-specific receptor mRNA is present in pheochromocytomas. In the present study, the mRNA expressions of ADM and its specific receptor RAMP2/CRLR were detected by reverse transcriptase polymerase chain reaction (RT-PCR) in pheochromocytoma. Its effect on the proliferation of pheochromocytoma cells was assayed by 3-(4,5-dimethylthiazol-2-yl) 2,5- diphenyl tetrazolium bromide (MTT).

MATERIALS AND METHODS

Patients

The pheochromocytoma samples confirmed by pathological examination for RT-PCR were taken from 18 patients undergoing tumor resection in the Department of Urology in PUMC Hospital from 2000–2003; this included 12 cases in males and 6 cases in females with a mean age of 39 ± 16 years. The adrenal tissues were obtained from 8 normal subjects who had died in accidents and donated kidneys for transplantation. Informed consent was obtained from family members of the kidney donors.

RT-PCR

The tissues were removed and immediately frozen in liquid nitrogen and stored at −70°C. Total RNA was isolated from 50 mg of the frozen pheochromocytoma and normal adrenal medulla tissues by the Trizol method. cDNA was synthesized by standard method (all of the reagents were from Promega Corp., Madison, WI). PCR was carried out in a final volume of 25 μL using specific primers for ADM, RAMP2, and CRLR, which produced 410 base pairs (bp), 283 bp, and 497 bp, respectively. The primers for ADM, RAMP2, and CRLR were designed on the basis of previous studies.[5–7] The primers for ADM were: sense AAGAAGTGGAATAAGTGGGCT, antisense TGGCTTAGAAGACACCAGAGT; for RAMP2: sense GGACGGTGAAGAACTATGAG, antisense TCATGGCCAGGAGTACATC; for CRLR: sense TGCTCTGTGAAGGCATTTAC, antisense CAGAATTGCTTGAACCTCTC; and for glycerol aldehyde phosphate dehydrogenase (GAPDH) (coamplified as an internal standard): sense GGTCGGAGTCAACGGATTTG, antisense ATGAGGTCCACCACCCTGTT. Glyceroldehyde-3-phosphate dehydrogenase (GAPDH) product was 969 bp. All experiments were performed three times. PCR protocols were as follows: For ADM: one cycle of denaturation at 94°C for 5 min, 30 cycles of denaturation for 45 s at 94°C, primer annealing for 1 min at 62°C, and primer extension for 1 min at 72°C, followed by one cycle of primer extension for 10 min at 72°C. For RAMP2: one cycle of denaturation at 94°C for 5 min, 28 cycles of denaturation for 30 s at 94°C, primer annealing for 45 s at 63°C, and primer extension for 45 s at 72°C, followed by one cycle of primer extension for 5 min at 72°C. For CRLR: one cycle of denaturation at 94°C for 5 min, 35 cycles of denaturation for 45 s at 94°C, primer annealing for 30 s at 63°C, and primer extension for 45 s at 72°C, followed by one cycle of primer extension for 10 min at 72°C.

PCR products were analyzed and sequenced. The ratios of ADM/GAPDH, RAMP2/GAPDH, and CRLR/GAPDH were used as an index to evaluate the quantity of the expression of ADM, RAMP2, and CRLR mRNA.

Cell Proliferation Assay

Pheochromocytoma tissues were obtained immediately after surgical removal, and the human pheochromocytoma cells were isolated by sequential collagenase type IA digestion from pheochromocytoma tissues as previously described.[8] Cells were seeded at 10^4 cells/well in 96-well plates, grown in Dulbecco's modified Eagle's medium (DMEM)-15% fetal calf serum (FCS) for 3 days, replaced with DMEM-1%FCS for 24 h, and further incubated with and without human ADM ($10^{-11}-10^{-7}$mmol/L) for 24 h. Then the cell proliferation was examined by the MTT assay. All experiments were performed three times.

Statistics

Data were analyzed by SPSS11.0 software (SPSS Inc., Chicago, IL), all values were expressed as mean ± SD, differences between two groups were analyzed by an unpaired *t*-test, and differences between more than two groups were examined by one-way analysis of variance test. Values of $P < 0.05$ were considered significant.

RESULTS

The mRNA Expression of ADM, RAMP2, and CRLR

Gel electrophoresis of the RT-PCR products with specific primers revealed expected size bands and GAPDH band simultaneously in the normal adrenal medulla and pheochromocytoma (FIG. 1). Sequence analysis of products confirmed that these RT-PCR products were the fragments of human ADM, RAMP2, and CRLR mRNA. The mRNA expression of ADM and RAMP2/CRLR are higher in pheochromocytoma than those of normal adrenal medulla (TABLE 1). The ADM mRNA expression was higher in extra-adrenal tumors than in intra-adrenal pheochromocytoma, and it is greater in malignant pheochromocytomas than in benign tumors. However, the difference of

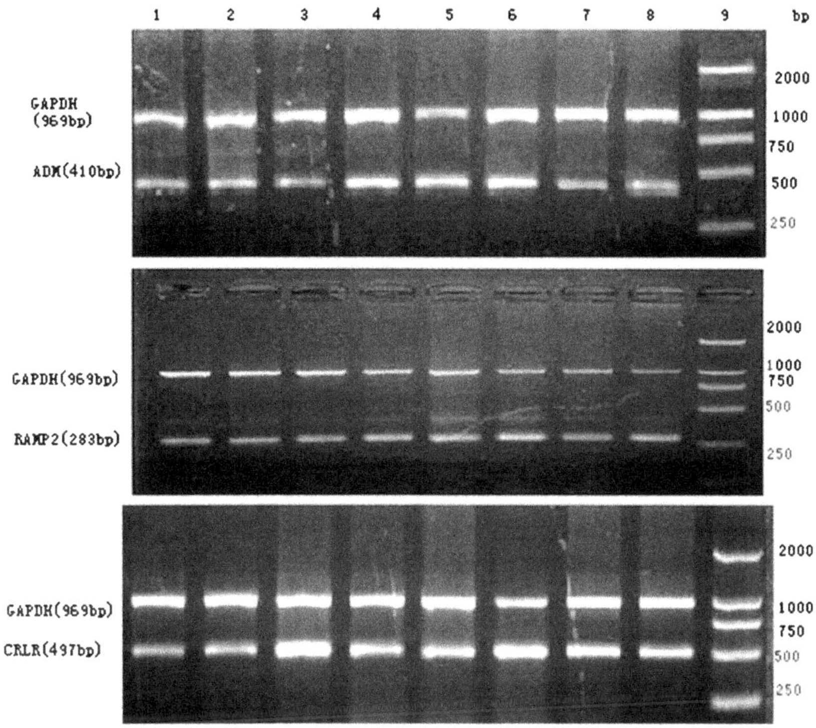

FIGURE 1. Gel electrophoresis analysis of ADM mRNA and RAMP2/CRLR mRNA. 1, 2: normal adrenal medulla tissues; 3–8: pheochromocytoma; 9: marker.

ADM mRNA expression between single and multiple pheochromocytomas, tumors in patients with persistent and paroxysmal hypertension, and tumors of different sizes and catecholamine secretion patterns did not achieve statistical significance. The expression of RAMP2/CRLR mRNA had no significant difference between pheochromocytomas of different clinical features (TABLES 2 and 3).

Effects of ADM on the Proliferation of Pheochromocytoma Cells

Treatment with ADM for 24 h significantly decreased the cell number with ADM concentration of 0.1 nM and greater (FIG. 2), suggesting that ADM inhibited the proliferation of pheochromocytoma cells.

DISCUSSION

The preliminary studies suggested that the concentrations of ADM varied significantly in the pheochromocytoma tissues, but the reason for this

TABLE 1. Primers for RT-PCR

Genes		Primers (5′–3′)	Size (bp)
ADM	Sense	AAGAAGTGGAATAAGTGGGCT	410
	Antisense	TGGCTTAGAAGACACCAGAGT	
RAMP2	Sense	GGACGGTGAAGAACTATGAG	283
	Antisense	ATCATGGCCAGGAGTACATC	
CRLR	Sense	TGCTCTGTGAAGGCATTTAC	497
	Antisense	CAGAATTGCTTGAACCTCTC	
GADPH	Sense	GGTCGGAGTCAACGGATTTG	969
	Antisense	ATGAGGTCCACCACCCTGTT	

ABBREVIATIONS: ADM = adrenomedullin; RAMP2 = recetor activity modifying protein 2; CRLR = calcitonin receptor-like receptor.

is unclear at present.[9–11] Previous immunohistochemistry studies from our laboratory demonstrated that the number of pheochromocytoma cases with positive staining of immunoreactive (ir)-ADM in the paroxysmal hypertensive group was higher than that in the sustained hypertensive group. It is suggested that ADM may be correlated with the diversity of blood pressure in patients with pheochromocytoma, but it should be further investigated at the level of molecule and receptor.[12]

In the present study, our findings revealed that ADM and RAMP2/CRLR mRNA were present in the normal adrenal medulla and pheochromocytoma. mRNA expression was evaluated by semiquantitative RT-PCR, which showed that ADM and RAMP2/CRLR mRNA were significantly higher in pheochromocytoma than in normal adrenal medulla. The coexpression of both ADM and RAMP2/CRLR mRNA implies that ADM exerts a possible autocrine and/or paracrine effect in the adrenal. To clarify the effect of ADM on the different clinical types of pheochromocytomas, we categorized the pheochromocytoma according to the clinical features. The findings suggested that the ADM mRNA expression was higher in extra-adrenal tumors than in intra-adrenal pheochromocytoma, and it was greater in malignant pheochromocytomas than in benign tumors. However, the difference of ADM mRNA expression between single and multiple pheochromocytomas, tumors with persistent and paroxysmal hypertension, and tumors of different sizes and catecholamine secretion patterns did

TABLE 2. Expression of ADM, RAMP2, and CRLR mRNA in tissues of normal adrenal medulla and pheochromocytoma ($x \pm s$)

Group	n	ADM/GAPDH	RAMP2/GAPDH	CRLR/GAPDH
N	8	$0.48 + 0.09$	0.79 ± 0.12	0.40 ± 0.08^a
P	18	0.75 ± 0.24^a	1.29 ± 0.30^a	0.87 ± 0.22^a

ABBREVIATIONS: N = normal adrenal medulla; P = pheochromocytoma.
[a] $P < 0.05$ compared with normal adrenal medulla.

TABLE 3. Expression of ADM, RAMP2, and CRLR mRNA in pheochromocytoma tissues with different clinical features ($x \pm s$)

Group	n	ADM/GAPDH	RAMP2/GAPDH	CRLR/GAPDH
Tumor				
Benign	13	0.69 ± 0.14	1.31 ± 0.34	0.91 ± 0.23
Malignant	5	1.01 ± 0.26[a]	1.26 ± 0.16	0.76 ± 0.15
Tumor location				
Intra-adrenal	11	0.64 ± 0.11	1.25 ± 0.28	0.85 ± 0.15
Extra-adrenal	7	0.95 ± 0.22[b]	1.37 ± 0.32	0.90 ± 0.31
Tumor number				
Single	12	0.74 ± 0.23	1.28 ± 0.35	0.83 ± 0.16
Multiple	6	0.80 ± 0.22	1.31 ± 0.1	0.94 ± 0.31
Blood pressure				
Paroxysmal	6	0.67 ± 0.13	1.21 ± 0.16	0.83 ± 0.13
Sustained	9	0.73 ± 0.12	1.32 ± 0.21	0.89 ± 0.26
Secretion hormone				
Epinephrine	8	0.86 ± 0.25	1.27 ± 0.31	0.77 ± 0.15
Narepinephrine	8	0.87 ± 0.26	1.39 ± 0.30	0.93 ± 0.26
Tumor size				
Diameter < 5cm	11	0.78 ± 0.22	1.25 ± 0.3	0.91 ± 0.21
Diameter ≥ 5cm	7	0.58 ± 0.19	1.32 ± 0.3	0.86 ± 0.18

[a] $P < 0.05$ compared with extra-adrenal tumors.
[b] $P < 0.05$ compared with malignant tumors.

not achieve statistical significance. The expression of RAMP2/CRLR mRNA had no significant difference between pheochromocytomas of different clinical features.

This study showed that ADM inhibited the proliferation of human pheochromocytoma cells by MTT. The mRNA expression of ADM and its receptor was

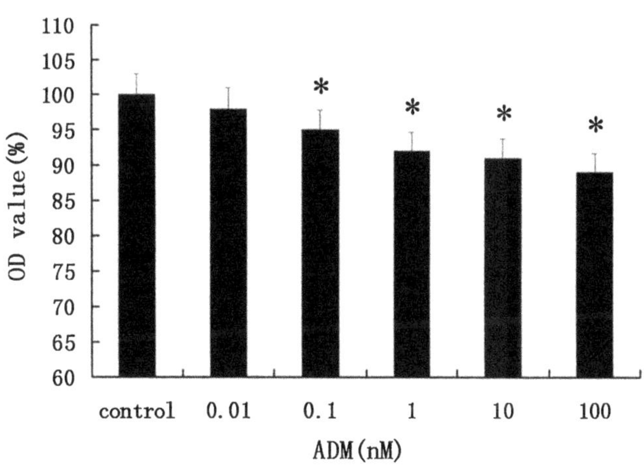

FIGURE 2. Effects of ADM with different concentrations on the proliferation of human pheochromocytoma cells. ($n = 6$, N = 3) Optical density (OD) value of control group is considered as 100%. * $P < 0.05$ vs. control group.

greater than that of normal adrenal medulla. Taken together, these results reveal that ADM may have a functional role in the compensatory mechanisms and that it exerts a possible autocrine or paracrine effect in the adrenal. In conclusion, the study suggests that ADM is probably involved in the pathogenesis of pheochromocytoma. However, further investigation is needed to elucidate the roles from the mechanism and clinical use.

REFERENCES

1. KITAMURA, K. *et al.* 1993. Adrenomedullin: a novel hypotensive peptide isolated from human pheochromocytoma. Biochem. Biophys. Res. Commun. **192:** 553–560.
2. MCLATCHIE, L.M. *et al.* 1998. RAMPs regulate the transport and ligand specificity of the calcitonin-receptor-like receptor. Nature **393:** 333–339.
3. KUWASAKO, K. *et al.* 2004. Adrenomedullin receptors: pharmacological features and possible pathophysiological roles. Peptides **25:** 2003–2012.
4. MUFF, R. *et al.* 2003. Adrenomedullin selectivity of calcitonin-like receptor/receptor activity modifying proteins. Hypertens. Res. **26** (Suppl. l)**:** S3–S8.
5. MILLER, M.J. *et al.* 1996. Adrenomedullin expression in human tumor cell lines. J. Biol. Chem. **271:** 23345–23351.
6. SAMS, A. *et al.* 1998. Expression of calcitonin receptor-like receptor and receptor-activity-modifying proteins in human cranial arteries. Neurosci. Lett. **258:** 41–44.
7. LINSCHEID, P. *et al.* 2005. Autocrine/paracrine role of inflammation-mediated calcitonin gene-related peptide and adrenomedullin expression in human adipose tissue. Endocrinology **146:** 2699–2708.
8. TONG, A.L. *et al.* 2003. The primary culture and identification of human pheochromocytoma cells. Basic Med. Clin. **23:** 447–450.
9. LIU, J. *et al.* 1997. Adrenomedullin gene expression and its different regulation in human adrenocortical and medullary tumors. J. Endocrinol. **155:** 483–490.
10. ICHIKI, Y. *et al.* 1994. Distribution and characterization of immunoreactive adrenomedullin in human tissue and plasma. FEBS Lett. **138:** 6–10.
11. SATOH, F. *et al.* 1997. Immunoreactive adrenomedullin in human adrenal glands and adrenal tumors. Cancer Detect. Prev. **21:** 51–54.
12. LU, L. *et al.* 2003. Immunohistochemical identification of adrenomedullin in adrenal diseases. Chin. J. Intern. Med. **42:** 1–4.

Expression and Effect of Transforming Growth Factor-α and Tumor Necrosis Factor-α in Human Pheochromocytoma

AN-LI TONG,[a] ZHENG-PEI ZENG,[a] HAN-ZHONG LI,[b] DI YANG,[c] LIN LU,[a] AND MING LI[a]

[a]*Departments of Endocrinology,* [b]*Urology, and* [c]*Pathology, Peking Union Medical College Hospital, Chinese Academy of Medical Sciences & Peking Union Medical College, 100730 Beijing, China*

ABSTRACT: This study observed the expression of transforming growth factor-α (TGF-α) and tumor necrosis factor-α (TNF-α) in pheochromocytoma (PHEO) tissue and examined their effects on the proliferation and apoptosis of human PHEO cells. The mRNA and protein expressions of TGF-α and TNF-α were higher in PHEO tissues than in normal adrenal medullary tissues, and their expressions varied with pathological features. TGF-α and TNF-α stimulated the proliferation of primary human PHEO cells, but had no effect on the cell apoptosis. Both TGF-α and TNF-α might be involved in the pathogenesis of human PHEO. TNF-α needs to be further investigated before its treatment of PHEO can be realized in clinical practice.

KEYWORDS: pheochromocytoma; TGF-α; TNF-α; proliferation; apoptosis; expression

INTRODUCTION

Pheochromocytomas (PHEOs) arise from the adrenal medulla and extra-adrenal chromaffin tissues. Cytokines released from the chromaffin cells are in close relation with and regulate the growth and function of the adrenal medulla. Although previous studies have revealed that cytokines are involved in the development of many other tumors, little is known about their roles in the pathogenesis of PHEO.

Transforming growth factor-α (TGF-α) is a potent mitogenic polypeptide and is overexpressed in hepatocellular and bladder carcinoma,[1,2] and their expression was closely related to the malignancy of the tumors and prognosis

Address for correspondence: Zheng-Pei Zeng, M.D., Department of Endocrinology, Peking Union Medical College Hospital, 100730 Beijing, China. Voice: 86-10-65295071; fax: 86-10-65230460.
e-mail: zengzhengpei@yahoo.com.cn

Ann. N.Y. Acad. Sci. 1073: 277–283 (2006). © 2006 New York Academy of Sciences.
doi: 10.1196/annals.1353.031

of the patients. Reports on TGF-α expression in PHEO are limited. TGF-α immunoreactivity was found in all of the six PHEO tissues, but only in one of three normal adrenal medullary tissues, indicating an increased expression of TGF-α in PHEO.[3] So far, no further investigations of TGF-α expression in transcription level in PHEO and its effect on human PHEO cells have been reported.

Tumor necrosis factor-α (TNF-α) is a polypeptide hormone with a wide range of biological activities; it is involved in cell proliferation, differentiation and apoptosis, and plays an important role in tumor progression. It has been reported that TNF-α was cytocidal or cytostatic for some tumor cell lines in tissue culture, and TNF-α has been considered to have anticancer activity. On the other hand, TNF-α can also stimulate the growth of normal cells as well as certain cancer cells *in vitro*. Because TNF-α can be constitutively produced by malignant cells, its expression could contribute to the progression and spread of tumors.[4–6] Until now, no study of the role of TNF-α in human PHEO is available. Furthermore, the value of TNF-α in PHEO treatment is still in doubt.

In this study, we therefore compared the expressions of TGF-α and TNF-α in transcription and protein levels in human PHEO tissues with those in normal adrenal medullary tissues, and studied the association between their expressions in PHEO tissues and clinicopathological characteristics of patients. We first observed the effect of these two cytokines on the proliferation and apoptosis of human PHEO cells.

MATERIALS AND METHODS

Detection of Cell Proliferation and Apoptosis

The human PHEO cells were collected with sequential collagenase (type I) digestion from PHEO tissue.[7] Cells were plated into 96-well plates at an initial concentration of 10^4 cells/well, in DMEM-15% FCS (GIBCO, Grand Island, NY). Cells were allowed to adhere and resume full growth pattern under standard conditions. Four days after the culture, cells were starved in culture medium with 1% FCS for 24 h. Then, the medium was replaced with 1% FCS containing rhTGF-α, rhTNF-α (both from PeproTech, London, UK) or with their vehicles (controls). Cells were incubated for 36 h, and then the cell proliferation rate was detected by using the 3-(4,5-dimethylthiazol-2-yl)-2,5-diphenyl-2H-tetrazolium bromide (MTT) assay.[8]

For the study of apoptosis, the cells were plated at a density of 4×10^5 cells/well in 6-well plates. And in the logarithmic growth period, the cells were washed in serum-free DMEM and treated with rhTGF-α or rhTNF-α (the concentration of each cytokine was 100 U/mL). After incubation for 72 h, apoptosis was measured by flow cytometry and Hoechst 33342 staining.[9]

RT-PCR and Immunohistochemistry

Human PHEO tissues were obtained during operations performed at PUMC hospital over the period from 1997 to 2002. Detailed clinicopathological data on each patient were recorded. The tumor identity was pathologically established for each case. Normal adrenal gland tissues were obtained from renal carcinoma operation in PUMC hospital.

Total RNA was extracted from 22 PHEOs or 18 normal adrenal medullary tissues and cDNA was synthesized by employing standard methods (all of the reagents were from Promega, Corp., Madison, WI). Polymerase chain reaction (PCR) was performed using specific primer pairs for TGF-α, TNF-α, and housekeeping gene β-actin (Bioasia Life Technologies, Inc., Shanghai, China). Primer sequences for TGF-α were 5′-GTCCCATTTTAATGACTGCCCA-3′ and 5′-GAGGTCCGCATGCTCACAGCGT-3′, which produced a 139-base-pair band. The TNF-α primers were 5′-CAGAGGGAAGAGTCCCCCAG-3′ and 5′-CCTTGGTCTGGTAGGAGACG-3′, which produced a 325-base-pair band. The β-actin primers were 5′-GTGGGGCGCCCCAGGCACCA-3′ and 5′-CTTCCTTAATGTCACGCACGATTTC-3′, which produced a 540-base-pair band. Each target gene and β-actin were amplified in a system which was performed in 25 μL of reaction solution containing 1.5 mM $MgCl_2$, 200 μM dNTP (TaKaRa, Otsu, Japan), 0.5 μM of each primer, and 1 U *Taq* DNA polymerase (TaKaRa). The PCR reaction was performed in a thermal cycler (FTG02TD, Techne, Cambridge, UK) with an initial denaturation step of 5 min at 94°C, and subsequently various cycles (32 cycles for TGF-α, 28 cycles for TNF-α) of denaturation (1 min at 94°C), annealing (1 min at 64°C for TGF-α, and 40 sec at 58°C for TNF-α), and extension (1 min at 72°C), followed by a final step of 10 min at 72°C. PCR products were analyzed by electrophoresis on a 1.5% agarose gel containing ethidium bromide. All experiments were repeated three times. The relative expression levels were calculated as the density of the product of the respective target genes divided by that of β-actin from the same cDNA.

Paraffin sections from 27 PHEOs and 14 normal adrenals were dewaxed and subjected to microwave antigen retrieval by immersion in citrate buffer (PH 6.0). Protein immunostaining was detected with the standard Envision technique (DAKO, Kyoto, Japan). The diluted concentration of TGF-α and TNF-α (both from Santa Cruz Biotechnology, Inc., Santa Cruz, CA) monoclonal antibodies was 1:50. Negative control (using PBS in place of primary antibody PBS) and positive controls (staining of normal human dermal cells for TGF-α and breast cancer cells for TNF-α) were utilized.

Statistical Analysis

The values from proliferation and apoptosis were expressed as the mean ± SD. The data were compared by using the analysis of variance (ANOVA) method. For data of RT-PCR products showed as median (25%, 75%), the nonparametric test of Mann-Whitney U was employed. Chi-square test was used for the statistical evaluation of enumeration data. Any $P < 0.05$ was considered to be statistically significant.

RESULTS

Effects of TGF-α and TNF-α on Cell Proliferation/Apoptosis

FIGURE 1 shows the effects of TGF-α and TNF-α on the proliferation of human PHEO cells. Both cytokines had a significant effect on cell proliferation at the concentration of 0.1–100 ng/mL. But they did not affect the apoptosis rate of the cells. The apoptosis rate of controls, TGF-α, and TNF-α groups were 3.98 ± 0.30%, 4.63 ± 1.56%, and 4.25 ± 2.28%, respectively. With Hoechst 33342 staining, the nuclei of both control and treated cells were stained uniformly, indicating that the nuclei were intact and the cells were viable.

RT-PCR and Immunohistochemical Analysis of TGF-α and TNF-α

Quantified by scanning the bands and normalized to the β-actin levels, TGF-α mRNA levels in human PHEO tissues and normal adrenal medulla were 0.060 (0.023, 0.121) and 0.395 (0.152, 0.520), and TNF-α mRNA in the two tissues were 0.200 (0.025, 0.786) and 0.498 (0.160, 1.160), respectively. mRNA levels of both cytokines were higher in PHEO tissue than in normal adrenal medulla ($P < 0.05$) (FIG. 2).

Twenty-six of 27 PHEO tissues demonstrated TGF-α-positive cytoplasm, with occasional nuclear staining, while 3 of 14 normal adrenal medullary tissues were positively stained for TGF-α. Positive TNF-α immunostaining was detected in cytoplasm in 8 of the 27 cases of PHEO, while the staining was negative in all of the normal adrenal medullary tissues. There were significant differences in the TGF-α and TNF-α staining between the two tissues ($P < 0.01$ and $P < 0.05$, respectively).

Intensive positive staining for TGF-α was detected in 9 of 13 extra-adrenal PHEOs, which was significantly higher than that in adrenal PHEOs (4/14) ($P < 0.05$). The rate of positive staining for TNF-α was higher in the malignant (6/9), or extra-adrenal (6/13), or multiple (7/9) tumors than that in the benign (2/18), or adrenal (2/14), or single (1/18) tumors ($P < 0.05$ for all). And their expressions were not related to the other clinicopathologic features, such as the weight and size of tumor.

DISCUSSION

TGF-α is a potent stimulator for many normal and tumorous cells and its overexpression is immediately related to tumor progression. TGF-α has also

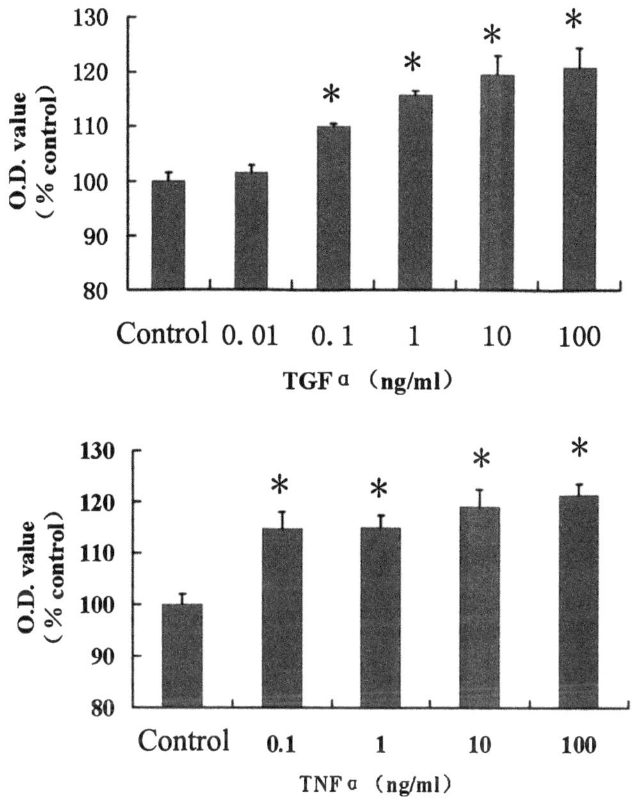

FIGURE 1. Effect of TGF-α and TNF-α of different concentrations on the proliferation of human pheochromocytoma cells ($n = 6$; $N = 3$); $^*P < 0.05$ vs. control group.

been reported to be overexpressed in some human neuroendocrine tumors, such as medullary thyroid carcinoma.[10] The present study documented an increased expression of TGF-α in PHEO, which is consistent with previous findings. TGF-α can stimulate proliferation of human PHEO cells and has no significant effect on the cell apoptosis. This study indicated that TGF-α might serve as a paracrine and autocrine growth factor in the pathogenesis of PHEO. TGF-α immunostaining is found in almost all PHEOs, including benign and malignant tumor, and tumors of different size and weight, suggesting that the overexpression of TGF-α may be a relatively early event in tumor development. We observed a higher level of TGF-α expression in extra-adrenal tumors than that in adrenal ones, indicating that pathogenesis for adrenal and extra-adrenal PHEO was different.

The present study also demonstrated that TNF-α expression was higher in PHEO than in normal adrenal medulla. Although no TNF-α expression was found in normal adrenal medulla, TNF-α receptors exist in chromaffin

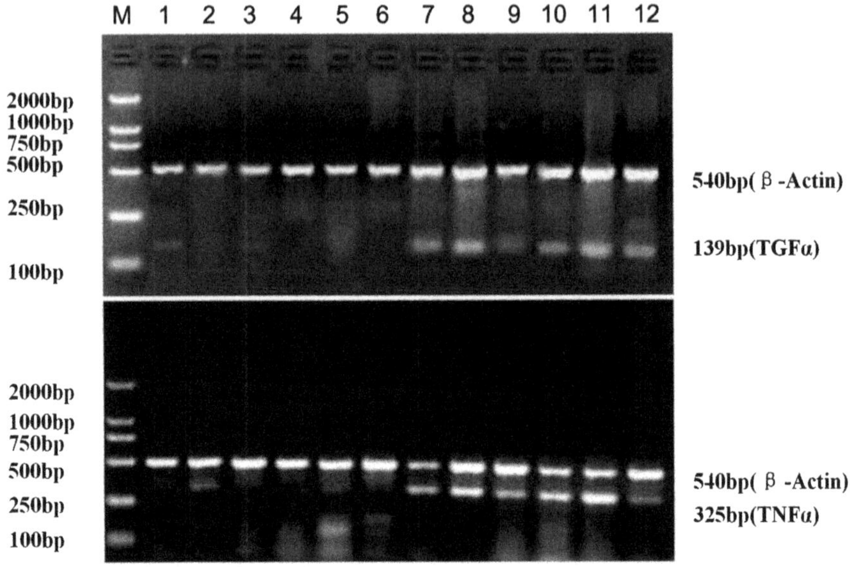

FIGURE 2. RT-PCR analysis of TGF-α and TNF-α mRNA with β-actin as an internal control. M, marker; 1–6, normal adrenal medulla; 7–14, pheochromocytoma.

cells. Exogenous TNF-α can affect the secretion of chromaffin cells *in vitro*.[11,12] We also observed that TNF-α increased PHEO cell proliferation and had no effect on the cell apoptosis, indicating that TNF-α promotes the growth of these cells. TNF-α is cytotoxic or cytostatic for some but not all tumor cells. The growth of neoplastic B cells, astrocytoma cells, and human osteosarcoma cells can also be stimulated by TNF-α. The growth of human cervical carcinoma cell lines is inhibited by high concentrations of TNF-α, but is stimulated by low concentrations. TNF-α is overexpressed in some tumors, such as ovarian cancer, and at the same time it stimulates the tumor cells' growth in an autocrine manner.[13] The present study on PHEO suggested that TNF-α may play an important role in tumor growth. TNF-α needs to be further investigated before its use in treating of PHEO can be realized in clinical practice. TNF-α expression is distinct in PHEOs with different clinicopathologic characteristics, which indicates that it is involved in the development of PHEO.

REFERENCES

1. KOBAYASHI, K. *et al.* 2000. Immunohistochemical localization of transforming growth factor alpha in chemically induced rat hepatocellular carcinomas with reference to differentiation and proliferation. Toxicol. Pathol. **28:** 664–667.
2. KEE, K.H. *et al.* 2001. Oncoprotein changes in the flat lesions with atypia and invasive neoplasms of the urinary bladder. Oncol. Rep. **8:** 579–583.

3. DRIMAN, D.K. *et al.* 1992. Transforming growth factor-α in normal and neoplastic human endocrine tissues. Hum. Pathol. **23:** 1360–1365.
4. MOCELLIN, S. *et al.* 2005. Tumor necrosis factor, cancer and anticancer therapy. Cytokine Growth Factor Rev. **16:** 35–53.
5. WU, S. *et al.* 1993. Tumor necrosis factor α as an autocrine and paracrine growth factor for ovarian cancer: monokine induction of tumor cell proliferation and tumor necrosis factor α expression. Cancer Res. **53:** 1939–1944.
6. ROLFE, M. *et al.* 1997. Tumor necrosis factor α (TNF α) suppresses apoptosis and induces DNA synthesis in rodent hepatocytes: a mediator of the hepatocarcinogenicity of peroxisome proliferators? Carcinogenesis **11:** 2277–2280.
7. TONG, A.L. *et al.* 2003. The primary culture and identification of human pheochromocytoma cells. Basic Med. Clin. **23:** 447–450.
8. FASSNACHT, M. *et al.* 2003. N-terminal proopiomelanocortin acts as a mitogen in adrenocortical tumor cells and decreases adrenal steroidogenesis. J. Clin. Endocrinol. Metab. **88:** 2171–2179.
9. AKAO, Y. *et al.* 2002. Ceramide accumulation is independent of camptothecin-induced apoptosis in prostate cancer LNCaP cells. Biochem. Biophys. Res. Commun. **294:** 363–370.
10. NILSSON, O. *et al.* 1995. Expression of transforming growth factor alpha and its receptor in human neuroendocrine tumors. Int. J. Cancer **60:** 645–651.
11. CALL, G.B. *et al.* 2000. Bovine adrenal cells secrete interleukin-6 and tumor necrosis factor in vitro. Gen. Comp. Endocrinol. **118:** 249–261.
12. ROBERT, L.E. *et al.* 1992. Interleukin-1α and tumor necrosis factor-α differentially regulate enkephalin, vasoactive intestinal polypeptide, neurotensin, and substance P biosynthesis in chromaffin cells. Endocrinology **130:** 2252–2258.
13. WU, S. *et al.* 1992. Stimulation of ovarian tumor cell proliferation with monocyte products including interleukin-1, interleukin-6, and tumor necrosis factor-α. Am. J. Obstet. Gynecol. **166:** 997–1007.

The Effects of Urotensin-II on Proliferation of Pheochromocytoma Cells and mRNA Expression of Urotensin-II and Its Receptor in Pheochromocytoma Tissues

ZHENG-PEI ZENG,[a] GUO-QIANG LIU,[a] HAN-ZHONG LI,[b] XIN-RONG FAN,[b] DONG-MEI LIU,[a] AN-LI TONG,[a] XIN ZHENG,[a] AND CHANG LIU[a]

[a]*Department of Endocrinology, Peking Union Medical College Hospital, Chinese Academy of Medical Sciences & Peking Union Medical College, Beijing 100730, China*

[b]*Department of Urology, Peking Union Medical College Hospital, Chinese Academy of Medical Sciences & Peking Union Medical College, Beijing 100730, China*

ABSTRACT: This study was conducted to investigate the effects of urotensin-II (UII) on the proliferation of pheochromocytoma cells and the mRNA expression of UII and its receptor G protein–coupled receptor 14 (GPR14) in normal adrenal and human pheochromocytoma tissues. The effects on the cell proliferation by different UII concentrations and at different time were observed with the MTT method in both rat pheochromocytoma cell line (PC12 cell) and human pheochromocytoma cells. The mRNA expression of UII and GPR14 was evaluated by RT-PCR. UII had no significant effect on the proliferation in PC12 cells, but promoted the proliferation of human pheochromocytoma cells. The mRNA expression of UII and GPR14 in pheochromocytoma was lower than that in normal adrenal tissues. But mRNA expression of UII and GPR14 in adrenal pheochromocytomas was lower than that in extra-adrenal pheochromocytomas. Thus, UII and its receptor GPR14 exert a possible effect in the pathogenesis of pheochromocytoma.

KEYWORDS: urotensin II; G protein–coupled receptor 14; pheochromocytoma

INTRODUCTION

Urotensin-II (UII) is a cyclic peptide initially isolated from the caudal neuroendocrine system and urophysis in the spinal cord of teleost fish. It is the most

Address for correspondence: Zheng-Pei Zeng, M.D., Department of Endocrinology, Peking Union Medical College Hospital, Beijing 100730, China. Voice: 86-10-65295071; fax: 86-10-65230460. e-mail: zengzhengpei@yahoo.com.cn

Ann. N.Y. Acad. Sci. 1073: 284–289 (2006).
doi: 10.1196/annals.1353.032

potent vasoconstrictor identified so far in mammals. Its vasoconstriction effect is 16-fold more potent than that of endothelin-1 in rat.[1] G protein–coupled receptor 14 (GPR14) is its specific receptor.[1]

Pheochromocytoma is an endocrine disease with hypertension as the main manifestation. The role of UII in the pathogenesis of pheochromocytoma has rarely been reported. In this study, we investigated the effects of UII on the proliferation of pheochromocytoma cells and the mRNA expression of UII and GPR14 in pheochromocytoma tissues.

MATERIALS AND METHODS

Effect of UII on the Proliferation of PC12 Cells

Resuscitated rat pheochromocytoma cells (PC12 cells line) were maintained in RPMI 1640 medium supplemented with 10% horse serum and 15% fetal bovine serum until logarithmic growth phase, and were then plated in a 96-well plate with 100 μL (10^4 cells) per well for 24 h. The culture medium was changed to RPMI 1640 with 2% horse serum and 2% fetal bovine serum. After 24 h further incubation with different UII concentrations (10^{-10}, 10^{-9}, 10^{-8}, 10^{-7}, and 10^{-6} M) was carried out in the culture medium. Proliferation of PC12 cells was examined by 3-(4,5-dimethylthiazol-2-yl) 2,5-diphenyl-ZH tetrazolium bromide (MTT) assay stimulated by 10^{-7} M UII at 12, 24, 36, 48, 60, and 72 h. Tumor necrosis factor (TGF) and transforming growth factor (TNF-α) were used as the positive control.

Effect on the Proliferation of Human Pheochromocytoma Cells by UII

Human pheochromocytoma tissues were obtained after surgically removing, the tumor, and they were digested by sequential 0.2% collagenase type IA. The cells were seeded at 10^4 cells/well in 96-well plates, and grown in Dulbecco's modified eagle medium (DMEM) supplemented with 15% fetal bovine serum for 72 h. This was replaced by DMEM with 1% bovine serum for the next 24 h. Then the cells were further incubated with UII at different concentrations (10^{-10}, 10^{-9}, 10^{-8}, 10^{-7}, 10^{-6} M) for 24 h. The MTT method was applied to evaluate the cell proliferation.

RT-PCR

Pheochromocytoma tissues were obtained from 19 patients in PUMC hospital from 2001 to 2003, including 14 males and 5 females, with an average age of 38.4 ± 14.4 years. According to clinical manifestation, patients with pheochromocytoma were classified into different types, including 13 cases of adrenal and 6 cases of extra-adrenal pheochromocytoma, 14 benign and 5 malignant tumors, 14 single tumor and 5 multiple tumors, and 11 in patients with persisting hypertension and 8 in patients with paroxysmal hypertension. Nine normal adrenal tissues were obtained at operation for renal carcinoma in PUMC hospital as the control samples. PC12 cell line was offered by the PUMC Cell Lines Center.

Total RNA was extracted with trizol reagent. After reverse transcription, primers for UII and internal control GAPDH, and primers for GPR14 and internal control β-actin were added for PCR amplification, respectively. The primers for UII were sequenced as a sense 5′-CTTTCAACTCTCAGCACCT CAT-3′ and an anti-sense 5′-CTTAGTTTTCTCCACACTGTT-3′. The sense and anti-sense primers for GAPDH were designed as 5′-GGTCGGAGTC AACGGATTTG-3′ and 5′-ATGAGGTCCACCACCCTGTT-3′, respectively. PCR for UII was performed in a total 25 μL volume containing 0.25 mmol/L dNTP, 2 mmol/L $MgCl_2$, 0.4 μmol/L UII primer, 0.12 μmol/L GAPDH primer, 1.5 u Taq DNA polymerase, and 2 μL cDNA. After preheating at 94°C for 2 min, denaturation was carried out at 94°C for 15 sec, annealing at 58°C for 60 sec, and elongation at 72°C for 90 sec, respectively, and 40 cycles were repeated for the reaction followed by 72°C for 5 min. The primers of UII and GAPDH were 385 bp and 969 bp, respectively. The PCR for GPR14 was performed using a sense primer 5′-CCCCAACGCAACCCTCAACA-3′ and an anti-sense primer 5′-GGTCGCGGTAGTTCCTGGTGA-3′. The primers of sense and anti-sense for β-actin were as 5′-GTGGGGGCGCCCCAGGCACCA-3′ and 5′-CTTCCTTAATGTCACGCACGATTTC-3′, respectively. The PCR was performed in a total 25 μL volume containing 0.4 mmol/L dNTP, 2.5 mmol/L $MgCl_2$, 0.25 μmol/L GPR14 and β-actin primers, 1 U Taq DNA polymerase, and 1 μL cDNA. After preheating at 94°C for 5 min, denaturation, annealing, and elongation were carried out at 94°C for 30 sec, 62°C for 30 sec, and 72°C for 120 sec, respectively, and the reaction were repeated for 40 cycles, followed by a final extension step at 72°C for 5 min. The primers of GPR14 and β-actin were 896 bp and 540 bp, respectively. Semiquantitative analysis of the mRNA expression level of UII and GPR14 was carried out using the ratio of UII/GAPDH and GPR14/β-actin.

RESULTS

The Effect of UII on the Proliferation in PC12 Cell Line

Neither treatment by UII at different concentrations nor treatment by 10^{-7} M UII with different times had an effect on proliferation in PC12 cell lines, while positive control has shown that 100 ng/mL TGF-α could stimulate the proliferation of PC12 cells, and 100 ng/mL TNF-α could suppress the cell proliferation.

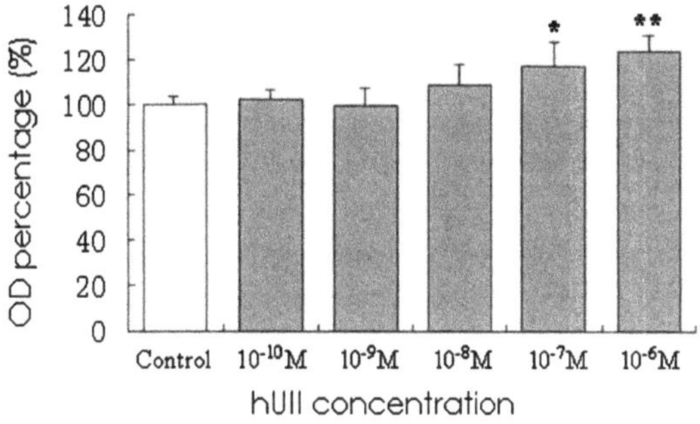

FIGURE 1. Effects on the proliferation of UII at different concentrations in cultured human pheochromocytoma cells ($n = 12$). *$P < 0.05$, **$P < 0.01$ vs. control. OD = optical density.

The Effect of UII on the Proliferation of Human Pheochromocytoma Cells

Both 10^{-7} M and 10^{-6} M UII could promote cell proliferation in primary culture for human pheochromocytoma in a dose-dependent manner (FIG. 1).

mRNA Expression of UII and GPR14

PCR products were analyzed and sequenced. The ratios of UII/GAPDH in normal adrenal cortex, medulla, and human pheochromocytoma were used as an index to evaluate the quantity of the mRNA expression of UII and GPR14 as 0.820 ± 0.134, 0.694 ± 0.292, and 0.216 ± 0.175, respectively. The ratios of GPR14/β-actin in the aforementioned three tissues were 1.687 ± 0.749, 1.123 ± > 0.407, and 0.639 ± 0.421, respectively. There were no significant differences of UII/GAPDH and GPR14/β-actin between normal adrenal cortex and medulla, while the foregoing ratios in the human pheochromocytoma tissues were significantly lower than those in the normal adrenal cortex and medulla ($P < 0.05$) (FIGS. 2 and 3).

The ratios of UII/GAPDH in adrenal or extra-adrenal pheochromocytoma were 0.168 ± 0.161 and 0.319 ± 0.171 ($P = 0.08$), respectively, while the ratios of GPR14/β-actin were 0.505 ± 0.306 and 0.930 ± 0.514 (FIG. 4). The

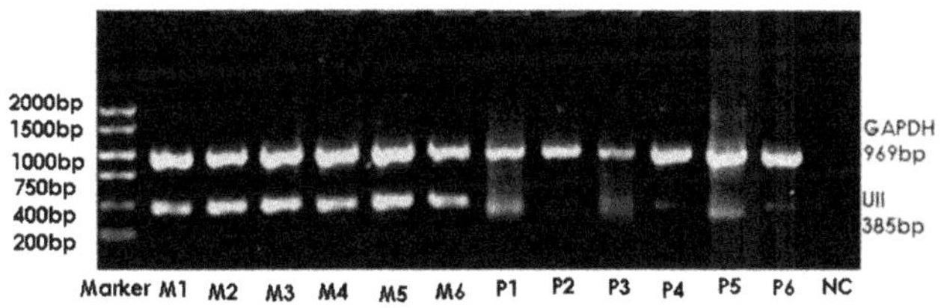

FIGURE 2. RT-PCR for UII mRNA in tissues of normal adrenal medulla and pheochromocytoma. M = normal adrenal medulla; P = pheochromocytoma; NC = negative control.

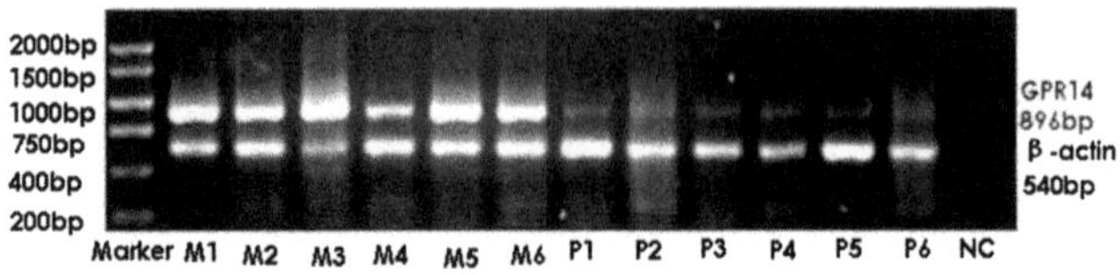

FIGURE 3. RT-PCR for GPR14 mRNA in tissues of normal adrenal medulla and pheochromocytoma. M = normal adrenal medulla; P = pheochromocytoma; NC = negative control.

mRNA expression of GPR14 in adrenal pheochromocytoma was lower than that in extra-adrenal pheochromocytoma ($P < 0.05$).

The ratios of UII/GAPDH and GPR14/β-actin showed no significant differences between benign and malignant tumors, single and multiple tumors, tumor diameters ≥5 cm and <5 cm, and tumors in patients with tumors sustained versus paroxysmal hypertension.

DISCUSSION

In 1998, the human UII gene was cloned by Coulouarn *et al.*[2] In 1999, Ames *et al.* discovered that the orphan receptor, GPR14, is the specific receptor of UII.[1] Many researchers proved that UII is the most potent vasoconstrictor ever found.[1]

Pheochromocytoma is a neuroendocrine tumor with high blood pressure as its main manifestation; the tumor can secrete different hormones. Takahashi *et al.* proved that UII and GPR14 mRNA were expressed in pheochromocytoma tissues ($n = 7$), but only qualitative analysis has been done.[3] Our results demonstrated that the UII and GPR14 mRNA were expressed in normal adrenal cortex, medulla and pheochromocytoma tissues, but that there is no mRNA expression of significant difference between the normal adrenal cortex and the medulla. The mRNA expression of UII in pheochromocytoma tissues is significantly lower than that in normal tissues of adrenal cortex and medulla. The reason for lower expression of UII and its receptor in pheochromocytoma tissues is unknown, while UII may stimulate catecholamine secretion and cell proliferation in pheochromocytoma.

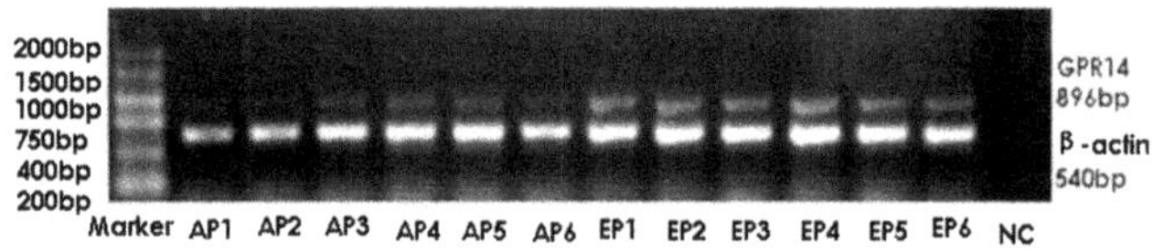

FIGURE 4. RT-PCR for GPR14 mRNA in tissues of adrenal pheochromocytoma and extra-adrenal pheochromocytoma. AP = adrenal pheochromocytoma; EP = extra-adrenal pheochromocytoma; NC = negative control.

Our study shows that the mRNA expression of GPR14 in extra-adrenal pheochromocytoma is significantly higher than that in adrenal pheochromocytoma, which is obviously related to the site of the tumors. We guess that in addition to catecholamine, other adrenal hormones, such as glucocorticoid hormone may have some effect on the synthesis and secretion of UII.

There is a cyclic structure with six amino acids at the C terminal of UII. This region related to biological activities is highly conserved in the evolution from rodent to mammals. Research has shown that 10^{-7} mol/L human UII could cause cell proliferation of myocardium in newborn rats, as well as cell proliferation of arterial smooth muscles in rats. Our result showed human UII could not stimulate proliferation for rat pheochromocytoma cell line (PC12 cell). This may be mainly due to difference in molecular structure of UII between human and rat, and in the process of establishing and generating cell line, the characteristics of PC12 cells may have changed.

UII has a potent effect on vasoconstriction[4] and the level of UII rises in patients with hypertension.[5] UII probably plays a certain role in the pathogenesis of vascular complications in patients with hypertension. The decrease of mRNA expression of UII and its receptor in pheochromocytoma tissue may be as a kind of self-protecting mechanism of the body in response to the elevated blood pressure. There are still few reports about the effects of UII on proliferation of human pheochromocytoma cells and rat pheochromocytoma cells. Our research shows that UII can stimulate cell proliferation of human pheochromocytoma cells cultured *in vitro.* UII may play a role in the pathogenesis and development of pheochromocytoma.

REFERENCES

1. AMES, R.S. *et al.* 1999. Human urotensin-II is a potent vasoconstrictor and agonist for the orphan receptor GPR14. Nature **402:** 898–912.
2. COULOUARN, Y. *et al.* 1998. Cloning of the cDNA encoding the UII precursor in frog and human reveals intense expression of the UII gene in motoneurons of the spinal cord. Proc. Natl. Acad. Sci. USA **95:** 15803–15808.
3. TAKAHASHI, K. *et al.* 2003. Expression of urotensin α and its receptor in adrenal tumors and stimulation of proliferation of cultured tumor cells by urotensin α. Peptides **24:** 301–306.
4. BENNETT, R.T. *et al.* 2004. Vasoconstrictive effects of endothelin-1, endothelin-3, and urotensin α in isolated perfused human lungs and isolated human pulmonary arteries. Thorax **59:** 401–407.
5. TOTSUNE, K. *et al.* 2003. Increased plasma U α levels in patients with diabetes mellitus. Clin. Sci. **104:** 65–67.

Gene Expression Profiling of Rat Pheochromocytoma

ABDEL G. ELKAHLOUN,[a] JAMES F. POWERS,[b] ABRAHAM NYSKA,[c] GRAEME EISENHOFER,[d] AND ARTHUR S. TISCHLER[b]

[a]*Genome Technology Branch, National Human Genome Research Institute, National Institutes of Health, Bethesda, Maryland 20892, USA*

[b]*Department of Pathology, Tufts-New England Medical Center, Boston, Massachusetts 02111, USA*

[c]*National Institute of Environmental Health Sciences, National Institutes of Health, Research Triangle Park, North Carolina, USA*

[d]*Clinical Neurocardiology Section, National Institute of Neurological Disorders and Stroke, National Institutes of Health, Bethesda, Maryland 20892, USA*

ABSTRACT: Sporadic and syndrome-associated human pheochromocytomas exhibit a spectrum of common and distinctive phenotypic markers. Animal models may contribute to understanding of common denominators leading to development and progression of pheochromocytoma, and to mechanisms that underlie distinctive phenotypes. Rat pheochromocytomas are common, in contrast to their human counterparts, and their frequency is increased by a variety of genotoxic or nongenotoxic agents. Toxicological studies of rats are therefore a potentially rich source of information on pheochromocytoma biology. To compare the molecular profiles of rat and human pheochromocytomas and to identify pathways potentially involved in pathogenesis of rat pheochromocytomas, we conducted a gene expression profiling study comparing 31 pheochromocytomas obtained from the National Toxicology Program to normal adult rat adrenal medulla. The microarray chips were generated from 31,769-oligomer set representing over 27,200 unique Mouse Ensembl genes. The analysis showed over 1,900 genes that were up- or downregulated in the tumors. More than half of the former are involved in protein synthesis and signal transduction, including oncogenes of the RAS family and several heat shock proteins and chaperones. Downregulated genes included receptors and tumor-suppressor genes, including NF2 and Dmbt1. Specific genes related to neuroendocrine function were either upregulated or downregulated in subsets of tumors. Cross-comparison with a human pheochromocytoma database showed greater than 60% correlation. Re-

Address for correspondence: Dr. Abdel. G. Elkahloun, Genome Technology Branch, National Human Genome Research Institute, National Institutes of Health, Bldg. 50, 50 South Drive, Bethesda, MD 20892, USA. Voice: 301-402-3170; fax: 301-480-1241.
e-mail: abdel@mail.nih.gov

Ann. N.Y. Acad. Sci. 1073: 290–299 (2006).
doi: 10.1196/annals.1353.033

sults of this study reveal both generic and specific parallels between rat and human pheochromocytomas.

KEYWORDS: **pheochromocytoma; phenylethanolamine N-methyltransferase; ret proto-oncogene; microarray; heat-shock proteins**

INTRODUCTION

Considerable data now available from gene expression profiling studies distinguish human pheochromocytomas from normal human adrenal medulla and identify subsets of the tumors with different expression profiles. However, deciphering the functional significance of the differentially expressed genes and their roles in tumorigenesis, invasiveness, and metastasis is hampered by the fact that human pheochromocytomas are rare tumors. In contrast, pheochromocytomas occur frequently in rats and are often encountered in toxicological studies, both in aging control animals and in test animals treated with a variety of drugs, food additives, or other chemicals.[1] Toxicological studies of rats are therefore a potentially rich source of information on pheochromocytoma biology, but the relevance of the rat tumors to their human counterparts is unclear.

In the present investigation we searched for common denominators distinguishing rat pheochromocytomas from normal adult rat adrenal medulla using microarray-based gene expression profiling. In addition, we compared expression profiles of the rat tumors to profiles in a human pheochromocytoma database.

MATERIALS AND METHODS

Rat Pheochromocytoma Tissues

Rat pheochromocytoma tumor tissue (31 tumors) was procured from the National Toxicology Program. Total RNA from tumor and normal adrenal medulla was extracted using the Trizol method (Clonetech, Inc., Carlsbad, CA).

Microarray Preparation, Probe Labeling, and Analysis

Oligonucleotide microarray chips were generated from 31,769 70mer probes set obtained from the Qiagen Mouse Genome Oligo Set Version 3.0. The set represents over 24,729 unique Refseq genes, over 25,152 unique Ensembl genes, and over 22,346 unique Unigene genes. Supplemental information can be accessed through our web site: http://magic2.nhgri.nih.gov/microarray/index.shtml. Each tumor RNA was compared to the same reference,

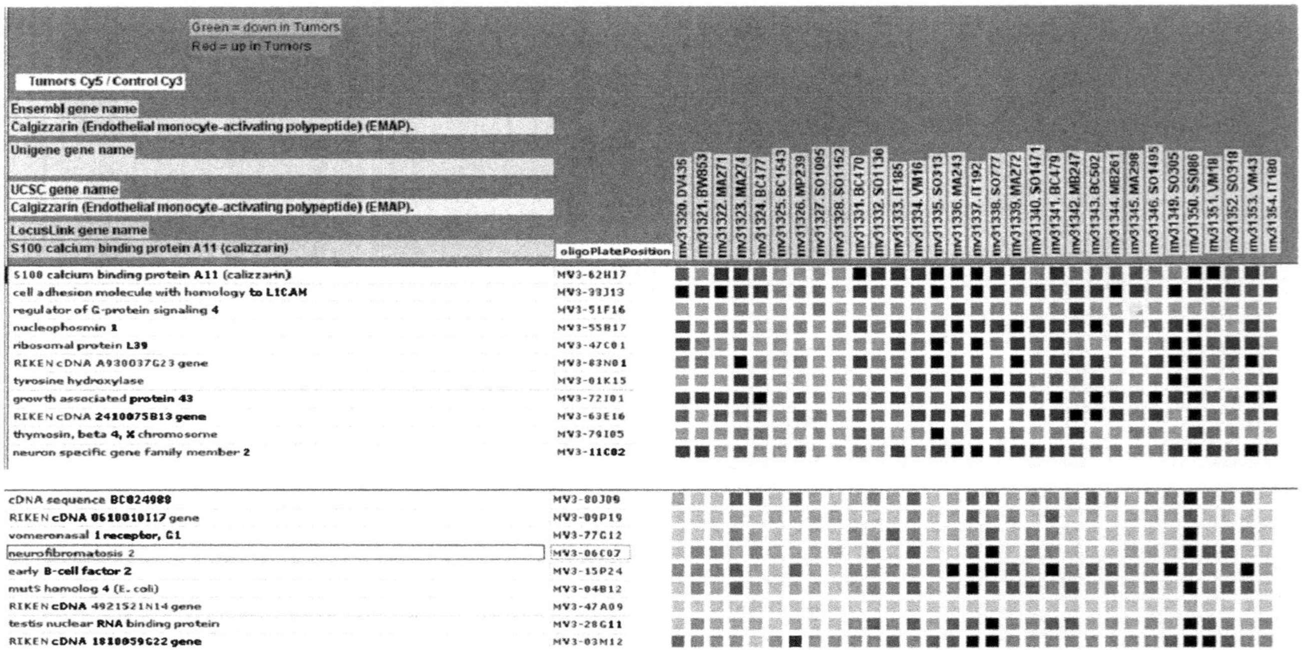

FIGURE 1. Subsets of genes differentially expressed in rat pheochromocytomas. The figure shows also the similar expression profiles of Ret, ribosomal genes, and heat-shock protein, indicating a possible pathway involving these genes.

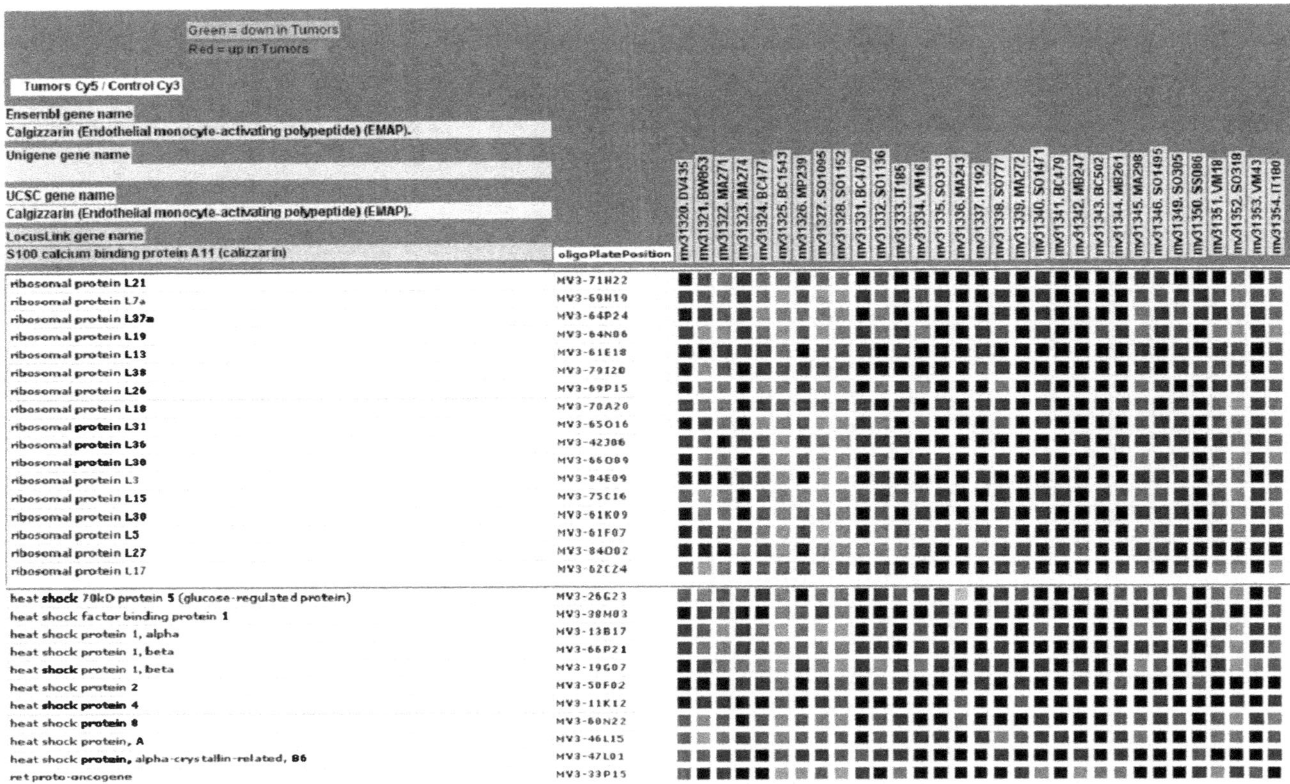

FIGURE 1. *Continued.*

which consists of an equimolar total RNA mixture of normal adrenal medulla from male and female. The details of the whole protocol can be accessed through the web site: http://magic2.nhgri.nih.gov/microarray/index.shtml. The fluorescence intensities at the target locations on the scanned array were measured using the DEARRAY software (BD Biosciences, Rockville, MD; www.scanalytics.com). After background subtraction, average intensities at each oligo in the sample hybridization were divided by the average intensity of the corresponding oligo in the reference hybridization. The ratios were normalized on the basis of the distribution of ratios of all targets on the array. Low-quality spot measurements were excluded from the analysis and were treated as missing values.[2]

Data were subject to a set of filtering criteria, statistical analysis, and gene selection based on a difference in P value of less than 0.001 as described elsewhere.[3] First, the average spot quality score (which ranges from 0 [worst] to 1 [best]) over all samples in the study was required to be at least 0.5.[2] Second, the normalized ratio to reference RNA was required to be above 2 or below 0.5 in three or more experiments. The resulting data were analyzed by generation of a weighted list of genes followed by random permutation analysis, as described elsewhere.[4,5] The tools and the statistical methods used for this particular analysis are posted at https://arrayanalysis.nih.gov/Main.do.

RESULTS

Differential Gene Expression in Rat Pheochromocytoma

To compare the molecular profile of rat and human pheochromocytomas, we conducted a gene expression profiling study comparing 31 pheochromocytomas obtained from the National Toxicology Program to normal adult rat adrenal medulla. After background subtraction and data normalization, the ratios were averaged for all the tumors. At a cutoff of twofold up- and downregulation and a quality of 0.95 or above, there were 530 oligo probes upregulated and 71 oligo probes downregulated. At a cutoff of 1.5-fold change, there were 2,223 oligo probes upregulated and 1,239 oligo probes downregulated. These 3,463 oligo probes represent 1,945 unique Unigene genes. Of these upregulated genes, some were upregulated in most of the tumors, for example, the lectin, galactose binding, soluble 1, and the regulator of G protein–signaling 4 (average ratio 6.72). Also, there were genes for which average ratios were low because some tumors had the gene upregulated and other tumors had it downregulated (Gnas and Rgs4). Similarly, there were genes that were downregulated in most of the tumors (e.g., NF 2 and Ing3), or only in a subset of tumors (e.g., Pias3 gene)(FIG. 1).

An unsupervised analysis of gene expression in all 31 rat pheochromocytomas based on the ratios did not reveal significant clustering of the tumors on the basis of the chemical and pathological characteristics of the tumors (data not shown), most probably due to the heterogeneity and the small number of tumors for each subgroup (there were 11 different chemicals used in 19 tumors).

However, the supervised t-statistic/f-statistics gene selection based on the microarray gene expression of phenylethanolamine N-methyltransferase (PNMT) revealed 255 genes with a P value <0.001. At least two of the top 10 functionally known genes encodes the adrenomedullin and purinergic receptor P2Y, proteins known to be involved in pheochromocytoma and adrenal tissue function.[6,7]

The ret proto-oncogene was overexpressed in 14 tumors and interestingly those tumors also showed the highest overexpression of ribosomal genes (FIG. 1), several heat-shock proteins, and oncogenes (e.g. Myc-like oncogene, s-Myc, and the Nmyc1). It has been well documented that N-Myc and c-Myc induce the expression of ribosomal genes.[8,9]

Gene Expression in Human Compared to Rat Pheochromocytomas

To investigate the correlation between human and rat pheochromocytomas, we compared the list of genes differentially regulated in our 31 rat tumors to a human database of gene expression profiles generated from over 110 pheochromocytoma and paraganglioma tumors.[10] The 601 oligo probes that are up- or downregulated by more than twofold in rat tumors represent 345 unique genes, of which 82 represent ribosomal genes, 78 are expressed sequence tags (ESTs) and Riken cDNA clones. The remaining 185 are named genes with some functional annotation. Of those 185 genes, 114 (61.6%) are also differentially expressed in human pheochromocytomas with a P value <0.009. Those rat genes that correlate with human genes cover different pathways related to multiple endocrine neoplasia Type 2 (MEN2), von Hippel–Lindau (VHL), SDHB, adrenergic/noradrenergic phenotypes, and metastasis. A total of 38 of the 114 rat genes are significantly involved in human pheochromocytomas that undergo metastasis.[10] Interestingly, several heat-shock proteins, including HSPCB and HSP8, are also differentially expressed in human tumors that are associated with metastasis ($P < 0.006$) independently of the adrenergic/noradrenergic status of the tumors (TABLE 1).

DISCUSSION

We have demonstrated sets of genes that are differentially expressed in rat pheochromocytomas. Among the differentially expressed genes between normal adrenal medulla and pheochromocytomas, we identified a subset of upregulated genes coding for secreted proteins and signaling cell-surface molecules, two sets of molecules of interest for diagnostic and drug development, respectively (e.g., A2m, Sfrp2, Spp1, Sectm1, Lgals1, Npy, Ptn, Ccr4, Gna13, Gng12, Gng10)(TABLE 1).

TABLE 1. List of representative up- and downregulated genes in rat pheochromocytomas with a human counterpart that are also up- or downregulated in human pheochromocytomas

Gene name	Average tumor ratios	Locus Link	Prot ID	Unigene ID
Neurofibromatosis 2	0.39	18016	NM_010898	Mm.297109
ATP-binding cassette, subfamily A (ABC1)	0.43	268379	NA	Mm.39270
Survivor of motor neuron protein interacting 1	0.43	66603	NM_025656	Mm.35353
Dermatopontin	0.44	56429	NM_019759	Mm.28935
Spermine oxidase	0.45	228608	NM_145533	Mm.136586
Docking protein 5	0.46	76829	NM_029761	Mm.41633
Endothelin 3	0.46	13616	NM_007903	Mm.9478
Hydrocephalus inducing	0.46		NA	Mm.108652
Lysosomal acid lipase 1	0.46		NA	Mm.157545
Ribulose-5-phosphate-3-epimerase	0.47	66646	NM_025683	Mm.240912
Interleukin-15 receptor, alpha chain	0.49	16169	NM_008358	Mm.200196
inhibitor of growth family, member 3	0.5	71777	NM_023626	Mm.39999
Neuropilin (NRP) and tolloid (TLL)-like 1	0.5	246317	NM_144946	Mm.329578
Pleiotrophin	2.01	19242	NM_008973	Mm.279690
Heat-shock protein 8	2.03	433302	NA	Mm.336743
Heat-shock protein, A	2.03		NM_010481	Mm.209419
Neural cell adhesion molecule 1	2.04	17967	NM_010875	Mm.4974
Transmembrane 4 superfamily member 4	2.04	229302	NM_145539	Mm.26618
Ret proto-oncogene	2.05	19713	NM_009050	Mm.57199
Calmodulin 2	2.19	270596	NA	Mm.329243
Cell adhesion molecule with homology to L1CAM	2.2	12661	NM_007697	Mm.251288
Regulator of G protein signaling 5	2.21	19737	NM_009063	Mm.20954
Heat-shock protein 1, beta	2.27	15516	NM_008302	Mm.2180
Ubiquitin carboxy-terminal hydrolase L1	2.32	22223	NM_011670	Mm.29807
DnaJ (HSP40) homolog, subfamily A, 4	2.36	58233	NM_021422	Mm.52319
TUBULIN, beta 3	2.36	22152	NM_023279	Mm.40068
Neurotransmitter transporter, noradrenalin	2.51	20538	NM_009209	Mm.57040
Nuclear DNA binding protein	2.52	57316	NM_020558	Mm.287982
S100 calcium binding protein A11	2.54	20195	NA	Mm.280038
Delta-like 1 homolog (*Drosophila*)	2.55	13386	NM_010052	Mm.157069

TABLE 1. *Continued*

Gene name	Average tumor ratios	LocusLink	Prot ID	Unigene ID
Eukaryotic translation elong factor 2	2.56		NM_007907	Mm.289431
Endothelial PAS domain protein 1	2.58	13819	NM_010137	Mm.1415
Beta-2 microglobulin	2.62	12010	NM_009735	Mm.163
Chromogranin B	2.98	12653	NM_007694	Mm.255241
Tubulin, alpha 1	2.98	22142	NA	Mm.301259
Neuritin 1	3.05	68404	NM_153529	Mm.232930
Tyrosine hydroxylase	3.1	21823	NM_009377	Mm.1292
Lectin, galactose binding, soluble 1	4.1	16852	NM_008495	Mm.43831
Diacylglycerol kinase, eta	4.24	380921	XM_358465	Mm.102293
Transmembrane 4 superfamily member 1	4.37	17112	NM_008536	Mm.856
Membrane protein, palmitoylated 6	5.5	56524	NM_019939	Mm.41288
Regulator of G protein signaling 4	6.72	19736	NM_009062	Mm.347490

The genes differentially expressed in rat pheochromocytomas are involved in several pathways that may be related to different clinico-pathological characteristics of the tumors. Of interest is the number of heat-shock proteins, ribosomal genes, and several oncogenes (e.g., ret proto-oncogene) that share similar expression profiles and may indicate a new pathway involving RET-HSPCB genes. Ribosomal genes are known to be upregulated by N-Myc.[8,9] Several of these ribosomal genes, such as RPL4, RPL3, bind to Annexin A2 and/or CDK4 inhibitor (CDKN2A) which are also upregulated in RET-expressing tumors. Moreover, HSPCB gene expression has been shown to be enhanced by N-Myc,[11] CDKN2A,[12] and p53.[13] HSPCA and HSPCB, which form the HSP90 complex, bind to several proteins including ARNT, AHR, NOS1, and AKT1 (genes also differentially expressed in our RET-expressing tumors) and are involved in several pathways with differential expression described in several other malignancies.[13] However, the well-known HSP90 inhibitors, geldanamycin and radicicol, have not yet been tested on pheochromocytomas. Inhibition of HSP90 with geldanamycin (17-AAG) reduces RET/PTC1 protein level,[14] decreases expression of c-Raf, reduces proliferation, and induces apoptosis.[15]

Cross-correlation with human pheochromocytomas shows over 60% gene expression similarities with the rat pheochromocytomas. This correlation may be higher if we take into account the large number of ESTs and genes that do not yet have any functional annotation. Correlations have also been found at the DNA level by array-based comparative genomic hybridization between mouse and human pheochromocytomas.[16]suggesting that similarities of pheochromocytoma genesis may exist across species at multiple levels. These results demonstrate relevance of the rat pheochromocytoma as an animal model for human pheochromocytomas. Potential applications include basic pathobiology and drug development.

ACKNOWLEDGMENTS

This research was supported by NIH Grant CA48017 to AST and the Intramural Research Program of the NIH, National Human Genome Research Institute, the National Institute of Neurological Disorders and Stroke, and the National Institute of Environmental Health Science.

REFERENCES

1. Tischler, A.S. *et al.* 200 models of pheochromocytoma. Histology **19:** 883–895.
2. Chen, Y. *et al.* 2002. Ratio statistics of gene expression levels and applications to microarray data analysis. Bioinformatics. **18:** 1207–1215.
3. Eisenhofer, G. *et al.* 2004. Distinct gene expression profiles in norepinephrine- and epinephrine-producing hereditary and sporadic pheochromocytomas: activation of hypoxia-driven angiogenic pathways in von Hippel-Lindau syndrome. Endocr. Relat. Cancer **11:** 897–911.
4. Allander, S.V. *et al.* 2003. Gastrointestinal stromal tumors with KIT mutations exhibit a remarkably homogeneous gene expression profile. Cancer Res. **61:** 8624–8628.
5. Kees, U.R. 2003. Gene expression signatures in lymphoid tumors. 2003. Immunol. Cell Biol. **82:** 154–160.
6. Letizia, C. *et al.* 2001. Plasma adrenomedullin concentrations in patients with adrenal pheochromocytoma. Horm. Metab. Res. **33:** 290–294.
7. Pooler, A.M. *et al.* 2005. Uridine enhances neurite outgrowth in nerve growth factor-differentiated pheochromocytoma cells. Neuroscience **134:** 207–214
8. Boon, K. *et al.* 2001. N-Myc enhances the expression of a large set of genes functioning in ribosome biogenesis and protein synthesis. EMBO J. **20:** 1383.
9. Kim, S. *et al.* 2000. Induction of ribosomal genes and hepatocyte hypertrophy by adenovirus-mediated expression of c-Myc *in vivo*. Proc. Natl. Acad. Sci. USA **97:** 11198.
10. Brouwers, F.M. *et al.* 2005. Gene expression profiling of human pheochromocytomas. Ann. N. Y. Acad. Sci. This Issue.
11. Teng, S.C. *et al.* 2004. Direct activation of *HSP90A* transcription by c-Myc contributes to c-Myc-induced transformation. J. Biol. Chem. **279:** 14649–14655.
12. Sherr, S.J. *et al.* 1999. CDK inhibitors: positive and negative regulators of G1-phase progression. Genes Dev. **13:** 1501.
13. Walerych, D. *et al.* 2004. Hsp90 chaperones wild-type p53 tumor suppressor protein. J. Biol. Chem. **279:** 48836–48845.

14. MARSEE, D.K. *et al.* 2004. Inhibition of heat shock protein 90, a novel Ret/PTC1-associated protein, increases radioiodide accumulation in thyroid cells. J. Biol. Chem. **279:** 43990–43997.
15. PARK, J.W. *et al.* 2003. The heat shock protein 90-binding geldanamycin inhibits cancer cell proliferation, down-regulates onco-proteins, and inhibits epidermal growth factor-induced invasion in thyroid cancer cell lines. J. Clin. Endocrinol. Metab. **88:** 3346–3353.
16. POWERS, J.F. *et al.* 2005. Microarray-based comparative genomic hybridization of pheochromocytoma cell lines from neurofibromatosis knockout mice reveals genetic alterations similar to those in human pheochromocytomas. Cancer Genet. Cytogenet. **159:** 27–31.

Animal Models of Pheochromocytoma Including NIH Initial Experience

SHOICHIRO OHTA,[a] EDWIN W. LAI,[a] SHUN'ICHIRO TANIGUCHI,[b] ARTHUR S. TISCHLER,[c] SALVATORE ALESCI,[d] AND KAREL PACAK[a]

[a]*Reproductive Biology and Medicine Branch, National Institute of Child Health and Human Development, Bethesda, Maryland 20892, USA*

[b]*Department of Molecular Oncology, Institute on Aging and Adaptation, Shinshu University Graduate School of Medicine, Matsumoto, Japan*

[c]*Department of Pathology, Tufts New England Medical Center, Tufts University School of Medicine, Boston, Massachusetts 02111, USA*

[d]*National Institute of Mental Health, Bethesda, Maryland 20892, USA*

ABSTRACT: Mouse models have been used to study the mechanisms underlying the carcinogenesis of a wide variety of human cancer. A considerable number of mouse and rat models, used for the study of elementary tumorgenic mechanisms, were found to develop pheochromocytomas. Some of these models resemble hereditary syndrome-related pheochromocytoma in humans and some may serve as a new starting point for human pheochromocytoma research. Recently, we generated a model of catecholamine-producing metastatic pheochromocytoma in athymic nude mice using tail-vein injection of mouse pheochromocytoma cells (MPCs). This and alternative animal models of metastatic pheochromocytoma are promising avenues in preclinical studies to evaluate new therapeutic approaches for malignant pheochromocytoma.

KEYWORDS: pheochromocytoma; animal model; 17-dimethylamino-17-demethoxygeldanamycin (17-DMAG)

ANIMAL MODELS

Up to about 36% of sporadic pheochromocytomas undergo malignant transformation, with an overall 5-year survival of about 50%.[1,2] Once pheochromocyotma has metastasized, there is no curative therapy. The ability to develop effective treatments requires the availability of relevant preclinical models to test new agents and approaches for their ability to kill tumor cells. The

Address for correspondence: Karel Pacak, M.D., Ph.D., D.Sc., Unit on Clinical Neuroendocrinology, RBMB, NICHD, NIH, Building 10, CRC, Room 1E-3141, 10 Center Drive MSC-1109, Bethesda, MD 20892-1109, USA. Voice: +1-301-402-4594; fax: +1-301-402-4712.
e-mail: karel@mail.nih.gov

Ann. N.Y. Acad. Sci. 1073: 300–305 (2006).
doi: 10.1196/annals.1353.034

establishment of relevant animal models of metastatic pheochromocytoma is important to meet this need.

The nerve growth factor–responsive PC12 cell line, established from a rat pheochromocytoma, has served for almost 30 years as a research tool for many aspects of neurobiology involving normal and neoplastic conditions. Recently developed pheochromocytoma cell lines from neurofibromatosis knockout mice supplement the PC12 line and have generated additional applications. Advantages of the mouse lines include expression of substantial levels of the epinephrine-synthesizing enzyme, phenylethanolamine N-methyltransferase, and expression of high levels of the receptor tyrosine kinase, ret, which is characteristic of sporadic and familial human pheochromocytomas but not of PC12 cells. Disadvantages include an apparently less stable phenotype. Overall, it is difficult to establish pheochromocytoma cell lines from any species, although the tumor cells persist in culture for many months.[3,4]

The attempt to develop metastatic pheochromocytoma has been first established using PC12 cells. However, metastatic lesions of the liver, a commonly seen site in patients with poor prognosis, was only achieved after intrasplenic injection of a selected PC12 cell variant (TABLE 1).

In the early 1990s, adrenal medullary neoplasms were reported in transgenic mice carrying SV40 or polyoma viral T-antigens driven by a variety of promoters, including those for tyrosine hydroxylase (TH) and phenylethanolamine-N-methyltransferase (PNMT). Better-differentiated-appearing pheochromocytomas have subsequently been reported to occur with high frequency in transgenic mice (TABLE 1). Later, transgenic and knockout mechanisms were tried to establish a new pheochromocytoma model. For example, better-differentiated-appearing pheochromocytomas and "hyperplastic nodules" have subsequently been reported to occur with high frequency in transgenic mice expressing *c-mos*[5,6] or multiple endocrine neoplasia (MEN)2B type mutant *ret* (Met 918),[7] and *Rb*,[8] *Pten*[9], or *Nf1*[10] knockouts. Unfortunately, some of these

TABLE 1. Murine models of pheochromocytoma

Type	Location	Animal	Frequency	Reference
Adrenal				
Rb±	Adrenal	Mouse	71%	[8]
Rb−/−p130−/−	Adrenal	Mouse	55%	[8]
p18 (Ink4c)−/−p27–Kip1)−/−	Adrenal	Mouse	91%	[15]
PTEN±	Adrenal	Mouse	24%	[9]
PTEN±p27(Kip1)−/−	Adrenal	Mouse	100%	[9]
NF±	Adrenal	Mouse	20%	[10]
c-mos transgenic	Adrenal	Mouse	58%	[5,6]
Metastatic				
Intrasplenic injection—PC12 Variant	Liver	Nude mouse	100%	[3]
Tail-vein injection—PC12 variant	Lung	Nude mouse	30%	[3]
Tail-vein injection—MPC	Liver	Nude mouse	92%	NIH model

mice have not been maintained and may be permanently lost as experimental models.

Recently, pheochromocytomas were developed in genetically engineered mice well resembling their naturally occurring counterparts.[11] A mosaic-like pattern formed by areas of cells with varied cytologic features may be seen. Tumor cells bordering vascular channels occasionally acquire columnar morphology with basal nuclei.[5] Immunohistochemically, tumors are consistently and diffusely positive for TH, but variably and sometimes only focally positive for PNMT. PNMT expression is absent or greatly reduced in tumors associated with viral T-antigens[5] and in a small series of MEN2B tumors,[7] but positive in pheochromocytomas associated with aging[5] or toxic chemicals and in tumors from *Nf1* knockout mice.[10] In both the *c-mos* and *Nf1*models, pheochromocytomas develop only in animals outbred to create a mixed genetic background.[6,10] Pheochromocytomas occur with increased frequency in mice with a heterozygous knockout mutation of exon 31 of the murine *Nf1* gene,[10] but not in other neurofibromatosis mouse models.[10] They are not known to be similarly inducible in other species, but arise with increased frequency in transgenic and knockout mice that to varying degrees recapitulate human tumor syndromes.

Here, we describe the establishment of an animal model of metastatic malignant pheochromocytoma, using mouse pheochromocytoma cells (MPC) cells that reproducibly metastasize to the liver and result in physiological effects similar to those seen in clinically advanced metastatic pheochromocytoma in patients.

To establish a new model of metastatic pheochromcytoma, unanesthetized mice underwent injection of 10×10^6 cells suspended in a volume of 100 μL PBS (phosphate-buffered saline solution) (Sigma Chemical Co., St. Louis, MO) using 1 mL tuberculin syringes with 30-gauge hypodermic needles. Mice were then examined daily for evidence of tumor development. Cell concentration was chosen as previously described.[11] Control mice were injected with 100 μL of PBS. After injection, the mice were examined daily for tumor development. The characteristics of tumor development and metastasis for the various injection methods and mouse strain are summarized in TABLE 1. Injection (i.p.) in nude mice produced the most rapidly growing tumors after weeks 3–5. A bloody peritoneal effusion was observed in all i.p injected mice and liver metastasis were seen in 5 of 11 (45%) mice. The s.c. injection generated local lesions in 100% of s.c. injected mice, but no distinct metastatic lesions.

In this new model, we found no evidence of metastatic tumors during the first 3 weeks, followed by the sudden appearance and rapid growth of metastatic tumors between weeks 4 and 5. Excellent detection of these tumors was advanced by using MicroCT together with molecularly targeted contrast agents. DHOG liver tumors as small as 0.35 mm in these animals were detected. All mice with hepatic metastases also developed elevated systolic blood pressure. The success rate of obtaining liver metastatic lesions was about 92% in mice injected in the tail vein. This model offers the advantages that it is easily reproducible, rapidly progressing, minimally invasive, and does not require surgery. In contrast, metastatic lesions appeared only in 5 of 11 mice when MPC cells were injected i.p. and no metastatic lesion appeared when MPC cells were injected s.c.

Tail-vein injection models have recently been established in neuroblastoma, melanoma, and pancreatic cancer . Neuroblastoma cells were injected in the nude rat tail vein and micrometastatic lesions spread to liver and femur. These experiments reveal possible mechanisms responsible for the development of metastatic lesions and include optimal homing conditions of the endothelium and a microenvironment that supports tumor growth.[6] Similarly our mouse model of metastatic pheochromocytoma may be extrapolated to patients with metastatic pheochromocytoma in liver. Tail-vein injection of neuroblastoma cells causes predominantly liver metastases, which reflect clinical scenario where children with neuroblastoma typically present with huge adrenal gland tumors and multiple small metastases in the liver. Thus, although we did not succeed developing a model with different organ lesions, mice with liver metastatic lesions are most valuable because they reflect the group of patients with the worst prognosis with metastatic pheochromocytoma.

The NIH animal model is promising and can be to be used for *in vivo* preclinical imaging studies and evaluation of new therapeutic approaches to malignant pheochromocytoma. Using previous microarray data as well as previously established results about which genes can be involved in pathogenesis of pheochromocytoma, we will attempt to use experimental approaches to treat metastatic pheochromocytoma using our model together with microarray data.[12]

For example, the heat-shock protein (HSP) class of chaperones has emerged as a molecular target candidate.[13] HSP90 was found to be increased in malignant pheochromocytomas, but was also expressed at a lower level in benign tumors.[14]

17-Dimethylamino-17-demethoxygeldanamycin (17-DMAG) is a unique agent in that, although it is directed toward a specific molecular target (HSP90), simultaneously inhibits multiple signaling pathways on which cancer cells depend for growth and survival. Many of these targets are involved in signaling pathways used by tumor cells, including pheochromocytoma cells, to protect against both endogenous and exogenous signals that induce several different modes of cell death. Therefore, we will examine 17-DMAG in our model can be one of promising avenue to treat metastatic pheochromocytoma in the future.

However, such new therapeutic approaches require relevant *in vivo* models and our mouse model of pheochromocytoma may facilitate various pre-clinical trials.

ACKNOWLEDGMENTS

This study is supported in part by NIH Grant P01 NS 37685 (A.S.T.). This research was also supported by the Intramural Research Program of the NIH, NICHD.

REFERENCES

1. John, H., W.H. Ziegler, D. Hauri, *et al.* 1999. Pheochromocytomas: can malignant potential be predicted? Urology **53:** 679–683.
2. Ohta, S., E.W. Lai, A.L. Pang, *et al.* 2005. Downregulation of metastasis suppressor genes in malignant pheochromocytoma. Int. J. Cancer **114:** 139–144.
3. Zielke, A.R., S. Bresalier, A.E. Siperstein, *et al.* 1998. A unique allogenic model of metastatic pheochromocytoma: PC12 rat pheochromocytoma xenografts to nude mice and establishment of metastases-derived PC12 variants. Clin. Exp. Metastasis **16:** 341–352.
4. Tischler, A.S., J.F. Power & J. Alroy. 2004. Animal models of pheochromocytoma. Histol. Histopathol. **19:** 883–895.
5. Schulz, N., F. Propst, M.M. Rosenberg, *et al.* 1992. Patterns of neoplasia in c-mos transgenic mice and their relevance to multiple endocrine neoplasia. Henry Ford Hosp. Med. J. **40:** 307–311.
6. Schulz, N., F. Propst, M.P. Rosenberg, *et al.* 1992. Pheochromocytomas and C-cell thyroid neoplasms in transgenic cmos mice: a model for the human multiple endocrine neoplasia type 2 syndrome. Cancer Res. **52:** 450–455.
7. Smith-Hicks, C.L., K.C. Sizer, J.F. Powers, *et al.* 2000. C-cell hyperplasia, pheochromocytoma and sympathoadrenal malformation in a mouse model of multiple endocrine neoplasia type 2B. EMBO J. **19:** 612–622.
8. Williams, B.O., E.M. Schmitt, L. Remington, *et al.* 1994. Extensive contribution of Rbdeficient cells to adult chimeric mice with limited histopathological consequences. EMBO J. **13:** 4251–4259.
9. You, M.J., D.H. Castrillon, B.C. Bastian, *et al.* 2002. Genetic analysis of Pten and Ink4a/Arf interactions in the suppression of tumorigenesis in mice. Proc. Natl. Acad. Sci. USA **99:** 1455–1460.
10. Powers, J.F., M.J. Evinger, P. Tsokas, *et al.* 2000. Pheochromocytoma cell lines from heterozygous neurofibromatosis knockout mice. Cell Tissue Res. **302:** 309–320.
11. Tischler, A.S., W. Sheldon & R. Gray. 1996. Immunohistochemical and morphological characterization of spontaneously occurring pheochromocytomas in the aging mouse. Vet. Pathol. **33:** 512–520.
12. Eisenhofer, G., T.T. Huynh, K. Pacak, *et al.* 2004. Distinct gene expression profiles in norepinephrine- and epinephrine-producing hereditary and sporadic pheochromocytomas: activation of hypoxia-driven angiogenic pathways in von Hippel-Lindau syndrome. Endocr. Relat. Cancer **11:** 897–911.
13. Bisht, K.S., C.M. Bradbur, D. Mattson, *et al.* 2003. Geldanamycin and 17-allylamino-17-demethoxygeldanamycin potentiate the in vitro and in vivo radiation response of cervical tumor cells via the heat shock protein 90-mediated intracellular signaling and cytotoxicity. Cancer Res. **63:** 8984–8995.

14. Boltze, C., H. Lehnert, R. Schneider-Stock, *et al.* 2003. HSP90 is a key for telomerase activation and malignant transition in pheochromocytoma. Endocrine **22:** 193–201.
15. Huang, X., M. Di Liberto, A.F. Cunningham, *et al.* 2004. Homeostatic cell cycle control by BLyS: induction of cell-cycle entry but not G1/S transition in opposition to p18INK4c and p27Kip1. Proc. Natl. Acad. Sci. USA **21:** 17789–17794.

DHEA Reduces NGF-Mediated Cell Survival in Serum-Deprived PC12 Cells

CHRISTIAN G. ZIEGLER, FLAVIE SICARD, SIMONE SPERBER, MONIKA EHRHART-BORNSTEIN, STEFAN R. BORNSTEIN, AND ALEXANDER W. KRUG

Carl Gustav Carus University Hospital, Medical Clinic III, University of Dresden, Dresden, Germany

ABSTRACT: Adrenocortical androgens, including dehydroepiandrosterone (DHEA), are produced in the inner zone of the adrenal cortex that is in direct contact with the neural crest–derived catecholamine-producing chromaffin cells. DHEA has recently been identified as a crucial regulator of neuronal stem cell proliferation. Thus, DHEA might play a hitherto unknown role in intra-adrenal tissue formation. In the present study, we examined the influence of DHEA on nerve growth factor (NGF)–mediated survival in serum-deprived PC12 cells and analyzed the influence of DHEA on NGF-induced ERK1/2 mitogen-activated protein (MAP) kinase activation by enzyme-linked immunosorbent assay (ELISA). Cell survival promoted by NGF in serum-deprived PC12 cells and neurite outgrowth was reduced by DHEA, pointing toward a role of DHEA in the differentiation process of chromaffin cells. Furthermore, NGF-induced ERK 1/2 activation was significantly inhibited by DHEA. Hence, we speculate that DHEA might influence NGF-mediated chromaffin differentiation processes using the ERK1/2 MAP kinase pathway during adrenal tissue development.

KEYWORDS: dehydroepiandrosterone (DHEA); nerve growth factor (NGF); PC12 cells; mitogen-activated protein kinases (MAPK)

INTRODUCTION

The adrenal gland comprises two embryological tissues of different origin. In the inner layer of the adrenal cortex, the *zona reticularis*, androgens are produced, predominantly dehydroepiandrosterone (DHEA), which is the most abundant hormone in the human body. DHEA has recently been identified as an important regulator of neuronal stem cell proliferation, neurogenesis, and neuronal survival.[1–3] Thus, in the course of the development of the adrenal

Address for correspondence: Stefan R. Bornstein, M.D., Ph.D., Department of Medicine, Carl Gustav Carus University Hospital, University of Dresden, Fetscherstrasse 74, 01307 Dresden, Germany. Voice: +49 351-458-5955; fax: +49 351-458-6398.
e-mail: stefan.bornstein@uniklinikum-dresden.de

**Ann. N.Y. Acad. Sci. 1073: 306–311 (2006). © 2006 New York Academy of Sciences.
doi: 10.1196/annals.1353.035**

gland, DHEA might significantly influence the neighboring, neuronal crest–derived chromaffin cells that are tightly intermingled with the adrenocortical cells. Furthermore, studies with glucocorticoid receptor knockout mice have suggested that glucocorticoids are not as essential for the development of the neuroendocrine phenotype of chromaffin cells as previously thought.[4]

The rat PC12 cell line is a well-characterized model of mitotic- and proliferation-competent chromaffin cells. After administration of nerve growth factor (NGF) or the glucocorticoid dexamethasone (DEX), these cells demonstrate a more neuronal or neuroendocrine differentiation, respectively.[5] The aim of the present study was to analyze the effect of DHEA on NGF-mediated survival of serum-deprived PC12 cells, providing possible insights in the role of DHEA in the development of adrenal tissue. In a next step, we analyzed the influence of DHEA on NGF-induced ERK1/2 MAP kinase activation. ERK1/2 is crucially involved in differentiation and proliferation processes in PC12 cells.

MATERIALS AND METHODS

Cell Culture

Rat PC12 cells were sustained in Keighn's modified Ham's F-12 medium (ATCC) with 2 mmol/L L-glutamine and 1,500 mg/L sodium bicarbonate supplemented with 15% horse serum, 2.5% bovine calf serum, and 20U/mL penicillin–streptomycin (Gibco) in a 5% CO_2/95% O_2 air-humidified atmosphere at 37°C. The culture medium was changed every 2 days. Before experiments, cells were grown in this culture medium for 72 h and then left in serum-free medium for the next 12–16 h. Cell number was measured using a Coulter Counter.

Quantification of ERK1/2 Phosphorylation by ELISA

For quantification of ERK1/2 phosphorylation we performed ELISA as described by us previously.[6] In brief: cells were seeded in 96-well plates at a density of 20,000 cells/0.32 cm^2. After reaching 70–80% of confluence cells were equilibrated in 1 × HEPES-Ringer solution (pH 7.4) at 37 °C for 30 min and then stimulated in the same buffer plus the respective vehicle (ethanol or DMSO) or the hormones and growth factors of interest for 5 min and subsequently fixed with 4% formaldehyde in PBS for 20 min at room temperature. Cells were incubated overnight with an anti-pERK1/2 primary antibody (1:1,000) (Cell Signaling, 9101S) in PBS/Triton containing 5% bovine serum albumin at 4°C. The next day, cells were incubated with an HRP-conjugated anti-rabbit secondary antibody (1:3,000) (Cell Signaling, 7074) in PBS/Triton containing 5% bovine serum albumin for 1 h at room temperature. Subsequently, cells were incubated in 50 μL of chemiluminescence working solution in the dark, supplied by the manufacturer (Active Motif, Rixensart, Belgium).

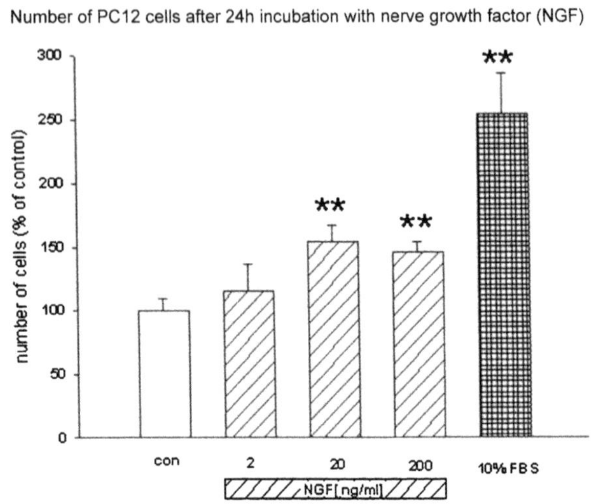

FIGURE 1. Cell number, determined with a Coulter Counter, after 24-h treatment of PC12 cells w/wo NGF (2–200 ng/mL). NGF dose-dependently (2–200 mg/mL) promoted cell survival in PC12 cells after serum withdrawal. ($n = 6$; **: $P < 0.02$ compared to control; values represent mean ± SEM).

Chemiluminescence signals were read within 10 min with a multiplate reader (Mithras, Berthold Technologies, Bad Wildberg, Germany). The wells were air-dried for 5 min at room temperature and then stained with 100 μL of crystal violet solution (25% in PBS) for 30 min. Afterward 100μL of 1% SDS solution was added and incubated on a shaker for 1 h at room temperature. After subsequent washing, 100 μL of 1% SDS solution was added and the plate was incubated on a shaker for 1 h at room temperature. Finally, the absorbance was measured at 595 nm.

Statistics

The data are presented as means ± SE. Significance of difference was tested by paired or unpaired Student's *t*-test or analysis of variance (ANOVA) as applicable. Differences were considered significant if P was < 0.05. Cells from at least two different passages were used for each experimental series. n represents the number of cells or tissue culture dishes investigated.

RESULTS

Influence of DHEA on NGF-Mediated Survival of Serum-Deprived PC12 Cells

Upon NGF stimulation chromaffin cells reversibly differentiate into neurons.[7] As expected, NGF (2–200 ng/mL) promoted cell survival in a

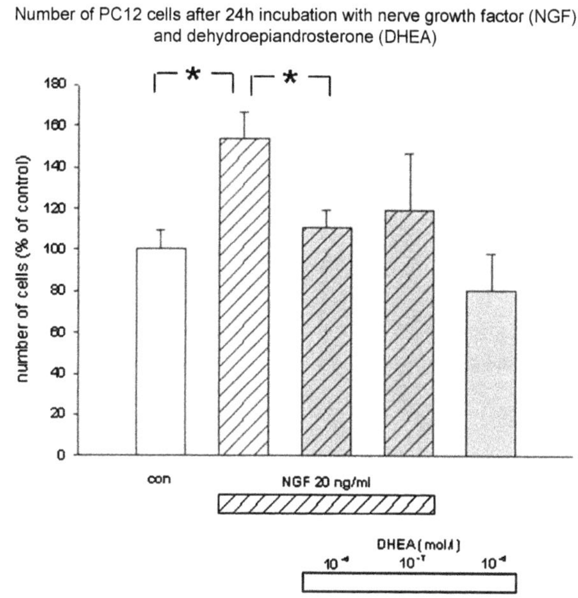

FIGURE 2. Cell number after 24-h treatment of PC12 cells with 20 ng/mL NGF together with DHEA. 10^{-6} mol/L DHEA significantly reduced NGF-mediated cell survival whereas DHEA alone did not have an effect. ($n = 6$; **: $P < 0.02$ compared to control; values represent mean ± SEM).

dose-dependent manner (FIG. 1) with PC12 cells exhibiting enhanced neurite outgrowth (not shown). Cell number was determined after 24 h. Incubation of PC12 cells with NGF (20 ng/mL) together with DHEA (10^{-6} mol/L) showed a significant reduction of NGF-mediated cell survival and reduced neurite outgrowth of the cells (not shown). DHEA (10^{-6} mol/L) alone did not significantly affect PC12 cell number as compared to control (under serum-free conditions) (FIG. 2).

Influence of DHEA on NGF-Induced ERK1/2 Phosporylation

Mitogen-activated protein (MAP) kinase signaling plays a crucial role in the differentiation as well as proliferation processes in PC12 cells. Especially the temporal activation pattern of extracellular signal-regulated kinases (ERKs) like ERK 1/2 is known to distinguish proliferation from differentiation processes.[8] NGF dose-dependently induces ERK1/2 phosphorylation in our cell model after 5-min stimulation (FIG. 3) as measured by ELISA. This effect is inhibited by DHEA (10^{-6} mol/L) and could selectively be inhibited by the MAPK pathway inhibitor U0126 (10 μmol/L).

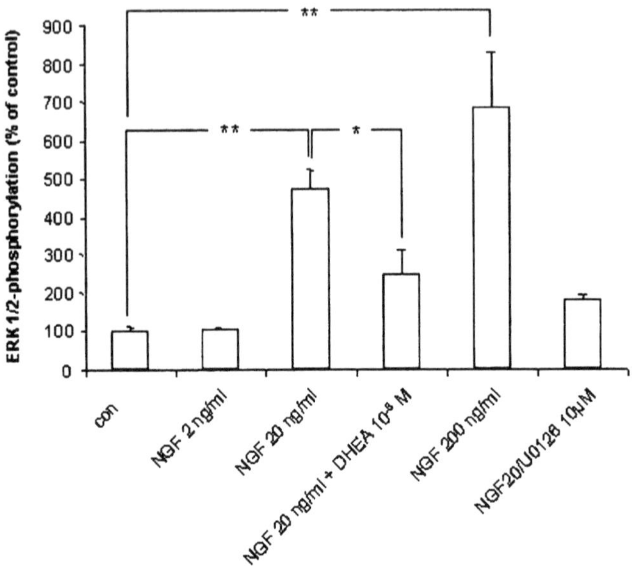

FIGURE 3. 5-min stimulation with NGF (20-200 ng/mL) induces ERK 1/2 phosphorylation in PC12 cells in a dose-dependent manner indicated by phospho-specific ELISA. This effect is significantly reduced by DHEA (10^{-6} mol/L). As expected, the MAPK inhibitor U0126 (10 μmol/L) blocks NGF-induced ERK1/2 phosphorylation ($n = 3$; ** $P < 0.02$,* $P < 0.05$ compared to control; values represent mean ± SEM).

DISCUSSION

Our results show that DHEA could reduce NGF-mediated cell survival and inhibit neurite outgrowth in chromaffin PC12 cells, indicating that possibly NGF-induced differentiation processes are counterbalanced by DHEA in the process of adrenal tissue formation. Furthermore, our data indicate that DHEA might exert this effect by influencing the ERK1/2 MAPK signaling pathway.

ACKNOWLEDGMENTS

This work was supported by a grant from the Deutsche Forschungsgemeinschaft (SFB 655/1-05) to S.R.B. and M.E.B.

REFERENCES

1. CHARALAMPOPOULOS, I. *et al.* 2004. Dehydroepiandrosterone and allopregnanolone protect sympathoadrenal medulla cells against apoptosis via antiapoptotic Bcl-2 proteins. Proc. Natl. Acad. Sci. USA **101:** 8209–8214.

2. SUZUKI, M. *et al.* 2004. Mitotic and neurogenic effects of dehydroepiandrosterone (DHEA) on human neural stem cell cultures derived from the fetal cortex. Proc. Natl. Acad. Sci. USA **101:** 3202–3207.
3. KARISHMA, K.K. & J. HERBERT. 2002. Dehydroepiandrosterone (DHEA) stimulates neurogenesis in the hippocampus of the rat, promotes survival of newly formed neurons and prevents corticosterone-induced suppression. Eur. J. Neurosci. **16:** 445–453.
4. FINOTTO, S. 1999. Analysis of mice carrying targeted mutations of the glucocorticoid receptor gene argues against an essential role of glucocorticoid signalling for generating adrenal chromaffin cells. Development **126:** 2935–2944.
5. BEAUJEAN, D. *et al.* 2003. Combinatorial code of growth factors and neuropeptides define neuroendocrine differentiation in PC12 cells. Exp. Neurol. **184:** 348–358.
6. KRUG, A.W. *et al.* 2002. Human epidermal growth factor receptor-1 expression renders Chinese hamster ovary cells sensitive to alternative aldosterone signaling. J. Biol. Chem. **277:** 45892–45897.
7. XIAO, J. *et al.* 2002. Variant PC12 cell line that spontaneously differentiates and extends neuritic processes. J. Neurosci. Res. **69:** 104–109.
8. STORCK, P.J.S. 2005. Directing NGF's action: it's a rap. Nat. Cell. Biol. **7:** 338–339.

Role of DHEA and Growth Factors in Chromaffin Cell Proliferation

F. SICARD, A.W. KRUG, C.G. ZIEGLER, S. SPERBER, M. EHRHART-BORNSTEIN, AND S.R. BORNSTEIN

Carl Gustav Carus University Hospital, Medical Clinic III, University of Dresden, Dresden, Germany

ABSTRACT: Dehydroepiandrostreone (DHEA) is a neuroactive steroid produced by the inner layer of the adrenal cortex close to the adrenomedullary cells. Chromaffin cell growth and proliferation are under the control of insulin-like growth factor II (IGF-II) and basic fibroblast growth factor (bFGF). The aim of the present study was to examine the role of DHEA on chromaffin cell proliferation induced by IGF-II and bFGF. In our model, DHEA significantly decreased IGF-II-induced proliferation by 48.7%, whereas it did not affect the proliferation induced by bFGF. These data suggest that DHEA exerts a paracrine function in the control of chromaffin cell growth.

KEYWORDS: dehydroepiandrostreone (DHEA); bovine chromaffin cell; proliferation; basic fibroblast growth factor (bFGF); insulin-like growth factor II (IGF-II)

INTRODUCTION

Earlier studies suggest that adrenocortical secretion affects not only the metabolism of distant target organs, but also the function of the adjacent adrenal medulla.[1,2] These effects are thought to distinguish chromaffin cells of the adrenal medulla from the other neuronal counterparts of the ectodermal neural crest.[3] Dehydroepiandrosterone (DHEA) is a neurosteroid with potential effects on neurogenesis, neuronal survival, and neuronal stem cell proliferation. Previous work has shown that adrenal androgens exert opposite effects to glucocorticoids in normal chromaffin cells and pheochromocytoma cells.[4,5] The DHEA-producing adrenocortical cells and the adrenomedullary chromaffin cells are tightly intermingled and provide ample contact surfaces for paracrine interactions. Interestingly, chromaffin cells are able to proliferate throughout the life span,[6] unlike the closely related sympathetic neurons.

Address for correspondence: Stefan R. Bornstein, M.D., Ph.D., Department of Medicine, Carl Gustav Carus University Hospital, University of Dresden, Fetscherstrasse 74, 01307 Dresden, Germany. Voice: +49-351-458-5955; fax: +49-351-458-6398.
e-mail: stefan.bornstein@uniklinikum-dresden.de

**Ann. N.Y. Acad. Sci. 1073: 312–316 (2006). © 2006 New York Academy of Sciences.
doi: 10.1196/annals.1353.036**

Furthermore, chromaffin cells and their tumor counterparts, the pheochromocytoma cells, synthesize, store, and release a large number of growth factors, which can act as local factors.[7,8] The aim of the present study was to examine the effect of DHEA on normal chromaffin cell proliferation induced by basic fibroblast growth factor (bFGF) and insulin-like growth factor-II (IGF-II).

EFFECT OF DHEA ON IGF-II AND bFGF-INDUCED PROLIFERATION

IGF I and II act as neurotrophic factors in various parts of the developing and adult nervous system. IGF II mRNA and protein have been detected in adrenal medulla and seem to be increased significantly in pheochromocytoma cells.[9,10] It has been shown that IGF-II stimulates DNA synthesis and mitosis of chromaffin cells cultured from neonatal, adolescent, and adult rats[11] and increases proliferation of rat PC12 cells.[12,13]

bFGF acts as a mitogen or proliferative signal for several cell types, including fibroblasts, smooth muscle cells, and endothelial cells and is also involved in the angiogenic process and in the formation of mesenchyme. bFGF is secreted by chromaffin cells. It has been shown, that bFGF stimulates DNA synthesis and mitosis of chromaffin cells cultured from neonatal and adult rats.[11]

In this study, chromaffin cells from young bovine animals were isolated as previously described.[14] The cells were then stimulated with graded concentrations of the various growth factors in serum-free medium. After 4 days' incubation, proliferation was quantified using a MTS tetrazolium assay. Contamination of our cell culture with overgrowth fibroblasts was excluded by staining chromaffin

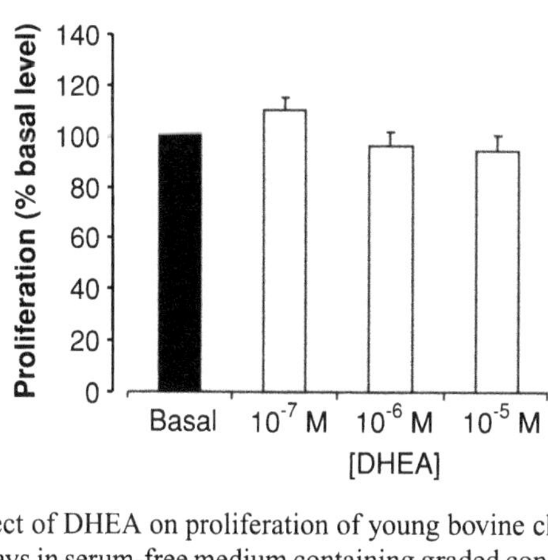

FIGURE 1. Effect of DHEA on proliferation of young bovine chromaffin cells. Cells were cultured for 4 days in serum-free medium containing graded concentrations of DHEA. Proliferation was quantified by Promega CellTiter 96 Aqueous One Solution Proliferation Assay. Values represent mean ± SEM. Each measurement was performed as least in quadruplicate.

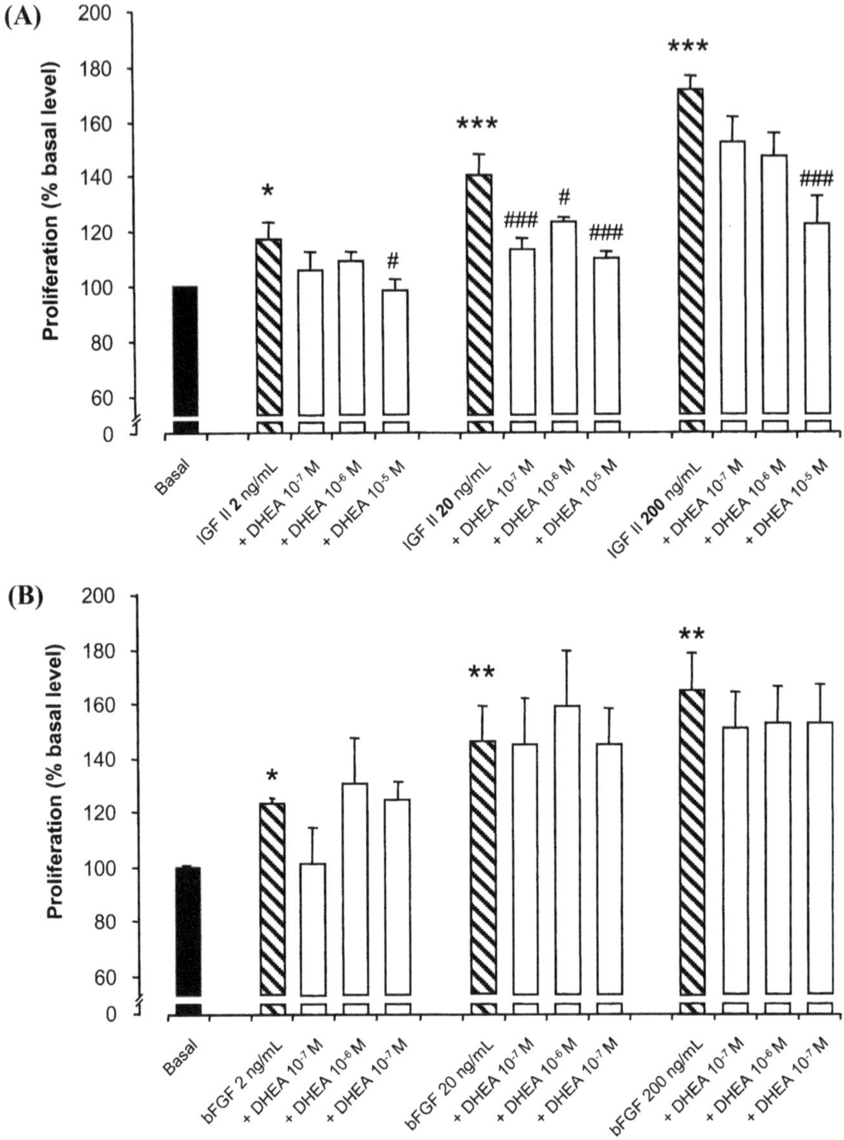

FIGURE 2. Effect of DHEA on proliferation of chromaffin cells induced by IGF-II (**A**) or bFGF (**B**). Cells were cultured for 4 days in serum-free medium containing graded concentrations of growth factors (*hatched columns*) or in combination with graded concentrations of DHEA (*open columns*). Cells cultured in the absence of growth factors served as control (*black columns*). Proliferation was quantified by Promega CellTiter 96 Aqueous One Solution Proliferation Assay. Values represent mean ± SEM. Each measurement was performed at least in triplicate. $^{\#,*}$, $P < 0.05$; $^{\#\#,**}$, $P < 0.01$; $^{\#\#\#,***}$, $P < 0.001$ (One-way analysis of variance (ANOVA) followed by Tukey post-test).

cells with antibodies against PNMT and chromogranin A (data not shown). As previously shown, bFGF and IGF-II stimulated the proliferation of chromaffin cells in a dose-dependent manner. DHEA by itself did not affect chromaffin cell proliferation (FIG. 1). In contrast, DHEA decreased significantly the cell proliferation induced by IGF-II by 48.7% ± 10.4, $P < 0.05$ (FIG. 2A). bFGF-induced proliferation was not affected by DHEA (FIG. 2B).

The important role of glucocorticoids in the development of chromaffin cells, particularly by dexamethasone, is well documented.[15,16] However, a recent publication revealed the presence of mature chromaffin cells in glucocorticoid-receptor knockout mice,[17] suggesting that glucocorticoids are not essential for neuroendocrine differentiation of chromaffin progenitor cells. On the other hand, the fetal adrenal gland does not secrete primarily glucocorticoids, but essentially DHEA and DHEAS. So far, little is known about the effect of these androgens on chromaffin cell differentiation and proliferation. A recent report shows that DHEA exerts a strong, dose-dependent antiapoptotic effect on rat primary serum-deprived adrenomedullary cells as well as PC-12 cells.[18] This protective effect involved the antiapoptotic Bcl-2 proteins. Besides, Frödin and Gammeltoft have demonstrated that, in neonatal and adult rat chromaffin cells, IGF-II and bFGF act synergically to promote chromaffin cell proliferation.[11] These data suggest that divergent signals at receptor levels may be involved in the response of chromaffin cells to these growth factors. Taken together, these results suggest that in bovine chromaffin cells, DHEA inhibits proliferation induced by IGF-II by interacting with any signaling pathways that differ from the bFGF-mediated signal transduction.

CONCLUSION

In conclusion, these data suggest that DHEA exerts a paracrine function in the control of growth of chromaffin cells. Therefore, DHEA may interact with growth factors involved in the control of adrenal medullary hyperplasia and/or tumor formation.

ACKNOWLEDGMENTS

This work was supported by a grant from the Deutsche FORSCHUNSGEME in schaft (SFB 655/1-05) to S.R.B. and M.E.B.

REFERENCES

1. WURTMAN, R.J. *et al.* 1972. Adrenocortical control of the biosynthesis of epinephrine and proteins in the adrenal medulla. Pharmacol. Rev. **24:** 411–425.

2. Pohorecky, L.A. & R.J. Wurtman. 1971. Adrenocortical control of epinephrine synthesis. Pharmacol. Rev. **23:** 1–235.
3. Anderson, D.J. 1989. Cellular "neoteny": a possible developmental basis for chromaffin cell plasticity. Trends Genet. **5:** 174–178.
4. Lai, G. & D.P. McCobb. 2002. Opposing actions of adrenal androgens and glucocorticoids on alternative splicing of Slo potassium channels in bovine chromaffin cells. Proc. Natl. Acad. Sci. USA **99:** 7722–7727.
5. Brown, J.W. *et al.* 1998. Studies of the neuronal transdifferentiation process in cultured human pheochromocytoma cells: effects of steroids with differing functional groups on catecholamine content and cell morphology. Steroids **63:** 587–594.
6. Unsicker, K. 1993. The chromaffin cell: paradigm in cell, developmental and growth factor biology. J. Anat. **183:** 207–221.
7. Lachmund, A. *et al.* 1994. Trophic factors from chromaffin granules promote survival of peripheral and central nervous system neurons. Neuroscience **62:** 361–370.
8. Unsicker, K. 1993. The trophic cocktail made by adrenal chromaffin cells. Exp. Neurol. **123:** 167–173.
9. El-Badry, O.M. *et al.* 1989. Autonomous growth of a human neuroblastoma cell line is mediated by insulin-like growth factor II. J. Clin. Invest. **84:** 829–839.
10. Suzuki, T. *et al.* 1989. IGF-II-like immunoreactivity in human tissues, neuroendocrine tumors, and PC12 cells. Diabetes Res. Clin. Pract. **7**(Suppl 1): S21–S27.
11. Frodin, M. & S. Gammeltoft. 1994. Insulin-like growth factors act synergistically with basic fibroblast growth factor and nerve growth factor to promote chromaffin cell proliferation. Proc. Natl. Acad. Sci. USA **91:** 1771–1775.
12. Dahmer, M.K. & R.L. Perlman. 1988. Insulin and insulin-like growth factors stimulate deoxyribonucleic acid synthesis in PC12 pheochromocytoma cells. Endocrinology **122:** 2109–2113.
13. Nielsen, F.C. & S. Gammeltoft. 1988. Insulin-like growth factors are mitogens for rat pheochromocytoma PC 12 cells. Biochem. Biophys. Res. Commun. **154:** 1018–1023.
14. Haidan, A. *et al.* 1998. Basal steroidogenic activity of adrenocortical cells is increased 10-fold by coculture with chromaffin cells. Endocrinology **139:** 772–780.
15. Doupe, A.J. *et al.* 1985. Environmental influences in the development of neural crest derivatives: glucocorticoids, growth factors, and chromaffin cell plasticity. J. Neurosci. **5:** 2119–2142.
16. Seidl, K. & K. Unsicker.1989. The determination of the adrenal medullary cell fate during embryogenesis. Dev. Biol. **136:** 481–490.
17. Finotto, S. *et al.* 1999. Analysis of mice carrying targeted mutations of the glucocorticoid receptor gene argues against an essential role of glucocorticoid signalling for generating adrenal chromaffin cells. Development **126:** 2935–2944.
18. Charalampopoulos, I. *et al.* 2004. Dehydroepiandrosterone and allopregnanolone protect sympathoadrenal medulla cells against apoptosis via antiapoptotic Bcl-2 proteins. Proc. Natl. Acad. Sci. USA **101:** 8209–8214.

Analysis of PTEN Mutation in Non-familial Pheochromocytoma

JANUSZ PUC,[a,b] GRZEGORZ PLACHA,[b] BOZENNA WOCIAL,[b] KATRINA PODSYPANINA,[a] RAMON PARSONS[a] AND ZBIGNIEW GACIONG[b]

[a]*Institute for Cancer Genetics, Columbia University, New York, New York 10032, USA*

[b]*Department of Internal Diseases and Hypertension, Medical University of Warsaw, 02-097 Warsaw, Poland*

ABSTRACT: PTEN, a tumor suppressor gene, is frequently mutated in a variety of human tumors. In mice, monoallelic inactivation of this gene predisposes animals to neoplasia of multiple organs. Interestingly, Pten heterozygous mice develop bilateral hyperplasia of the adrenal medulla. In this report we demonstrate that these neoplasms are hormonally active pheochromocytomas that secrete increased amounts of bioactive catecholamines: norepinephrine and epinephrine. To test a possibility that PTEN might be one of the genes responsible for human sporadic pheochromocytoma, we performed mutation analysis of DNA obtained from tumors of 29 patients. However, direct sequencing of all nine exons of the PTEN gene, including the splice junctions, revealed no mutations. Examination of protein expression by immunohistochemistry using 8 normal adrenals and 11 sporadic pheochromocytomas showed no decrease in the PTEN protein expression in the tumor tissue, but upregulation of insulin-like growth factor II, a peptide implicated in growth of adrenal tissue, was observed in four cases (36%).

KEYWORDS: PTEN; pheochromocytoma; IGF II

INTRODUCTION

Pheochromocytoma is a rare catecholamine-secreting tumor, typically arising in approximately 85% of cases from adrenomedullary tissue and in about 15% from extra-adrenal chromaffin cells. Excessive growth of medullary chromaffin cells is demonstrated by increased production of bioactive catecholamines, resulting in the elevation of blood pressure. According to different statistical studies, pheochromocytoma accounts for approximately 0.05 to

Address for correspondence: Janusz Puc, Ph.D., Department of Molecular Medicine, University of California, San Diego, 9500 Gilman Drive, La Jolla, CA 92093-0648. Voice: 858-534-0758; fax: 858-534-8180.
e-mail: jpuc@ucsd.edu

Ann. N.Y. Acad. Sci. 1073: 317–331 (2006).
doi: 10.1196/annals.1353.037

0.1% of patients with any degree of sustained hypertension.[1] It is not surprising that the genetic causes of the disease are under continuous investigation. As a result of advances made in the field of molecular genetics, it has become possible to localize and clone genes responsible, at least in part, for onset of pheochromocytoma. Particularly useful were studies focusing on hereditary cancer syndromes. Linkage analyses, conducted in families in which prevalence of pheochromocytoma amongst their members was particularly high, resulted in cloning and characterization of the disease-associated genes.

Pheochromocytoma occurs in three familial cancer syndromes: neurofibromatosis type 1 (NF 1),[2,3] multiple endocrine neoplasia type 2 (MEN 2),[4,5] and von Hippel–Lindau disease (VHL).[6] In addition, its prevalence is associated with mutations in SDHB[7] and SDHD genes.[8,9] However, the large majority of pheochromocytoma is of sporadic nature and other critical genes involved in pathogenesis of the disease are yet to be identified.

PTEN/MMAC1/TEP1[10–12] is a tumor-suppressor gene located on chromosome 10q23. Somatic deletions or mutations of PTEN have been identified in breast,[13,14] prostate,[15,16] endometrial cancer,[17,18] as well as in glioblastoma[19,20] and melanoma.[21,22] In addition, PTEN mutations were found in individuals with rare familial cancer predisposition syndromes: Cowden's disease[23] and Bannayan-Zonana.[24]

Pten heterozygous mice develop neoplasia of many organs, suggesting that PTEN is an important tumor suppressor.[25,26] Interestingly, mice generated by Podsypanina *et al.*[27] develop bilateral adrenal hyperplasia by the age of 26 weeks. We decided to characterize these growths and showed these neoplasms to be hormonally active pheochromocytomas. This, in turn, prompted us to investigate PTEN mutation status in human sporadic pheochromocytomas.

MATERIALS AND METHODS

Generation of Pten ± Mice

Pten heterozygous animals were generated as described by Podsypanina *et al.* (1999).[26]

Analysis of Plasma and Tissue Catecholamines in Pten +/+ and ± Mice

Pten +/+ ($n = 6$) and ± ($n = 6$) mice, mean age 45 weeks, were euthanized by CO_2 inhalation. Blood was drawn directly from the heart using an 18 GG needle, transferred to a 1.7-mL conical tube, and allowed to clot. The sample was spun down at 2000 × *g* for 10 min at room temperature. Plasma was carefully aspirated, transferred to a fresh tube and snap-frozen in methanol/dry ice. HPLC Plasma Catecholamine Kit (Bio-Rad, Hercules, CA) was used as per manufacturer's recommendations to quantify catecholamines. To measure tissue amine levels, adrenal glands from Pten +/+ ($n = 9$) and ± ($n = 9$) mice were washed with ice-cold phosphate-buffered saline (pH 7.4) and snap-frozen in methanol/dry ice. Subsequently, tissues were homogenized in 10 ml of 0.4 M perchloric acid, and further steps were carried out as with plasma.

Statistics

Statistical analysis was performed by using the Mann–Whitney test.

PTEN Mutation Analysis of Human Sporadic Pheochromocytomas

A total of 29 matched normal–tumor pairs of sporadic pheochromocytoma used for this study were obtained from patients (20 females, 9 males, age 21–69 years) who underwent adrenalectomy at the Central Clinical Hospital, Warsaw, Poland, between 1987 and 1999. The diagnosis was based on increased secretion of catecholamines and their metabolites, as well as histological evaluation of the adrenal tissue itself. Excluded from the study were patients with invasive form of pheochromocytoma and those diagnosed with multiple endocrine neoplasia type 2 (MEN2). Blood used for isolation of mononuclear cells was collected from the same patients at the time of surgery.

High molecular weight DNA was extracted from two 10-μM-thick paraffin-embedded sections, or from frozen tissue, when available. Paraffin-embedded tissue sections were de-paraffinized in xylene, washed in 100% ethanol, and digested overnight in 300 μL of the digestion buffer (1% SDS, 0.5 mg/ml Proteinase K, 500 mM Tris, 20 mM EDTA, 10 mM NaCl, pH 8.9) at 58°C. The mixture was then boiled for 10 min., allowed to cool down for 15 min, and extracted with equal volume of phenol/chloroform/isoamyl alcohol (25:24:1, v/v/v). The aqueous phase was collected and DNA was precipitated by addition of 650 μL of 100% ethanol, 180 μL of 10 M ammonium acetate, and 5 μL of 20 mg/ml glycogen. The tubes were spun down at 10,000 × *g* for 10 min at room temperature. The DNA pellet was washed twice with 500 μL of 70% ethanol, air-dried, and dissolved in 10 mM Tris-HCl, pH 8.5.

For extraction from frozen tissue, two 10-μM-thick, cryostat-sliced sections were digested in the digestion buffer and phenol/chloroform-extracted and precipitated. Matched normal DNA sample for each tumor was obtained from peripheral blood lymphocytes by using QiaAmp DNA Mini Kit (Qiagen, Valencia, CA).

Intronic primer pairs were designed to amplify and sequence each of the nine exons of the PTEN gene, including the splice junctions. The sequences of primers used are as follows:

Exon 1, PCR set: GAG GAT TAT TCG TCT TCT CCC/ACT ACG GAC ATT TTC GCA TC, sequencing: ACT ACG GAC ATT TTC GCA TC (R)

Exon 2, PCR set: GTT TGA TTG CTG CAT ATT TCA G/TCT AAA TGA AAA CAC AAC ATG AA, sequencing: GGC TTA GAA ATC TTT TCT AAA TG (R)

Exon 3, PCR set: ATT TCA AAT GTT AGC TCA TTT TG/TTT AGA AGA TAT TTC AAG CAT AC, sequencing: AAT GTT AGC TCA TTT TGT TAA TG (F)

Exon 4, PCR set: CAT TAT AAA GAT TCA GGC AAT G/GAC AGT AAG ATA CAG TCT ATC, sequencing: GAT TCA GGC AAT GTT TGT TAG (F)

Exon 5, PCR set: ACC TGT TAA GTT TGT ATG CAA C/TCC AGG AAG AGG AAA GGA AA, sequencing: AAT CTG AGG TTA TCT TTT TAC C (F)

Exon 6, PCR set: CAT AGC AAT TTA GTG AAA TAA CT/GAT ATG GTT AAG AAA ACT GTT C, sequencing: CCA ATA CAT GGA AGG ATG AG (R)

Exon 7, PCR set: TGA CAG TTT GAC AGT TAA AGG/GGA TAT TTC TCC CAA TGA AAG, sequencing: CAG TTA AAG GCA TTT CCT GTG (F)

Exon 8, PCR set: CTC AGA TTG CCT TAT AAT AGT C/TCA TGT TAC TGC TAC GTA AAC, sequencing: GTA AAT ACA TTC TTC ATA CCA G (F), TTA AAG TAA GTA CTA GAT ATT CC (R)

Exon 9, PCR set: AAG GCC TCT TAA AAG ATC ATG/TTT TCA TGG TGT TTT ATC CCT C, sequencing: AGT AGA GGA GCC GTC AAA TC (F)

Fifty to one hundred nanograms of template genomic DNA were amplified by the polymerase chain reaction (PCR). Initially, the DNA was denatured at 94° C for 5 min, and then the reactions were run for 35–40 cycles (depending on the exon amplified) at 94°C for 30 s, 54°C for 1 min, and 72°C for 1 min, followed by a final extension step at 72°C for 5 min, using Hybaid OmniGene Thermal Cycler (Hybaid, Ashford, Middlesex, United Kingdom). The reactions were performed in 50 μL volume containing: 1 μL target DNA, 37.5 μL water, 5 μL 10 × PCR buffer, 1 μL 25 mM dNTPs, 3 μL DMSO, 0.5 μL (2.5 U) Platinum Taq Polymerase (Invitrogen), 1 μL of the forward primer (350 ng), and 1 μL of the reverse primer (350 ng). Ten microliters of the reaction were run on 0.8% agarose gel to verify amplification of the product. The remaining product was column-purified using QIAquick PCR Purification Kit (Qiagen, Valencia, CA). Cycle sequencing was performed directly on purified PCR products, using a nested sequencing primer and the ABI Prism Dye Terminator Cycle Sequencing Ready Reaction Kit, and analyzed on an ABI 377 automated DNA sequencer using the GeneScan 2.1.1 application program (Perkin-Elmer, Norwalk, CT).

Immunohistochemical Staining

Eight healthy human adrenals were obtained from kidney donors who gave consent for their organs to be used for transplantation at the Department of Transplantation Surgery, Central Clinical Hospital, Warsaw. Eleven sporadic pheochromocytoma tumors were obtained from patients who underwent adrenalectomy. All tissues were formalin-fixed and paraffin-embedded. Five-micrometer sections were stained with hematoxylin–eosin for initial histological evaluation. Additional sections were used for immunohistochemistry. Sections were de-paraffinized in xylene, and then immersed in decreasing concentrations of ethanol, ranging from 100% to 20%, 3 min each treatment, followed by a re-hydration step in distilled water. Antigen retrieval was achieved by boiling the slides in 1mM EDTA for 10 min followed by a slow simmer for 15 min and gradual cooling at RT for 60 min. DNAse I (Gibco, Gaithersburg, MD) treatment was carried out in Tris-buffered saline (TBS), pH 7.5, containing 2.5 μg/mL of the enzyme, for 30 min at room temperature. The tissue sections were then blocked in 1% human serum (Sigma-Aldrich, St. Louis, MO) in TBS for 15 min. Primary antibody hybridization was performed overnight at room temperature in TBS supplemented with 0.1% bovine serum albumin (BSA; Sigma-Aldrich) and appropriate dilution of the primary antibody. PTEN antibody was purchased from NeoMarkers (Fremont, CA) and used at 1:500 dilution. Insulin-like growth factor II (IGF II) rabbit polyclonal antiserum was obtained from GroPep (Adelaide, Australia) and used at 1:3000 dilution. The following day, the slides were washed twice with TBS containing 0.1% Tween-20 (TBST), and then hybridized for 60 min in TBS supplemented with BSA to final concentration of 0.1%, and 1:600 dilution of the biotin-conjugated secondary antibody (Pierce, Rockford, IL). The slides were washed again in two changes of TBST. Endogenous peroxidase activity was blocked by incubating the sections for 30 min in TBST containing 3% hydrogen peroxide and 0.1% sodium azide. After three washes in TBST, signal was amplified by incubating the sections in TBST + 1:400 dilution of the avidin/horseradish peroxidase (Sigma-Aldrich) for 30 min at room temperature. After three washes in TBST, the slides were developed in aminoethylcarbazole (AEC, Sigma-Aldrich) dissolved in acetate buffer (10.5 mM acetic acid, 39.3 mM sodium acetate, pH 5.5) for 15–30 min. Finally, the tissue sections were washed three times with deionized water and counterstained with Mayer's hematoxylin for 1 min. After extensive washing with deionized water, the slides were mounted with glycerol/gelatin (Sigma-Aldrich). Stained section images were acquired at 100× magnification by digital SPOT camera mounted to a Nikon Eclipse E300 microscope using Adobe Photoshop software.

RESULTS

To create an *in vivo* model of the disease, mice deficient in one copy of the Pten gene were created.[26,27] Pten deletion subjects mice to tumors of multiple organs, of which many are seen in human patients. Interestingly, deletion of one copy of the gene predisposes almost 100% of the animals to adrenal neoplasia by the age of 26 weeks. For comparison, normal architecture of the

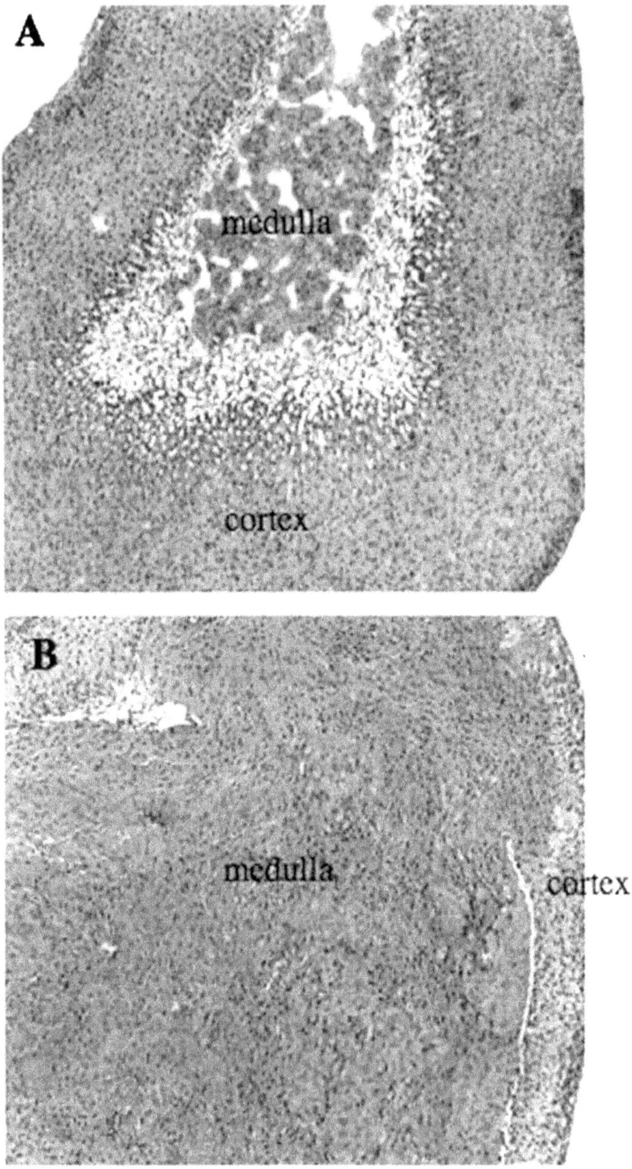

FIGURE 1. H&E staining of murine adrenals. Representative Pten wild-type (**A**) and heterozygous (**B**) adrenal tissue is shown. Abnormal architecture of (**B**) is evident.

adrenal gland is shown in Figure 1A. In contrast, heterozygous mice display an abnormal organization of the adrenal (FIG. 1B) with overgrown medullary tissue. This observation prompted us to postulate that these neoplasms might be of pheochromocytoma nature.

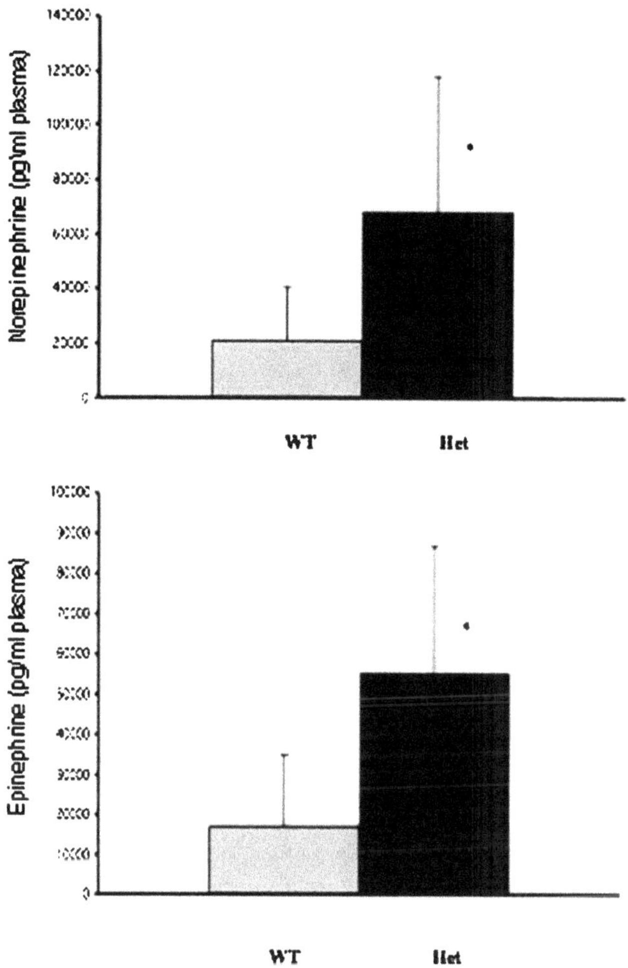

FIGURE 2. Analysis of plasma catecholamine levels in Pten heterozygous (Het) mice. Pten heterozygotes circulate increased levels of norepinephrine and epinephrine. $P < 0.05$.

Analysis of plasma catecholamine levels from Pten wild type ($n = 6$) and heterozygous animals ($n = 6$) showed significant elevation of these agents in the heterozygous animals.

Plasma norepinephrine and epinephrine levels were 20755 ± 19891 for the wild-type versus 68203 ± 49880 for the heterozygous and 17056 ± 18062 for the wild-type versus 55177 ± 316661 for the heterozygous, respectively (FIG. 2). These values were statistically significant. In addition, evaluation of catecholamine levels in the adrenal tissue itself, revealed increased levels of these amines in heterozygous animals (data not shown). Thus biochemical evaluation of active amines confirmed that adrenal neoplasms seen in Pten heterozygous mice are hormonally active pheochromocytomas. We wished to see whether a murine adrenal model of the disease could be extrapolated to humans. We therefore hypothesized that mutation of human PTEN gene may lead to neoplastic transformation of otherwise normal adrenal tissue. Since linkage analysis did not implicate chromosomal region 10q23, in which PTEN gene is located in the familial form of the disease, we decided to examine sporadic pheochromocytoma samples for somatic mutations in the PTEN gene.

DNA was extracted from tumors and entire coding sequence of the PTEN gene was analyzed by direct sequencing. However in a set of 29 samples no point mutations were found.

An alternative mechanism of gene inactivation is by means of promoter hypermethylation. This process occurs on CpG islands of the gene promoter and can be responsible for silencing the gene, even in the absence of mutation. For instance, Sato *et al.*[28] showed PTEN inactivation in one case of 58 primary gastric cancers by this very mechanism and Damman *et al.*[29] demonstrated that 8% of analyzed non-familial pheochromocytomas displayed PTEN promoter hypermethylation. To determine PTEN protein by immunohistochemistry, we performed immunostaining on 11 human sporadic pheochromocytomas and 8 normal adrenals, but no significant difference in the PTEN protein expression between normal (FIG. 3A) and pheochromocytoma (FIG. 3B) tissue could be observed.

Insulin-like growth factor II (IGF II) has been implicated in growth of pheochromocytoma. For instance, Gelato and Vassalotti,[30] in their analysis of seven human pheochromocytomas, measured the content of the IGF II peptide in these tumors and found it considerably elevated, when compared to the normal tissue (2.8–41 μg/g for tumor versus 0.225 ± 0.005 μg for normal). Suzuki *et al.*[31] showed increased immunoreactivity of IGF II antibody toward pheochromocytoma cells, but not toward cells of the normal adrenal medulla. This link seemed very important to investigate, as there was a possibility that Pten loss could be causally correlated with an increased expression of IGF II in human pheochromocytomas. However, first we wished to see whether Pten loss could be linked to IGF II expression in the mouse adrenal tissue. We therefore stained a representative pheochromocytoma derived from a heterozygous mouse for Pten (FIG. 4A) and IGF II (FIG. 4B). Interestingly, PTEN downregulation resulted in increased immunoreactivity of the IGF II antibody toward these cells. In addition, analysis of human sporadic pheochromocytomas for expression of IGF II revealed increased staining for the IGF II peptide in 4 of 11 pheochromocytomas. Representative samples are shown in FIGURES 3C–E.

DISCUSSION

Human PTEN gene is frequently mutated in tissues of many organs. Somatic mutations of PTEN have been reported in tumors of the brain, endometrium,

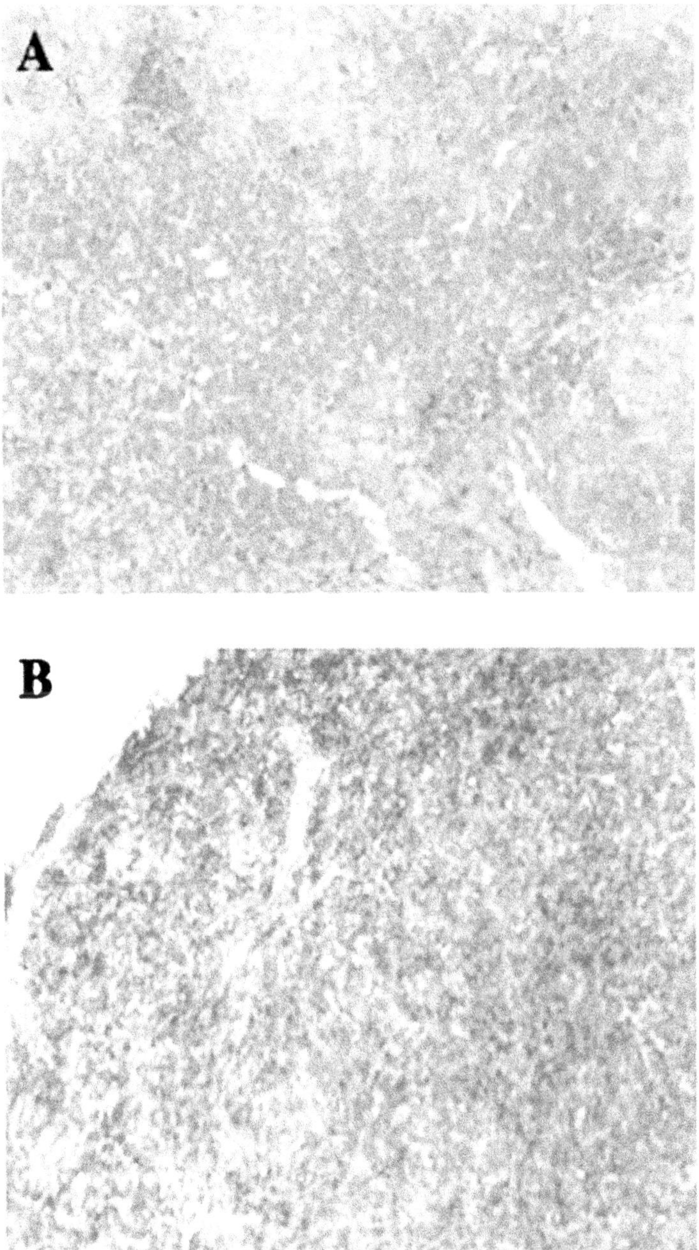

FIGURE 3. PTEN protein expression levels in non-familial pheochromocytoma. Normal human adrenal (**A**) and a pheochromocytoma tissue (**B**) were stained with PTEN antibody. Representative samples are shown. There is no apparent difference in protein expression levels between normal and tumor tissue.

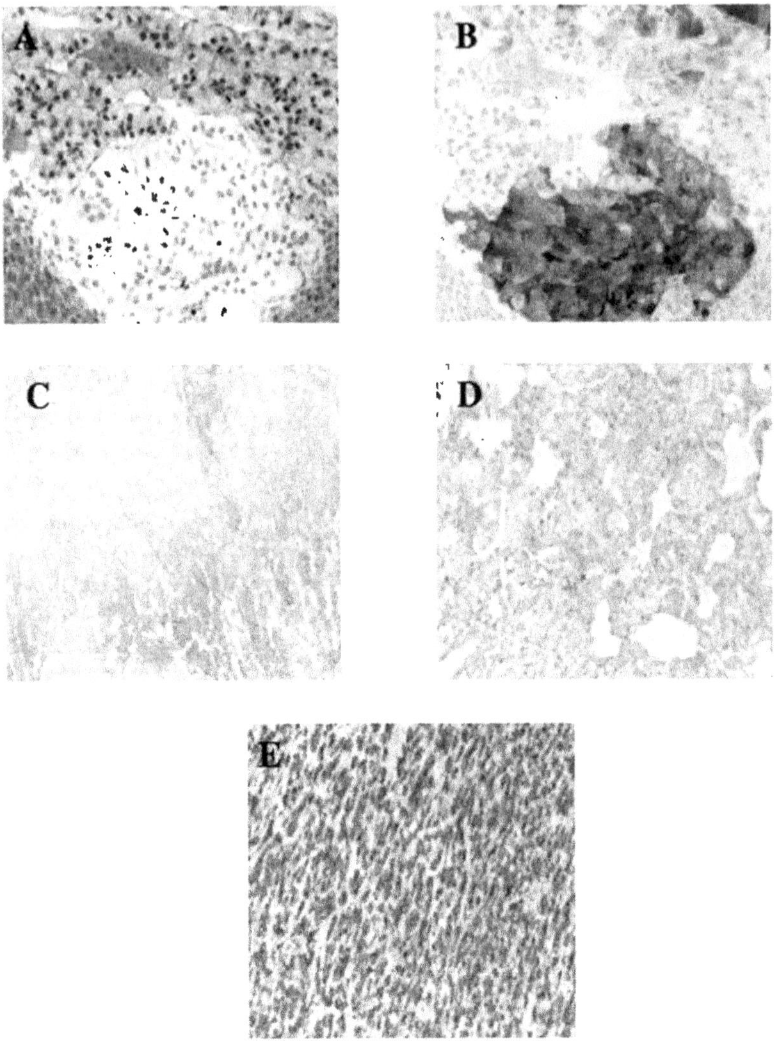

FIGURE 4. IGF II protein expression in adrenal tissue. Serial sections of an adrenal gland harvested from a Pten heterozygous mouse were stained for Pten (**A**) and Igf II (**B**). Downregulation of Pten leads to upregulation of Igf II. Staining for IGF II in normal human adrenal (**C**) and pheochromocytoma tissue (**D, E**). Increased expression of IGF II is seen in (**E**).

prostate, breast, and skin. In addition, PTEN alterations were found to be associated with familial cancer predisposition syndromes: Cowden disease and Bannyan-Zonana. The presence of cutaneous benign hamartomas, as well as visible phenotypic developmental changes in patients suffering from these syndromes, suggested that PTEN haploinsufficiency could affect cell growth during development.

Different mutations were introduced into murine embryonic stem cells to develop a model of tumor progression.[25,26,32] Heterozygous mice generated by Podsypanina *et al.*, exhibited neoplasms in multiple organs including the endometrium, liver, prostate, gastrointestinal tract, thyroid, thymus, and the adrenal glands. Interestingly, many of these abnormalities are also seen in human subjects with established PTEN mutation status. Neoplasia of the thyroid and the adrenal gland was of particular interest since it phenotypically resembled gross pathological changes seen in patients diagnosed with multiple endocrine neoplasia type 2. In addition to that, pheochromocytoma is a characteristic feature of the von Hippel–Lindau disease and neurofibromatosis type I.

One striking phenotype of the heterozygous animals was that almost 100% of them developed bilateral adrenal hyperplasia by the age of 26 weeks. Histologically, these growths resembled pheochromocytoma tumors.

The adult adrenal is composed of two parts: the cortex, which is the outer part, and the inner medulla. The adrenomedullary chromaffin cells synthesize and secrete neurotransmitters and neuropeptides under splanchnic control. Similarly to the architecture of the human adrenal gland, Pten wild-type mice exhibit normal histological patterning of the gland, with small adrenal medulla engulfed by intermediate zone, and the outside tissue of the cortex. However, in Pten heterozygous mice, the medulla is largely overgrown, making the intermediate zone disappear, and pushing the cortex to the outside of the gland (FIG. 1B).

Pheochromocytomas differ from the normal adrenal medulla in that the tumors mainly secrete norepinephrine, whereas the predominant catecholamine secreted by the adrenal medulla is epinephrine. It is norepinephrine that is, therefore, more consistently elevated in patients with pheochromocytoma. Pheochromocytoma-associated elevations in only epinephrine are infrequent[3].

In the analysis of plasma catecholamine levels, norepinephrine was significantly increased in blood of heterozygous animals. Similarly, plasma epinephrine was elevated as well (FIG. 2).

Our study provided evidence that adrenomedullary tumors spontaneously occurring in Pten heterozygous mice are hormonally active pheochromocytomas.

Traditionally, tumor-suppressor genes are isolated because of certain patterns of chromosome loss in families in which prevalence of an inherited cancer predisposition syndrome is high. In pheochromocytoma, loss of heterozygosity occurs frequently on chromosome 17p, 17q, or 3p, implicating p53, NF1, or VHL genes in the disease.

The PTEN gene is mutated in a vast array of sporadic and inherited forms of cancer. No other gene, except the famed p53, has such a high frequency of mutation. One may expect that inactivation of such an essential gene might cause genetic instability, which in due time would subsequently lead to neoplastic transformation of the cell in which the mutation occurred. Inactivation of Pten in the germline of mice, subjects these animals to multiple tumors, including those affecting the adrenal gland. Of knockout mice generated in the past by many groups, only very few develop pheochromocytomas. For instance, animals heterozygous for Nf1 develop this type of cancer in about 50% of the cases.[33] Taking into consideration conservation of key regulatory pathways among species, but also bearing in mind certain differences existing therein, one could hypothesize that the human PTEN gene might be altered in sporadic pheochromocytoma. This alteration might occur through simple inactivation of both copies of the gene, either by a gross deletion of a chromosomal fragment containing one copy of the gene and subtle mutation of the other allele, or mutation of both alleles. However no gross chromosomal aberrations occur within the PTEN locus in pheochromocytoma. To test whether PTEN point mutations might be, at least in part, responsible for pathogenesis of pheochromocytoma, 29 sporadic tumors, for which normal tissue was available, were analyzed for mutations within coding sequence of the PTEN gene. However, analysis of the assembled open reading frame revealed no mutations within PTEN. One possible explanation is that the number of samples used for analysis was too small to reveal any mutations. For example, Brauch *et al.*[34] investigated 62 German patients with pheochromocytoma without a history of hereditary disease, and found VHL mutations in only 2 patients (3%); no mutations were found in the RET gene. Bar *et al.*[35] studied 27 sporadic cases. Only 1 patient, with atypical clinical presentation, had a VHL germline mutation, and none had a RET mutation. Both groups concluded that sporadic pheochromocytomas are rarely associated with germline mutations in either of these genes. The mutation rate of PTEN in sporadic pheochromocytoma may be even lower, thus explaining our inability to identify any mutations in the studied DNA samples.

To investigate a possibility of PTEN downregulation by mechanisms other than mutation, we looked at PTEN protein levels by immunohistochemistry. Even though we did not observe any difference in PTEN protein expression in the set of 11 sporadic pheochromocytomas, we did see upregulation of IGF II expression in 4 samples.

Overexpression of the IGF II peptide is a frequent event in human pheochromocytoma, as well as other types of cancer. In human hepatoma cells and in gastric cancer PTEN downregulates IGF II expression.[36,37] Interestingly, we found that upregulation of IGF II peptide was present even in cells expressing normal PTEN protein levels. In contrast to human tissue, in mouse adrenal lesions, the area of PTEN loss corresponds to the area of IGF II overexpression (FIG. 4A and B). It is not clear why the same phenomenon is not true for human adrenal tissue. It seems that in spite of many similarities existing between mouse and human genetics and physiology, signaling in which PTEN is a player does not seem to be equally conserved in the adrenal tissue of the two species. This could be exemplified by a link between PTEN loss and human brain tumor formation. PTEN loss in glioblastoma multiforme is as high as 60% of tumors with loss of heterozygosity.[19] In contrast, mice heterozygous for Pten do not develop brain tumors.

Another likely explanation for the absence of PTEN mutations in the analyzed group of 29 tumors is that inactivation of PTEN in human sporadic pheochromocytoma is such an unusually infrequent event that it is very difficult to detect. Alternatively, mechanisms other than mutation in just one tumor-suppressor gene may be responsible for development of sporadic pheochromocytoma. One rationale for generating tumor-suppressor mutant mice is that they may serve as a useful model for the corresponding human disease. A number of explanations may be provided to rationalize the lack of correlation between mouse and human disease. The species-specific differences could be a result of relatively subtle differences in growth control pathways in mouse and human cells of particular tissues. Also, the differences could also be explained by species-dependent dissimilarities in susceptibility to loss of the remaining wild-type tumor suppressor allele. In conclusion, our results show that in spite of many similarities between murine and human physiology, in humans PTEN does not seem to be a major gene involved in pathogenesis of pheochromocytoma.

REFERENCES

1. MANGER, W.M. & R.W. GIFFORD. 1996. Clinical and Experimental Pheochromocytoma. Blackwell Science. Cambridge, MA.
2. WALLACE, M.R. *et al.* 1990. Type 1 neurofibromatosis gene: identification of a large transcript disrupted in three NF1 patients. Science. **249:** 181–186.
3. PACAK, K. *et al.* 2001. Pheochromocytoma. *In* Adrenal Disorders. A.N. Margioris & G.P. Chrousos, Eds.: 379–413. Humana Press. Totowa, NJ.
4. CARLSON, K.M. *et al.* 1994. Single missense mutation in the tyrosine kinase catalytic domain of the RET protooncogene is associated with multiple endocrine neoplasia type 2B. Proc. Natl Acad. Sci. US A **91:** 1579–1583.
5. ENG, C. *et al.* 1994. Point mutation within the tyrosine kinase domain of the RET proto-oncogene in multiple endocrine neoplasia type 2B and related sporadic tumours. Hum. Mol. Genet. **3:** 237–241.
6. ENG, C. *et al.* 1995. Mutations in the RET proto-oncogene and the von Hippel-Lindau disease tumour suppressor gene in sporadic and syndromic phaeochromocytomas. J. Med. Genet. **32:** 934–937.
7. GIMENEZ-ROQUEPLO, A.P. *et al.* 2002. Functional consequences of a SDHB gene mutation in an apparently sporadic pheochromocytoma. J. Clin. Endocrinol. Metab. **87:** 4771–4774.
8. GIMM, O. *et al.* 2000. Somatic and occult germ-line mutations in SDHD, a mitochondrial complex II gene, in nonfamilial pheochromocytoma. Cancer Res. **60:** 6822–6825.
9. NEUMANN, H.P. *et al.* 2002. Germ-line mutations in nonsyndromic pheochromocytoma. N. Engl. J. Med. **346:** 1459–1466.
10. LI, J. *et al.* 1997. PTEN, a putative protein tyrosine phosphatase gene mutated in human brain, breast, and prostate cancer. Science. **275:** 1943–1947.
11. STECK, P.A. *et al.* 1997. Identification of a candidate tumour suppressor gene, MMAC1, at chromosome 10q23.3 that is mutated in multiple advanced cancers. Nat. Genet. **15:** 356–362.

12. LI, D.M. & H. SUN. 1997. TEP1, encoded by a candidate tumor suppressor locus, is a novel protein tyrosine phosphatase regulated by transforming growth factor beta. Cancer Res. **57:** 2124–2129.
13. FEILOTTER, H.E. *et al.* 1999. Analysis of the 10q23 chromosomal region and the PTEN gene in human sporadic breast carcinoma. Br. J. Cancer. **79:** 718–723.
14. RHEI, E. *et al.* 1997. Mutation analysis of the putative tumor suppressor gene PTEN/MMAC1 in primary breast carcinomas. Cancer Res. **57:** 3657–3659.
15. CAIRNS, P. *et al.* 1997. Frequent inactivation of PTEN/MMAC1 in primary prostate cancer. Cancer Res. **57:** 4997–5000.
16. WANG, S.I., R. PARSONS & M. ITTMANN. 1998. Homozygous deletion of the PTEN tumor suppressor gene in a subset of prostate adenocarcinomas. Clin. Cancer Res. **4:** 811–815.
17. TASHIRO, H. *et al.* 1997. Mutations in PTEN are frequent in endometrial carcinoma but rare in other common gynecological malignancies. Cancer Res. **57:** 3935–3940.
18. RISINGER, J.I. *et al.* 1997. PTEN/MMAC1 mutations in endometrial cancers. Cancer Res. **57:** 4736–4738.
19. WANG, S.I. *et al.* 1997. Somatic mutations of PTEN in glioblastoma multiforme. Cancer Res. **57:** 4183–4186.
20. CHIARIELLO, E. *et al.* 1998. PTEN/MMAC1 mutations in primary glioblastomas and short-term cultures of malignant gliomas. Oncogene. **16:** 541–545.
21. GULDBERG, P. *et al.* 1997. Disruption of the MMAC1/PTEN gene by deletion or mutation is a frequent event in malignant melanoma. Cancer Res. **57:** 3660–3663.
22. REIFENBERGER, J. *et al.* 2000. Allelic losses on chromosome arm 10q and mutation of the PTEN (MMAC1) tumour suppressor gene in primary and metastatic malignant melanomas. Virchows Arch. **436:** 487–493.
23. LIAW, D. *et al.* 1997. Germline mutations of the PTEN gene in Cowden disease, an inherited breast and thyroid cancer syndrome. Nat Genet. **16:** 64–67.
24. MARSH, D.J. *et al.* 1997. Germline mutations in PTEN are present in Bannayan-Zonana syndrome. Nat. Genet. **16:** 333–334.
25. DI CRISTOFANO, A. *et al.* 1998. Pten is essential for embryonic development and tumour suppression. Nat. Genet. **19:** 348–355.
26. PODSYPANINA, K. *et al.* 1999. Mutation of Pten/Mmac1 in mice causes neoplasia in multiple organ systems. Proc. Natl Acad. Sci. USA **96:** 1563–1568.
27. PODSYPANINA, K. *et al.* 2001. An inhibitor of mTOR reduces neoplasia and normalizes p70/S6 kinase activity in Pten± mice. Proc. Natl Acad. Sci. USA **98:** 10320–10325.
28. SATO, K. *et al.* 2002. Analysis of genetic and epigenetic alterations of the PTEN gene in gastric cancer. Virchows Arch. **440:** 160–165.
29. DAMMANN, R. *et al.* 2005. Frequent promoter methylation of tumor-related genes in sporadic and men2-associated pheochromocytomas. Exp. Clin. Endocrinol. Diabetes. **113:** 1–7.
30. GELATO, M.C. & J. VASSALOTTI. 1990. Insulin-like growth factor-II: possible local growth factor in pheochromocytoma. J. Clin. Endocrinol. Metab. **71:** 1168–1174.
31. SUZUKI, T. *et al.* 1992. Immunocytochemical demonstration of IGF-II immunoreactivity in human phaeochromocytoma and extra-adrenal abdominal paraganglioma. J. Pathol. **167:** 199–203.

32. SUZUKI, A. *et al.* 1998. High cancer susceptibility and embryonic lethality associated with mutation of the PTEN tumor suppressor gene in mice. Curr. Biol. **8:** 1169–1178.
33. VISKOCHIL, D. *et al.* 1990. Deletions and a translocation interrupt a cloned gene at the neurofibromatosis type 1 locus. Cell. **62:** 187–192.
34. BRAUCH, H. *et al.* 1997. Sporadic pheochromocytomas are rarely associated with germline mutations in the VHL tumor suppressor gene or the ret protooncogene. J. Clin. Endocrinol. Metab. **82:** 4101–4104.
35. BAR, M. *et al.* 1997. Sporadic phaeochromocytomas are rarely associated with germline mutations in the von Hippel-Lindau and RET genes. Clin. Endocrinol. (Oxf). **47:** 707–712.
36. HWANG, P.H. *et al.* 2005. PTEN/MMAC1 enhances the growth inhibition by anticancer drugs with downregulation of IGF-II expression in gastric cancer cells. Exp. Mol. Med. **37:** 391–398.
37. KANG-PARK, S. & Y.I. LEE. 2003. PTEN modulates insulin-like growth factor II (IGF-II)-mediated signaling; the protein phosphatase activity of PTEN downregulates IGF-II expression in hepatoma cells. FEBS Lett. **545:** 203–208.

Biochemical Diagnosis and Localization of Pheochromocytoma

Can We Reach a Consensus?

ASHLEY GROSSMAN,[a] KAREL PACAK,[b] ANNA SAWKA,[c] JACQUES W. M. LENDERS,[d] DEBRA HARLANDER,[e] ROBERT T. PEASTON,[f] RODNEY REZNEK,[g] JAMES SISSON,[h] AND GRAEME EISENHOFER[i]

[a]*Department of Endocrinology, St. Bartholomew's Hospital, West Smithfield, London, UK*

[b]*Reproductive Biology and Medicine Branch, National Institute of Child Health and Human Development, National Institutes of Health, Bethesda, Maryland 20892, USA*

[c]*Department of Medicine, University of Toronto, Toronto, Ontario, Canada*

[d]*Department of General Internal Medicine, St. Radboud University Hospital, Nijmegen, the Netherlands*

[e]*Pheochromocytoma Support Group, Camden, New York 13316, USA*

[f]*Department of Clinical Biochemistry, Freeman Hospital, Newcastle upon Tyne, UK*

[g]*Division of Radiology, St. Bartholomew's Hospital, West Smithfield, London, UK*

[h]*Department of Radiology, University of Michigan Hospitals, Ann Arbor, Michigan 48109, USA*

[i]*Clinical Neurocardiology Section, National Institute of Neurological Disorders and Stroke, National Institutes of Health, Bethesda, Maryland 20892, USA*

ABSTRACT: **Pheochromocytomas can have a highly variable presentation, making diagnosis challenging. To think of the tumor represents the crucial initial step, but establishing the diagnosis requires biochemical evidence of excessive catecholamine production and imaging studies to localize the source. Currently, however, there exist no generally agreed upon guidelines based on which tests and testing algorithms should be used to confirm and locate or exclude a suspected pheochromocytoma. Choice of biochemical tests and imaging studies instead usually depends on institutional experience. At the First International Symposium on Pheochromocytoma (ISP2005), held in Bethesda in October 2005, a panel of experts and patient representatives discussed current problems and available options for tumor diagnosis and localization and formulated**

Address for correspondence: Ashley Grossman, M.D., F.R.C.P., FMed. Sci., Department of Endocrinology, St. Bartholomew's Hospital, West Smithfield, London, EC1A 7BE, UK. Voice: 44 20 760 18343, fax: 44 20 760 18505.
e-mail: a.b.grossman@qmul.ac.uk

Ann. N.Y. Acad. Sci. 1073: 332–347 (2006). © 2006 New York Academy of Sciences.
doi: 10.1196/annals.1353.038

recommendations, which were subsequently agreed upon by those in attendance at the meeting. This article summarizes the discussion and recommendations derived from that session.

KEYWORDS: pheochromocytoma; biochemical diagnosis; metanephrines; catecholamines; localization; computed tomography; magnetic resonance imaging; MIBG; positron emission tomography

INTRODUCTION

Pheochromocytomas, although a rare cause of hypertension, are dangerous but usually surgically curable tumors that require consideration among large numbers of patients, at considerable cost to healthcare systems. Among overall numbers of patients tested for pheochromocytoma, less than 1% actually harbor the tumor, but, based on autopsy studies, probably as many cases or more are missed than are diagnosed.[1–3] Thus, although frequently searched for and rarely found, the tumor remains an overlooked clinical entity.

As discussed by Dr. William Manger (New York University Medical Center, New York) in the keynote address at the First International Symposium on Pheochromocytoma (ISP2005), diagnosis of the tumor first requires recognition of the varied clinical conditions and situations where pheochromocytoma should be considered. To consider the possibility of the tumor represents the crucial initial step, but confirming the diagnosis requires biochemical measurements of catecholamines and catecholamine metabolites in urine or plasma, followed by imaging studies to localize the source preparatory to surgical removal.

A major problem in reaching or excluding the diagnosis of pheochromocytoma is that there are no generally agreed upon guidelines about how and which biochemical tests and imaging studies should best be carried out, interpreted, and followed-up. Practices vary among different centers, and recommendations are more often based on institutional experience than on evidence-based medicine. Representatives of patient support groups at ISP2005 also indicated that there was a need for improved education of clinicians in how to recognize, diagnose, and localize the tumor, and they expressed frustration that progress seemed hampered by lack of agreement and conflicting views from experts in the field.

A "breakout session" was therefore held during ISP2005 with the aim of fostering resolution of issues and problems associated with biochemical diagnosis and localization of pheochromocytoma. More than 40 participants, including leading experts in the field and representatives from patient support groups, attended the session. Under the guidance of impartial moderators (Dr. Ashley Grossman, St Bartholomew's Hospital, London, UK, and Dr. Hendrik Lehnert, University of Warwick, UK), participants were asked to formulate recommendations that were subsequently discussed and agreed upon at a final general session of this symposium where all attendees could be present. Recommendations were based on answers to a series of questions, as detailed below.

- What are the preferred biochemical tests or testing algorithms for confirming or excluding pheochromocytoma and what cost–benefit factors should be considered?
- What precautions should be considered to minimize or avoid false-positive results or drug interference during biochemical testing and imaging procedures?
- What evidence for the presence of a tumor justifies imaging studies?
- What imaging strategies are appropriate for localization of pheochromocytoma and in what order should they be applied?

This report reviews the discussion held at the breakout session, where possible outlines generally agreed upon recommendations, and where not possible seeks to account for why there may be no clear answer and what future advances may assist in reaching an answer. Because the presentation of pheochromocytoma can be variable and complex,[4] which exerts a subsequent impact on the choice of biochemical tests and imaging strategies, outlined recommendations are not intended as strict guidelines, but as complements to sound clinical judgment.

BIOCHEMICAL DIAGNOSIS

An important recommendation agreed upon by all attending participants at the breakout and final discussion sessions of ISP2005 was that initial biochemical testing for pheochromocytoma should include measurements of plasma concentrations or urinary excretion of fractionated metanephrines (separate measurements of normetanephrine and metanephrine) wherever these tests are available. Importantly, this recommendation does not exclude the additional use of other tests (e.g., urinary or plasma catecholamines) or measurements of both plasma and urinary fractionated metanephrines during initial testing for the tumor. Whereas other tests are used during initial testing, these should be used in conjunction with measurements of fractionated metanephrines in plasma or urine.

The importance of measurements of urinary or plasma fractionated metanephrines for the diagnosis of pheochromocytoma is principally based on research by National Institutes of Health (NIH) investigators establishing that pheochromocytomas contain catechol-*O*-methyltransferase, the presence of which results in the metabolism of catecholamines to metanephrines within tumor cells.[5–7] It is further proposed that production of metanephrines within tumor cells is continuous and more accurately reflects tumor mass than release of catecholamines, which can occur episodically or not at all in nonsecretory tumors. Consistent with these concepts, it has now been established by four independent groups of investigators that measurements of plasma

TABLE 1. Sensitivity and specificity of measurements of plasma fractionated metanephrines for diagnosis of pheochromocytoma

	Study Cohort (n)		URL (nmol/L)		Diagnostic Performance	
Center	Pheo	No pheo	NMN	MN	Sensitivity	Specificity
Vienna[9]	17	14	0.66	0.31	100%	100%
NIH[10]	214	644	0.61	0.31	99%	89%
			2.19	1.20	79%[a]	100%
Mayo Clinic[12]	56	445	0.90	0.50	96%	85%
University of Essen[13]	24	126	0.69	0.19	96%	80%
Freeman Hospital[b]	11	114	0.90	0.55	100%	91%
Cleveland Clinic[c]	32	0	0.90	0.50	97%	—
			2.19	1.20	84%[a]	—
All centers	354	1,343			98%	87%

URL = upper reference limits of reference intervals; NMN = normetanephrine; MN = metanephrine.

[a]Denotes values of diagnostic sensitivity calculated using upper reference limits adjusted to provide 100% specificity; indicates percentage of patients where there is close to 100% probability of a pheochromocytoma.

[b]Peaston, R.T., Neely, R.D.G. 2005. Biochemical diagnosis of pheochromocytoma: the role of plasma metanephrines. Proceedings of the First International Symposium on Pheochromocytoma [abstract]. 150.

[c]Bravo, E.L., Bravo, T. 2005. Clinical characteristics of incidentally discovered pheochromocytoma from an analysis of 50 proven cases. Proceedings of the First International Symposium on Pheochromocytoma [abstract] 27. This volume.

metanephrines provides superior diagnostic sensitivity over measurements of plasma or urinary catecholamines for the detection of pheochromocytoma.[8–13] A further study presented at ISP2005 by Dr. Robert Peaston (Freeman Hospital, Newcastle upon Tyne, UK) provided documentation by a fifth group that measurements of plasma metanephrines provide improved accuracy over urinary catecholamines for the diagnosis of the tumor (TABLE 1).

Several studies involving measurements of urinary fractionated metanephrines have similarly indicated that these tests provide superior diagnostic sensitivity over urinary or plasma catecholamines, urinary vanillylmandelic acid, or total metanephrines, the latter measured as the combined sum of normetanephrine and metanephrine by early spectrophotometric methods.[10,14–17] Taken together, the weight of accumulating evidence clearly indicates that measurements of fractionated metanephrines in urine or plasma provide superior diagnostic sensitivity over urinary or plasma measurements of catecholamines and other catecholamine metabolites.

There was no consensus at the meeting as to whether measurements of plasma or urinary fractionated metanephrines offer the preferred test, although evidence by two different groups has indicated that the plasma test may offer diagnostic advantages over the urine test.[10,13] Against this, Dr. Emmanuel Bravo (Cleveland Clinic, OH) presented evidence at ISP2005 that measurements of urinary fractionated metanephrines were superior to plasma-free

TABLE 2. Relative merits and demerits of measurements of urinary fractionated and plasma-free metanephrines for the diagnosis of pheochromocytoma

Urinary Fractionated Metanephrines	Plasma-Free Metanephrines
Well-established, widely available test	Relatively new test with limited availability
Urinary concentrations (200–2,000 nmol) make analysis relatively easy	Plasma concentrations (0.1–0.5 nmol) can make analysis difficult
Easy for clinicians to implement with minimal expenditure of time and effort	Blood collections require some time and effort by medical staff
Twenty-four-hour collections can be inconvenient for patients	Blood sampling relatively more convenient for patients
Problems with reliability of incomplete timed urine collections	Collection and handling of blood samples can be better regulated
Difficult to control dietary and daily life influences on sympathoadrenal function	Influences of diet and sympathoadrenal function more easily controlled
In children 24-h collections are difficult and results are difficult to interpret without age-appropriate reference intervals	In children blood sampling may be stressful, but results are more easily interpreted without age-appropriate reference intervals
Urine collections may be inappropriate in patients with renal failure	Test is applicable in patients with renal failure

metanephrines for the diagnosis of incidentally discovered pheochromocytomas; the urinary test returned positive results in 96% of patients with the tumor compared to 84% for the plasma test. The latter value, however, was obtained using upper limits of reference intervals identical to those described elsewhere that had been adjusted to provide 100% specificity.[10] Thus, the results of the study by Bravo may be reinterpreted to indicate that 84% of the patients with pheochromocytoma had elevations of plasma metanephrines of sufficiently high magnitude to provide close to 100% probability of a tumor. When results were re-examined using the appropriate laboratory-derived reference intervals, diagnostic sensitivity was 97% (TABLE 1).

Any differences in overall diagnostic accuracy of plasma compared to urinary fractionated metanephrines are probably relatively small compared to differences of either test of metanephrines with tests of plasma or urinary catecholamines. Choice of either plasma or urinary fractionated metanephrines may benefit from consideration of additional factors as outlined in TABLE 2.

Dr. Anna Sawka (University of Toronto, Toronto, Canada), who described the experience of investigators at the Mayo Clinic in the diagnosis of pheochromocytoma, contended that while plasma measurements of metanephrines offered high diagnostic *sensitivity*, the test was not widely available and has lower *specificity* compared with some other tests, which has a negative impact on cost-effectiveness.[18] Dr. Karel Pacak (NIH, Bethesda, MD) countered that cost–benefit projections should take into account the potential costs of missing the diagnosis due to use of tests with inadequate sensitivity.

It was further indicated by Dr. Graeme Eisenhofer (NIH, Bethesda, MD) that because missing a pheochromocytoma can have deadly consequences, one of the most important considerations in the choice of initial test is a high level of reliability that the test will provide a positive result in that rare patient with the tumor. In other words, the initial screening test should be of very high sensitivity. This conversely also provides confidence that a negative result reliably excludes the tumor, thus avoiding the need for multiple or repeat biochemical testing or even costly and unnecessary imaging studies to rule out the tumor, aspects that also should be considered in any cost–benefit analysis. There was general agreement with the conclusions reached by Dr. Sawka in her decision analysis that it was not cost-effective to screen all hypertensives for pheochromocytoma, at least using currently available biochemical tests. In contrast, for individuals genetically predisposed to syndromic pheochromocytoma or identified with an adrenal incidentaloma, the risk or pretest probability of disease is so high that biochemical testing is usually warranted for all such patients.

It was recognized that while measurements of plasma or urinary metanephrines may fail to detect some tumors that synthesize only small amounts of catecholamines or exclusively dopamine, patients with such tumors have an atypical clinical presentation that can benefit from consideration of other testing strategies. As originally established by Dr. Morris Brown (University of Cambridge, Cambridge, UK), present at the breakout session, urinary dopamine is mainly derived from renal extraction of circulating dihydroxyphenylalanine and local conversion to dopamine by aromatic amino-acid decarboxylase.[19] Thus, measurements of plasma dopamine or its *O*-methylated metabolite, methoxytyramine (which may be measured in urinary and plasma assays of metanephrines), provide better methods for detecting dopamine-producing tumors than measurements of urinary dopamine.[20] In general, though, it should be emphasized that in any test the sensitivity and specificity are inter-related, and dependent on reference intervals. Assessment of diagnostic efficacy is therefore most appropriately achieved by combined examination of sensitivity and specificity in a given clinical context.

A second recommendation arising from the discussions related to the above considerations at the breakout session was that reference intervals for initial tests of urinary or plasma-fractionated metanephrines should be established primarily to ensure optimum diagnostic sensitivity, with specificity being a secondary consideration. Suboptimal diagnostic specificity was nevertheless agreed to present a significant problem. To address the problem of false-positive results, it was further recommended that testing algorithms should not simply rely on a binary approach for test interpretation (i.e., consideration of whether a test yields a positive or negative result), but should take advantage of the continuous nature of biochemical test results (FIG. 1). For example, while a single elevation of urinary or plasma normetanephrine slightly above the upper reference intervals may only marginally increase the pre- to post-test probability of pheochromocytoma, an elevation of more than fourfold above

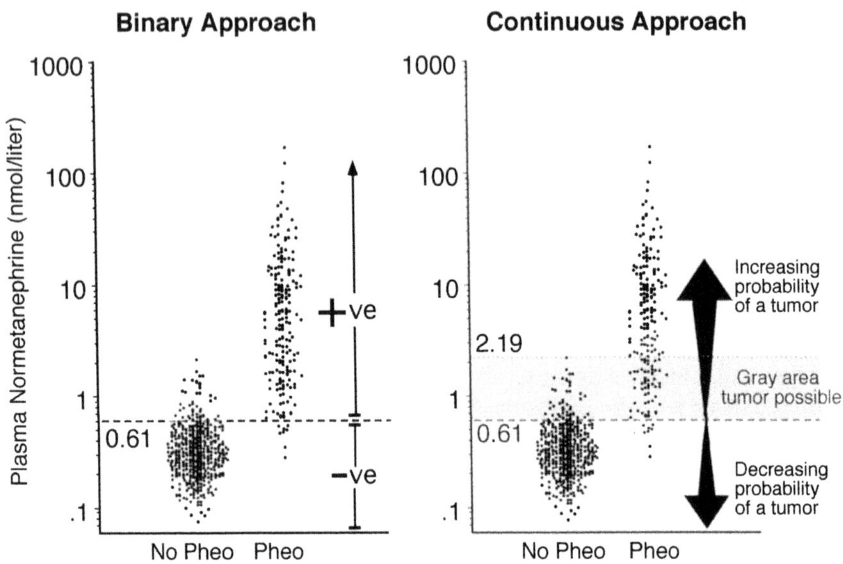

FIGURE 1. The binary versus continuous approach for the interpretation of biochemical test results is illustrated using measurements of plasma normetanephrine. The *horizontal dashed line* in both panels illustrates the upper reference limits (0.61 nmol/L) used to determine whether a plasma concentration of normetanephrine is normal or elevated (negative vs. positive test results according to the binary approach). With some exceptions, noted as follows, pheochromocytoma may be excluded when plasma levels of normetanephrine fall below that level. Exceptions where plasma values in patients with pheochromocytoma fall below the upper reference limit include patients with isolated elevations of plasma metanephrine (metabolite of epinephrine) or methoxytyramine (metabolite of dopamine) or patients with small or microscopic tumors and no other biochemical evidence or signs or symptoms of catecholamine excess. The *horizontal dotted line* in the panel on the right illustrates the level of plasma normetanephrine (2.19 nmol/L) above which the test provides 100% diagnostic specificity. Results that are situated between the two levels (*gray area*) indicate a tumor is possible, with the probability increasing the higher the value of the test result. Levels above 2.19 nmol/L provide close to 100% probability of a tumor.

these intervals is associated with close to 100% probability of the tumor. In the latter situation more emphasis may be placed on immediately locating the tumor, whereas in the former situation involving test results in the "gray area," there is more of a need to first exclude a false-positive result. Again, some idea of the diagnostic overlap that is seen in weighing sensitivity against specificity is shown by the results in FIGURE 1.

The above recommendations followed lengthy discussion at the breakout session centering on reference intervals, and this was clearly contingent upon the form of sample collection and the appropriate methods for blood sampling. Ms. Debra Harlander (Camden, NY), representing the Pheochromocytoma Support Group, outlined how highly variable instructions for blood sampling from various laboratories and institutions were causing confusion among patients and clinicians. At some centers blood sampling was done after 20 min of supine rest using an indwelling i.v. cannula with patients fasting and avoiding acetaminophen (paracetamol). In contrast, elsewhere instructions were inconsistent, with sampling usually carried out with patients seated.

The issue of seated versus supine blood sampling was addressed by Jacques Lenders (St. Radboud University Hospital, Nimegen, the Netherlands), who presented evidence at ISP2005 that blood sampling in the seated position resulted in 25–30% increases in plasma metanephrines compared to sampling after 20 min of supine rest. It was further shown that use of reference intervals established from blood samples collected in the seated position resulted in reduced diagnostic sensitivity, while testing for pheochromocytoma in seated patients using reference intervals established from samples collected in the supine position substantially reduced diagnostic specificity. It was therefore agreed by all present that reference intervals for plasma free metanephrines should be established using samples collected with the patient in the supine position. To minimize false-positive results, it was further recommended that blood samples for the diagnosis of pheochromocytoma should ideally be collected after 20 min of supine rest. A caveat to this recommendation was the recognition that blood sampling is usually done by phlebotomists licensed to carry out the procedure according to specific practices. It was therefore proposed that where blood sampling in the seated position returns positive results in the "gray area," repeat testing should be carried out with blood samples collected after 20 min of supine rest, and where necessary carried out by clinical staff not subject to the same restrictions as phlebotomy technicians.

The use of appropriate normotensive versus hypertensive reference populations,[21] including (as pointed out by Dr. Sawka) requirements for age adjustments,[22] and by Dr. Eisenhofer, gender influences,[23] represented other issues touched upon during the breakout session that may assist in interpretation of biochemical tests of catecholamine excess. Taking into account such variables, together with the continuous nature of test results, to calculate changes in pre- to post-test probabilities of disease for individual patients may be facilitated by advances in test reporting to provide improved approaches to guide clinical decision making for the future. Irrespective of such advances, difficulties in distinguishing true- from false-positive results for tests of catecholamine excess will almost certainly persist, particularly when emphasis is placed on diagnostic sensitivity over specificity.

There was general agreement at the breakout session that imaging studies to search for a suspected tumor should usually not be initiated until biochemical or other evidence of a pheochromocytoma is reasonably compelling. The possibility of false-positive biochemical test results should first be considered and wherever possible excluded. Medications represent common causes of false-positive results, either through direct analytical interference with techniques used to measure catecholamines and catecholamine metabolites, or through pharmacological influences on actual plasma or urinary levels.

The former causes tend to be method-specific and vary from laboratory to laboratory, making general recommendations on what medications to avoid largely inappropriate. Among the latter causes, tricyclic antidepressants and the α-adrenoceptor blocker, phenoxybenzamine, were described in one study as responsible for close to 50% of all false-positive elevations of plasma and urinary norepinephrine and normetanephrine.[24] Repeat testing after discontinuation of suspect medications can be used to exclude these as causes of false-positive results. Use of confirmatory follow-up tests, such as urinary fractionated metanephrines to support patterns of increases in initial measurements of plasma metanephrines, or *vice versa*, were outlined as other approaches to exclude false-positive results, particularly where there is concern about analytical validity.

In all approaches involving multiple tests of catecholamine excess, due consideration should also be given to the inter-dependence of the various analytes that may compromise Bayesian approaches to clinical decision making. A false-positive elevation of urinary normetanephrine due to sympathetic activation is also likely to be associated with false-positive elevations of urinary and plasma norepinephrine and plasma normetanephrine. Thus, while elevations in the latter analytes measured in follow-up tests may serve to confirm the validity of the initial elevated urinary normetanephrine, those additional positive test results do not always provide increased evidence of a pheochromocytoma any more than they provide increased evidence for sympathetic activation. In such situations suppression tests using clonidine or pentolinium can be useful for distinguishing true-positive results due to a pheochromocytoma from false-positive results due to sympathetic activation.[25,26] Such tests, although originally developed to distinguish true- from false-positive elevations of plasma catecholamines, may also be applied to distinguish true- from false-positive elevations of urinary metanephrines[27] or plasma normetanephrine.[24]

TUMOR LOCALIZATION

Several recent advances in our understanding of pheochromocytoma are now important for physicians to consider when deciding on which imaging modality to use for localization of pheochromocytoma. As outlined at ISP2005 by Dr. Hartmut Neumann (University of Freiburg, Freiburg, Germany) and Dr. Anne-Paule Gimenez-Roqueplo (Université Paris-Descartes, Paris, France), between 12% and 24% of patients with apparently sporadic pheochromocytoma may in fact be carriers of germline mutations, indicating hereditary disease with a predisposition for bilateral adrenal, extra-adrenal, or multiple tumors.[28,29] Malignant pheochromocytoma, although rare in multiple endocrine neoplasia type 2 (MEN 2) and von Hippel-Lindau (VHL) syndrome, is common in patients with succinate dehydrogenase B (SDHB) mutations, and is present in about 10% of patients overall at presentation.[29–31] Further, as outlined at the meeting by Dr. Pierre-François Plouin (Université Paris-Descartes, Paris, France), about 11% of pheochromocytomas recur as malignant disease. Furthermore, improved biochemical diagnosis of pheochromocytoma requires imaging techniques to locate increasingly smaller tumors (often around 1 cm in size). In addition, the more frequent use of imaging techniques is leading to increased recognition of "adrenal incidentalomas" as an important clinical finding, requiring follow-up to distinguish functional tumors (e.g., pheochromocytomas) from the more common benign cortical adenomas.[32,33] Well-defined biochemical phenotypes of adrenal versus extra-adrenal pheochromocytomas and relationships of biochemical findings with tumor mass may further help guide the proper use of anatomical and functional imaging studies.[34]

Below are outlined some of the more important considerations and recommendations on the use of anatomical and functional imaging studies (including their advantages and disadvantages) as discussed during the breakout session. Careful selection of imaging studies should decrease costs and radiation exposure, as well as time and effort required for correct diagnostic localization of tumors.

Anatomical Imaging Studies

In general, participants felt strongly that localization of pheochromocytoma should only be initiated once the clinical evidence for the tumor is reasonably compelling. For most patients when initial suspicion is based on signs and symptoms, such evidence may include strongly positive biochemical test results (e.g., as illustrated in FIGURE 1) or, when results are not strongly positive, repeated testing after ruling out causes of false-positive results. Imaging studies may be warranted in patients in whom the risk of pheochromocytoma is high because of a hereditary predisposition or a previous history of the tumor, even when biochemical evidence of a pheochromocytoma is less than compelling. In some such patients, imaging studies may be appropriate as part of a periodic surveillance plan, not only for pheochromocytoma, but also to check for other tumors (e.g., kidney tumors in VHL syndrome).

Except for children and pregnant women or rarely in patients with allergies to contrast medium, there was no consensus about whether to use computed tomography (CT) or magnetic resonance imaging (MRI) for the initial localization of a tumor. It was concluded that this depends largely on institutional preference and expertise. Both imaging modalities have excellent sensitivity for the detection of adrenal tumors, but lack adequate specificity for unequivocally confirming a mass as a pheochromocytoma. Neither CT nor MRI can distinguish with clear certainty a functional from a nonfunctional tumor.

Overall, the sensitivity of contrast-enhanced CT in the localization of pheochromocytoma is about 90–95%.[35–37] Adrenal pheochromocytoma of 1 cm or larger or metastatic tumors at least 1.0–2.0 cm in size can be easily detected by CT using narrow collimation. CT densitometry using Hounsfield units (HU) is helpful to distinguish between benign adrenal adenomas and other tumors (often functioning) including metastatic lesions. Thus, a homogeneous mass with a density measurement of less than 10 HU on an unenhanced CT is almost certainly an adenoma. The appearance of homogeneity with soft-tissue density (approximately 40–50 HU) and showing uniform enhancement following intravenous injection of contrast medium is suggestive of a pheochromocytoma, but again it is important to note that it does not distinguish a functional tumor from a nonfunctional one. Larger pheochromocytomas may undergo hemorrhage or necrosis, which results in an inhomogeneous appearance both before and after intravenous injection of contrast medium. Calcification occurs in about 10–15% of cases.

The advantages of CT in the localization of pheochromocytoma are the moderate cost and excellent detection of structures surrounding a pheochromocytoma. Data from several different institutions suggest that new nonionic contrast media do not pose a significant risk of a hypertensive crisis.[38] Consequently, several attendees indicated that they no longer use or recommend α-adrenoceptor blockade for such imaging. The recent development of multidetector computed tomography (MDCT) effectively allowing "volume" acquisition of data using 16, 64, or even more detectors has revolutionized CT. Images can now be acquired at great speed, viewed at very fine space intervals, and reformatted to produce multiplanar or 3D images. This is likely to prove useful, particularly in the identification of small and extra-adrenal tumors.

MRI is also widely used for the diagnosis of adrenal, extra-adrenal, or metastatic pheochromocytoma and has similar sensitivity to CT.[37,39] The hypervascularity of pheochromocytomas characteristically makes them appear to have a high or intermediate signal intensity on T2-weighted sequences.[40] However, it should be noted that such intense signals can be elicited by hemorrhage or hematomas, adenomas, and carcinomas, so an overlap with these tumors and pheochromocytoma must be considered. Moreover, MRI is also a very good imaging modality for the detection of extra-adrenal pheochromocytomas such as intracardiac, juxtacardiac, and juxtavascular pheochromocytoma. This is in part due to the superior contrast resolution of MRI, but also because of the multiplanar acquisition of data without the need for reformatting. MRI can be carried out with or without using intravenous contrast agents, and without requiring α-adrenergic blockade. MRI is the preferred initial imaging procedure for pheochromocytoma in children, during pregnancy, or in patients with known allergy to contrast agents.

Functional Imaging Studies

There is debate about whether functional imaging is necessary once a tumor is located by CT or MRI. The functional imaging test of choice is currently [^{123}I]-metaiodobenzylguanidine (MIBG) scintigraphy,[41,42] but as outlined above, several considerations may have an impact on the use of such tests. Participants agreed that additional functional imaging studies should be performed in most cases of biochemically proven pheochromocytoma for two main reasons: (1) to prove that the tumor is indeed a pheochromocytoma; and (2) to correctly detect any extension of disease that is not identified by anatomic imaging (e.g., presence of multifocal or bilateral disease or metastatic lesions), which may guide an appropriate therapeutic plan. It should be noted that this recommendation was based on expert opinion, as data for or against the use of routine functional imaging are limited. As reviewed by Dr. James Sisson (University of Michigan, Ann Arbor, MI), a unilateral lesion shown on CT or MRI in the absence of a family history or any evidence of malignancy usually does not reveal additional disease on [^{123}I]-MIBG scintigraphy.[43] Nevertheless, exceptions do occur and [^{123}I]-MIBG scintigraphy may be specially useful when the biochemical evidence for a pheochromocytoma is unequivocal, but CT or MRI fails to identify the source.

Decisions for imaging should also take into account prior knowledge of the patient. For example, in some patients at risk for extra-adrenal tumors due to germline mutations of SDHB and succinate dehydrogenase D (SDHD) genes or a previous history of paraganglioma, it may be appropriate to include [^{123}I]-MIBG scintigraphy with CT or MRI as part of the initial imaging evaluation. As indicated by Dr. Karel Pacak, exceptions where [^{123}I]-MIBG scintigraphy may not be necessary include solitary adrenal masses of less than 5 cm associated with elevations of plasma or urinary epinephrine or its metabolite, metanephrine. This suggestion was based on the perception that malignant disease mainly occurs in association with large norepinephrine-predominant tumors, as well as findings that practically all epinephrine-producing pheochromocytomas—including those in patients with MEN 2—are found in the adrenal gland or are recurrences of previously resected adrenal tumors.[34]

Although no firm recommendations were directed to the use of other functional imaging modalities, these should nevertheless be mentioned because they hold considerable promise, and in certain situations they have already been demonstrated to be of value in the localization of certain cases of the tumor. Such functional positron emission tomography (PET) imaging approaches include use of several imaging agents: 6-[^{18}F]-fluorodopamine, [^{18}F]-dihydroxyphenylalanine, [^{11}C]-hydroxyephedrine, and [^{11}C]epinephrine.[44–48] All these imaging modalities are highly specific for pheochromocytoma because they depend on uptake into tumor cells by norepinephrine transporters or other transport and storage mechanisms uniquely expressed in chromaffin tissues, including pheochromocytoma tumor cells. Thus, positive results obtained by these methods as well as [^{123}I]-MIBG scintigraphy detect pheochromocytoma with almost 100% specificity.

[^{18}F]-fluorodeoxyglucose ([^{18}F]-FDG) PET scanning is another approach used to localize pheochromocytoma. [^{18}F]-FDG, however, is a nonspecific imaging agent with localization dependent on the higher metabolic rate of tumors compared to surrounding normal tissue. Therefore, the use of this imaging modality should be reserved for those patients in whom either pheochromocytoma cannot be localized by other imaging methods or in patients with rapidly growing tumors that have a high metabolic rate, which often results in excellent detection of those tumors. A disadvantage of PET is that most of the radiopharmaceuticals (except FDG) are not widely available and patients must be referred to a specialized medical center.

Another promising method to localize pheochromocytomas is somatostatin receptor scintigraphy ("OctreoScan").[49,50] Although the method appears to have limited use for the localization of solitary pheochromocytomas, it can be useful in patients with metastatic disease or extra-adrenal paragangliomas.

Finally, some of those present at the breakout session indicated, in selected instances, that venous catheterization and sampling studies may add information not readily obtainable by other techniques.[51] This would include sampling from the adrenal veins in patients with elevated catecholamine or catecholamine metabolites and in whom imaging studies have been uninformative, particularly those with a background of hereditary disease. Reversal of the normally high epinephrine-to-norepinephrine ratio in adrenal venous blood can be particularly useful in such cases for pointing to an intra-adrenal tumor.[51] Measurements of metanephrines in blood obtained during venous catheterization can provide further advantages over measurements of the parent catecholamines.[52]

In summary, in most patients localization and confirmation of pheochromocytoma should be attempted using at least two imaging modalities. It was generally agreed that anatomical imaging studies (CT or MRI) should be combined with functional (nuclear medicine) imaging studies for optimal localization of primary, recurrent, multiple, or metastatic pheochromocytomas. CT or MRI of the abdomen and pelvis should usually be used first and if they are found to be negative, then CT or MRI of chest and neck and functional imaging should follow. The functional imaging test of choice is [^{123}I]-MIBG scintigraphy, which may be further used to confirm a tumor as a pheochromocytoma and to check for additional multifocal or malignant disease. If MIBG scintigraphy is negative, the diagnosis should be reconsidered, particularly in the light of drug-related false-positive results or the sleep apnea syndrome. Further localization studies should be carried out in major centers and can include PET with specific radiopharmaceuticals, octreotide scintigraphy, or selective venous sampling. If suspicion of a poorly differentiated pheochromocytoma remains, imaging with [^{18}F]FDG PET may be appropriate.

ACKNOWLEDGMENTS

The input of all participants in the breakout and final general discussion sessions at ISP2005 is gratefully appreciated. Particular thanks are extended to Drs. Stephen Ball, Morris Brown, and Emmanuel Bravo for their valuable suggestions during the preparation of this manuscript. This work was supported in part by the Intramural Research Program of the NIH, National Institute of Neurological Disorders and Stroke, and National Institute of Child Health and Human Development.

REFERENCES

1. PLATTS, J.K., P.J. DREW & J.N. HARVEY. 1995. Death from phaeochromocytoma: lessons from a post-mortem survey. J. Roy. Coll. Physicians Lond. **29:** 299–306.
2. LO, C.Y. *et al.* 2000. Adrenal pheochromocytoma remains a frequently overlooked diagnosis. Am. J. Surg. **179:** 212–215.
3. MCNEIL, A.R. *et al.* 2000. Phaeochromocytomas discovered during coronial autopsies in Sydney, Melbourne and Auckland. Aust. N. Z. J. Med. **30:** 648–652.
4. KALTSAS, G.A., D. PAPADOGIAS & A.B. GROSSMAN. 2004. The clinical presentation (symptoms and signs) of sporadic and familial chromaffin cell tumours (phaeochromocytomas and paragangliomas). Front. Horm. Res. **31:** 61–75.
5. SJOERDSMA, A. *et al.* 1959. Studies on the biogenesis and metabolism of norepinephrine in patients with pheochromocytoma. J. Clin. Invest. **38:** 31–38.
6. CROUT, J.R. & A. SJOERDSMA. 1964. Turnover and metabolism of catecholamines in patients with pheochromocytoma. J. Clin. Invest. **43:** 94–102.
7. EISENHOFER, G. *et al.* 2003. Pheochromocytoma: rediscovery as a catecholamine-metabolizing tumor. Endocr. Pathol. **14:** 193–212.
8. EISENHOFER, G. *et al.* 1999. Plasma normetanephrine and metanephrine for detecting pheochromocytoma in von Hippel-Lindau disease and multiple endocrine neoplasia type 2. N. Engl. J. Med. **340:** 1872–1879.
9. RABER, W. *et al.* 2000. Diagnostic efficacy of unconjugated plasma metanephrines for the detection of pheochromocytoma. Arch. Intern. Med. **160:** 2957–2963.
10. LENDERS, J.W. *et al.* 2002. Biochemical diagnosis of pheochromocytoma: which test is best? JAMA **287:** 1427–1434.
11. SAWKA, A.M. *et al.* 2003. A comparison of biochemical tests for pheochromocytoma: measurement of fractionated plasma metanephrines compared with the combination of 24-hour urinary metanephrines and catecholamines. J. Clin. Endocrinol. Metab. **88:** 553–558.
12. SAWKA, A.M. *et al.* 2004. A systematic review of the literature examining the diagnostic efficacy of measurement of fractionated plasma free metanephrines in the biochemical diagnosis of pheochromocytoma. BMC Endocr. Disord. **4:** 2.
13. UNGER, N. *et al.* 2006. Diagnostic value of various biochemical parameters for the diagnosis of pheochromocytoma in patients with adrenal mass. Eur. J. Endocrinol. **154:** 409–417.
14. GARDET, V. *et al.* 2001. Lessons from an unpleasant surprise: a biochemical strategy for the diagnosis of pheochromocytoma. J. Hypertens. **19:** 1029–1035.
15. GERLO, E.A. & C. SEVENS. 1994. Urinary and plasma catecholamines and urinary catecholamine metabolites in pheochromocytoma: diagnostic value in 19 cases. Clin. Chem. **40:** 250–256.
16. DAVIDSON, D.F. 2002. Phaeochromocytoma with normal urinary catecholamines: the potential value of urinary free metadrenalines. Ann. Clin. Biochem. **39:** 557–566.

17. GULLER, U. *et al.* 2006. Detecting pheochromocytoma: defining the most sensitive test. Ann. Surg. **243:** 102–107.
18. SAWKA, A.M. *et al.* 2004. The economic implications of three biochemical screening algorithms for pheochromocytoma. J. Clin. Endocrinol. Metab. **89:** 2859–2866.
19. BROWN, M.J. & D.J. ALLISON. 1981. Renal conversion of plasma DOPA to urine dopamine. Br. J. Clin. Pharmacol. **12:** 251–253.
20. EISENHOFER, G. *et al.* 2005. Biochemical and clinical manifestations of dopamine-producing paragangliomas: utility of plasma methoxytyramine. J. Clin. Endocrinol. Metab. **90:** 2068–2075.
21. ROSS, G.A. *et al.* 1993. Plasma and 24 h-urinary catecholamine concentrations in normal and patient populations. Ann. Clin. Biochem. **30** (Pt. 1)**:** 38–44.
22. SAWKA, A.M. *et al.* 2005. Measurement of fractionated plasma metanephrines for exclusion of pheochromocytoma: can specificity be improved by adjustment for age? BMC Endocr. Disord. **5:** 1.
23. EISENHOFER, G. *et al.* 1995. Plasma metadrenalines: do they provide useful information about sympatho-adrenal function and catecholamine metabolism? Clin. Sci. (Lond.) **88:** 533–542.
24. EISENHOFER, G. *et al.* 2003. Biochemical diagnosis of pheochromocytoma: how to distinguish true- from false-positive test results. J. Clin. Endocrinol. Metab. **88:** 2656–2666.
25. BROWN, M.J. *et al.* 1981. Increased sensitivity and accuracy of phaeochromocytoma diagnosis achieved by use of plasma-adrenaline estimations and a pentolinium-suppression test. Lancet **1:** 174–177.
26. BRAVO, E.L. *et al.* 1981. Clonidine-suppression test: a useful aid in the diagnosis of pheochromocytoma. N. Engl. J. Med. **305:** 623–626.
27. MULINARI, R.A. *et al.* 1987. The clonidine test for the diagnosis of pheochromocytoma: the usefulness of urinary metanephrine measurements. Braz. J. Med. Biol. Res. **20:** 43–46.
28. NEUMANN, H.P. *et al.* 2002. Germ-line mutations in nonsyndromic pheochromocytoma. N. Engl. J. Med. **346:** 1459–1466.
29. AMAR, L. *et al.* 2005. Genetic testing in pheochromocytoma or functional paraganglioma. J. Clin. Oncol. **23:** 8812–8818.
30. REMINE, W. *et al.* 1974. Current management of pheochromocytoma. Ann. Surg. **179:** 740–748.
31. TRONCONE, L. *et al.* 1990. The diagnostic and therapeutic utility of radioiodinated metaiodobenzylguanidine (MIBG): 5 years of experience. Eur. J. Nucl. Med. **16:** 325–335.
32. PEPPERCORN, P.D., A.B. GROSSMAN & R.H. REZNEK. 1998. Imaging of incidentally discovered adrenal masses. Clin. Endocrinol. (Oxford) **48:** 379–388.
33. GRUMBACH, M.M. *et al.* 2003. Management of the clinically inapparent adrenal mass ("incidentaloma"). Ann. Intern. Med. **138:** 424–429.
34. EISENHOFER, G. *et al.* 2005. Pheochromocytoma catecholamine phenotypes and prediction of tumor size and location by use of plasma free metanephrines. Clin. Chem. **51:** 735–744.
35. FRANCIS, I. & M. KOROBKIN. 1996. Pheochromocytoma. Adv. Uroradiol. **34:** 1101–1112.
36. GOLDSTEIN, R.E. *et al.* 1999. Clinical experience over 48 years with pheochromocytoma. Ann. Surg. **229:** 755–764; discussion 764–766.

37. SAHDEV, A. *et al.* 2005. CT and MR imaging of unusual locations of extra-adrenal paragangliomas (pheochromocytomas). Eur. Radiol. **15:** 85–92.
38. MUKHERJEE, J.J. *et al.* 1997. Pheochromocytoma: effect of nonionic contrast medium in CT on circulating catecholamine levels. Radiology **202:** 227–231.
39. QUINT, L.E. *et al.* 1987. Pheochromocytoma and paraganglioma: comparison of MR imaging with CT and I-131 MIBG scintigraphy. Radiology **165:** 89–93.
40. VARGHESE, J.C. *et al.* 1997. MR differentiation of phaeochromocytoma from other adrenal lesions based on qualitative analysis of T2 relaxation times. Clin. Radiol. **52:** 603–606.
41. FURUTA, N. *et al.* 1999. Diagnosis of pheochromocytoma using [123I]-compared with [131I]-metaiodobenzylguanidine scintigraphy. Int. J. Urol. **6:** 119–124.
42. ILIAS, I., B. SHULKIN & K. PACAK. 2005. New functional imaging modalities for chromaffin tumors, neuroblastomas and ganglioneuromas. Trends Endocrinol. Metab. **16:** 66–72.
43. MISKULIN, J. *et al.* 2003. Is preoperative iodine 123 meta-iodobenzylguanidine scintigraphy routinely necessary before initial adrenalectomy for pheochromocytoma? Surgery **134:** 918–922; discussion 922–923.
44. HOEGERLE, S. *et al.* 2002. Pheochromocytomas: detection with 18F DOPA whole body PET: initial results. Radiology. **222:** 507–512.
45. PACAK, K. *et al.* 2001. 6-[18F]fluorodopamine positron emission tomographic (PET) scanning for diagnostic localization of pheochromocytoma. Hypertension **38:** 6–8.
46. SHULKIN, B.L. *et al.* 1999. Pheochromocytomas: imaging with 2-[fluorine-18]fluoro-2-deoxy-D-glucose PET. Nucl. Med. **212:** 35–41.
47. MANN, G.N. *et al.* 2006. [(11)C]metahydroxyephedrine and [(18)F]Fluorodeoxyglucose positron emission tomography improve clinical decision making in suspected pheochromocytoma. Ann. Surg. Oncol. **13:** 187–197.
48. TRAMPAL, C. *et al.* 2004. Pheochromocytomas: detection with 11C hydroxyephedrine PET. Radiology **230:** 423–428.
49. MEDIAVILLA GARCIA, J.D. *et al.* 1999. A comparative study of 9 cases of adrenal pheochromocytoma and 11 cases of extra-adrenal pheochromocytoma. Rev. Clin. Esp. **199:** 343–348.
50. KALTSAS, G. *et al.* 2001. Comparison of somatostatin analog and meta-iodobenzylguanidine radionuclides in the diagnosis and localization of advanced neuroendocrine tumors. J. Clin. Endocrinol. Metab. **86:** 895–902.
51. CHEW, S.L. *et al.* 1994. Bilateral phaeochromocytomas in von Hippel-Lindau disease: diagnosis by adrenal vein sampling and catecholamine assay. Q. J. Med. **87:** 49–54.
52. PACAK, K. *et al.* 2001. A "pheo" lurks: novel approaches for locating occult pheochromocytoma. J. Clin. Endocrinol. Metab. **86:** 3641–3646.

Diagnostic Value of Biochemical Parameters in the Differential Diagnosis of an Adrenal Mass

STEPHAN PETERSENN,[a] NICOLE UNGER,[a] MARTIN K. WALZ,[b] AND KLAUS MANN[a]

[a]*Division of Endocrinology, Medical Centre, University of Duisberg-Essen, Essen, Germany*

[b]*Department of Surgery and Center of Minimally Invasive Surgery, Kliniken Essen-Mitte, Essen, Germany*

Abstract: In patients with an adrenal mass, hormonally active tumors including pheochromocytomas as well as aldosterone- and cortisol-secreting adenomas need to be considered. Several studies have demonstrated that metanephrines, which are the metabolites of catecholamines, are reliable parameters for the diagnosis of pheochromocytoma. In patients with an adrenal mass, we found plasma metanephrines, measured by a newly available radioimmunoassay, to be highly sensitive and specific for pheochromocytomas, with a better accuracy than any other biochemical parameter.The plasma aldosterone concentration (PAC) to plasma renin activity (PRA) ratio is an established screening tool for primary hyperaldosteronism. However, determination of active renin concentration (ARC) in contrast to PRA may offer advantages in regard to processing and standardization. We found a PAC to ARC ratio of >62 in patients with PAC levels >200 ng/L to be a reliable screening method for primary hyperaldosteronism in patients with adrenal masses.The screening for hypercortisolism relies on excess urinary cortisol secretion, loss of the physiological feedback during dexamethasone challenge, and loss of the circadian rhythm. Because urinary-free cortisol may not identify subclinical Cushing's syndrome, in which hypercortisolism is still mild, the 1-mg dexamethasone suppression test has been recommended in all patients with incidentally detected masses. Alternatively, late-night cortisol levels in saliva have been found to have a high sensitivity and specificity for the diagnosis of Cushing's syndrome. In summary, in patients with an adrenal mass, hormonally active adrenal tumors can be excluded with high certainty using a few highly reliable biochemical parameters.

Keywords: adrenal mass; pheochromocytoma; metanephrines; primary hyperaldosteronism; renin; hypercortisolism; hypertension

Address for correspondence: Dr. Stephan Petersenn, Division of Endocrinology, Medical Center, University of Duisburg-Essen, Hufelandstr. 55, 45122 Essen, Germany. Voice: 0049-201-723-2822; fax: 0049-201-723-5187.

e-mail: stephan.petersenn@uni-essen.de

Ann. N.Y. Acad. Sci. 1073: 348–357 (2006). © 2006 New York Academy of Sciences. doi: 10.1196/annals.1353.039

INTRODUCTION

Because of the improved MRI or CT techniques and a frequent use of these tools, adrenal tumors are increasingly recognized. Therefore, reliable and simple parameters are required to exclude hormonally active tumors in these patients. The clinically most important entities include pheochromocytomas, aldosterone-producing tumors, and cortisol-producing tumors. In this review, various methods for the biochemical diagnosis of adrenal masses are discussed.

Biochemical Parameters for the Diagnosis of Pheochromocytoma

An undiagnosed pheochromocytoma might result in life-threatening consequences. Therefore, highly sensitive biochemical assays are essential to avoid false-negative results. The diagnosis of pheochromocytoma is based on the overproduction of catecholamines. Determinations of plasma and in particular 24-h urinary epinephrine and norepinephrine levels are established diagnostic tools. A handicap is that they may be falsely negative in patients with a biochemically silent or periodically secreting pheochromocytoma.[1] On the other hand they may be falsely elevated in patients with panic disorder or congestive heart failure.[1]

Metanephrines, which are metabolites of catecholamines (FIG. 1), have been suggested as an alternative diagnostic tool.[2–4] Previous studies provided thresholds with sensitivities between 97% and 100% and specificities >85% and 96%.[5,6] In a recent study, we prospectively compared catecholamines and metanephrines in plasma and urine for the diagnosis of pheochromocytoma in patients with adrenal tumors.[7] Of 92 subjects operated upon for various reasons, histological investigation proved a pheochromocytoma in 24 patients. Considering histology the gold standard, ROC analysis was employed to provide biochemical thresholds with an optimal balance between sensitivity and specificity. Whereas catecholamines were determined by HPLC, plasma and urinary metanephrines were measured by radioimmunoassay. Our study revealed plasma normetanephrine as the best single parameter (TABLE 1). Using a threshold of 125.5 pg/mL, only two patients had falsely negative findings. Considering two respective parameters, plasma metanephrine and normetanephrine were the best biochemical combination compared to the other tests (FIG. 2). Similarly, Raber *et al.* studied patients with pheochromocytoma in comparison to 14 patients with other adrenal tumors[8] (TABLE 2). In that study, normal values for plasma catecholamines and metanephrines were adapted from previous studies.[5] The authors demonstrated a sensitivity and specificity of 100% each for plasma normetanephrine. An explanation for the potential superiority of metanephrines compared to catecholamines was provided by a recent study.[9] Pheochromocytomas contain high amounts of catechol-O-methyltransferase

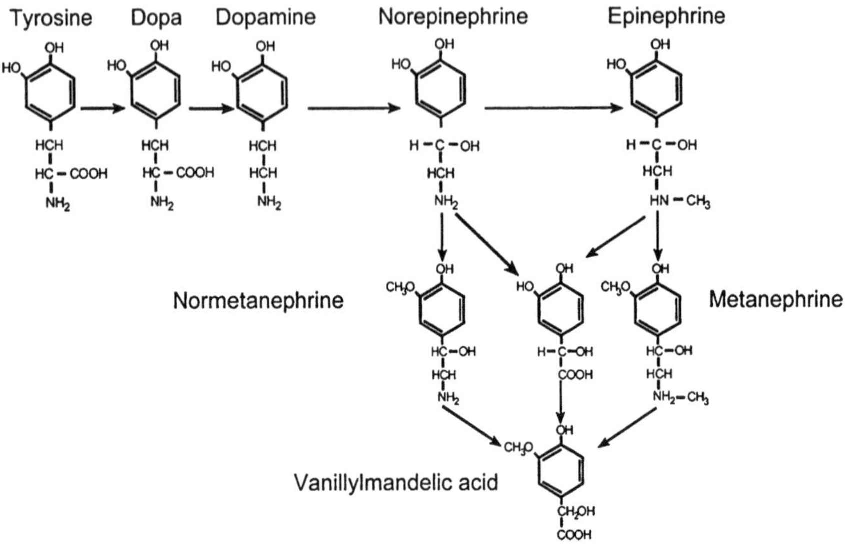

FIGURE 1. Synthesis and metabolism of catecholamines.

(COMT), an enzyme metabolizing catecholamines into free metanephrines. Rapid metabolism of catecholamines into metanephrines within the tumor may result in a continued high secretion of the metabolites, but an episodic and low secretion of the parent amines.

Our study, for the first time, measured plasma metanephrines by radioimmunoassay, while previous studies employed chromatographic procedures. Use of a radioimmunoassay provides standardization and savings of time, but may require different thresholds. Whereas our threshold of 125.5 pg/mL for normetanephrine is quite similar to those of the previous studies using HPLC (range: 112–165 pg/mL), a threshold of 38 pg/mL for metanephrine is rather

TABLE 1. Optimal thresholds of various biochemical parameters and their sensitivity and specificity for the diagnosis of pheochromocytomas, as determined by Unger *et al.*

		Threshold	Sens (%)	Spec (%)	AUC
Urine	E (μg/day)	2.5	73.3	64.2	0.78
	NE (μg/day)	68.1	73.3	84.9	0.87
	MN (μg/day)	110.7	80.0	82.7	0.86
	NMN (μg/day)	436.5	93.3	86.5	0.96
Plasma	E (pg/mL)	24.5	40.0	88.7	0.64
	NE (pg/mL)	219.5	60.0	72.6	0.73
	MN (pg/mL)	38.0	70.8	79.4	0.76
	NMN (pg/mL)	125.5	91.7	95.6	0.96

E = epinephrine; NE = norepinephrine; MN = metanephrine; NMN = normetanephrine.

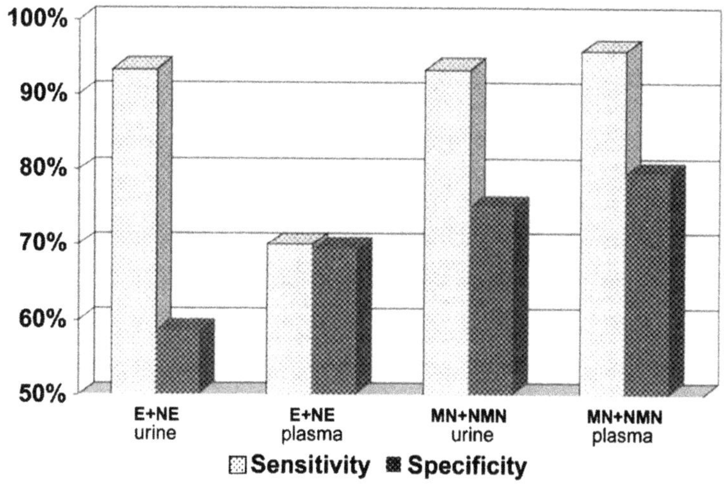

FIGURE 2. Sensitivity and specificity of various combinations of biochemical parameters for the diagnosis of pheochromocytomas, as determined by Unger *et al.*[7] E = epinephrine, NE = norepinephrine, MN = metanephrine, NMN = normetanephrine.

low compared to thresholds between 59 pg/mL and 99 pg/mL in previous studies.

In most studies, urinary fractionated metanephrines demonstrated a slightly lower sensitivity and specificity than their plasma counterparts. Urinary metanephrines largely reflect sulfate-conjugated metabolites, which are formed in gastrointestinal tissue. Therefore, they are not only related to the pheochromocytoma, which may explain the reduced accuracy compared to plasma metanephrines.[10,11] Previous studies relied mostly on the measurement of total urinary metanephrines. Opposite to a separate determination of

TABLE 2. Comparison of various studies investigating the diagnostic value of plasma metanephrines for the diagnosis of pheochromocytomas

Reference	Study cohort	Method	Parameter	Threshold (pg/mL)	Sens (%)	Spec (%)
Eisenhofer *et al.* [13]	208 pheo, 648 controls	HPLC	MN	61	53	95
			NMN	112	96	92
Sawka *et al.* [6]	33 pheo, 316 controls	HPLC	MN	99	n.s.	n.s.
			NMN	165	87	94
Raber *et al.* [8]	17 pheo, 14 controls	HPLC	MN	60	71	100
			NMN	121	100	100
Unger *et al.* [7]	24 pheo, 126 controls	RIA	MN	38	71	79
			NMN	126	92	96

MN = metanephrine; NMN = normetanephrine.

metanephrine and normetanephrine in urine, total metanephrines describe the combined measurement of metanephrine and normetanephrine in a single assay. Urinary total metanephrines demonstrated sensitivities between 65–89% and specificities from 89–95%.[5,12–14] Determination of fractionated metanephrines measured by HPLC in previous studies resulted in higher sensitivities from 88–97%, but impaired specificities from 69–85%.[12,14]

During the diagnostic workup of pheochromocytomas, the possible influence of drugs on the levels of catecholamines and their metabolites has to be considered.[13] Nonselective alpha-blockers may be associated with higher plasma and urinary levels of norepinephrine and normetanephrine, but not epinephrine and metanephrine. Beta-blockers to a much lower extent may be responsible for elevated levels of plasma metanephrines and urinary catecholamines and metanephrines.

In conclusion, determination of plasma metanephrine and normetanephrine, as measured by HPLC or RIA, is a reliable test for the diagnosis of pheochromocytoma, especially in patients with adrenal tumors of unknown etiology.

Biochemical Parameters for the Diagnosis of Primary Hyperaldosteronism

Primary hyperaldosteronism is classically characterized by a combination of hypertension, hypokalemia, suppressed renin, and an elevated nonsuppressible plasma aldosterone concentration (PAC). Measurement of these single parameters does not allow a reliable diagnosis. Normokalemia is noted in patients with primary hyperaldosteronism,[15–17] as well as suppressed renin in hypertensive patients.[18,19] In contrast to single measurement of either PAC or plasma renin activity (PRA), the PAC to PRA ratio seems independent from diurnal and day-to-day variations, salt intake, and diuretics. It was demonstrated as a reliable and convenient screening tool for ambulatory conditions, independent of body posture.[20] An NIH consensus statement suggests a PAC to PRA ratio $\geq$300 (ng/L to ng/mL per h) and PAC $\geq$200 ng/L for the diagnosis of primary hyperaldosteronism.[21] However, a recent study revealed a low reproducibility of the ratio in patients with aldosterone-producing adrenal adenoma under random conditions.[22] PRA is determined by radioimmunological measurement of angiotensin-1 generated from angiotensinogen during *in vitro* incubation with plasma renin. Therefore, determination is limited to physiological angiotensinogen levels. Conditions with decreased angiotensinogen levels, (e.g., liver cirrhosis, severe cardiac failure) result in underestimation of renin.[23,24] In contrast, estrogen treatment increases angiotensinogen levels, resulting in an overestimation of renin.[25,26] The lack of standardization is another methodical disadvantage. Processing of plasma samples, especially in regard to incubation time, pH, and dilution varies among different laboratories. In patients with suppressed renin, the ratio is depending on the lower detection limit.

To avoid these disadvantages, generation of monoclonal antibodies against active renin allowed direct measurement of active renin concentration (ARC) independent from angiotensinogen levels. Standardization of ARC measurement by calibration against a WHO standard enables improved comparability among different laboratories. Furthermore, automated methods for determination of ARC provide savings of time. The accuracy of determination has improved by development of immunoradiometric and immunoluminometric assays.[27] In a recent study, we prospectively compared PRA and ARC under random conditions to investigate the use of ARC for the diagnosis of primary hyperaldosteronism in patients with aldosterone-producing adenomas.[28] Fifty patients with an adrenal mass including 10 patients with aldosterone-secreting adenomas were investigated by both methods. A threshold value of 90 for the PAC to ARC ratio provided a high sensitivity and specificity for the diagnosis of primary hyperaldosteronism. By additional consideration of PAC $\geq$200 ng/L, a ratio threshold of 62 was established with improved specificity. Trenkel *et al.* studied 17 patients with primary hyperaldosteronism (9 adrenal adenomas, 8 cases of idiopathic hyperaldosteronism), 146 hypertensive patients on various medications, and 37 normotensive subjects.[29] A PAC to ARC ratio cut-off value of 50 revealed a sensitivity of 89% and a specificity of 96%. In contrast to our study, sensitivity decreased to 84% and specificity increased to 100% by consideration of PAC $\geq$200 ng/L as an additional criterion. The high proportion of idiopathic hyperaldosteronism, which is probably susceptible for lower aldosterone levels, might explain the lower threshold in that study.

The influence of antihypertensive medication for the accuracy of PAC to PRA and ARC ratio, respectively, is discussed controversially. Gallay *et al.* showed no significant correlation between different values of the PAC to PRA ratio and numbers or types of antihypertensive medications.[16] Moreover, several studies that discontinued antihypertensive treatment revealed a PAC to PRA ratio nearly similar to those results of studies with continued antihypertensive medication. However, Seifarth *et al.* found some influence of antihypertensive medication on the PAC to ARC ratio.[30] β-blockers significantly increased the ratio, while ACE inhibitors, aldosterone antagonists and AT^1 receptor antagonists significantly decreased the ratio.

In summary, the PAC to ARC ratio is a reliable screening method for primary hyperaldosteronism in patients with adrenal masses.

Biochemical Parameters for the Diagnosis of Adrenal Hypercortisolism

Medical history and clinical examination may raise suspicion of Cushing's syndrome (CS) in patients with an adrenal mass. The cardinal biochemical features are excess endogenous integrated cortisol secretion, loss of the physiological feedback of the HPA axis, and disturbed circadian rhythm of the cortisol secretion.[31] Collection of 24-h urinary-free cortisol (UFC) is widely used as a screening test.[32] It gives an index of the free (unbound) cortisol that circulated in the blood during that time period. In contrast to plasma cortisol levels, which measure total (unbound and bound) cortisol, it is not influenced by factors that alter cortisol-binding globulin (CBG) levels. The adequacy of collection is a major problem, and therefore written instructions should be provided to the patient with at least two 24-h urine collections being performed. In one study, UFC measurement was shown to have a very high sensitivity and specificity of 100% and 98%, respectively, in the differentiation of patients with hypercortisolism from various control subjects.[33] However, mild elevations of UFC may also be found in various conditions, such as depression and alcoholism (pseudo-Cushing). The recent introduction of immunoassays for the measurement of UFC in most laboratories poses some new problems, as reference ranges have not been established in sufficient detail and measurement is influenced by various metabolites of cortisol and some synthetic glucocorticoids. In contrast, chromatographic methods like HPLC allow the separation of various urinary steroids, but are time-consuming, costly, and influenced by occasional interfering substances like carbamazepin or digoxin.

Because UFC may not identify subclinical CS in which hypercortisolism is still mild, the 1-mg dexamethasone suppression test has been recommended in all patients with incidentally detected masses.[21] It consists of the oral intake of 1 mg dexamethasone between 2300 and 2400 h, followed by measurement of fasting cortisol between 0800 and 0900 h the next morning. For overt CS, a sensitivity of 98% has been reported, whereas specificity ranges between 80.5 and 98.9%.[34] The reported threshold levels for suppression of cortisol range from 100–200 nmol/L (3.6–7.2 μg/dL).[31] However, a recent extensive review suggests that suppression of cortisol ≤50 nmol/L after dexamethasone very effectively excludes CS that may be more favorable for a screening test.[35]

Whereas patients with CS often have morning cortisol levels within or slightly above the normal range, they lack a normal circadian rhythm. The midnight sleeping cortisol has a very high sensitivity for CS, when applying a threshold of 50 nmol/L (1.8 μg/dL).[36] However, the test requires in-patient admission, the samples need to be withdrawn within 10 min of waking the patient, and the specificity of this test has not been established. Late-night (2300 h) salivary samples may be used alternatively. Cortisol levels in saliva are highly correlated with free plasma cortisol, independent of salivary flow, and stable at room temperature for 1 week.[32] They have been found to have a high sensitivity and specificity for the diagnosis of CS.[37,38] The normal reference ranges are assay-dependent, and therefore need to be established for each laboratory. In a recent study on 120 patients with Cushing's disease and 100 control subjects, we determined a 2200 h salivary cortisol threshold of

1.9 μg/L with a sensitivity and specificity of 97.6% and 100%, respectively, measured by a radioimmunoassay.[39]

Once hypercortisolism is established, ACTH may be measured to confirm ACTH-independent CS in patients with an adrenal mass. ACTH is rapidly degraded by plasma proteases, and therefore blood needs to be withdrawn in prechilled EDTA tubes, placed on ice, and rapidly centrifuged. When highly sensitive immunoradiometric assays are used, ACTH levels <10 pg/mL at 0900 h suggest an ACTH-independent cause, whereas levels >20 pg/mL suggest an ACTH-dependent cause.[32]

SUMMARY

In patients with an adrenal mass, collection of a single blood sample is sufficient to screen for autonomous secretion of catecholamines and aldosterone. Autonomous cortisol secretion in these patients may be excluded by 1-mg dexamethasone testing or measurement of late-night salivary cortisol.

REFERENCES

1. EISENHOFER, G. *et al.* 2000. Plasma metanephrines: a novel and cost-effective test for pheochromocytoma. Braz. J. Med. Biol. Res. **33:** 1157–1169.
2. EISENHOFER, G. 2003. Editorial: biochemical diagnosis of pheochromocytoma—is it time to switch to plasma-free metanephrines?. J. Clin. Endocrinol. Metab. **88:** 550–552.
3. RODEN, M. 2002. How to detect pheochromocytomas?—the diagnostic relevance of plasma free metanephrines. Wien. Klin. Wochenschr. **114:** 246–251.
4. SAWKA, A.M. *et al.* 2004. A systematic review of the literature examining the diagnostic efficacy of measurement of fractionated plasma free metanephrines in the biochemical diagnosis of pheochromocytoma. BMC Endocr. Disord. **4:** 2–11.
5. LENDERS, J.W. *et al.* 1995. Plasma metanephrines in the diagnosis of pheochromocytoma. Ann. Intern. Med. **123:** 101–109.
6. SAWKA, A.M. *et al.* 2003. A comparison of biochemical tests for pheochromocytoma: measurement of fractionated plasma metanephrines compared with the combination of 24-hour urinary metanephrines and catecholamines. J. Clin. Endocrinol. Metab. **88:** 553–558.
7. UNGER, N. *et al.* 2006. Diagnostic value of various biochemical parameters for the diagnosis of pheochromocytoma in patients with adrenal mass. Eur. J. Endocrinol. **154:** 409–417.
8. RABER, W. *et al.* 2000. Diagnostic efficacy of unconjugated plasma metanephrines for the detection of pheochromocytoma. Arch. Intern. Med. **160:** 2957–2963.
9. EISENHOFER, G. *et al.* 1998. Plasma metanephrines are markers of pheochromocytoma produced by catechol-O-methyltransferase within tumors. J. Clin. Endocrinol. Metab. **83:** 2175–2185.
10. EISENHOFER, G. 2001. Free or total metanephrines for diagnosis of pheochromocytoma: what is the difference? Clin. Chem. **47:** 988–989.

11. EISENHOFER, G. *et al.* 2001. Understanding catecholamine metabolism as a guide to the biochemical diagnosis of pheochromocytoma. Rev. Endocr. Metab. Disord. **2:** 297–311.
12. LENDERS, J.W. *et al.* 2002. Biochemical diagnosis of pheochromocytoma: which test is best? JAMA **287:** 1427–1434.
13. EISENHOFER, G. *et al.* 2003. Biochemical diagnosis of pheochromocytoma: how to distinguish true- from false-positive test results. J. Clin. Endocrinol. Metab. **88:** 2656–2666.
14. GARDET, V. *et al.* 2001. Lessons from an unpleasant surprise: a biochemical strategy for the diagnosis of pheochromocytoma. J. Hypertens. **19:** 1029–1035.
15. HIRAMATSU, K. *et al.* 1981. A screening test to identify aldosterone-producing adenoma by measuring plasma renin activity. Results in hypertensive patients. Arch. Intern. Med. **141:** 1589–1593.
16. GALLAY, B.J. *et al.* 2001. Screening for primary aldosteronism without discontinuing hypertensive medications: plasma aldosterone-renin ratio. Am. J. Kidney Dis. **37:** 699–705.
17. LOH, K.C. *et al.* 2000. Prevalence of primary aldosteronism among Asian hypertensive patients in Singapore. J. Clin. Endocrinol. Metab. **85:** 2854–2859.
18. FISHMAN, L.M. *et al.* 1968. Incidence of primary aldosteronism uncomplicated "essential" hypertension. A prospective study with elevated aldosterone secretion and suppressed plasma renin activity used as diagnostic criteria. JAMA **205:** 497–502.
19. DISTLER, A. *et al.* 1977. Low renin hypertension. Contrib. Nephrol. **8:** 69–80.
20. MCKENNA, T.J. *et al.* 1991. Diagnosis under random conditions of all disorders of the renin-angiotensin-aldosterone axis, including primary hyperaldosteronism. J. Clin. Endocrinol. Metab. **73:** 952–957.
21. GRUMBACH, M.M. *et al.* 2003. Management of the clinically inapparent adrenal mass ("incidentaloma"). Ann. Intern. Med. **138:** 424–429.
22. TANABE, A. *et al.* 2003. Variability in the renin/aldosterone profile under random and standardized sampling conditions in primary aldosteronism. J. Clin. Endocrinol. Metab. **88:** 2489–2494.
23. ARNAL, J.F. *et al.* 1991. Recent advances in the investigation of the renin-angiotensin and cardiac natriuretic systems in patients with chronic heart insufficiency. Arch. Mal. Coeur Vaiss. **84:** 1273–1280.
24. PLOUIN, P.F. *et al.* 1990. Immunoradiometric assay of active renin versus determination of plasma renin activity in the clinical investigation of hypertension, congestive heart failure, and liver cirrhosis. Horm. Res. **34:** 138–141.
25. GORDON, D.B., I.N. SACHIN & V.N. DODD. 1976. Heterogeneity of renin substrate in human plasma: effect of pregnancy and oral contraceptives. Proc. Soc. Exp. Biol. Med. **153:** 314–318.
26. DERKX, F.H. *et al.* 1986. Immunoreactive renin, prorenin, and enzymatically active renin in plasma during pregnancy and in women taking oral contraceptives. J. Clin. Endocrinol. Metab. **63:** 1008–1015.
27. SIMON, D. *et al.* 1992. Two-site direct immunoassay specific for active renin. Clin Chem. **38:** 1959–62.
28. UNGER, N. *et al.* 2004. Comparison of active renin concentration and plasma renin activity for the diagnosis of primary hyperaldosteronism in patients with an adrenal mass. Eur. J. Endocrinol. **150:** 517–523.

29. TRENKEL, S. *et al.* 2002. Ratio of serum aldosterone to plasma renin concentration in essential hypertension and primary aldosteronism. Exp. Clin. Endocrinol. Diabetes **110:** 80–85.
30. SEIFARTH, C. *et al.* 2002. Influence of antihypertensive medication on aldosterone and renin concentration in the differential diagnosis of essential hypertension and primary aldosteronism. Clin. Endocrinol (Oxf). **57:** 457–465.
31. NEWELL-PRICE, J. *et al.* 1998. The diagnosis and differential diagnosis of Cushing's syndrome and pseudo-Cushing's states. Endocr. Rev. **19:** 647–672.
32. ARNALDI, G. *et al.* 2003. Diagnosis and complications of Cushing's syndrome: a consensus statement. J. Clin. Endocrinol. Metab. **88:** 5593–5602.
33. MENGDEN, T. *et al.* 1992. Urinary free cortisol versus 17-hydroxycorticosteroids: a comparative study of their diagnostic value in Cushing's syndrome. Clin. Investig. **70:** 545–548.
34. CRAPO, L. 1979. Cushing's syndrome: a review of diagnostic tests. Metabolism **28:** 955–977.
35. WOOD, P.J. *et al.* 1997. Evidence for the low dose dexamethasone suppression test to screen for Cushing's syndrome—recommendations for a protocol for biochemistry laboratories. Ann. Clin. Biochem. **34:** 222–229.
36. NEWELL-PRICE, J. *et al.* 1995. A single sleeping midnight cortisol has 100% sensitivity for the diagnosis of Cushing's syndrome. Clin. Endocrinol (Oxf). **43:** 545–550.
37. PAPANICOLAOU, D.A. *et al.* 2002. Nighttime salivary cortisol: a useful test for the diagnosis of Cushing's syndrome. J. Clin. Endocrinol. Metab. **87:** 4515–4521.
38. RAFF, H., J.L. RAFF & J.W. FINDLING. 1998. Late-night salivary cortisol as a screening test for Cushing's syndrome. J. Clin. Endocrinol. Metab. **83:** 2681–2686.
39. TRILCK, M. *et al.* 2005. Salivary cortisol measurement—a reliable method for the diagnosis of Cushing's syndrome. Exp. Clin. Endocrinol. Diabetes **113:** 225–230.

Multicenter Study on the Diagnostic Value of a New RIA for the Detection of Free Plasma Metanephrines in the Work-Up for Pheochromocytoma

TOMAS LENZ,[a,g] JOACHIM ZORNER,[a] CARL KIRCHMAIER,[b] DANIELE PILLITTERI,[b] KLAUS BADENHOOP,[c] CHRISTINE BARTEL,[d] HELMUT GEIGER,[d] KATRIN HASSELBACHER,[e] ULRICH TUSCHY,[e] JÜRGEN WESTERMANN,[f] AND LOTHAR SALEWSKI[f]

[a]*Kuratorium für Dialyse und Nierentransplantation e.V. (KfH) Kidney Center, Maxstrasse 48, 67059 Ludwigshafen, Germany*

[b]*Deutsche Klinik für Diagnostik, Department of Hemostasiology, Aukammallee 33, 65191 Wiesbaden, Germany*

[c]*University Hospital, Medical Clinic I, Theodor Stern Kai 7, 60590 Frankfurt, Germany*

[d]*University Hospital, Medical Clinic III, Theodor Stern Kai 7, 60590 Frankfurt, Germany*

[e]*HELIOS-Klinikum, Medical Clinic 2, Nordhäuserstrasse 74, 99089 Erfurt, Germany*

[f]*IBL GmbH, Flughafenstrasse 52 a, 22335 Hamburg, Germany*

[g]*Institute for the Prevention of Kidney Diseases and Hypertension (IPNH), Maxstrasse 48, 67059 Ludwigshafen, Germany*

ABSTRACT: Available laboratory test methods for the detection of elevated concentrations of catecholamines and their metabolites in urine and/or plasma are not always sensitive enough for the detection of pheochromocytoma. High-quality immunoassays for these compounds appear to be as accurate as high-pressure liquid chromatography (HPLC) or gas chromatography/mass spectrometry (GC-MS). Therefore, the current project aims to establish a new sensitive radioimmunoassay (RIA) for the measurement of free metanephrines in the plasma of patients in the work-up for pheochromocytoma. We report first results of an ongoing multicenter clinico–chemical evaluation study in hypertensive patients and normotensive volunteers. After an overnight fast plasma samples were collected on ice in EDTA- and heparin-coated tubes after

Address for correspondence: Tomas Lenz, M.D., Institute for the Prevention of Kidney Diseases and Hypertension (IPNH), c/o KfH Nierenzentrum, Maxstrasse 48, 67059 Ludwigshafen, Germany. Voice: +49 621-68599722; fax: +49 621-68599752.

e-mail: Tomas.Lenz@kfh-dialyse.de

**Ann. N.Y. Acad. Sci. 1073: 358–373 (2006). © 2006 New York Academy of Sciences.
doi: 10.1196/annals.1353.040**

insertion of an indwelling venous line and resting in the supine (patients) or sitting position (normal volunteers) for 30 min. Plasma metanephrines were measured by a newly developed RIA from IBL, Hamburg, Germany. Good agreement of the assay with the tandem mass spectrometry (LC-MS/MS) method for normetanephrine ($r^2 = 0.975$) and for metanephrine ($r^2 = 0.985$) could be demonstrated. Both specimens, EDTA and heparin plasma, can be used with the same results. The RIA has a good precision of <15% in the normal range and of <10% in the elevated concentration range. Our preliminary data suggest a high validity of the newly developed RIA for measuring free metanephrine and normetanephrine in hypertensive subjects in both EDTA and heparin plasma. Further work is required to determine the accuracy of the test in larger patient populations and in patients with pheochromocytoma.

KEYWORDS: **pheochromocytoma; immunoassay; free plasma metanephrines; LC-MS/MS; heparin; EDTA**

INTRODUCTION

The catecholamines epinephrine (adrenalin), norepinephrine (noradrenalin), and dopamine are synthesized in the adrenal medulla, the sympathetic nervous system, and the brain. As they influence virtually all tissues and are involved with other hormonal and neuronal systems in the regulation of a wide variety of physiological processes, they are subjects of great scientific interest and clinical applications.

The concentrations of catecholamines and their metabolites are elevated in urine and plasma in several diseases and are of clinical interest, especially in the diagnosis of pheochromocytoma, neuroblastoma, and ganglioneuroma.[1]

Pheochromocytoma is a life-threatening tumor of the sympathetic nervous system and occurs mostly in the adrenal medulla. Correct diagnosis of the condition can result in the successful removal of the tumor in 90% of cases. However, if it is not correctly diagnosed, it is invariably fatal. Even today misdiagnosis is frequent, so that approximately one in three pheochromocytomas is only identified post mortem.[2–4]

Pheochromocytoma can produce an excess of adrenalin, noradrenalin, dopamine, metanephrines, and vanillylmandelic acid (VMA). The detection of these substances forms the basis of pheochromocytoma diagnosis.[5,6] Currently, there is no consensus as to which test is the most suitable for the biochemical identification of pheochromocytoma or what type of sample should be used.

In recent retrospective multicenter studies the usefulness of the different analytes has been investigated. Among laboratory assays the measurement of urinary VMA was the most frequently used screening method. However, this was also the method with the lowest diagnostic sensitivity,[7–9] and should be considered as obsolete, to be replaced by more specific tests.

The diagnostic problem with regard to pheochromocytoma is to separate pheochromocytoma patients with only moderate biosynthetic activity of the tumor from patients with unspecific stimulated sympathetic nervous system activity, that is, patients with essential, neurogenic or renovascular hypertension. Furthermore, measurements of catecholamines and their metabolites in the plasma and urine may reveal normal values when the tumor only secretes periodically. Therefore, commonly used investigations of urinary or plasma catecholamines and/or their metabolites and other biochemical tests, such as measurement of plasma chromogranin A levels, are not always able to reliably confirm or reject the diagnosis.

Recent studies suggest that the determination of plasma-free metanephrines (determination with high-pressure liquid chromatography [HPLC]) provides 100% sensitivity for the detection of a pheochromocytoma compared to only 82% when plasma and urinary catecholamines were determined.[10] It therefore appears that measurement of the plasma levels of free normetanephrine and metanephrine has even higher sensitivity than other biochemical tests for the diagnosis of both familial and sporadic pheochromocytoma. A larger increase and a longer persistence of metanephrines than catecholamines in plasma may contribute to their greater diagnostic accuracy.[11] The measurement of free plasma metanephrines today is mostly done by labor- and cost-intensive methods like HPLC and tandem mass spectrometry (LC-MS/MS). Besides these methods immunoassays can also be applied to the measurement of metanephrines.

In this article we present first results of a multicenter study on the diagnostic value of a newly developed radioimmunoassay for the detection of free plasma metanephrines in the work-up for pheochromocytoma.

MATERIALS AND METHODS

Chemicals

All fine chemicals and biochemicals were purchased from Sigma (Munich, Germany) or Merck (Darmstadt, Germany), unless otherwise stated. The C18 reverse phase extraction columns were from Waters (Eschborn, Germany). All reagents used for the radioimmunoassay kit are provided by the manufacturer (IBL GmbH, Hamburg, Germany). The anti-*N*-acylmetanephrine and anti-*N*-acylnormetanephrine antisera used for the kit were produced by immunizing rabbits with bovine serum albumin conjugates using a conventional immunization technique, as previously described.[12] Catechol-o-methyltransferase (COMT) (E.C. No. 2.1.1.6.) was prepared from pig liver, as reported by Tilgmann and Kalkkinen.[13] *N*-succinimidyl-Biotin (NHS-Biotin) and amino-phenyl-boronic acid affinity gel were synthesized by the manufacturer (IBL GmbH).

Patient Samples

Patients and normal volunteers were enrolled from the outpatient clinics of the University Hospital in Frankfurt am Main and the Deutsche Klinik für Diagnostik (DKD) in Wiesbaden, all Germany. The study was approved by the local ethical committees. Informed consent was obtained from all subjects. The patient and normal subject characteristics were as follows: hypertensive patients: $n = 49$ (23 females, 26 males; mean age 52 years, range 22–82 years), on standard antihypertensive medications (mean 2.8 meds per patient); average blood pressure $157 \pm 24/90 \pm 16$ mm Hg; mean creatinine value 1.11 mg/dL. Normotensive volunteers: $n = 53$ (10 females, 43 males; mean age 52 years, range 30–80 years); normal blood pressure and normal kidney function.

After an overnight fast plasma samples were collected in polyethylene tubes containing EDTA or heparin as anticoagulant after insertion of an indwelling venous line and resting in the supine (patients) or sitting (normal volunteers) position for 30 min. The plasma was separated by centrifugation (3000 *g* at 4°C for 20 min) and then stored aliquoted at −80°C until use.

Radioimmunoassay for Free Metanephrine and Normetanephrine

Since the metanephrines as such do not possess sufficient immunogenic properties, making it difficult to raise specific antibodies against them, use is being made of their *N*-acyl-hemisuccinates derivatives. Specific antibodies against these derivatives can be produced in rabbits by coupling both metanephrines to bovine serum albumin. By reaction with I125-Bolton–Hunter reagent [3-(*p*-hydroxyphenyl) propionic acid *N*-hydroxysuccinimide ester] the radioactive tracer was synthesized, whereas the standards and samples are derivatized with NHS-Biotin.

As source for standards and tracer the biological active L-form was produced by the use of COMT. The L-form of epinephrine and norepinephrine was converted to the corresponding L-metanephrines with pig liver COMT and S-adenosyl-methionine as coenzyme. The catechols are used in excess and afterward removed with amino-phenyl-boronic acid affinity gel. The produced L-metanephrines were extracted and further purified.

The kits are on the basis of the following principle: After extraction of the samples with reverse phase C18 extraction columns and elution of the metanephrines with methanol/ethanol, a chemical derivatization step with NHS-Biotin follows. After evaporation of the organic solvent and reconstitution of the remaining acylated metanephrines with assay buffer the samples are ready for the assay. The evaporation in a vacuum centrifuge is the used standard procedure. Drying the sample by blowing with N_2, as an alternative method, was as good as the standard procedure ($r = 0.9987$).

The assay procedure is on the basis of the basic principle of a competitive RIA: the competition between a Bolton–Hunter-labeled tracer and the *N*-acylated antigens of the samples for a fixed number of antibody-binding sites (rabbit-anti-metanephrine or rabbit anti-normetanephrine). After separation of the bound from the free antigen by precipitation with a goat-anti-rabbit antibody and centrifugation, the amount of bound radioactivity of the precipitates is measured in a gamma counter. Results of samples can be determined directly using the standard curve.

Analytical Procedure of Radioimmunoassay

For a detailed description of the analytical procedure (both for metanephrine and normetanephrine) we refer to the booklets supplied by the manufacturer and included in each test kit. Here we present a shortened version describing the different analytical steps in less detail.

Column Conditioning

One milliliter of methanol (undiluted) was added to the columns. The solvent was passed through the column by centrifugation for 1 min at 120 *g*. After the addition of 1 mL of bidist. water to the columns and passing through the column by centrifugation the columns are ready for sample application. Proceeding with sample application was without delay in order to avoid drying of columns.

Sample Application

Standards, controls, and samples (0.5 mL) were pipetted to the columns together with 0.5 mL bidist. water each and centrifuged.

Washing: Washing was performed with 1 mL of bidist. water. The solvent was passed through by spinning and discarded.

Elution of Extract

The columns were placed into new, correspondingly marked acylation tubes (coated with acylation reagent). For elution 0.5 mL of 50%/50% (v/v) methanol and ethanol were used. The derivatization reaction starts immediately after elution.

Evaporation and Reconstitution of Extract

Evaporation of the solvent to dryness was done by use of an evaporator centrifuge. This will take approximately 90 min.

Alternative: Use of N2 for evaporation. This will take approximately 45 min. Reconstitute samples with 0.5 mL of reconstitution buffer. We vortex all tubes at least 1 min.

Radioimmunoassay

One hundred microliter of each extracted standard, control, and plasma sample was pipetted into the respective tubes. For non-specific binding (NSB) 100 μL of reconstitution buffer was used.

Fifty microliter of metanephrine or normetanephrine 125I-tracer was added to all tubes. Afterward 50 μL of metanephrine or normetanephrine antiserum followed and was allowed to stand at room temperature overnight (at least 14 h). On the next day 1 mL of precipitating antiserum was added and incubated for 15 min. Centrifugation of 15 min at 3000 *g* at room temperature was used for separation. The supernatants were decanted and the precipitates were measured for 1 min in a gamma counter.

Calculation of results and used software calculations were performed with the computer program "Microwin" distributed by Mikrotek (Krefeld, Germany) with four-parameter logistic. Both for the calibrators and for the patient samples the mean of the obtained duplicate cpm readings was taken and radioactive counts as percentage of the value of the zero calibrator were calculated (Tables 1 and 2). To obtain a calibration curve, the absorbance percentages (*y* values) of the calibrators were plotted against the logarithms of the concentrations of the calibrators (x axis, see FIGS. 1 and 2 for typical standard curves). From these calibration curves, concentrations, and the calculated percentages of the patient samples, metanephrine or normetanephrine

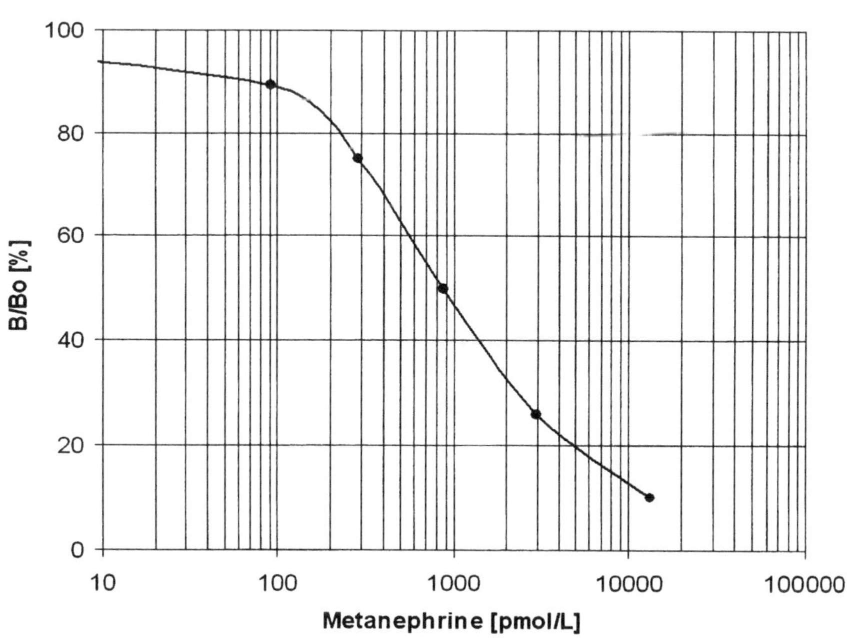

FIGURE 1. Typical standard curve for metanephrine.

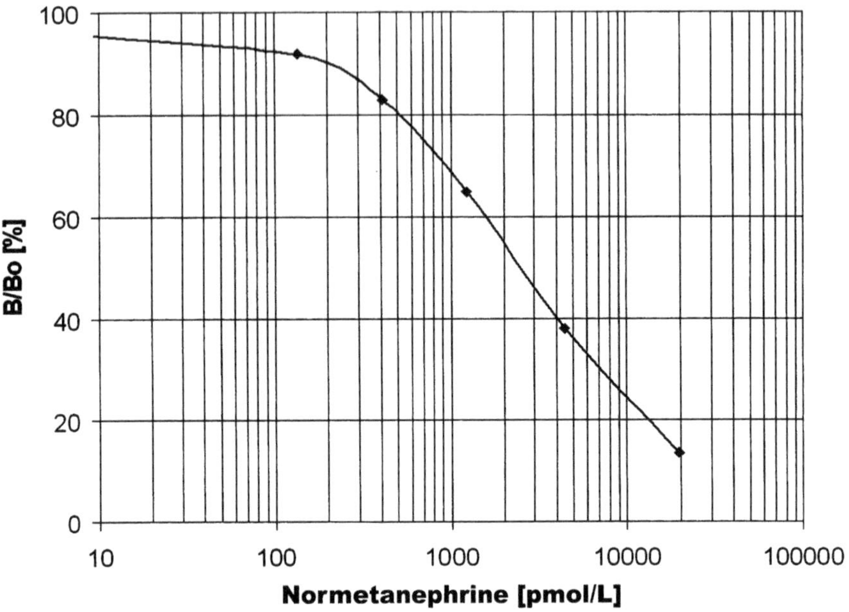

FIGURE 2. Typical standard curve for normetanephrine.

concentrations in these samples were derived. The gamma counter used in the present investigation was from Berthold Technologies (Bad Wildbad, Germany). The counter was linked via the serial port to a computer. Statistical calculations were performed according to Davies.[14] All data were processed using Microsoft Excel or Winstat (Kalmia Co. Inc., Cambridge, MA). The slope of the calibration curves was calculated according to Nix.[15]

Statistics

Results of comparisons between measurements by RIA and LC-MS/MS were obtained by method comparison statistics according to Passing and Bablok.[16] Correlation coefficients were calculated on the basis of usual least-squares (Pearson) linear regression analysis.

RESULTS

Specificity of the Antisera

The specificity of the rabbit anti-*N*-acylmetanephrine and anti-*N*-acylnormetanephrine antisera was evaluated by determining cross-reactivity at 50% displacement of various compounds, listed in TABLES 3 and 4, which

TABLE 1. Typical calibration curve for metanephrine

Standard	Metanephrine [pmol/L]	[cpm]	B/T [%]	B/B0 [%]	CV [%]
Total activity		56,647			3.54
NSB		425	0.8		11.16
Std. A	0	20,777	35.9	100	0.33
Std. B	91	18,556		89	1.45
Std. C	284	15,680		75	0.80
Std. D	862	10,596		50	0.87
Std. E	2,966	5,699		26	2.18
Std. F	13,182	2,485		10	1.85

are structurally related to the intended analytes, and may therefore potentially interfere with the assays. All compounds tested showed a cross-reaction below 0.6%. In all cases the interference by these compounds in the RIA is insignificant.

Interference of Blood Components

Hemoglobin, bilirubin, and triglycerides were evaluated for possible interference in plasma metanephrine and normetanephrine determination with the RIA. Hemoglobin was tested at concentrations from 0.06 to 1.0 mg/mL, bilirubin from 0.06 to 1 mg/mL, and triglycerides from 0.3 to 10.0 mg/mL. Each of these compounds was added to aliquots of two different plasma samples at 10% of the total sample volume. Controls were prepared similarly by adding phosphate-buffered saline only. Spiked samples and controls were assayed and the metanephrine and normetanephrine contents evaluated (data not shown). No significant interference was seen by addition of hemoglobin, bilirubin, or triglycerides. All calculated recoveries of metanephrine and normetanephrine from hemoglobin, bilirubin, and triglycerides-spiked plasma were in the range of 80–120%.

TABLE 2. Typical calibration curve for normetanephrine

Standard	Normetanephrine [pmol/L]	[cpm]	B/T [%]	B/B0 [%]	CV [%]
T		57,858			1.01
NSB		623	1.1		2.84
Std. A	0	9,532	15.4	100	0.22
Std. B	137	8,806		92	0.94
Std. C	410	7,885		82	0.58
Std. D	1,229	6,463		66	2.93
Std. E	4,423	3,894		37	1.53
Std. F	19,656	1,837		14	0.15

TABLE 3. Cross-reactivity for metanephrine

Compound	Max. added conc [μmol/L]	Cross-reactivity [%]
Metanephrine	—	100
Adrenaline	32,751	0.5
Normetanephrine	27,310	0.3
4-hydroxy-3-methoxy-phenylglycol	26,397	0.01
3-methoxy-tyramine	29,455	<0.01
Noradrenalin	35,461	<0.01
Vanillicmandelic acid	30,272	<0.01
Homovanillic mandelic acid	10,977	<0.01
Dopamine	31,646	<0.01
3-methoxy-tyrosine	28,409	<0.01
L-tyrosine	27,561	<0.01
Tryptophane	29,383	<0.01
4-hydroxy-3-methoxy-phenylpyruvic acid	11,893	<0.01
L-dopa	30,426	<0.01
4-hydroxy-3-methoxy-phenyllactic acid	25,619	<0.01
Caffeic acid	27,747	<0.01
Ferula acid	38,620	<0.01

Precision

Intra-assay and interassay variation of the two RIA were investigated by assaying a number of plasma samples from controls within a series of measurements and in different runs. The results are listed in TABLE 5.

TABLE 4. Cross-reactivity for normetanephrine

Compound	Max. added conc [μmol/L]	Cross-reactivity [%]
Normetanephrine	—	100
Metanephrine	25,674	0.6
3-methoxy-tyramine	29,455	0.4
4-hydroxy-3-methoxy-phenylglycol	26,397	0.15
Noradrenalin	35,461	<0.05
Homovanillic mandelic acid	10,977	<0.02
4-hydroxy-3-methoxy-phenylpyruvic acid	11,893	<0.01
Adrenaline	32,751	<0.01
Vanillicmandelic acid	30,272	<0.01
Dopamine	31,646	<0.01
3-methoxy-tyrosine	28,409	<0.01
L-tyrosine	27,561	<0.01
Tryptophane	29,383	<0.01
L-dopa	30,426	<0.01
4-hydroxy-3-methoxy-phenyllactic acid	25,619	<0.01
Caffeic acid	27,747	<0.01
Ferula acid	38,620	<0.01

TABLE 5. Precision

Sample	No. of measurements	Mean ± SD [pg/mL]	CV [%]
1	20	37 ± 4	10
2	20	64 ± 9	14
3	20	109 ± 10	9
Interassay variation for metanephrine			
Sample	No. of runs	Mean ± SD [pg/mL]	CV [%]
1	16	36 ± 5	13.4
2	16	125 ± 8	6.5
3	16	648 ± 51	7.9
Intra-assay variation for normetanephrine			
Sample	No. of measurements	Mean ± SD [pg/mL]	CV [%]
1	20	84 ± 10	12
2	20	141 ± 9	7
3	20	244 ± 13	5
Interassay variation for normetanephrine			
Sample	No. of runs	Mean ± SD [pg/ml]	CV [%]
1	12	76 ± 12	15.6
2	12	161 ± 21	12.8
3	12	285 ± 27	9.4
4	12	822 ± 72	8.7

Linearity

Two plasma samples having high concentration of metanephrine/normetanephrine were serially diluted with standard A and assayed. Each dilution was measured in duplicates in one assay run. The results are shown in TABLE 6. No relevant deviation of the expected linearity was observed. The mean recovery of the diluted metanephrine samples was 98% and the mean recovery of the diluted normetanephrine samples was 92%.

Recovery Measurements

We estimated the analytical recovery of metanephrine and normetanephrine in MetCombi RIA (plasma) in three different samples. Increasing amounts of metanephrine/normetanephrine were added to plasma samples. All samples (spiked and unspiked) were assayed in one run. The concentration of metanephrine/normetanephrine was measured and the percentage recovery rates were calculated. The results are shown in TABLE 7. The mean recovery for metanephrine was 96% (range 89–104%) and for normetanephrine was 93% (range 81–118%). The ratio between expected and measured concentrations of metanephrine and normetanephrine did not significantly deviate over the concentration range studied.

Analytical Sensitivity

The analytical sensitivity for metanephrine as well as normetanephrine determinations was calculated from the mean absorbance values minus three

TABLE 6. Linearity

Sample	Dilution factor	Measured value [pg/mL]	Expected value [pg/mL]	Recovery [%]
Linearity of metanephrine samples				
Sample 1	1:1	824	824	100
	1:2	356	412	86
	1:4	183	206	89
	1:8	96	103	93
	1:16	37	52	73
	1:32	24	26	92
Sample 2	1:1	190	190	100
	1:2	113	95	119
	1:4	53	47	112
	1:8	26	24	112
	1:16	12	12	102
Linearity of normetanephrine samples				
Sample 1	1:1	3,599	3,599	100
	1:2	1,740	1,800	97
	1:4	912	900	101
	1:8	430	450	96
	1:16	199	225	88
	1:32	90	112	80
Sample 2	1:1	897	897	100
	1:2	395	449	88
	1:4	180	224	80
	1:8	111	112	99
	1:16	47	56	84
	1:32	26	28	92

times the standard deviation SD of the zero calibrator of 20 replicate analyses. The values were determined to be 12 pmol/L (2.4 pg/mL) for metanephrine and 58 pmol/L (10.7 pg/mL) for normetanephrine.

Influence of Different Anticoagulation Agents

To test the influence of heparin and EDTA as anticoagulants we have sampled pairs of both plasma kinds. The samples were measured in one run and compared. The statistical analysis was made with specimen from normal values to highly pathological ones. We found a good agreement between both specimens for metanephrine ($r = 0.985$) and normetanephrine ($r = 0.992$). Therefore we decided to establish a common reference range for EDTA and heparin plasma.

Reference Ranges for Free Metanephrine and Normetanephrine

The concentration of metanephrine and normetanephrine was measured in 178 plasma samples of apparently healthy volunteers with radioimmunoassay. The results are summarized in TABLE 8. The results in plasma samples from

TABLE 7. Recovery

Sample	Original concentration [pg/mL]	Spiked concentration [pg/mL]	Final concentration [pg/mL]	Measured concentration [pg/mL]	Recovery [%]
Recovery of metanephrine in plasma					
QCP1	32	1,045	1,077	1,007	93.5
	32	298	330	328	99.4
	32	99	131	123	93.9
	32	33	65	66	101.5
QCP8	135	1,045	1,180	1,075	91.1
	135	298	433	426	98.4
	135	99	234	244	104.3
	135	33	168	160	95.2
QCP9	268	1,045	1,313	1,162	88.5
	268	298	566	525	92.8
	268	99	367	344	93.7
	268	33	301	285	94.7
Recovery of normetanephrine in plasma					
QCP1	63	1,347	1,410	1,175	83.3
	63	385	448	404	90.2
	63	128	191	204	106.7
	63	43	106	86	81.3
QCP8	141	1,347	1,488	1,235	83.0
	141	385	526	498	94.7
	141	128	269	277	102.9
	141	43	184	171	93.1
QCP9	259	1,347	1,606	1,313	81.8
	259	385	644	761	118.2
	259	128	387	350	90.4
	259	43	302	270	89.5

hypertensive subjects tended to be slightly higher, however, not statistically significant, than in the apparently healthy volunteers (data not shown).

Method Comparison: IBL Metanephrine and Normetanephrine RIA (Plasma) Versus LC-MS/MS

The normetanephrine content of 25 EDTA plasma samples was determined in-house with IBL RIA and by LC-MS/MS performed by Dr. Eric Grouzmann at the Vaudois Center University Hospital, Division of Clinical Pharmacology

TABLE 8. Reference ranges plasma

Samples	N	Median [pg/mL]	Percentile 95% [pg/mL]	Percentile 97.5% [pg/mL]	Percentile 99% [pg/mL]	Range [pg/mL]
Reference range for free metanephrine in plasma						
Plasma	178	22	66	75	80	10–100
Reference range for free normetanephrine in plasma						
Plasma	178	46	151	161	169	15–170

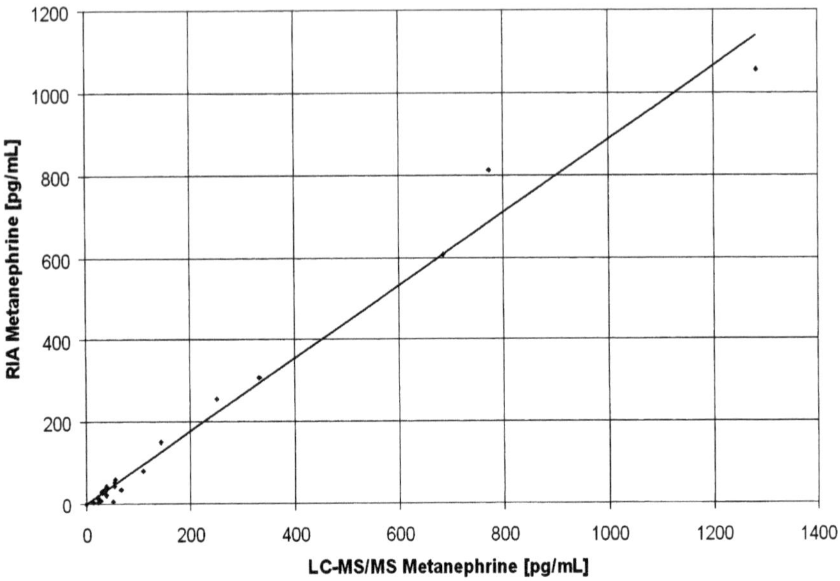

FIGURE 3. Method comparison metanephrine.

and Toxicology, Hospital De Beaumont, Lausanne, Switzerland. Results obtained by applying the RIA and LC-MS procedure were compared and graphically displayed in FIGURES 3 and 4. The obtained parameters from the statistical analyses are:

$$\text{metanephrine IBL-Assay} = 0.888 \times [\text{LC-MS/MS}] + 0.32 \text{ r2} = 0.985; \text{n} = 25$$

$$\text{normetanephrine IBL-Assay} = 1.018 \times [\text{LC-MS/MS}] - 44.0 \text{ r2} = 0.975; \text{n} = 25$$

From FIGURES 3 and 4 and the given parameters it can be concluded that an acceptable correlation between both methods exists.

DISCUSSION

Several different analytical techniques, such as spectrophotometry and fluorometry, have been used in the past for the determination of catecholamines. Toward the end of the 1970s the introduction of HPLC with electrochemical detection for the measurement of urinary catecholamines was considered to be a major advance.[10] Several modifications to improve the sensitivity of the method in order to obtain reliable results for plasma catecholamines have been subsequently described.[11] However, all these methods are very time consuming and cumbersome so that their use is limited to highly specialized laboratories.

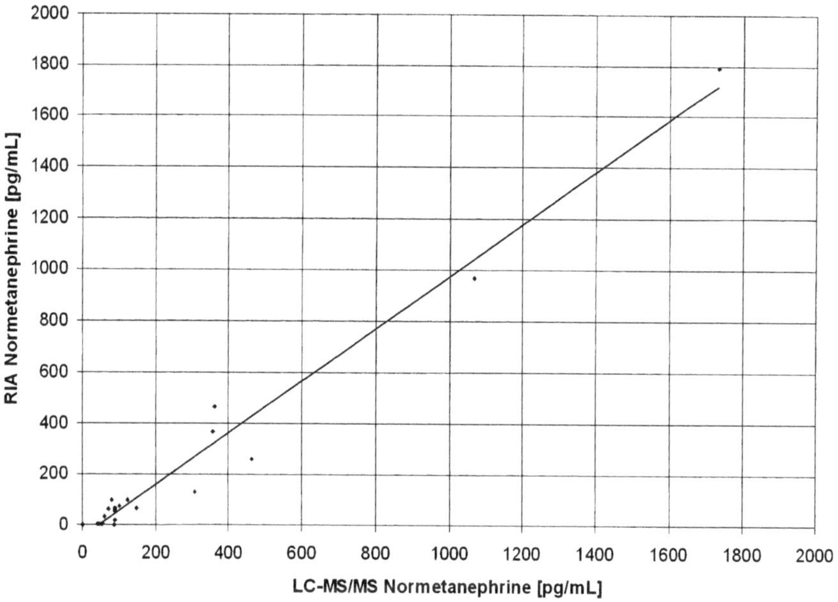

FIGURE 4. Method comparison normetanephrine.

The HPLC methods used differ between laboratories and some methods are prone to interference, often by antihypertensive agents (e.g., angiotensin-converting enzyme inhibitors, β-blockers, calcium channel blockers, and diuretics), which patients with suspected pheochromocytoma often receive.[17,18] This important issue must be taken into account when comparing the results of different methods,[17] or when examining the catecholamine plasma levels (using the HPLC method) from patients receiving sympathomimetic and sympatholytic agents in the intensive care unit and operating room.[19] Recent reports on the determination of plasma-free metanephrines by HPLC have shown an interference with paracetamol.[20]

Another concern in HPLC measurement is the influence of caffeic acid and ferula acid, the metabolite of COMT action on caffeic acid. Both substances were tested in the immunoassay and have shown no cross-reactivity with the antibody used (see TABLE 4).

The detection of interference of drugs in immunoassays is more difficult than in HPLC because no visual hardcopy of the measured end product is produced. Wassell *et al.*[17] studied the influence of angiotensin-converting enzyme inhibitors, ß-blockers, calcium channel blockers, diuretics, statins, α-methyldopa, and α-receptor antagonists in immunoassay and HPLC. They found that none of the drugs examined showed significant interferences in the immunoassay, but interferences were found in the HPLC system. They argue that this seems to be the result of the use of highly specific antibodies in the immunoassay (see TABLES 3 and 4 for specificity).

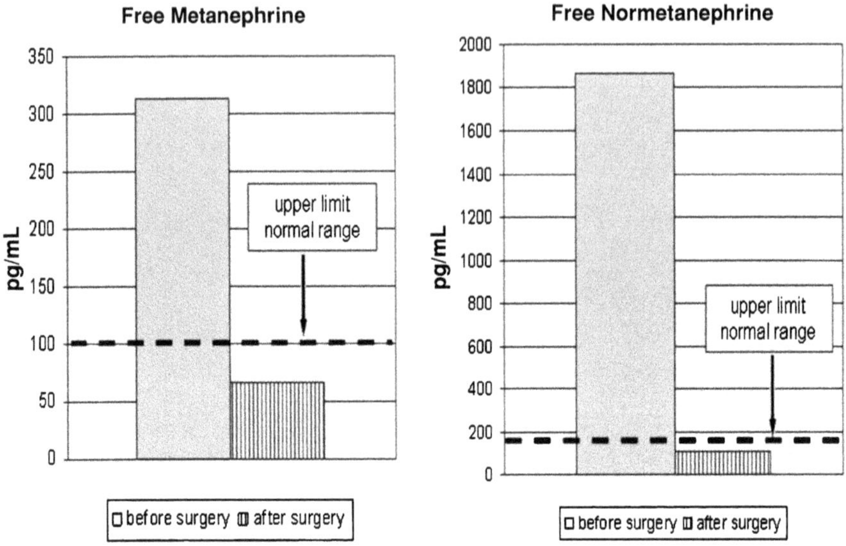

FIGURE 5. Plasma metanephrines in a patient with pheochromocytoma before and after removal of the tumor (upper reference range for metanephrine was 100 pg/mL and for normetanephrine 170 pg/mL).

In our multicenter study, hypertensive patients on different medications were included and we found no abnormal or no plausible elevations of free metanephrines in the plasma of these individuals. In a first patient from another cooperating outpatient center with proven pheochromocytoma measurement of free plasma metanephrines using our newly developed radioimmunoassay demonstrated vastly elevated plasma concentrations before surgical removal of the tumor and values within the normal reference range thereafter (FIG. 5).

In summary, our preliminary results from this clinical study suggest that the new immunoassay that is presented here is as accurate as LC-MS/MS and that tube coating with EDTA or heparin leads to similar results. We believe that highly sophisticated methods, such as HPLC are not really required anymore for routine diagnostic purposes and that immunoassays for free metanephrines are most likely becoming the standard tests of the future. Of course, future studies on larger patient numbers will be necessary to substantiate the diagnostic role of immunoassays for the measurement of free plasma metanephrines in the work-up for pheochromocytoma.

ACKNOWLEDGMENTS

The authors thank Mrs. Susan Sina, Mrs. Doris Schwarz, and Mrs. Schlegel from Frankfurt University Hospital for technical and logistical support.

REFERENCES

1. ROSANO, T.G. *et al.* 1991. Advances in catecholamine and metabolite measurements for diagnosis of pheochromocytoma. Clin. Chem. **37:** 1854–1867.
2. SUTTON, J. *et al.* 1981. Prevalence of clinically unsuspected pheochromocytoma. Review of 50-year autopsy series. Mayo Clin. Proc. **56:** 354–360.
3. PLATTS, J. *et al.* 1995. Death from pheochromocytoma: lessons from a post mortem survey. J. R. Coll. Physicians Lond. **29:** 299–306.
4. LO, C. *et al.* 2000. Adrenal pheochromocytoma remains a frequently overlooked diagnosis. Am. J. Surg. **179:** 212–215.
5. POMARES, F. *et al.* 1998. Differences between sporadic and multiple endocrine neo-plasia type 2A pheochromocytoma. Clin. Endocrinol. **48:** 195–200.
6. GRAHAM, P. *et al.* 1993. Laboratory diagnosis of pheochromocytoma: which analytes should we measure? Ann. Clin. Biochem. **30:** 129–134.
7. LUCON, A. *et al.* 1997. Pheochromocytoma: study of 50 cases. J. Urol. **157:** 1208–1212.
8. MANELLI, M. *et al.* 1999. Pheochromocytoma in Italy: a multicentric retrospective study. Eur. J. Endocrinol. **141:** 619–624.
9. GERLO, E. & C. SEVENS. 1994. Urinary and plasma catecholamines and urinary catecholamine metabolites in pheochromocytoma: diagnostic value in 19 cases. Clin. Chem. **40:** 250–256.
10. RABER, W. *et al.* 2000. Diagnostic efficacy of unconjugated plasma metanephrines for the detection of pheochromocytoma. Arch. Intern. Med. **160:** 2957–2963.
11. GROUZMANN, E. *et al.* 2001. Disappearance rate of catecholamines, total metanephrines, and neuropeptide Y from the plasma of patients after resection of pheochromocytoma. Clin. Chem. **47:** 1075–1082.
12. WESTERMANN, J. *et al.* 2002. Simple, rapid and sensitive determination of epinephrine and norepinephrine in urine and plasma by non-competitive enzyme immunoassay, compared with HPLC method. Clin. Lab. **48:** 61–71.
13. TILGMANN, C. & N. KALKKINEN. 1990. Purification and partial characterization of rat liver soluble catechol-o-methyltransferase. FEBS Lett. **264:** 95–99.
14. DAVIES, C. 1994. Technical performance concepts. *In* The Immunoassay Handbook. D. Wild, Ed.: 83–100. Stockton Press. New York.
15. NIX, B. 1994. Calibration curve-fitting. *In* The Immunoassay Handbook. D. Wild, Ed.: 117–123. Stockton Press. New York.
16. PASSING, W. & H. BABLOK. 1983. A new procedure for testing the equality of measurements from two methods. J. Clin. Chem. Clin. Biochem. **21:** 709–720.
17. WASSELL, J. *et al.* 1999. Freedom from drug interference in new immunoassays for urinary catecholamines and metanephrines. Clin. Chem. **45:** 2216–2223.
18. BOULOUX, P. & M. FAKEEH. 1995. Investigation of pheochromocytoma. Clin. Endocrinol. **43:** 657–664.
19. WEISSMAN, C. *et al.* 1995. Do synthetic adrenergic agents interfere with the measurement of endogenous plasma catecholamine concentrations? J. Crit. Care **10:** 72–77.
20. LENDERS, J.W.M. *et al.* 2005. Phaeochromocytoma. Lancet **366:** 665–675.

Current Trends in Functional Imaging of Pheochromocytomas and Paragangliomas

BARRY L. SHULKIN,[a] IOANNIS ILIAS,[b] JAMES C. SISSON,[c] AND KAREL PACAK[d]

[a]*Division of Nuclear Medicine, Department of Radiological Sciences, St. Jude Children's Research Hospital, Memphis, Tennessee 38105-2794, USA*

[b]*Department of Pharmacology, Medical School, University of Patras, Rion-GR-26504, Greece*

[c]*Division of Nuclear Medicine, Department of Radiology, University of Michigan Medical Center, 1500 East Medical Center Drive, UH B1G 505D, Ann Arbor, Michigan 48109-0028, USA*

[d]*Reproductive Biology and Medicine Branch, National Institute of Child Health and Human Development, National Institutes of Health, Bethesda, Maryland 20892-1109, USA*

ABSTRACT: Most pheochromocytomas/paragangliomas should be evaluated with anatomical imaging (computed tomography or magnetic resonance imaging) followed by functional imaging (nuclear medicine modalities). Functional imaging assures that the tumor is indeed a pheochromocytoma/paraganglioma and enables more thorough localization, especially detecting as many lesions as possible (in particular for metastatic disease). Functional imaging for pheochromocytomas/paragangliomas, can use radiolabled ligands specific for pathways of synthesis, metabolism, and inactivation of catecholamines or nonspecific ligands. In an overview of the available nuclear medicine modalities, we summarize the accumulated experience and recommend when functional imaging should be applied to patients with pheochromocytoma/paraganglioma.

KEYWORDS: nuclear medicine methods; radionuclide imaging; positron emission tomography; pheochromocytoma diagnosis

Address for correspondence: Karel Pacak, M.D., Ph.D., Section on Medical Neuroendocrinology, Reproductive Biology and Medicine Branch, National Institute of Child Health and Human Development, National Institutes of Health, Building 10, CRC, 1 East, Room 1-3140, 10 Center Drive, MSC-1109, Bethesda, MD 20892-1109. Voice: 301-402-4594; fax: 301-402-4712.
e-mail: karel@mail.nih.gov

**Ann. N.Y. Acad. Sci. 1073: 374–382 (2006). © 2006 New York Academy of Sciences.
doi: 10.1196/annals.1353.041**

INTRODUCTION

Although pheochromocytomas are predominantly sporadic, about 24% of patients with apparent sporadic pheochromocytoma may be carriers of germline mutations that entail a predisposition for extra-adrenal and often multifocal disease.[1] About 26–35% of these tumors are metastastic,[2–5] and about 10% present with metastatic disease at initial diagnosis.[6] In the context of the clinical evaluation of pheochromocytoma/paraganglioma, anatomical imaging with computed tomography (CT) or magnetic resonance (MR) should be done in all patients. After anatomical imaging is performed, functional (nuclear medicine) modalities are used to prove that the tumor is indeed pheochromocytoma/paraganglioma, as well as to detect as many lesions as possible (for metastatic disease) and to choose the appropriate therapeutic plan. Nuclear medicine modalities can be categorized into those that are specific for the catecholamine synthesis/secretion pathway and those that are nonspecific, that is, they reflect other aspects of tumor pathophysiology.

Most pheochromocytoma/paraganglioma cells (chromaffin cells) are distinguished from other tumor cells in that they express the norepinephrine transport system (hNET).[7] The latter is responsible for the uptake of norepinephrine and epinephrine from the synaptic cleft into the presynaptic neuron of the sympathetic nervous system. hNET thus not only terminates neural transmission by removal of the neurotransmitter norepinephrine but also enables specific functional imaging. In this manuscript we will review the results of imaging of pheochromocytoma obtained with various radiotracers. We begin by describing several radiotracers that depend upon hNET for transport to pheochromocytoma cells followed by tracers whose uptake and retention are independent of hNET (FIG. 1).

SPECIFIC FUNCTIONAL IMAGING

Attempts to image pheochromocytoma by specific radiotracer techniques began with the development of meta-iodobenzylguanidine (m-IBG) by Wieland and colleagues at the University of Michigan.[8] Sisson and colleagues reported successful localization of pheochromocytomas using m-IBG.[9] Initially, m-IBG was labeled with iodine-131. m-IBG labeled with iodine-123 has become more common because of the characteristics of I-123, which makes it a better radiolabel than iodine-131 for diagnostic evaluation of pheochromocytoma. Relative to I-131, I-123 has a shorter half-life (13.2 h vs. 8 days), a principal emission photon energy much closer to the 140 kEv of Tc-99m, around which gamma cameras are designed (159 kEv I-123 vs. 364 kEv I-131), and lack of beta particulate emission, which adds to the radiation burden and limits the activity that can be administered. Because of the higher emitted photon flux, I-123 m-IBG images contain about tenfold the number of

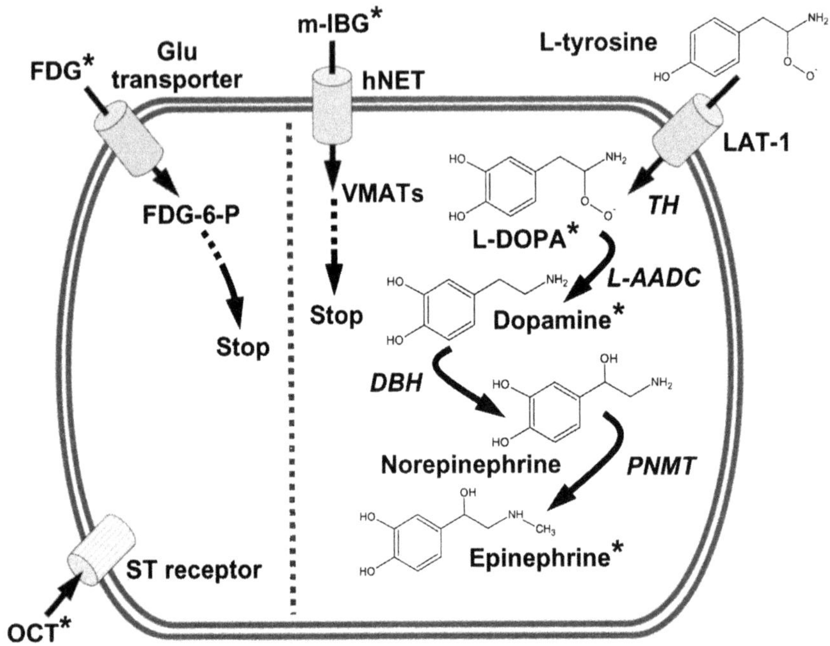

FIGURE 1. Targets for functional imaging of pheochromocytomas/paragangliomas. On the right are shown steps and molecules involved in the synthesis of catecholamines; these are targets for radioligands specific for such cells. On the left are nonspecific targets. Molecules with asterisks are radiolabeled to be used for functional imaging. TH: tyrosine hydroxylase; hNET: human norepinephrine transporter (responsible for re-uptake of catecholamines); m-IBG: meta-iodobenzylguanidine; VMATs: vesicular monoamine transporters (they transport m-IBG into norepinephrine and epinephrine storage vesicles); LAT-1: large neutral amino acid transporter; L-DOPA: L-dihydroxyphenylalanine; L-AADC: aromatic-L-amino acid decarboxylase; DBH: dopamine beta-hydroxylase; PNMT: phenylethanolamine-N-methyltransferase; ST: somatostatin; OCT: octreotide; Glu: glucose; FDG: 18-F-fluorodeoxyglucose; FDG-6-P: FDG-6-phosphate; Stop: not further metabolized.

acquired counts as do those obtained with I-131 m-IBG; they are of much higher quality; and tomographic images (SPECT – single photon emission computed tomography) can be obtained for further localization (FIG. 2).

m-IBG is useful in localizing pheochromocytomas in any part of the body. It is especially valuable in localizing extra-adrenal sites of pheochromocytoma, and pheochromocytoma in areas of the body previously operated upon, where anatomic imaging is compromised by distortion of anatomy and the presence of metallic clips that degrade anatomic-based images. a-IBG (amino-iodobenzylguanidine) was synthesized as a kit-based formula that would allow local production of the radiolabeled compound.[10] Although pheochromocytomas were readily identified using this compound, lung accumulation of a-IBG was higher than that of m-IBG.

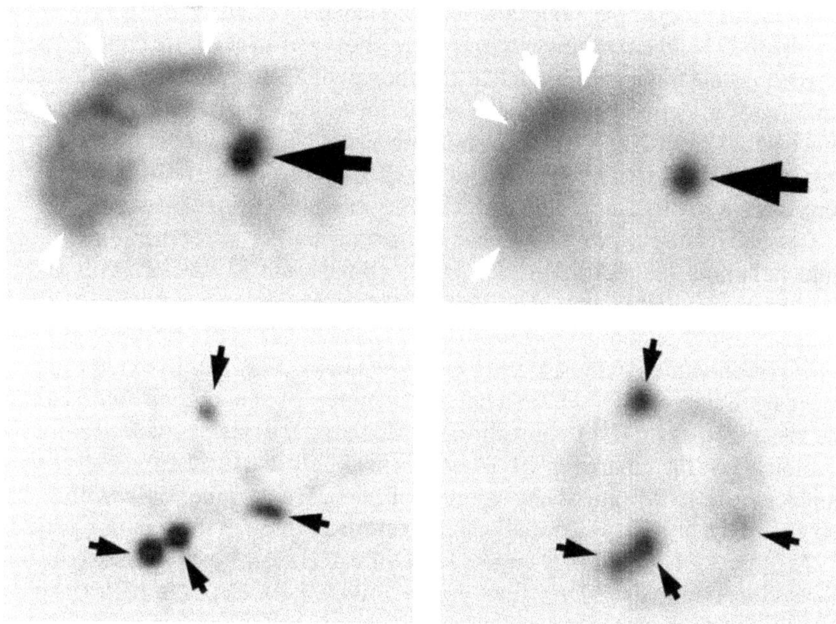

FIGURE 2. The upper left panel is a 11-C-hydroxyephedrine (HED) PET image at 40 min and the upper right panel is a I-123-m-IBG (meta-iodobenzylguanidine) SPECT image at 24 h of a 72-year-old patient with a mid-abdominal pheochromocytoma (hepatic uptake is indicated with small white arrows; the tumor is indicated with the large dark arrow). The lower left panel is a 11-C-HED PET image at 40 min and the lower right panel is a I-123-m-IBG SPECT image at 24 h of a 60-year-old patient with malignant pheochromocytoma (multiple foci of uptake are indicated with small dark arrows).

Positron emission tomography (PET) tracers present some advantages compared with single photon-emitting tracers. PET tracers utilize PET cameras, which inherently produce tomographic images with higher spatial resolution than conventional scintigraphic imaging. PET tracers utilize shorter-lived isotopes, enabling higher doses to be administered for a similar radiation exposure. Because of the short half-life, tracers that reflect different aspects of tumor biology could be administered in a single session.

The first positron-emitting tracer of the sympathetic nervous system suitable for administration in humans was m-hydroxyephedrine (HED). HED was designed to image the sympathetic innervation of the heart. Structurally, it resembles norepinephrine but is not susceptible to intracellular degradation by the enzyme monoamine oxidase. m-HED was shown to accumulate in myocardium by transport by the human norepinephrine transporter (hNET). It was labeled with the positron emitter, carbon-11. C-11 has a half-life of only 20 min, thus C-11 HED requires onsite synthesis as its short half-life precludes widespread distribution. Shulkin and colleagues showed that outstanding functional images of pheochromocytomas could be obtained using C-11 HED and a PET camera (FIG. 2).[11] Pheochromocytomas were localized in 9 of 10 patients with pheochromocytoma. High-quality functional images were acquired within minutes of injection, and tumor to nontumor ratios were more favorable than those of I-123 m-IBG. Trampal and colleagues have also reported excellent results with C-11 HED.[12] Because of the need for onsite synthesis, few centers have access to this compound and it is not yet widely utilized.

Closely related to the endogenous neurotransmitter norepinephrine is the catecholamine epinephrine. Like HED, epinephrine is labeled with C-11, requiring onsite synthesis. Unlike HED, epinephrine is a substrate for the catecholamine catabolic enzymes COMT (catechol-*O*-methyltransferase) and MAO (monoamine oxidase), and thus its retention in myocardium requires intact catecholamine storage vesicles. The majority of pheochromocytomas can be visualized using C-11 epinephrine.[13] However, the rate of successful localization is less than that of m-IBG, and it is not likely that C-11 epinephrine will replace m-IBG for functional imaging of pheochromocytoma. As with C-11 HED, uptake occurs quite rapidly and is sustained through the imaging period.

Another PET ligand that targets steps of catecholamine synthesis is F-18-fluorodopamine (F-18-DA) (FIG. 3). PET with F-18-DA was performed in 18 patients with metastatic pheochromocytoma and was compared to planar I-131-m-IBG scintigraphy. F-18-DA was superior to I-131-m-IBG: it localized pheochromocytomas in all patients and showed numerous foci that were not imaged with I-131-m-IBG scintigraphy.[14] In more recent studies, PET with F-18-DA was superior to I-123-m-IBG scintigraphy in imaging adrenal and/or benign pheochromocytomas and paragangliomas (Pacak *et al.*, unpublished data).[15]

Fluorodopa was developed to image the dopaminergic elements of the central nervous system. More recently it has been shown to provide functional images of pheochromocytoma. In 14 patients, 17 sites of pheochromocytoma were identified both by MRI and PET F-18 fluorodopa imaging.[16] In 4 patients, m-IBG scintigraphy was falsely negative. F-18 fluorodopa is presumably converted into fluorodopamine and then transported into pheochromocytomas by hNET, although the large neutral amino acid transporter may also contribute.

NONSPECIFIC FUNCTIONAL IMAGING

FDG (18-fluorodeoxyglucose) is used for the detection and management of many types of tumors in children and adults. FDG portrays the glucose metabolic activity of tumors, and its uptake and retention are unrelated to catecholamine uptake and storage. FDG is now widely available commercially. The first report of FDG uptake in pheochromocytoma involved two patients whose pheochromocytomas did not accumulate mIBG. Further studies showed that most benign and most malignant pheochromocytomas could be localized

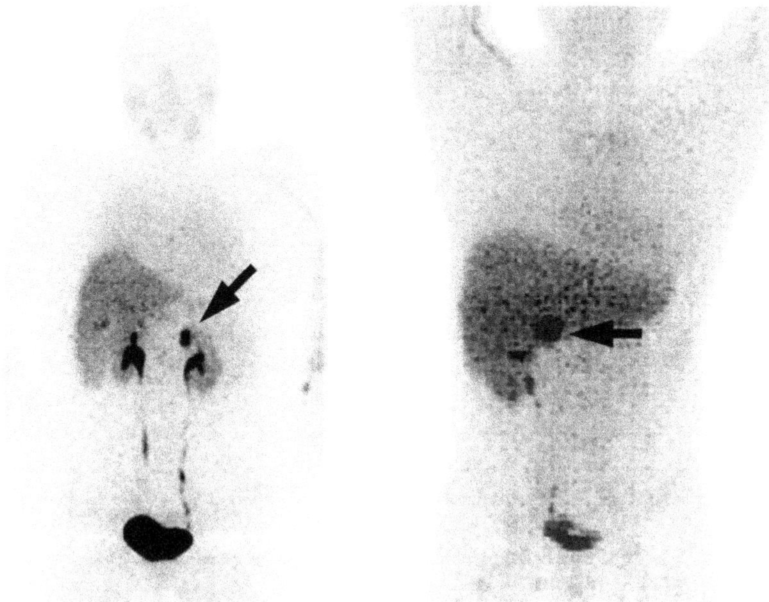

FIGURE 3. PET scans with F-18-fluorodopamine of patients with adrenal pheochromocytomas: left panel shows a left adrenal pheochromocytoma (dark arrow) and right panel shows a right adrenal pheochromocytoma (dark arrow).

with FDG PET.[17] FDG PET appears particularly valuable for the localization of pheochromocytomas that do not accumulate m-IBG or other tracers of the sympathetic nervous system.[17–19]

Somatostatin receptor scintigraphy is of limited value in the localization of pheochromocytoma. Both pheochromocytomas and paragangliomas express somatostatin receptors.[20–22] The octapeptide octreotide is an analogue of somatostatin that is chelated with diethylenetriaminepentaacetate (DTPA) and labeled with indium-111 for diagnostic imaging. We have not found it useful in the evaluation of pheochromocytomas in the abdomen because of its normal intense accumulation in the liver, spleen, and kidneys, and excretion into the gastrointestinal tract. It might be useful for identifying malignant/metastatic pheochromocytomas or paragangliomas;[23–29] such malignant/metastatic tumors can be candidates for radiolabeled somatostatin analogue therapy.

NEWER FUNCTIONAL IMAGING LIGANDS

Newer potential functional imaging modalities specific for pheochromocytomas/paragangliomas include PET with F-18-fluorobenzylguanidine.[30] New somatostatin receptor ligands, which are yet to be evaluated clinically, for

SPECT[31] or PET[32–37] have been developed (they are nevertheless nonspecific for pheochromocytomas/paragangliomas).

RECOMMENDATIONS AND PERSPECTIVES

In conclusion, regarding clinical practice, functional imaging evaluation should be done after anatomical imaging with CT or MRI. Furthermore, we propose that functional imaging be performed in all patients with extra-adrenal, metastatic, or multiple pheochromocytomas, norepinephrine-secreting pheochromocytomas, and epinephrine-secreting adrenal pheochromocytomas larger than 5 cm in diameter. Additionally, functional imaging modalities should be chosen in the postsurgical setting, when biochemical evaluation for pheochromocytoma is inconclusive and in particular when anatomical imaging is negative. Specific functional imaging modalities (m-IBG scintigraphy or PET with 18-F-DA, 18-F-DOPA, or 11-C-HED) are to be used first, and if these turn out to be negative, nonspecific modalities (somatostatin receptor scintigraphy or FDG-PET) should follow.

In future, we anticipate that at centers with PET departments and access to specific PET ligands, most functional imaging procedures for pheochromocytoma/paraganglioma may be PET studies.

REFERENCES

1. NEUMANN, H.P. *et al.* 2002. Germ-line mutations in nonsyndromic pheochromocytoma. N. Engl. J. Med. **346:** 1459–1466.
2. MUNDSCHENK, J. *et al.* 1998. Malignant pheochromocytoma. Exp. Clin. Endocrinol. Diabetes **106:** 373–376.
3. AVERBUCH, S.D. *et al.* 1988. Malignant pheochromocytoma: effective treatment with a combination of cyclophosphamide, vincristine and dacarbazine. Ann. Intern. Med. **109:** 267–273.
4. PROYE, C. *et al.* 1992. High incidence of malignant pheochromocytoma in a surgical unit: 26 cases out of 100 patients operated from 1971 to 1991. J. Endocrinol. Invest. **15:** 651–663.
5. TISCHLER, A. 1998. The adrenal medulla and extra-adrenal paraganglia. *In* Functional Endocrine Pathology. K. Kovacs & S. Asa, Eds.: 550–595. Blackwell. Oxford.
6. GOLDSTEIN, R.E. *et al.* 1999. Clinical experience over 48 years with pheochromocytoma. Ann. Surg. **229:** 755–766.
7. SCHULZ, C. *et al.* 2004. Principles of catecholamine biosynthesis, metabolism and release. Front. Horm. Res. **31:** 1–25.
8. WIELAND, D.M. *et al.* 1980. Radiolabeled adrenergic neuron-blocking agents: adrenomedullary imaging with [^{131}I]iodobenzylguanidine. J. Nucl. Med. **21:** 349–353.
9. SISSON, J.C. *et al.* 1981. Scintigraphic localization of pheochromocytoma. N. Engl. J. Med. **305:** 12–17.

10. SHULKIN, B. *et al.* 1986. 123I-4-Amino-3-iodobenzylguanidine (123I-AIBG), a new sympatho-adrenal imaging agent: comparison with 123I-meta-iodobenzylguanidine (123I-MIBG). J. Nucl. Med. **27:** 1138–1142.
11. SHULKIN, B.L. *et al.* 1992. PET scanning with hydroxyephedrine: an approach to the localization of pheochromocytoma. J. Nucl. Med. **33:** 1125–1131.
12. TRAMPAL, C. *et al.* 2004. Pheochromocytomas: detection with ^{11}C hydroxyephedrine PET. Radiology **230:** 423–428.
13. SHULKIN, B.L. *et al.* 1995. PET epinephrine studies of pheochromocytoma. J. Nucl. Med. **36:** 22P–23P.
14. ILIAS, I. *et al.* 2003. Superiority of 6-[^{18}F]-fluorodopamine positron emission tomography versus [^{131}I]-metaiodobenzylguanidine scintigraphy in the localization of metastatic pheochromocytoma. J. Clin. Endocrinol. Metab. **88:** 4083–4087.
15. ILIAS, I. *et al.* 2004. Comparison of 6-[^{18}F]-fluorodopamine positron emission tomography with [123In]-metaiodobenzylguanidine and [111In]-pentetreotide scintigraphy in the localization of pheochromocytoma, ENDO. 86th Annual Meeting of the American Endocrine Society, New Orleans, LA, The Endocrine Society**:** 452–453.
16. HOEGERLE, S. *et al.* 2002. Pheochromocytomas: detection with ^{18}F DOPA whole body PET—initial results. Radiology **222:** 507–512.
17. SHULKIN, B.L. *et al.* 1999. Pheochromocytomas: imaging with 2-[fluorine-18]fluoro-2-deoxy-D-glucose PET. Radiology **212:** 35–41.
18. MAMEDE, M. *et al.* 2005. Discordant localization of [18-F]-fluorodeoxyglucose, in [18-F]-fluorodopamine-negative metastatic pheochromocytoma sites. J. Nucl. Med. **46** (CD-ROM Suppl.)**:** 1324.
19. EZUDDIN, S. *et al.* 2005. MIBG and FDG PET findings in a patient with malignant pheochromocytoma: a significant discrepancy. Clin. Nucl. Med. **30:** 579–581.
20. HOFLAND, L.J. *et al.* 1999. Immunohistochemical detection of somatostatin receptor subtypes sst1 and sst2A in human somatostatin receptor positive tumors. J. Clin. Endocrinol. Metab. **84:** 775–780.
21. REUBI, J.C. *et al.* 1992. In vitro and in vivo detection of somatostatin receptors in pheochromocytomas and paragangliomas. J. Clin. Endocrinol. Metab. **74:** 1082–1089.
22. MUNDSCHENK, J. *et al.* 2003. Somatostatin receptor subtypes in human pheochromocytoma: subcellular expression pattern and functional relevance for octreotide scintigraphy. J. Clin. Endocrinol. Metab. **88:** 5150–5157.
23. VAN DER HARST, E. *et al.* 2001. [(123)I]metaiodobenzylguanidine and [(111)In] octreotide uptake in benign and malignant pheochromocytomas. J. Clin. Endocrinol. Metab. **86:** 685–693.
24. SCHMIDT, M. *et al.* 2002. Clinical value of somatostatin receptor imaging in patients with suspected head and neck paragangliomas. Eur. J. Nucl. Med. Mol. Imaging **29:** 1571–1580.
25. LAMBERTS, S.W. *et al.* 1990. Somatostatin-receptor imaging in the localization of endocrine tumors. N. Engl. J. Med. **323:** 1246–1249.
26. KRENNING, E.P. *et al.* 1993. Somatostatin receptor scintigraphy with [111In-DTPA-D-Phe1]- and [123I-Tyr3]-octreotide: the Rotterdam experience with more than 1000 patients. Eur. J. Nucl. Med. **20:** 716–731.
27. TELISCHI, F.F. *et al.* 2000. Octreotide scintigraphy for the detection of paragangliomas. Otolaryngol. Head Neck Surg. **122:** 358–362.

28. DUET, M. *et al.* 2003. Clinical impact of somatostatin receptor scintigraphy in the management of paragangliomas of the head and neck. J. Nucl. Med. **44:** 1767–1774.
29. BUSTILLO, A. *et al.* 2004. Octreotide scintigraphy in the head and neck. Laryngoscope **114:** 434–440.
30. BERRY, C.R. *et al.* 2002. Imaging of pheochromocytoma in 2 dogs using p-[18F] fluorobenzylguanidine. Vet. Radiol. Ultrasound. **43:** 183–186.
31. PLACHCINSKA, A. *et al.* 2003. Clinical usefulness of 99mTc-EDDA/HYNIC-TOC scintigraphy in oncological diagnostics: a preliminary communication. Eur. J. Nucl. Med. Mol. Imaging **30:** 1402–1406.
32. HOFMANN, M. *et al.* 2001. Biokinetics and imaging with the somatostatin receptor PET radioligand (68)Ga-DOTATOC: preliminary data. Eur. J. Nucl. Med. **28:** 1751–1757.
33. ANDERSON, C.J. *et al.* 2001. 64Cu-TETA-octreotide as a PET imaging agent for patients with neuroendocrine tumors. J. Nucl. Med. **42:** 213–221.
34. WESTER, H.J. *et al.* 2003. PET imaging of somatostatin receptors: design, synthesis and preclinical evaluation of a novel 18F-labelled, carbohydrated analogue of octreotide. Eur. J. Nucl. Med. Mol. Imaging **30:** 117–122.
35. SCHOTTELIUS, M. *et al.* 2004. First (18)F-labeled tracer suitable for routine clinical imaging of sst receptor-expressing tumors using positron emission tomography. Clin. Cancer Res. **10:** 3593–3606.
36. KOWALSKI, J. *et al.* 2003. Evaluation of positron emission tomography imaging using [68Ga]-DOTA-D Phe(1)-Tyr(3)-octreotide in comparison to [111In]-DTPAOC SPECT: first results in patients with neuroendocrine tumors. Mol. Imaging Biol. **5:** 42–48.
37. GABRIEL, M. *et al.* 2003. An intrapatient comparison of 99mTc-EDDA/HYNIC-TOC with 111In-DTPA-octreotide for diagnosis of somatostatin receptor-expressing tumors. J. Nucl. Med. **44:** 708–716.

Changes in Urinary Total Metanephrine Excretion in Recurrent and Malignant Pheochromocytomas and Secreting Paragangliomas

LAURENCE AMAR,[a] SÉVERINE PEYRARD,[b] PATRICK ROSSIGNOL,[a] FRANCK ZINZINDOHOUE,[c] ANNE-PAULE GIMENEZ-ROQUEPLO,[d] AND PIERRE-FRANÇOIS PLOUIN[a]

[a]*Hypertension Unit, Université Paris-Descartes, Faculté de Médecine; AP-HP, Hôpital Européen Georges Pompidou, 75908 Paris cedex 15, France*

[b]*Clinical Investigation Center, Université Paris-Descartes, Faculté de Médecine; AP-HP, Hôpital Européen Georges Pompidou, 75908 Paris cedex 15, France*

[c]*Department of Visceral Surgery, Université Paris-Descartes, Faculté de Médecine; AP-HP, Hôpital Européen Georges Pompidou, 75908 Paris cedex 15, France*

[d]*Department of Genetics, Université Paris-Descartes, Faculté de Médecine; AP-HP, Hôpital Européen Georges Pompidou, 75908 Paris cedex 15, France*

ABSTRACT: We quantified urinary excretion of total metanephrines (metanephrine plus normetanephrine) (UETM) in 261 patients with pheochromocytoma (PH) or secreting paraganglioma, before primary tumor resection. We then determined UETM 2 weeks after primary tumor resection and once per year thereafter. The tumor was considered benign in 242 patients and malignant in 19 patients. Patients with malignant tumors had higher UETM and tumor diameters, lower plasma epinephrine concentrations, and were more likely to have secreting paragangliomas than patients with benign tumors. In the 215 patients with a single-benign primary tumor, preoperative UETM and tumor diameter were significantly correlated. Thirty-six patients subsequently developed recurrences or new tumors, which were malignant in 18 cases. All recurrent or new tumors could be detected before the onset of symptoms, on the basis of an increase in metanephrine concentration. We followed one patient with von Hippel–Lindau disease and a new tumor for 50 months before reoperation and found that UETM and tumor diameter

Address for correspondence: Pierre-François Plouin, Hypertension Unit, Hôpital Européen Georges Pompidou, 20 rue Leblanc, 75908 Paris cedex 15, France. Voice: 33-1-56-09-3773; fax: 33-1-56-09-3791.
e-mail: pierre-francois.plouin@egp.aphp.fr

Ann. N.Y. Acad. Sci. 1073: 383–391 (2006).
doi: 10.1196/annals.1353.042

were significantly correlated. In patients with malignant tumors, the logarithm of UETM was significantly correlated with time, suggesting an exponential increase in tumor activity and, presumably, tumor burden. Urinary metanephrine excretion is a marker of tumor activity and a surrogate of tumor burden in patients with pheochromocytoma or secreting paraganglioma. UETM excretion could be used to assess treatment response in malignant cases.

KEYWORDS: **burden, tumor; catecholamine; metanephrine; neoplasm; malignant; paraganglioma; pheochromocytoma; recurrence**

Pheochromocytomas (PH) are catecholamine-secreting tumors that arise from the adrenal medulla. Catecholamine-secreting paragangliomas (CSP) may also develop in retroperitoneal, pelvic, or thoracic chromaffin paraganglia. PH and CSP expose the patient to the consequences of catecholamine hypersecretion—hypertension, arrhythmia, and diabetes—and to the consequences of tumor growth, including tumor recurrence and metastasis.[1]

Catecholamine (epinephrine and norepinephrine) secretion is usually episodic in patients with PH and CSP, whereas the O-methylated catecholamine metabolites metanephrine and normetanephrine are continually produced in tumors.[2,3] The determination of plasma concentration or urinary excretion of total metanephrines (metanephrine plus normetanephrine) (UETM) is therefore a better diagnostic index for PH and CSP than the determination of urinary or plasma catecholamines,[1–4] and metanephrine hypersecretion, rather than catecholamine hypersecretion, is closely related to primary tumor size.[5,6] About 10% of PH and CSP are malignant at presentation.[1,5,7–9] Malignant tumors are larger[5,8,10] and secrete more metanephrines[5,8] than benign tumors. Initially benign PH and CSP may recur, either as new tumors—particularly in cases of hereditary disease—or as true benign or malignant recurrences following complete eradication of the primary tumor.[5,7–9] The 10-year probability of recurrence is 15–20%, but increases with primary tumor size and it is higher for CSP than for adrenal PH.[5,7,10] Finally, patients with PH or CSP may ultimately die from the consequences of catecholamine hypersecretion or tumor growth, and UETM is significantly related to mortality.[11]

In this study, we analyzed the relationships between UETM and tumor burden in patients with PH or CSP. We investigated the relationship between UETM and tumor size in patients referred before initial surgery. We then considered changes in UETM and tumor size in patients with a new benign tumor, before reoperation. Finally, we examined changes in UETM over time in patients with malignant PH or CSP. Our data suggest that UETM is a useful surrogate of tumor burden in patients with recurrent or malignant tumors.

PATIENTS AND METHODS

Initial Assessment and Follow-Up

The procedures used for PH/CSP diagnosis and management were consistent with institutional guidelines and have been described elsewhere.[4,5,8] Patients gave informed written consent for participation in the study. UETM was determined by liquid chromatography.[12] In the late 1970s angiography was used to locate the tumors. Computed tomography and [^{123}I]MIBG scintigraphy were introduced in 1979 and 1983, respectively. Magnetic resonance imaging has replaced computed tomography since 1985 in some patients, mostly children and pregnant women. The size of primary tumors was determined from fresh specimens, during histological examination, and the size of other tumors was determined by computed tomography wherever possible. We measured tumor longest diameter (TLD) as a one-dimensional estimator of tumor size, as recommended by the Response Evaluation Criteria In Solid Tumors (RECIST) guidelines.[13]

Familial disease was diagnosed on the basis of family history or of phenotypic evidence of multiple endocrine neoplasia type 2 (MEN 2), von Hippel–Lindau disease (VHL), neurofibromatosis 1 (NF 1) or hereditary PGL. We screened for tumor persistence or recurrence by determining UETM 15 days and 6 months after the operation, and every other year thereafter. [^{123}I]MIBG scintigraphy was performed in all cases of high UETM during follow-up. Tumors were classified as malignant if there was histological evidence of tumor cells invading nonchromaffin organs or if computed tomography or MIBG scintigraphy detected distant metastases.[8,10] Tumors were considered to be persistent when biochemical and/or imaging tests revealed postoperative evidence of disease. Recurrence was defined as the reappearance of the disease after eradication of the tumor, confirmed by negative biochemical and imaging tests. Malignant recurrences were defined according to the malignancy criteria described above. Other recurrences were deemed benign.

Data Analysis

The values given are numbers of patients, medians [interquartile range], or means $\pm$ SD, as appropriate. The significance of differences between means was assessed by means of unpaired Student's t-tests or Mann–Whitney tests for two independent populations, or an ANOVA or the Kruskall–Wallis test for more than two independent populations, as appropriate. The chi-squared test or Fisher's exact test was used to compare qualitative variables. Correlations between UETM and tumor diameter were assessed with a linear regression model, after log transformation of the UETM values, and using Pearson's coefficient. SAS (version 8.2) statistical software was used for the statistical analysis. A P value <0.05 was considered significant.

RESULTS

From 1975 to the present, 308 patients (146 men) with PH and/or CSP were referred to this unit. Seventy-six (24.7%) had hereditary diseases (VHL in 25, NF 1 in 19, hereditary paraganglioma in 16, MEN 2 in 15, and unknown in 1). At presentation or during a recurrence, 58 patients had at least one CSP and 57 had malignant tumors. Overall, 63 patients had recurrences or new tumors during a median follow-up period of 8.5 (3.8–13.2) years after first operation.

UETM and TLD at First Operation

Preoperative UETM and TLD were determined in 261 patients referred before first operation. The tumor was considered benign in 242 patients and malignant in 19 patients. Selected characteristics of these patients are shown in TABLE 1. Patients with malignant tumors had higher UETM and TLD, lower plasma epinephrine concentrations, and were more likely to have CSP than patients with benign tumors.

In the 215 patients with a single benign tumor, the relationship between UETM (μmol/day) and TLD (mm) was $\ln(\text{UETM}) = 0.020\ \text{TLD} + 2.097$ ($r = 0.34$, $P < 0.0001$) (FIG. 1). In those with single right adrenal ($n = 113$), left adrenal ($n = 72$), or extra-adrenal tumors (i.e., CSP, $n = 30$), the relationship was $\ln(\text{UETM}) = 0.019\ \text{TLD} + 2.179$ ($r = 0.39$, $P < 0.0001$), $\ln(\text{UETM}) = 0.020\ \text{TLD} + 2.012$ ($r = 0.22$, $P < 0.0001$), and $\ln(\text{UETM}) = 0.030$ TLD diameter + 1.32 ($r = 0.31$, $P = 0.0009$), respectively. The slope of the regression line between ln(UETM) and TLD did not differ between patients with right adrenal, left adrenal, and extra-adrenal tumors ($P = 0.5082$).

Long-Term Follow-Up of Urinary Metanephrines

Thirty-six patients undergoing surgery subsequently developed recurrences or new tumors, which were malignant in 18 cases. All recurrent or new tumors could be detected before the onset of symptoms, on the basis of an increase in metanephrine levels. Detection was confirmed by computed tomography, magnetic resonance imaging, and/or [^{123}I]MIBG scintigraphy in all cases.

We detected a new left PH in a patient with VHL who had undergone resection of a right PH. He was asymptomatic, normotensive, and normoglycemic.

TABLE 1. Preoperative characteristics of patients referred before first operation, by tumor status (benign verses malignant)

		All, $n = 261$	Benign, $n = 242$	Malignant, $n = 19$	P*
Patients with familial disease		59 (22.6)	55 (22.7)	4 (21.1)	1.000
Males		124 (47.5)	112 (46.3)	12 (63.2)	0.156
Age, years		42.5 ± 15.0	42.4 ± 15.1	43.4 ± 14.0	0.770
Presence of hypertension		232 (88.9)	215 (88.8)	17 (89.5)	1.000
If yes, time from diagnosis of hypertension, years		2 [1;5]	2 [1;6]	1 [1;4]	0.231
Plasma epinephrine concentration, nmol/L		0.56 [0.10;2.02]	0.62 [0.12;2.29]	0.10 [0.00;0.58]	0.019
Plasma norepinephrine concentration, nmol/L		12.8 [3.8;34.4]	12.2 [3.7;31.9]	21.6 [10.3;69.1]	0.062
Urinary excretion of total metanephrine, μmol/day		23.1 [12.8;49.9]	22.1 [12.2;48.6]	46.1 [28.2;84.8]	0.004
Tumor longest diameter, mm		55.8 ± 29.0	53.7 ± 27.1	82.9 ± 38.0	0.004
Tumor site	Both adrenal glands	14 (5.4)	12 (5.0)	2 (10.5)	0.030
	Left adrenal gland	83 (31.8)	78 (32.3)	5 (26.3)	
	Right adrenal gland	125 (47.9)	120 (49.6)	5 (26.3)	
	At least one extra-adrenal tumor	39 (14.9)	32 (13.2)	7 (36.8)	

Values are numbers of patients (%), median (interquartile range), or mean ± SD, as appropriate. *Benign versus malignant tumors.

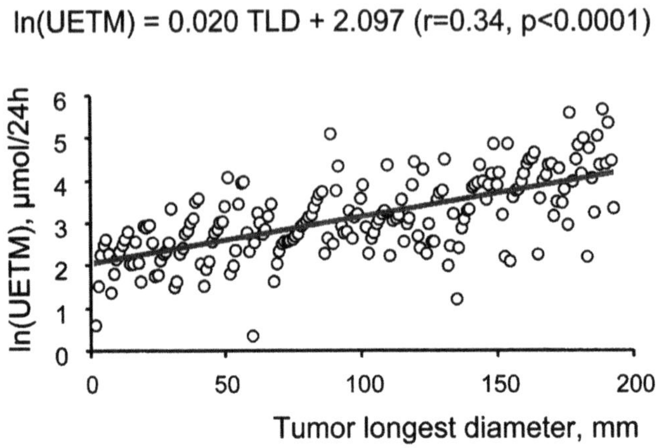

FIGURE 1. Relationship between UETM and TLD in patients with a single tumor.

He preferred to delay reintervention and biochemical tests and computed tomography were carried out periodically for 50 months. This patient ultimately underwent left adrenalectomy. UETM and TLD were significantly related during follow-up (FIG. 2).

In patients with malignant tumors, we determined UETM at least once yearly and standardized UETM according to urinary creatinine levels, to reduce intrapatient variation linked to incomplete urine collection.[12] UETM/creatinine ratio increased over time and the logarithm of this ratio was linearly related to time, indicating an exponential increase in UETM, and making it possible to calculate a UETM doubling time (doubling time in months is the ratio of ln(2) to the slope of the regression line). FIGURE 3 shows linear and semilogarithmic plots of the UETM to creatinine ratio over time from first operation to death in a patient with a malignant Zuckerkandl body CSP and an *SDHB* gene mutation.

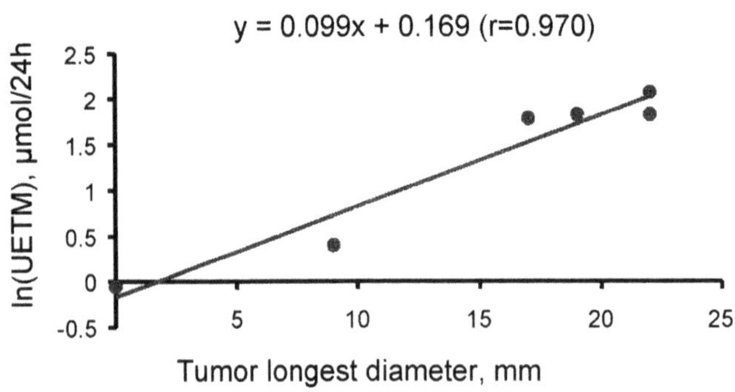

FIGURE 2. Relationship between urinary excretion of total metanephrines and TLD in a patient with von Hippel–Lindau disease and a new PH.

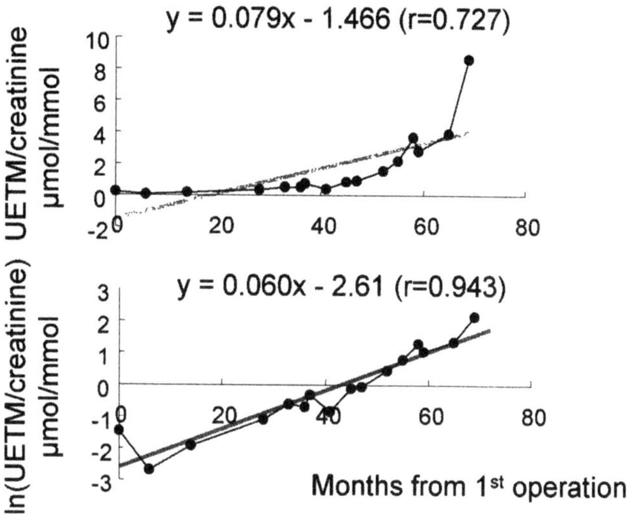

FIGURE 3. Changes in urinary total metanephrine (UTM) to creatinine ratio in a patient with a malignant secreting paraganglioma followed-up from first operation to death. Comparison of linear (upper panel) and logarithmic (lower panel) representations. The x axis represents the time in months from first operation. Urinary metanephrine excretion before resection of the primary tumor is not shown.

DISCUSSION

Benign PH and CSP are relatively large solid tumors that can be easily measured before surgery, by computed tomography or magnetic resonance imaging, and after surgery, during pathology examinations. Although they are usually larger than benign tumors,[8,10] malignant PH and CSP are more frequently cystic and associated with extensive local invasion,[10] which may render measurement unreliable.[13] Tumor persistence and malignant recurrence are usually associated with lymph node and/or bone mestastases,[14] or tumor extensions that are considered to be unmeasurable.[13] There is therefore a need for a tumor marker to assess tumor activity and tumor burden in malignant PH and CSP.

Primary tumor size and plasma or urinary metanephrine concentrations are significantly correlated in patients with catecholamine-secreting tumors.[5,6] Our work confirms this relationship in patients with adrenal (PH proper, $n = 185$) and extra-adrenal (CSP, $n = 30$) primary tumors (FIG. 1). Several studies have also reported a significant relationship between primary tumor size and plasma chromogranin A (CGA) concentration in patients with neuroendocrine tumors, including PH.[15–18] However, this relationship was reported for small series of patients, including a minority of patients with CSP. Indeed, the value of plasma CGA concentration determination for the diagnosis of CSP is unclear, as two reports concerning 25 and 6 patients with CSP found that 2 (8%) and 5 (83%) patients, respectively, had plasma CGA concentrations above normal levels. The poor sensitivity of CGA determination precludes its use as a surrogate of tumor size in CSP.

In this study, we found that serial determinations of UETM and tumor size were correlated in an individual patient with a new benign tumor (FIG. 2), suggesting that the relationship between UETM and tumor size remains stable during tumor growth in benign PH. In patients with malignant PH or CSP, we found that UETM increased exponentially over time, making it possible to determine a doubling time, quantifying tumor activity. Further work is required to determine whether UETM can be used for prognosis in malignant PH or CSP, like urinary excretion of 5-hydroxyindoleacetic acid in carcinoid tumors[19] and urinary excretion of paraprotein in multiple myeloma.[20]

Urinary metanephrine excretion is a marker of tumor activity and a surrogate of tumor burden in patients with PH or CSP. Monitoring UETM excretion could be used to assess treatment response in malignant cases.

ACKNOWLEDGMENTS

This study is supported by grant AOM 02 068 from the Assistance Publique-Hôpitaux de Paris, Délégation à la Recherche Clinique, for the COMETE (COrtico and MEdullo-surrenale: les Tumeurs Endocrines) network.

REFERENCES

1. LENDERS, J.W.M. *et al.* 2005. Phaeochromocytoma. Lancet **366:** 665–675.
2. CROUT, R. & A. SJOERDSMA. 1964. Turnover and metabolism of catecholamines in patients with pheochromocytoma. J. Clin. Invest. **43:** 94–102.
3. EISENHOFER, G. *et al.* 1998. Plasma metanephrines are markers of pheochromocytoma produced by catechol-O-methyltransferase within tumors. J. Clin. Endocrinol. Metab. **83:** 2175–2185.
4. PLOUIN, P.F. *et al.* 1981. Biochemical tests for diagnosis of phaeochromocytoma: urinary versus plasma determinations. Br. Med. J. **282:** 853–854.
5. AMAR, L. *et al.* 2005. Year of diagnosis, features at presentation, and risk of recurrence in patients with pheochromocytoma or secreting paraganglioma. J. Clin. Endocrinol. Metab. **90:** 2110–2116.
6. EISENHOFER, G. *et al.* 2005. Pheochromocytoma catecholamine phenotypes and prediction of tumor size and location by use of plasma free metanephrines. Clin. Chem. **51:** 735–744.
7. O'RIORDAIN, D.S. *et al.* 1996. Clinical spectrum and outcome of functional extraadrenal paraganglioma. World J. Surg. **20:** 916–921.
8. PLOUIN, P.F. *et al.* 1997. Tumor recurrence and hypertension persistence after successful pheochromocytoma operation. Hypertension **29:** 1133–1139.

9. GOLDSTEIN, R.E. *et al.* 1999. Clinical experience over 48 years with pheochromocytoma. Ann. Surg. **229:** 755–764.
10. LINNOILA, R.I. *et al.* 1990. Histopathology of benign versus malignant sympathoadrenal paragangliomas: clinicopathological study of 120 cases including unusual histologic features. Hum. Pathol. **21:** 1168–1180.
11. KHORRAM-MANESH, A. *et al.* 2005. Long-term outcome of a large series of patients surgically treated for pheochromocytoma. J. Intern. Med. **258:** 55–66.
12. HÉRON, E. *et al.* 1996. The urinary metanephrine to creatinine ratio in the diagnosis of pheochromocytoma. Ann. Intern. Med. **125:** 300–303.
13. THERASSE, P. *et al.* 2000. New guidelines to evaluate the response to treatment in solid tumors. European Organization for Research and Treatment of Cancer, National Cancer Institute of the United States, National Cancer Institute of Canada. J. Natl. Cancer Inst. **92:** 205–216.
14. SHAPIRO, B. *et al.* 1984. Malignant pheochromocytoma: clinical, biochemical and scintigraphic characterization. Clin. Endocrinol. **20:** 189–203.
15. NOBELS, F.R. *et al.* 1997. Chromogranin A as serum marker for neuroendocrine neoplasia: comparison with neuron-specific enolase and the alpha-subunit of glycoprotein hormones. J. Clin. Endocrinol. Metab. **82:** 2622–2628.
16. BAUDIN, E. *et al.* 1998. Neuron-specific enolase and chromogranin A as markers of neuroendocrine tumours. Br. J. Cancer **78:** 1102–1107.
17. D'HERBOMEZ, M. *et al.* 2001. Chromogranin A assay and (131)I-MIBG scintigraphy for diagnosis and follow-up of pheochromocytoma. J. Nucl. Med. **42:** 993–997.
18. TAUPENOT, L. *et al.* 2003. The chromogranin-secretogranin family. N. Engl. J. Med. **348:** 1134–1149.
19. KVOLS, L.K. *et al.* 1986. Treatment of the malignant carcinoid syndrome. Evaluation of a long-acting somatostatin analogue. N. Engl. J. Med. **315:** 663–666.
20. SINGHAL, S. *et al.* 1999. Antitumor activity of thalidomide in refractory myeloma. N. Engl. J. Med. **341:** 1565–1571.

Anatomical and Functional Imaging of Tumors in Animal Models

Focus on Pheochromocytoma

LUCIA MARTINIOVA,[a] SHOICHIRO OHTA,[a] PETER GUION,[b] DANIEL SCHIMEL,[c] EDWIN W. LAI,[a] BRENDA KLAUNBERG,[c] ELAINE JAGODA,[d] AND KAREL PACAK[a]

[a]*Reproductive Biology and Medicine Branch, National Institutes of Child Health and Human Development, Bethesda, Maryland 20892, USA*

[b]*Radiation Oncology Branch, National Cancer Institute, Bethesda, Maryland 20892, USA*

[c]*National Institute of Neurological Disorders and Stroke/Mouse Imaging Facility, Charles River Labs, Bethesda, Maryland 20892, USA*

[d]*Intramural Science PRGMS, National Institute of Biomedical Imaging and Bioengineering, Bethesda, Maryland 20892, USA*

ABSTRACT: This review focuses on anatomical (computed tomography, magnetic resonance imaging) and functional (positron emission tomography) imaging methods for tumor localization and identification of experimentally induced tumors in animal models, especially pheochromocytoma. Although anatomical imaging can precisely locate primary and metastatic tumors, functional imaging has high specificity for some tumors, especially those of endocrine origin. This is due to the fact that endocrine tumor cells take up hormone precursors, express hormone receptors and transporters, and synthesize, store, and release hormones. These characteristic properties of endocrine tumors enable investigators to create highly specific radiopharmaceuticals, particularly for positron emission tomography. For example, localization of pheochromocytoma involves [^{18}F]-6F-dopamine. It is a highly specific radiopharmaceutical since it uses the norepinephrine transporter system expressed in most pheochromocytoma cells. Here we review both anatomical and functional imaging methods that are used conjointly in order to localize and identify specific characteristics of tumors.

KEYWORDS: pheochromocytoma; anatomical imaging; functional imaging; animal model; [^{18}F]-6F-dopamine

Address for correspondence: Karel Pacak, M.D., Ph.D., D.Sc., Building 10, Room 1E3140, National Institutes of Health, 10 Center Drive MSC-1583, Bethesda, MD 20892-1583. Voice: 301-402-4594; fax: 301-402-4712.
e-mail: karel@mail.nih.gov

Ann. N.Y. Acad. Sci. 1073: 392–404 (2006).
doi: 10.1196/annals.1353.043

INTRODUCTION

Many traditional and clinically used imaging techniques, such as computed tomography (CT), magnetic resonance imaging (MRI), ultrasound (US), and single-photon emission computed tomography (SPECT) have been adapted in recent years for imaging of small laboratory animal models.[1] This is mainly due to the fact that genetically altered mice and rats have recently become available to study the development, progression, and treatment-induced responses of various tumors in these animals.[2] The above-mentioned imaging studies, although well suited to locate tumors precisely, are not able to describe any of their functional characteristics. Functional characteristics are based on pathophysiological features common to most malignancies, such as local blood flow (^{15}O-labeled water, ^{13}N-labeled ammonia),[3] apoptosis ([^{18}F]-annexin V),[4] protein synthesis ([^{11}C]-methionine, [^{11}C]-tyrosine),[5,6] hypoxia ([^{18}F]-fluoromisonidazole),[7] angiogenesis ([^{18}F]-galacto-arginine-glycine-aspartic acid),[8,9] and cellular proliferation or DNA synthesis ([^{11}C]-choline, [^{11}C]-thymidine, [^{18}F]-fluorothymidine).[10] These characteristics can be best evaluated by functional imaging techniques, such as positron emission tomography (PET).

Pheochromocytomas belong to the group of endocrine tumors that present with unique cell characteristics. For example, endocrine tumor cells take up hormone precursors, express hormone receptors and transporters, and synthesize, store, and release hormones, making these tumors an excellent target for functional imaging. Such findings have already been translated into clinical practice (e.g., the use of OctreoScan in the localization of endocrine various tumors,[11] [^{18}F]-6F-dopamine ([^{18}F]-6F-DA) PET in the localization of pheochromocytoma,[12] and [^{18}F]-2-fluoro dcoxy-D-glucose (FDG) in the localization of recurrent and metastatic thyroid cancer).[13] By making simultaneous use of anatomical imaging modalities with functional imaging approaches, the most accurate localization and functional assessment of these tumors can be made.

Recently, we introduced a new model of metastatic pheochromocytoma in nude mice, using the mouse pheochromocytoma cell (MPC) line administered intravenously.[14,15] In this model, liver metastatic lesions were found 4–5 weeks after MPC was injected intravenously into mice. Local subcutaneous tumors were generated if MPC cells were injected subcutaneously. This model, although not ideal, can serve as the starting point to apply novel functional imaging agents to this tumor and to study its behavior in response to experimental treatments.

ANATOMICAL IMAGING

Computed Tomography

Computed tomography (CT) is a three-dimensional data set comprising of a series of radiographic projections. As a miniaturized version of the traditional clinical CT imaging system, small animal microCT scanners are capable of providing excellent high resolution (37–91 μm) three-dimensional anatomical images of small laboratory animals (TABLE 1).

Typically in microCT machines, the X-ray source and detector rotate around the subject while collecting data. X-ray photons travel through the subject and then hit a detector on the opposite side. When the photons hit the detectors, the energy is converted into a visible signal to create the digital radiographic image. Bone tissue absorbs more photons than soft tissue and fat. Tumors surrounded by fat can be seen because of the contrast the fat creates, but a tumor within an organ or muscle would not be visible. Although this system was primarily used for bone imaging, applications[16] and the availability of different contrast materials make it now also possible to visualize soft tissue structures and sometimes tumors.

MicroCT is an accurate technique for the evaluation of the presence and extent of tumors in small animal tumor models. Generally, this technique provides several advantages over other imaging techniques, the ability to generate high spatial resolution images and to do so in a short amount of time.[17] MicroCT also has the potential to provide detailed anatomical imaging in small animals and serves as a means to monitor both tumor growth and regression.[18]

There are a few difficulties in the adoption of this method for use on living systems, however. The main problem is the low tumor-to-background ratio, which results in difficulty in the interpretation of some anatomical structures. This includes tumor localization, especially if no contrast agent is used. Thus, contrast agent is often required to localize either the tumor or the surrounding tissues near the tumor. Radiographic contrast agents absorb X-ray photons more efficiently than the tissue and gives contrast to the image. However, not all types of tumors can be affected by contrast materials. For example, liver tumors in the model of metastatic pheochromocytoma in nude mice cannot be localized without contrast agent (FIG. 1). Because microCT without contrast enhancement cannot accurately distinguish tumor from normal liver, a specific

TABLE 1. Comparison of individual imaging methods, according to the resolution and eligibility of each technique for pheochromocytoma

	Anatomical		Functional
Imaging method	*CT*	*MRI*	*PET*
Resolution (mm)	<0.07	<0.5	<1.8
Voxel dimension (mm)	0.04 × 0.04 × 0.04	0.5 × 0.5 × 0.5	0.56 × 0.56 × 1.125
Contrast agent	Fenestra™LC	–	radiocompound
Scanning time (min)	<20	<5	<45
Tumor localization	excellent	excellent	moderate
Suitability for pheochromocytoma	good	good	excellent

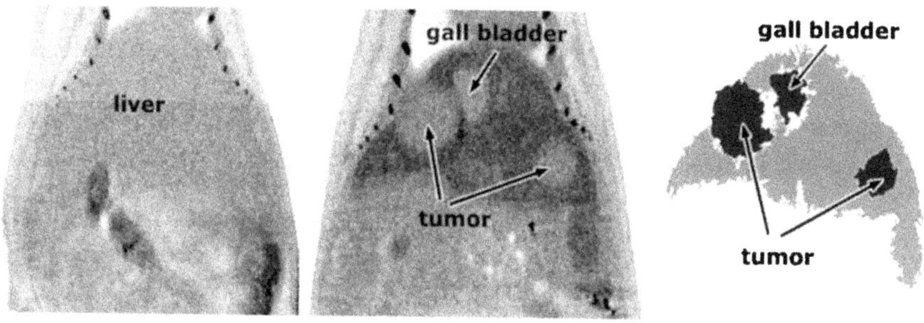

FIGURE 1. Comparison of noncontrast and contrast microCT in liver tumor animal model. There are coronal views (*left* and *middle* image) and two-dimensional reconstruction (*right* image) of metastatic tumors in liver, the 5th week after i.v. injection of approximately 10^7 MPC cells in nude mouse. The *arrows* indicate liver tumors and gall bladder.

contrast agent in order to localize liver tumors in animal model was used.[18] If a contrast agent is used, such as Fenestra™LC, tumors in these animals are visible. Thus, some contrast agents also provide visualization of the hepatobiliary system by using the endogenous lipid metabolism pathways.

Metastatic liver lesions were found 5 weeks after i.v. injection of approximately 1×10^7 MPC cells (FIG. 1). To achieve better tissue contrast, 0.3 mL of the hepatobiliary-specific contrast agent Fenestra™LC was injected through the tail vein 3 h before CT scanning to enhance the liver uptake. This particular contrast agent visualizes the liver tissue around tumors, making the tumors appear as dark spots. These pictures were obtained with 46-μm resolution.

The noncontrast CT scan shows uniform density of soft tissue structures (FIG. 1). It is not possible to distinguish between liver tissues, tumor, and gallbladder. The contrast agent provides the sharp edge contrast of tissue structures (images were evaluated using Admira software Version 3.1 (TGS, San Diego, CA)). This mouse was scanned *in vivo* with inhalation anesthesia on CT scanner (ImTek, Inc., microCAT II, Knoxville, TN).[19]

One must consider the effect of radiation doses on the animal with CT scanning. During one CT scanning procedure on a microCT machine, each animal typically receives 7–22 rem (the unit "rem" is the unit of dose equivalent which is numerically equal to the absorbed dose in rads multiplied by the quality factor distribution factor, and any other necessary modifying factors). The exact amount depends on the physical parameters of the set-up for each scan. To improve the spatial resolution of the images requires increasing the exposure to the animal. This is not feasible for repeated imaging exams of animals because of the high radiation they would receive. This would result in the increased probability of morbidity or even mortality of the experimental animals after a few CT scans in conjunction with several PET scans.

In summary, microCT is a convenient technique for tumor localization because it shows the results in a short period of time and can be also used for fusion (coregistration) with other imaging techniques (PET/CT, CT/SPECT for small animals). PET/CT devices are now commercially available and used in clinical practice, with the main objective to improve diagnostic accuracy.[20,21] The main drawback is the significant radiation exposure in experimental animals which is preventive to studying tumor growth over some period of time.

Magnetic Resonance Imaging

MRI is an imaging technique used primarily in medical settings to produce high-quality images of the human body. It is based on the principles of nuclear magnetic resonance (NMR).

Currently, MRI is also being used to study many lesions *in vivo* in small-animal models by use of conventional MR scanners for humans. A typical clinical scanner has a magnetic field strength of 1.5Tesla (1.5T) with a spatial resolution greater than or equal to 300 μm.[22] Clinical MRIs can produce high-resolution images of human subjects, but may not provide enough detail for smaller animals without specialized equipment. Clinical MR scanners are available in many institutions worldwide and are, therefore, easily accessible. Experimental and clinical MRI human scanners are also becoming available with higher magnetic fields (3T). They can generate images with a higher signal-to-noise ratio (SNR) and are ideal for small-animal imaging. A wide range of animal magnets are currently available, and a few have magnetic fields as high as 11.7 T.

There are several advantages of using MRIs for tumor localization in animal models. The first advantage is that it is possible to monitor tumor growth *in vivo* without having to inject any radiopharmaceutical or contrast agents to establish good imaging contrast. This is different from CT and PET, where such an approach is required. Thus, an animal is not exposed to any radiation (as is in CT and PET) and toxicity from contrast agent.

The second advantage is the relatively short scanning time. Although the actual time for a given scan depends on a number of parameters, most sequences can usually be set from a few minutes to an hour. This is convenient for scanning multiple experimental animals in a single hour or two, making it a very attractive imaging modality. By comparison, CT scans typically take 20 min (plus 3 h for contrast agent to be absorbed), PET scans 45 min, and MRI scans 5–10 min per animal scan. However, using an MRI to image a mouse heart *in vivo* requires at least 1 h of scan time, whereas a similar postmortem scan could provide the same information and could be conducted in minutes. The reason for this difference is that the hearts and lungs are moving in the living animal, and motion during MR imaging distorts the resulting images.[23]

As was mentioned before, it is possible to use an MRI designed primarily for humans to achieve sufficient and acceptable images with mice.[24] However, to study small structures, it is necessary to increase the SNR by use of high-magnetic-field scanners equipped with small radiofrequency (RF) coils and

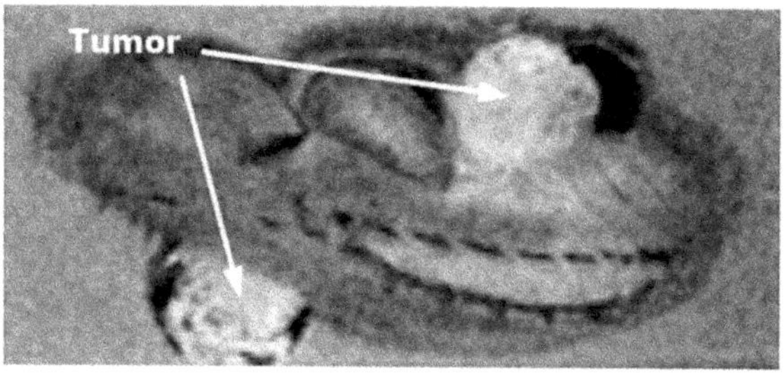

FIGURE 2. Horizontal slice of a subcutaneous tumor. This mouse was scanned *ex vivo* with no contrast agent on a 3 Tesla Philips Intera system. Image was analyzed on ImageJ software. This image was taken with a voxel resolution of 0.5 mm.

strong magnetic field gradients. This can only be done with the use of specific imaging coils developed for rodent imaging.[25] While it is advantageous not to be limited to animal-specific hardware, without such an imaging coil the SNR would be too low to acquire useful images.

The most significant advantage of MRI is its ability to show significant soft tissue contrast without the need for contrast agents. Recent tumor experiments demonstrated that MRI is an excellent imaging modality to detect metastatic lesions in the mouse pheochromocytoma model. FIGURE 2 shows an MR image of subcutaneous pheochromocytoma as a consequence of subcutaneous injection of MPC (FIG. 2). This mouse was scanned *ex vivo* without any contrast agent on a 3T Philips Intera MRI system. Subcutaneous tumors and surrounding tissue were easily identified in the MR image. The same tumors were not obvious with CT imaging due to the lack of soft tissue contrast.

One disadvantage of MRI is its inability to handle motion. Movement of the animal during imaging, such as respiratory motion, results in artifacts in the acquired images. The degree of severity of artifacts is proportional to the amount of movement. However, there are special probes that have been created that allow the MR scanner to acquire image data in portions of the breathing cycle with the least movement (gated imaging). In addition, the magnitude of a small animal's (especially mouse) respiratory movement is not large, and other movements are minimized with the proper application of anesthesia. Motion artifacts are also seen with CT imaging, but often do not affect the quality of the data.

FUNCTIONAL IMAGING

Positron Emission Tomography

PET is currently the most useful imaging technique for noninvasive, regional measurement of drug pharmacokinetics in a variety of tissues.[26] The most significant benefit of the microPET scanners compared to other traditional functional imaging methods, such as autoradiography and direct tissue counting (biodistribution), is that the animal can be scanned *in vivo*. This makes it possible to repeatedly image animals to monitor the progression of a disease or metabolic processes with sequential scans. This is obviously not possible in any *ex vivo* functional imaging procedures. The microPET technique allows researchers to determine responses to experimental treatment, monitor the biochemical metabolism of specific organs, and follow tumor growth over time.

The PET application that is usually employed first is *static imaging*, where the time-uptake information about a radio-tracer is not required. In *static imaging,* a single data set from a time-stationary tracer distribution is acquired. *Whole-body imaging* acquires static image data from several consecutive bed positions and automatically merges the data into a single whole-body image. In contrast, when it is important to know the time distribution of a radio-tracer and its behavior in tissue, *dynamic imaging* is employed to acquire data sets from dynamically varying tracer distributions using fixed frame durations. One of the unique attributes of PET is that the images display the spatial distribution of radiopharmaceutical in three dimensions. In dynamic studies, four-dimensional views can be acquired, whereas in CT it is not possible.

There are multiple physical parameters of the animal PET that are important for the correct interpretation of acquired scan images. Some of these include spatial resolution, sensitivity, contrast, and sources of error. As an example, when structures are scanned that are of a size that approximates the spatial resolution of the scanner (FWHM—full width at half maximum value), partial volume effects need to be considered. For structures smaller than the FWHM, the intensity of the voxels is mixed with the intensity of surrounding tissues.[27]

It is important to choose a suitable radiotracer for each individual study. For instance, the tumor localization requires an understanding of all biochemical processes in the tumor cells, their transporter systems, and behavior. As an example, we will consider the imaging of pheochromocytoma in an animal study. Pheochromocytomas were imaged by PET after the administration of [^{18}F]-6F-dopamine ([^{18}F]-6F-DA).[12,28,29] [^{18}F]-6F-DA enters cells via the membrane norepinephrine transporter. Thus, the animal model of metastatic pheochromocytoma is a relevant model of norepinephrine production in humans. Once inside the tumor cell, [^{18}F]-6F-DA is translocated via the vesicular monoamine transporter into storage vesicles where the radioactivity is concentrated. Alternatively, [^{18}F]-L-3,4-dihydroxyphenylalanine ([^{18}F]-DOPA) can also be used in PET for the localization of pheochromocytoma, because the cancer cells take up amino acids, transform them into biogenic amines (dopamine and serotonin) by decarboxylation, and store the amines in vesicles.[30,31]

Tumors in the mouse were found 6 weeks after i.v. injection of MPC (FIG. 3).[32] Five tumors were recognized in the live animal using 0.2 mCi of [^{18}F]-6F-DA. These same tumors were found on CT scan as well. The PET image data were collected on an Advanced Technology Laboratory Animal

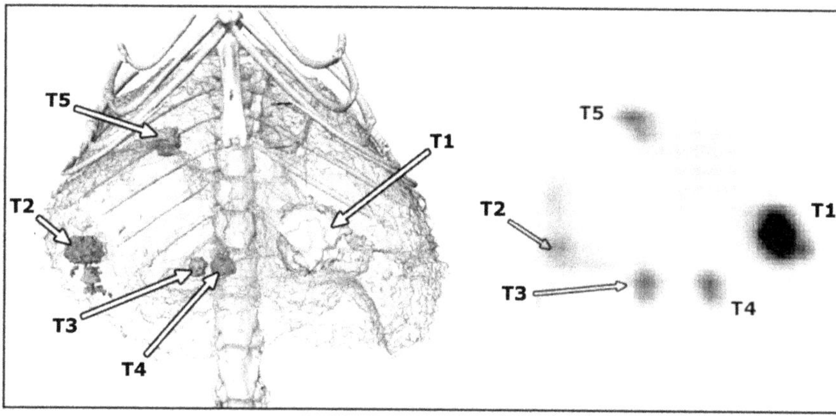

FIGURE 3. Comparison of tumors in liver 6 weeks after i.v. injection of MPC cells. CT scan–the liver of the same mouse scanned *in vivo* with microCT scanner (*left*) and with the microPET ATLAS scanner (*right*) 60 min after administering of 0.2 mCi of [^{18}F]-6F-DA. The microPET scan (*right*) was performed on ATLAS scanner 1 day after the CT (*left*).

Scanner (ATLAS). It is a single ring-type with an effective transverse field-of-view (FOV) of 6 cm and an axial FOV of 2 cm. The reconstructed voxel size is $0.56 \times 0.56 \times 1.125$ mm, which is important information when using the data analysis software. The spatial resolution of this system is 1.8 mm FWHM in the central FOV.[19] It is important to note that several metastases of sizes smaller than the scanner resolution may remain undetected.

PET uses short half-life radioisotopes for visualization of biochemical processes. The most convenient radioisotopes are ^{18}F with a half-life of 109.7 min and ^{11}C with a half-life of 20.4 min. The short half-life of PET radionuclides permits repetitive and longitudinal studies before and after experimental treatment.[26]

PET images are sometimes hard to interpret without anatomical landmarks; therefore a microCT scan of the same mouse, scanned 1 day prior to PET scan, is also necessary for precise localization of tumors (FIG. 3).

Furthermore, it should be noted, that when PET scanning is used, the activity of the radio-tracer has to be in the range of 100–300 μCi. The amount of the radiopharmaceutical is linearly proportional to the injected activity for a given specific concentration of radio-tracer.[33] The total amount of radioactivity is also limited by the maximum volume that can be injected into the specific laboratory animal. For instance, typically the total amount that can be safely injected in a mouse is approximately 10% of the total blood volume. This is typically about 0.25 mL, infused over the period of 2–3 min.[34] If a rat is used instead, the total blood volume is about 20 mL,[35] allowing a bolus injection of 1 mL or infusion of 2 mL within 2–3 min.

There are several disadvantages to PET scanning. One is the relatively longer scanning time. The actual time of a given scan will inversely depend on the concentration of radiopharmaceutical, with lower concentrations requiring longer scanning times. As a comparison, CT scans typically take 20 min and MRI scans may only take 5 min. The other disadvantage of PET is that it uses radioisotopes with short half-lives since the radioactivity lingering in the body is not desirable after a scanning. Consequently, it is necessary to have the cyclotron (which produces positron-emitters) available close to the PET imaging laboratory. Because PET imaging is a functional and not an anatomical imaging modality, the ability to analyze the tumor presented by PET is substantially enhanced if the images obtained by PET are fused with anatomical imaging.[36,37]

Bioluminescence

Reporter gene technology is a useful tool for tracking individual cell movement and cell function both *in vitro* or *in vivo*.[38] Reporter genes can be used for both anatomical and functional imaging in laboratory animals. There are many reporters available, but a useful one for animal cells is the firefly bioluminescence gene, which encodes for the enzyme luciferase. There are no endogenous luciferase genes in small animals, so the use of this reporter yields images with virtually no background noise.[39]

Luciferase can be used to label individual cell populations or entire transgenic animals. In order to visualize the location of luciferase-positive cells, the substrate luciferin must be added. For *in vivo* experiments, this involves a simple intraperitoneal injection of luciferin. In the presence of oxygen and ATP, luciferase catalyzes the oxydation reaction of luciferin and photons of light are given off as a product. A sensitive camera can detect and quantify the number of photons that hit the detectors and a computer converts the signal into an image. Luciferase is often used to label a particular population of cells with the reporter gene under the control of a ubiquitously expressed promotor (such as CMV). In this way, the gene is always "turned on" and able to be detected at any time. It is also possible to use this gene in a more functional assay. Luciferase can be constructed such that it is only expressed under inducible conditions (such as the presence of an antibiotic), or physiological conditions (such as changes in intracellular pH).[40] Not all of these methods are robust, but the technology provides exciting possibilities.

There are several advantages of using the luciferase reporter system. The simplicity of the reporter system is elegant. Because the gene is located within the cell's DNA, the reporter does not get diluted with cell proliferation. In fact, the reporter signal will strengthen as the numbers of positive cells increase. Furthermore, the bioluminescence detection programs are capable of quantifying the signals, so the number of photons detected can be compared over time or between samples. This makes luciferase a useful tool to monitor primary tumor growth or regression, as well as metastatic disease. The imaging device is simple to use and does not require a large amount of space. Additionally, the scan time is rapid (1–10 min and generates data in "real time." Luciferin is nontoxic, and the imaging is noninvasive, so the only risk to the animal is the short anesthetic procedure. The advantage of luciferase over other optical imaging methods (such as fluorescence) is its high sensitivity. There is almost no background noise to confound the final image, so the researcher can be confident that the signal detected is originating only from the source of interest.[41]

The disadvantages of luciferase imaging are few, but may be significant. Currently, bioluminescence imaging is limited to two-dimensional images. It is useful for anatomical locations, but it is currently not possible to make volumetric measurements. Also, any impedance to light emission may affect the results. One factor that can affect the photon pathways is the depth of the region of interest; the deeper the ROI (region of the interest), the more difficult it is for the photons to reach the detectors. Additionally, fur and pigmented tissue, such as melanocytes, can interfere with light emission. For this reason, many investigators choose to use nude animals for ease of imaging. Another disadvantage to reporter gene technology is that the reporter must be stably incorporated into the host genome. In theory this is a simple process, but one must realize that changing the host genome may affect the natural behavior and physiology of the cell. Lastly, although this reporter system is a sensitive *in vivo* assay, a minimum amount of photon emission is required for the signal to be detected. This amount varies with the biological systems in which it is being tested; however, it may be necessary to have approximately 10,000 cells before a signal can be detected *in vivo*.

The future applications of bioluminescence technology are vast and exciting. Although it is not currently being used for clinical *in vivo* applications, bioluminescence has been used for clinical diagnostics *in vitro*.[42] New devices are in development that will allow three-dimensional imaging. Also, as the sensitivity of detectors increases, smaller volumes of tissue will be able to be detected, thus perhaps allowing diagnosis of disease in the subclinical phase of development.

SUMMARY

Small-animal imaging is a rapid and effective method for the evaluation of tumor development, progression, and responses to various therapeutic modalities. Preclinical data generated from animal models are essential to support experimental clinical trials.

The microPET technique is an excellent method for studying functional characteristics of endocrine tumors. This also includes pheochromocytoma, where microPET imaging was found to localize liver metastatic lesions. MicroPET appears to have a high sensitivity for detection of these tumors and their proper localization on account of their specific norepinephrine transporter system.

Unlike microPET, microCT provides excellent images of contrast-adjusted tumor structures. Although microCT offers precise localization of primary and metastatic tumors, the high-dose exposure from X-radiation can be a limiting factor in some studies. Therefore, using MRI may be preferable to microCT for observing tumor growth or reduction over time periods of weeks or months.

ACKNOWLEDGMENTS

We would like to acknowledge valuable assistance of our colleagues. In particular, thanks are due to Ms. Shiromi Perera for her help with cell culturing and to Mr. Danny Solis for his continual assistance and advice. Special thanks go to Dr. Thomasson for introducing us to MRI and to Matus Martini, Hiroshi Yazawa, and Dr. Liow for their guidance and assistance. This research was supported (in part) by the Intramural Research Program of the NIH/NICHD.

REFERENCES

1. WEISSLEDER, R. & U. MAHMOOD. 2001. Molecular imaging. Radiology **219:** 316–333.
2. BUDINGER, T.F., D.A. BENARON & A.P. KORETSKY. 1999. Imaging transgenic animals. Annu. Rev. Biomed. Eng. **1:** 611–648.
3. THIEL, A. *et al.* 1998. Localization of language-related cortex with 15O-labeled water PET in patients with gliomas. Neuroimage **7:** 284–295.
4. BLANKENBERG, F.G. *et al.* 2000. Apoptosis: the importance of nuclear medicine. Nucl. Med. Commun. **21:** 241–250.
5. VAALBURG, W. *et al.* 1992. Amino acids for the measurement of protein synthesis in vivo by PET. Int. J. Rad. Appl. Instrum. B. **19:** 227–237.
6. WILLEMSEN, A.T. *et al.* 1995. In vivo protein synthesis rate determination in primary or recurrent brain tumors using L-[111C]-tyrosine and PET. J. Nucl. Med. **36:** 411–419.
7. LEWIS, J.S. & M.J. WELCH. 2001. PET imaging of hypoxia. Q. J. Nucl. Med. **45:** 183–188.
8. HAUBNER, R. *et al.* 2001. Noninvasive imaging of alpha(v)beta3 integrin expression using 18F-labeled RGD-containing glycopeptide and positron emission tomography. Cancer Res. **61:** 1781–1785.
9. COSTOUROS, N.G., F.E. DIEHN & S.K. LIBUTTI. 2002. Molecular imaging of tumor angiogenesis. J. Cell. Biochem. Suppl. **39:** 72–78.
10. GRIERSON, J.R. & A.F. SHIELDS. 2000. Radiosynthesis of 3′-deoxy-3′-[(18)F]fluorothymidine: [(18)F]FLT for imaging of cellular proliferation in vivo. Nucl. Med. Biol. **27:** 143–156.
11. CORLETO, V.D. *et al.* 1996. Somatostatin receptor localization of pancreatic endocrine tumors. World J. Surg. **20:** 241–244.
12. PACAK, K. *et al.* 2001. 6-[18F]fluorodopamine positron emission tomographic (PET) scanning for diagnostic localization of pheochromocytoma. Hypertension **38:** 6–8.

13. CHUNG, J.K. *et al.* 1999. Value of FDG PET in papillary thyroid carcinoma with negative 131I whole-body scan. J. Nucl. Med. **40:** 986–992.
14. PACAK, K. *et al.* 2001. Pheochromocytoma: progress in diagnosis, therapy, and genetics. *In* Adrenal Disorders, Vol. 1. A. Margioris & G.P. Chrousos, Eds.: 479–523. Humana Press. Totowa, NJ.
15. TISCHLER, A.S., J.F. POWERS & J. ALROY. 2004. Animal models of pheochromocytoma. Histol. Histopathol. **19:** 883–895.
16. BORAH, B. *et al.* 2001. Three-dimensional microimaging (MRmicroI and microCT), finite element modeling, and rapid prototyping provide unique insights into bone architecture in osteoporosis. Anat. Rec. **265:** 101–110.
17. LEWIS, J.S. *et al.* 2002. Small animal imaging current technology and perspectives for oncological imaging. Eur. J. Cancer **38:** 2173–2188.
18. WEBER, S.M. *et al.* 2004. Imaging of murine liver tumor using microCT with a hepatocyte-selective contrast agent: accuracy is dependent on adequate contrast enhancement. J. Surg. Res. **119:** 41–45.
19. SEIDEL, J. 2002. Features of the NIH ATLAS small animal PET scanner and its use with a coaxial small animal volume CT scanner. Proc IEEE International Symposium on Biomedical Imaging (ISBI'02) **TP-P14:** 545–548.
20. SCHODER, H., S.M. LARSON & H.W. YEUNG. 2004. PET/CT in oncology: integration into clinical management of lymphoma, melanoma, and gastrointestinal malignancies. J. Nucl. Med. **45(Suppl. 1)**: 72S–81S.
21. WAHL, R.A. 2004. Why nearly all PET of abdominal and pelvic cancers will be performed as PET/CT. J. Nucl. Med. **45:** 82S–95S.
22. FAYAD, Z.A. *et al.* 1998. Noninvasive in vivo high-resolution magnetic resonance imaging of atherosclerotic lesions in genetically engineered mice. Circulation **98:** 1541–1547.
23. BALABAN, R.S. & V.A. HAMPSHIRE. 2001. Challenges in small animal noninvasive imaging. ILAR J. **42:** 248–262.
24. DU, W. *et al.* 2005. Comparison of high-resolution echo-planar spectroscopic imaging with conventional MR imaging of prostate tumors in mice. NMR Biomed. **18:** 285–292.
25. HANSJŐ, G. 2003. Inductively coupled rf coils for examinations of small animals and objects in Standard whole-body MR scanners. Med. Phys. **30:** 1241–1245.
26. PAWELKE, B. 2005. Metabolite analysis in positron emission tomography studies: examples from food sciences. Amino Acids **29:** 377–388.
27. HUTCHINS, G.D. 2003. Small animal PET imaging. WSPC/trim size: 9 in × 6 in. Proceedings **November 30:** 381–390.
28. GOLDSTEIN, D.S., L. CORONADO & I.J. KOPIN. 1994. 6-[Fluorine-18]fluorodopamine pharmacokinetics and dosimetry in humans. J. Nucl. Med. **35:** 964–973.
29. CHIRAKAL, R. *et al.* 1996. Direct radiofluorination of dopamine: 18F-labeled 6-fluorodopamine for imaging cardiac sympathetic innervation in humans using positron emission tomography. Nucl. Med. Biol. **23:** 41–45.
30. HOEGERLE, S. *et al.* 2001. 18F-DOPA positron emission tomography for tumour detection in patients with medullary thyroid carcinoma and elevated calcitonin levels. Eur. J. Nucl. Med. **28:** 64–71.
31. HOEGERLE, S. *et al.* 2001. Whole-body 18F dopa PET for detection of gastrointestinal carcinoid tumors. Radiology **220:** 373–380.
32. OHTA, S. *et al.* 2005. Downregulation of metastasis suppressor genes in malignant pheochromocytoma. Int. J. Cancer **114:** 139–143.

33. HUME, S.P., R.N. GUNN & T. JONES. 1998. Pharmacological constraints associated with positron emission tomographic scanning of small laboratory animals. Eur. J. Nucl. Med. **25:** 173–176.
34. CHATZIIOANNOU, A.F. 2002. Molecular imaging of small animals with dedicated PET tomographs. Eur. J. Nucl. Med. Mol. Imaging **29:** 98–114.
35. MOORE, T.H. *et al.* 2000. Quantitative assessment of longitudinal metabolic changes in vivo after traumatic brain injury in the adult rat using FDG-microPET. J. Cereb. Blood Flow Metab. **20:** 1492–1501.
36. HAYAKAWA, N. *et al.* 2000. A PET-MRI registration technique for PET studies of the rat brain. Nucl. Med. Biol. **27:** 121–125.
37. VAQUERO, J.J. 2001. PET, CT and MRI image registration of the rat brain and skull. IEEE Trans. Nuc. Sci. **48:** 1440–1445.
38. MARX, J. 2003. Imaging. Animal models: live and in color. Science **302:** 1880–1882.
39. SATO, A., B. KLAUNBERG & R. TOLWANI. 2004. In vivo bioluminescence imaging. Comp. Med. **54:** 631–634.
40. ZHANG, N. *et al.* 2005. NF-kappaB and not the MAPK signaling pathway regulates GADD45beta expression during acute inflammation. J. Biol. Chem. **280:** 21400–21408.
41. CONTAG, P.R. *et al.* 1998. Bioluminescent indicators in living mammals. Nat. Med. **4:** 245–247.
42. CHIU, N.H. & T.K. CHRISTOPOULOS. 1999. Two-site expression immunoassay using a firefly luciferase-coding DNA label. Clin. Chem. **45:** 1954–1959.

Management and Treatment of Pheochromocytomas and Paragangliomas

MASSIMO MANNELLI

Department of Clinical Pathophysiology, Endocrinology Unit, University of Florence, Florence, Italy

ABSTRACT: Pheochromocytomas and paragangliomas are rare neural crest–derived tumors of sympathetic (generally catecholamine producing) or parasympathetic (rarely catecholamine producing) origin. Patients affected by these tumors present with a variable clinical picture, often making diagnosis troublesome. Surgery is the treatment of choice, but requires appropriate medical management before, during, and after tumor resection. Appropriate follow-up of patients is particularly important to identify recurrences, remaining disease, or developing malignancy. Currently, however, no firm guidelines exist about what form follow-up should take. There is also a general lack of prospective studies establishing the best approaches for management and treatment of the tumor. Choice of the many available different therapeutic options instead usually depends on institutional experience and clinical setting, which may vary for different groups of patients. At the First International Symposium on Pheochromocytoma (ISP2005), held in Bethesda in October 2005, a panel of experts addressed and discussed the many therapeutic options and problems associated with management and treatment of patients with pheochromocytoma, reporting their personal experience and sharing their opinions with those of patient representatives. The aim of this special Discussion Session was to reconcile differences of opinion and reach agreement about appropriate management and therapeutic options. This article summarizes the discussion and the recommendations derived from that session.

KEYWORDS: pheochromocytoma; paraganglioma; treatment; surgery; follow-up

INTRODUCTION

The clinical management of patients with pheochromocytoma is a multistep process, reliant on a strict collaboration among different specialists,

Address for correspondence: Prof. M. Mannelli, Endocrinology Section, Department of Clinical Physiopathology, University of Florence, Viale Pieraccini 6, 50139 Florence, Italy. Voice: ++39-055-4271428; fax: ++39-055-4271413.
e-mail: m.mannelli@dfc.unifi.it

Ann. N.Y. Acad. Sci. 1073: 405–416 (2006).
doi: 10.1196/annals.1353.044

including endocrinologists, oncologists, internists, anesthesiologists, surgeons, pediatricians, radiologists, and cardiologists.[1–7] In most patients the tumor is usually cured by surgical resection, but the success of this intervention also depends on appropriate medical therapy to prepare the patient for surgery and prevent or treat catecholamine-related cardiovascular and endocrine complications before, during, and after surgery. The patient is at risk before and during surgery for severe hypertensive crises and cardiac arrhythmias caused by spontaneous or provoked release of catecholamines by the tumor. In contrast, after the surgeon has clamped the tumor vessels, the patient is at risk for a severe hypotensive crisis on account of abrupt reversal of catecholamine-induced vasoconstriction. Subsequent hypotension may be more profound because of reduced vascular volume secondary to previous prolonged vasoconstriction. A priority of presurgical medical treatment is therefore to avoid or minimize occurrence of these adverse events.

There are many options for medical management of the patient with pheochromocytoma, but no randomized prospective studies establishing the optimal options. As reviewed elsewhere,[8] and as shown at the meeting by Dr. William Manger (New York University Medical Center), the high variability in the clinical presentation of pheochromocytoma makes it unlikely that any single medical management or treatment strategy will be optimal for every patient. This and international differences in medical approaches and available or approved therapies make strict standardized approaches to management and treatment of patients with pheochromocytoma largely inappropriate. Nevertheless, some general recommendations on management and treatment may be valuable for clinicians who do not routinely see patients with pheochromocytoma. A moderator-led Breakout Session was therefore held during this First International Symposium on Pheochromocytoma (ISP2005) to address the following issues:

1. What are the most appropriate strategies for the medical management of patients with pheochromocytoma before and during surgery? Which drugs and at what doses should these drugs be used? Which clinical parameters should be followed? Which surgical approaches or alternatives to surgery for different adrenal and extra-adrenal tumors should be considered?
2. What medical management should be considered for pregnant patients with pheochromocytoma or those who are asymptomatic and normotensive?
3. What is the appropriate follow-up of patients who have undergone surgical resection of a pheochromocytoma?

This report does not seek to establish a binding consensus or guidelines on the above issues, but rather intends to provide a review of the discussion, and, where possible, to outline recommendations based on the personal experience

TABLE 1. Recommendations for preoperative evaluation

Collaboration among different specialists, such as endocrinologists, anesthesiologists, surgeons, pediatricians, cardiologists, radiologists, internists, and oncologists.
An accurate preoperative cardiovascular examination should be carried out, especially to detect the presence of a cardiomyopathy or coronary artery disease.

of experts in the field, with assistance from patient representatives who were present at the session.

PREOPERATIVE MEDICAL EVALUATION

Exposure to high levels of circulating catecholamines, together with the concomitant hypertension, may predispose the patient with pheochromocytoma to impaired cardiovascular function, particularly involving the heart.[9,10] Such underlying conditions should be evaluated prior to surgery (TABLE 1). The most common pathological finding is arrhythmia, usually tachyarrhythmia. In some patients, especially those with large increases in plasma catecholamine levels or severe long-lasting hypertension, respective conditions of aseptic myocarditis or cardiomyopathy may be present.[11] Cardiomyopathy generally lessens after appropriate medical management, tumor removal, and treatment of hypertension.[12–14] Coronary artery disease, although not necessarily more common in patients with pheochromocytoma than in those without the tumor, when present may predispose the patient with the tumor to catecholamine-induced coronary vasospasm, with resultant angina or myocardial infarction. Thus, the panel of experts agreed that a preoperative accurate cardiologic evaluation is a wise precaution in patients with pheochromocytoma, regardless of blood pressure levels.

PREOPERATIVE MEDICAL TREATMENT

Some investigators have reported that on account of advances in anesthetic and monitoring techniques and improved availability of fast-acting drugs capable of treating acute hemodynamic changes, presurgical medical treatment may not always be necessary for patients with pheochromocytoma.[15] Nevertheless, the panel of experts recommended that preoperative administration of antihypertensive drugs was a prudent consideration for all patients with catecholamine-producing pheochromocytomas and paragangliomas (TABLE 2).

Alpha adrenoceptor antagonists are usually the treatment of choice,[16,17] but this is by no means universal. These drugs counteract the cardiovascular effects of catecholamines, thereby reducing peripheral vascular resistance, lowering blood pressure, reversing volume depletion, and α-adrenoceptor desensitization. Consequently, α-adrenoceptor antagonists improve hemodynamic

TABLE 2. Suggestions for preoperative medical treatment

Preoperative medical treatment of patients is recommended.
α-adrenoceptor antagonists are the drugs most widely used but other drugs, such as calcium-channel blockers, have been successfully employed.
Optimal doses of drugs are variable and should be titrated to the patients' needs.
Sometimes β-blockers should be added to α-adrenoceptor antagonists.
β-blockers should never be used alone.
Duration of treatment is variable and depends mainly on the effects obtained on the patient's blood pressure profile. The presence of cardiomyopathy or coronary artery disease may influence presurgical medical treatment.
Volume expansion on the days preceding surgery is also recommended.

stability, reducing both preoperative hypertensive and postoperative hypotensive crises.[18–20]

During the breakout session, there was general agreement that treatment should last at least 1 week, doses should be patient-titrated, and treatment efficacy assessed mainly from the patient's blood pressure profile.[21] In patients who are normotensive and asymptomatic, plasma catecholamines may be elevated and contribute to maintaining vascular resistances. Furthermore, even when both blood pressure and catecholamines are normal, it is likely that anesthetic and surgical procedures may provoke an otherwise dormant tumor to secrete catecholamines. Thus, as pointed out by Dr. Karel Pacak (National Institute of Health, Bethesda, Maryland), treatment remains important in normotensive patients. Exceptions where treatment may not be required for blood pressure control include patients with parasympathetic-derived head or neck paragangliomas that do not produce catecholamines or patients with very rare tumors producing only dopamine.[22,23]

The two most widely used α-adrenoceptor antagonists are phenoxybenzamine and doxazosin.[2] Phenoxybenzamine is a noncompetitive, nonselective antagonist, available in 10-mg capsules. Its plasma half-life is about 24 h, but because of noncompetitive binding to α-adrenoceptors and resistance to displacement by endogenous catecholamines, the actions of the drug are longer lasting. At correct doses, the drug provides good hemodynamic stability before tumor resection; however, the long-lasting properties of the drug may contribute to hypotension after clamping of tumor vessels and later well into the postoperative period.[24] Doses of 20 to 40 mg daily are generally adequate but doses may be increased for blood pressure control of up to 200 mg/day.[25] Side effects include orthostatic hypotension, fatigue, somnolence, diarrhea, retrograde ejaculation, nasal stiffness, and tachycardia, often requiring administration of β-blockers. Because β-adrenoceptors mediate vasodilation, it is recommended that β-blockers should not be administered to patients with pheochromocytoma without adequate pretreatment with α-antagonists. In fact, β-blockade without previous α-blockade may induce a hypertensive crisis.

Doxazosin is a selective α_1-antagonist, available in 1, 2, 4, or 8 mg tablets, with a plasma half-life of about 20 h.[26] Because the drug is a competitive antagonist, it can be displaced by endogenous catecholamines.[27] Doses ranging up to more than 20 mg/day may be required to control blood pressure. Doxazosin is preferred over phenoxybenzamine by some clinicians, because the drug does not cause reflex tachycardia (avoiding the need for β-blockers) and it has a shorter duration of action that permits rapid adjustments of dose before surgery with resultant minimal hypotension after surgery.[2,28] Other selective α1-antagonists, such as prazosin and terazosin, have shorter half-lives and therefore require more frequent administration than doxazosin or phenoxybenzamine.

As described by Dr. Emmanuel Bravo (Cleveland Clinic, Cleveland, Ohio), calcium channel blockers (the dihydropyridines) may also be suitable for control of blood pressure and symptoms in patients with pheochromocytoma.[29–34] Because these drugs do not cause orthostatic or postoperative hypotension, their use seems particularly appropriate in patients who are normotensive but who suffer from occasional hypertensive paroxysms. These drugs may also prevent norepinephrine-induced coronary vasospasms and myocarditis. Blood pressure control is not secondary to decreased catecholamine release by tumors,[35] but is secondary to vasodilation following inhibition of norepinephrine-induced intracellular calcium influx in smooth muscle cells of the arterial vasculature.[36] Effective doses of nifedipine range from 30 to 90 mg/day. Nicardipine infusion during surgery has been shown to control hemodynamic fluctuations. Calcium channel blockers can be safely used in combination with α1-antagonists to control more resistant cases of hypertension.

Alpha-methyl-para-tyrosine (methyltyrosine, Demser) reduces tumor catecholamine stores by inhibiting tyrosine hydroxylase, the rate-limiting step in catecholamine synthesis. Although mainly restricted to the medical treatment of patients with extensive metastatic pheochromocytoma, the drug can also be used in the preoperative period in selected patients.[37,38] Oral doses range from 0.5 to 4 g/day.[39] Use of the drug is limited by undesirable side effects.

Volume expansion achieved by saline infusion or increased water intake is recommended, in addition to vasodilators, to further decrease the risk of hypotension in the postsurgical period.

Although presurgical medical treatment limits cardiovascular instability, hypertensive crises remain possible during tumor manipulation. Control of blood pressure can then be achieved using i.v. phentolamine, sodium nitroprusside, nitroglycerine, magnesium sulfate, or urapidil.[1,2] Ventricular and supraventricular cardiac arrhythmias can be treated using lidocaine or short-acting β-blockers, such as esmolol.[1,2]

ANESTHESIA

Surgery, usually carried out with the patient under general anesthesia,[40] can benefit from a number of considerations unique to patients with catecholamine-producing tumors (TABLES 3 and 4). Premedication with a benzodiazepine is

TABLE 3. Suggestions for anesthesia

Sedation of patients on the day of surgery is recommended.
Induction and maintenance of anesthesia relies on the use of gaseous or i.v. anesthetics, such as isoflurane, sevoflurane, enflurane, propofol, and alfentanyl.
A myorelaxant, such as vecuronium, is usually appropriate.
Agents that cause catecholamine release such as ketamine, ephedrine, droperidol, atracurium, succinylcholine, tubocurarine, gallamine, curare, halothane, and desflurane should be avoided.

generally recommended to reduce anxiety.[41] Before induction of anesthesia, an intra-arterial catheter is appropriate for continuous blood pressure monitoring.

Induction of anesthesia is generally achieved by intravenous administration of such agents as propofol or thiopental.[40] Use of agents that can provoke catecholamine release or cause sympathetic stimulation—such as ketamine, ephedrine, morphine, meperidine, or droperidol—should be avoided.

Anesthesia is generally maintained with inhalation agents, such as sevoflurane,[1] isoflurane,[25] or enflurane.[42] Other agents such as desflurane and halothane are not recommended. Among the agents used to obtain muscle relaxation, vecuronium seems to be the safest.[25] Use of other myorelaxants, such as atracurium, succinylcholine, tubocurarine, gallamine, and curare is not recommended.[1]

Once the surgeon has clamped off the venous drainage of the tumor to the general circulation, the patient is at risk of hypotensive crises. Hypotension can be severe and long lasting if the patient has not been properly treated before surgery, usually by intravascular volume expansion.[16] Infusion of pressor agents, such as norepinephrine or phenylephrine, may be employed.[40–43] The use of vasopressin is controversial. Dr. Michael James (University of Cape Town, South Africa) reported his positive experience with the use of magnesium sulfate in the perioperative management of pheochromocytoma.[44,45]

SURGERY

Surgery is the therapy of choice (TABLE 5) and should be performed by an experienced surgeon, in conjunction with an experienced anesthesiologist.

TABLE 4. Suggestions for the treatment of intra- and postoperative complications

Intraoperative hypertensive crises may be promptly treated with i.v. administration of antihypertensive drugs, such as phentolamine, nitroprusside, nitroglycerine, MgSO4, and urapidil.
Intraoperative arrhythmias may be treated with antiarrhythmic drugs, such as short-acting β-blockers or lidocaine.
Intraoperative or postoperative hypotensive crises may be promptly treated with volume expansion, and i.v. administration of pressor agents, such as noradrenaline or phenylephrine. The use of vasopressin is controversial.

TABLE 5. Suggestions for surgical procedures

Surgical approach varies according to the type, site, and size of the tumor. When possible, video-assisted removal of the tumor is recommended.
Adrenal-sparing surgery should be considered in cases of bilateral or familial pheochromocytomas.

There was general agreement that pheochromocytomas or abdominal paragangliomas, when possible, should be removed using a laparoscopic approach.[46–50] This involves less postoperative pain and allows a shortened hospital stay, faster recovery, and less cosmetic damage. Open surgery is generally reserved for very large tumors and tumors in locations difficult to remove laparoscopically. Thoracic surgery is necessary for pheochromocytomas in the chest.

Also, resection of head and neck paragangliomas is best left to experienced surgeons. Since many of these tumors do not produce or secrete catecholamines, there is less concern about cardiovascular instability so that preoperative control of blood pressure may not be necessary. The main surgical risk, particularly for larger paragangliomas, is damage to local nerves and arteries. Damage to nerves can result in impairments to breathing, swallowing, speaking, hearing, and blood pressure control (e.g., baroreflex failure). The risk of local hemorrhage may be reduced by tumor embolization before surgery.

As discussed by Dr. S. Henning Dralle (Martin-Luther University, Halle-Wittemberg, Germany) and S. Jansson (Göteborg University, Göteborg, Sweden), adrenal-sparing surgery to avoid chronic hypoadrenalism should be considered whenever there may be bilateral adrenal involvement.[51–54] This usually involves patients with a familial syndrome where there is a high probability of contralateral adrenal gland involvement.

POSTOPERATIVE FOLLOW-UP

Patients should be monitored for 24–48 h after surgery for cardiovascular and metabolic instability (TABLE 6). Hypoglycemia can be a problem that should be promptly diagnosed and treated by infusion of 5% dextrose.[55,56]

TABLE 6. Suggestions for follow-up

A strict clinical control of the patient is recommended in the first 24 h after surgery to prevent possible complications, such as hypoglycemia and hypotension.
Repeat biochemical testing is recommended after about 14 days from surgery.
Recurrences, including subsequent development of metastases remain possible after successful resection of a pheochromocytoma so that all patients should be advised to undergo periodic follow-up biochemical testing for recurrent disease.
In patients with familial pheochromocytoma/paraganglioma a life-long clinical and biochemical follow-up is mandatory.

TABLE 7. Clues to pheochromocytoma in pregnancy

Diagnosis of pheochromocytoma in pregnancy is very difficult. Medical alertness is required to detect nonspecific signs and symptoms, which may resemble those of pre-eclampsia.
An early diagnosis has important clinical impact on survival of the mother and fetus.

There was general agreement that biochemical testing should be repeated after about 14 days from surgery in order to check for the remaining disease. If results of biochemical tests are entirely normal, resection is probably complete and those patients with sporadic disease are likely cured. Importantly, however, normal postoperative biochemical test results do not exclude remaining microscopic disease so that regular follow-up to check for recurrences remains necessary.[57] It is therefore misleading to inform patients who have undergone a successful resection that they are cured. As illustrated by several case reports from patient representatives, lack of recommendations for follow-up seems to remain a significant problem. In some of these cases involving subsequent development of extensive malignant disease, the patients or their surviving family members expressed views that the outcome might have been more favorable if appropriate information had been provided about the need for follow-up. A regular and long-lasting postoperative clinical follow-up was clearly articulated and advocated by one patient representative who recalled his clinical history during the Breakout Session. On the basis of his personal experience, he strongly recommended that each patient affected by a chromaffin cell tumor should be referred to a medical center with staff experienced in the treatment and follow-up of these tumors. Although follow-up is especially important for extra-adrenal or large (>5 cm) adrenal tumors, there is currently no method based on pathological examination of a resected tumor to establish potential for malignancy or recurrence. Thus, long-term periodic follow-up currently remains important for all cases of pheochromocytoma or paraganglioma.

As reported by Dr. Pierre-Francois Plouin (Université Paris-Descartes, Hôpital Européen G. Pompidou, Paris, France) in his series of 205 patients operated for a single chromaffin tumor, 34 (17%) had recurrent or new tumors, which were malignant in 18 (9%) cases. Measurements of urinary metanephrines, performed once a year, permitted prompt diagnosis of local recurrence or metastatic disease.

Moreover, as presented by Dr. Khorram-Manesh (Göteborg University, Göteborg, Sweden) increased risk of developing other malignancies in patients with pheochromocytoma, including a majority of sporadic cases, justifies a general clinical follow-up. Patients affected by a familial pheochromocytoma require life-long follow-up, with clinical and biochemical assessment every 6–12 months for early detection of recurrences, metastatic lesions, and other syndromic neoplasms.

PHEOCHROMOCYTOMA AND PARAGANGLIOMA IN PREGNANCY

The occurrence of chromaffin cell tumors during pregnancy is extremely rare, but very important to consider when there are signs and symptoms of hypercatecholaminemia.[58] As reported by Dr. H. Timmers (St. Radboud University Hospital, Nijmegen, the Netherlands), because signs and symptoms may resemble those of preeclampsia, diagnosis can be missed with devastating consequences. Pheochromocytoma should therefore be considered in any pregnant women with hypertension, especially if paroxysmal or labile (TABLE 7). Sonography or MRI can be used to locate pheochromocytomas during pregnancy, since it delivers no radiation. Data from the literature strongly suggest the therapeutic use of phenoxybenzamine, which has been demonstrated to be safe for the fetus.[59] Timing of surgery and delivery should be decided through a strict collaboration among obstetricians, endocrinologists, anesthesiologists, and surgeons. Pheochromocytoma in pregnancy remains a diagnostic and management challenge.[60]

ACKNOWLEDGMENTS

The author is indebted to Håkan Ahlman (University of Göteborg, Göteborg, Sweden), E.L. Bravo (Department of Nephrology and Hypertension, Cleveland, Ohio, USA), S. H. Dralle (Martin-Luther University, Halle-Wittemberg, Germany), J.W.M. Lenders (Department of Medicine, Radboud University Nijmegen Medical Center, Nijmegen, the Netherlands), W.M. Manger (New York University Medical Center, New York, USA), P.F. Plouin (Hôpital Européen G. Pompidou, Paris, France), R. Udelsman (Yale University School of Medicine, New Haven, Connecticut, USA), and W.F. Young, Jr., (Mayo Clinic, Rochester, Minnesota, USA) for their comments and suggestions in reviewing the manuscript. The author wishes to thank also the other colleagues and the patients who participated in the Breakout Session, particularly the patients' representative Mr. R. Karnell. This work was partly supported by grants from MIUR (Ministero dell'Istruzione, dell'Università e della Ricerca) (prot.2004069534) and Department of Clinical Pathophysiology, University of Florence.

REFERENCES

1. KINNEY, M.A.O. *et al.* 2002. Perioperative management of pheochromocytoma. J. Cardiothorac. Vasc. Anesth. **16:** 359–369.
2. PRYS-ROBERTS, C. 2000. Phaeochromocytoma: recent progress in its management. Br. J. Anaesth. **85:** 44–57.
3. LENDERS, J.W.M. *et al.* 2005. Phaeochromocytoma. Lancet **366:** 665–675.

4. Pacak, K. *et al.* 2001. Recent advances in genetics, diagnosis, localization and treatment of pheochromocytoma. Ann. Intern. Med. **134:** 315–329.
5. Bravo, E.L. & R. Tagle. 2003. Pheochromocytoma: state of the art and future prospects. Endocr. Rev. **24:** 539–553.
6. Werbel, S.S. & K.P. Ober. 1995. Phaeochromocytoma: update on diagnosis, localization, and management. Med. Clin. N. Am. **79:** 131–153.
7. Kebebew, E. & Q.Y. Duh. 1998. Benign and malignant phaeochromocytoma: diagnosis, treatment, and follow-up. Surg. Oncol. Clin. N. Am. **7:** 765–789.
8. Mannelli, M. *et al.* 1999. Phaeochromocytoma in Italy: a multicentric retrospective study. Eur. J. Endocrinol. **141:** 619–624.
9. Schurmeyer, T.H. *et al.* 2005. Cardiological effects of catecholamine-secreting tumors. Eur. J. Clin. Invest. **27:** 189–195.
10. Liao, W.B. *et al.* 2000. Cardiovascular manifestations of pheochromocytoma. Am. J. Emerg. Med. **18:** 622–625.
11. Quigg, R.J. & A. Om. 1994. Reversal of severe cardiac systolic dysfunction caused by pheochromocytoma in a heart transplant candidate. J. Heart Lung Transplant. **13:** 525–532.
12. Lam, J.B. *et al.* 1985. Reversible dilatation of hypertrophied left ventricle in pheochromocytoma: serial two-dimensional echocardiographic observations. Am. Heart J. **109:** 613–615.
13. Nanda, A.S. *et al.* 1995. Acute reversal of pheochromocytoma-induced catecholamine cardiomyopathy. Clin. Cardiol. **18:** 421–423.
14. Imperato-McGinley, J. *et al.* 1987. Reversibility of catecholamine-induced dilated cardiomyopathy in a child with pheochromocytoma. N. Engl. J. Med. **316:** 793–797.
15. Boutros, A.R. *et al.* 1990. Perioperative management of 63 patients with pheochromocytoma. Cleve. Clin. J. Med. **57:** 613–617.
16. Bravo, E.L. 1997. Pheochromocytoma. Curr. Ther. Endocrinol. Metab. **6:** 195–197.
17. Iseri, L.T. *et al.* 1951. Use of adrenolytic drug, regitine, in pheochromocytoma. Am. Heart J. **42:** 129–136.
18. Hull, C.J. 1986. Pheochromocytoma: diagnosis, pre-operative preparation, and anesthetic management. Br. J. Anaesth. **58:** 1453–1468.
19. Manger, W.M. & J.W. Gifford Jr. 1994. Pheochromocytoma: a clinical overview. *In* Textbook of Hypertension. J.D. Swales, Ed.: 941–958. Oxford. Blackwell Scientific.
20. Stenstom, G. *et al.* 1985. Influence of pre-operative treatment with phenoxybenzamine on the incidence of cardiovascular reactions during anaesthesia and surgery for pheochromocytoma. Acta Anaesthesiol. Scand. **29:** 797–803.
21. Roizen, M.F. *et al.* 1987. Anesthesia for patients with pheochromocytoma. Anesthesiol. Clin. N. Am. **5:** 269–275.
22. Awoke, S. & R.S. Perlstein. 1985. Dopamine and norepinephrine secreting intrapericardial pheochromocytoma in a normotensive patient. South Med. J. **78:** 994–998.
23. Mannelli, M. *et al.* 1989. Dopamine and pheochromocytoma. *In* Peripheral Dopamine Pathophysiology. F. Amenta, Ed.: 203–210. CRC Press, Boca Raton.
24. Bergman, S.M. *et al.* 1978. Postoperative management of patients with pheochromocytoma. J. Urol. **120:** 109–112.
25. Kinney, M.A. *et al.* 2000. Perianesthetic risks and outcomes of pheochromocytoma and paraganglioma resection. Anesth. Analg. **91:** 1118–1123.

26. BABAMOTO, K.S. & W.T. HIROKAWA. 1992. Doxazosin: a new α_1-adrenergic antagonist. Clin. Pharm. **11:** 415–427.
27. ELLIOT, H.L. *et al.* 1986. Clinical pharmacological studies with doxadosin. Br. J. Clin. Pharmacol. **21:** 27S–31S.
28. LEE, J.E. *et al.* 1996. Cortical sparing adrenalectomy for patients with bilateral pheochromocytoma. Surgery **120:** 1064–1070.
29. PROYE, C. *et al.* 1989. Exclusive use of calcium channel blockers in preoperative and intraoperative control of pheochromocytomas: hemodynamics and free catecholamine assays in ten consecutive patients. Surgery **106:** 1149–1154.
30. TAKAHASHI, S. *et al.* 1989. Effectiveness of long-acting nifedipine in pheochromocytoma. Jpn. Heart J. **30:** 751–757.
31. LENDERS, J.W. *et al.* 1985. Treatment of a phaeochromocytoma of the urinary bladder with nifedipine. Br. Med. J. Clin. Res. **290:** 1624–1625.
32. FAVRE, L. & M.B. VALLOTTON. 1986. Nifedipine in pheochromocytoma [letter]. Ann. Intern. Med. **104:** 125.
33. TOKIOKA, H. *et al.* 1988. Use of nicardipine hydrochloride to control circulatory fluctuations during resection of a phaeochromocytoma. Br. J. Anaesth. **60:** 582–587.
34. SERFAS, D. *et al.* 1983. Phaeochromocytoma and hypertrophic cardiomyopathy: apparent suppression of symptoms and noradrenaline secretion by calcium-channel blockade. Lancet **2:** 711–713.
35. MANNELLI, M. *et al.* 1986. Effect of verapamil on catecholamine secretion by human pheochromocytoma [letter]. Hypertension **8:** 813–814.
36. LEHMANN, H.U. *et al.* 1983. Hemodynamic effects of calcium antagonists [review]. Hypertension **5:** II66–II73.
37. PERRY, R.R. *et al.* 1990. Surgical management of pheochromocytoma with the use of metyrosine. Ann. Surg. **212:** 621–628.
38. STEINSAPIR, J. *et al.* 1997. Metyrosine and pheochromocytoma. Arch. Intern. Med. **157:** 901–906.
39. FARID, I.S. & J.E. TETZLAFF. 2000. Preoperative management of pheochromocytoma. Am. J. Anesthesiol. **27:** 156–160.
40. DESMONTS, J.M. & J. MARTY. 1984. Anaesthetic management of patients with phaeochromocytoma. Br. J. Anaesth. **56:** 781–789.
41. WARNER, M.A. & J.A. VAN HEERDEN. 1996. Pheochromocytoma: anesthetic and surgical management employed at the Mayo Clinic. *In* Clinical and Experimental Pheochromocytoma. W.M. Manger & R.W. Gifford Jr., Eds.: 388–407. Blackwell Science. Cambridge, MA.
42. JANECZKO, G.F. *et al.* 1977. Enflurane anesthesia for surgical removal of pheochromocytoma. Anesth. Analg. **56:** 62–67.
43. ROIZEN, M.F. 1998. Diseases of the endocrine system. *In* Anesthesia and Uncommon Diseases. J.L. Benumof, Ed.: 255–273. Saunders. Philadelphia, PA.
44. JAMES, M.F.M. 1989. Use of magnesium sulphate in the anaesthetic management of pheochromocytoma: a review of 17 anaesthetics. Br. J. Anaesth. **62:** 616–623.
45. JAMES, M.F.M. *et al.* 1988. The use of magnesium sulphate in the anaesthetic management of pheochromocytoma in pregnancy. Can. J. Anaesth. **35:** 178–182.
46. JANETSCHEK, G. *et al.* 1998. Laparoscopic surgery for pheochromocytoma: adrenalectomy, partial resection, excision of paragangliomas. J. Urol. **160:** 330–334.

47. WALZ, M.K. *et al.* 2002. Endoscopic treatment of solitary, bilateral, multiple, and recurrent pheochromocytomas and paragangliomas. World J. Surg. **26:** 1005–1012.
48. JAROSZEWSKI, D.E. *et al.* 2003. Laparoscopic adrenalectomy for pheochromocytoma. Mayo. Clin. Proc. **78:** 1501–1504.
49. HWANG, J. *et al.* 2004. Laparoscopic management of extra-adrenal pheochromocytoma. J. Urol. **171:** 72–76.
50. CHEAH, W.K. *et al.* 2002. Laparoscopic adrenalectomy for pheochromocytoma. World. J. Surg. **26:** 1048–1051.
51. NEUMANN, H.P. *et al.* 1999. Preserved adrenocortical function after laparoscopic bilateral adrenal sparing surgery for hereditary pheochromocytoma. J. Clin. Endocrinol. Metab. **84:** 2608–2610.
52. WALTHER, M.M. *et al.* 2000. Laparoscopic partial adrenalectomy in patients with hereditary forms of pheochromocytoma. J. Urol. **164:** 14–17.
53. BRAUCKHOFF, M. *et al.* 2004. Repeat adrenocortical-sparing adrenalectomy for recurrent hereditary pheochromocytoma. Surg. Today **34:** 251–255.
54. NEUMANN, H.P. *et al.* 1999. Adrenal-sparing surgery for phaeochromocytoma. Br. J. Surg. **86:** 94–97.
55. MEEKE, R.I. *et al.* 1985. Phaeochromocytoma removal and postoperative hypoglycemia. Anaesthesia **40:** 1093–1096.
56. COSTELLO, G.T. *et al.* 1988. Hypoglycemia following bilateral adrenalectomy for pheochromocytoma. Crit. Care Med. **16:** 562–563.
57. PLOUIN, P.F. *et al.* 1997. Tumor recurrence and hypertension persistence after successful pheochromocytoma operation. Hypertension **29:** 1133–1139.
58. MANNELLI, M. & D. BEMPORAD. 2002. Diagnosis and management of pheochromocytoma in pregnancy. J. Endocrinol. Invest. **25:** 567–571.
59. AHLAWAT, S.K. *et al.* 1999. Pheochromocytoma associated with pregnancy: case report and review of the literature. Obstet. Gynecol. Surv. **54:** 728–737.
60. MANGER, W.M. 2005. The vagaries of pheochromocytomas. Am. J. Hypertens. **18:** 1266–1270

Risk-Oriented Approach to Hereditary Adrenal Pheochromocytoma

ANDREAS MACHENS, MICHAEL BRAUCKHOFF, OLIVER GIMM, AND HENNING DRALLE

Department of General, Visceral and Vascular Surgery, Martin-Luther-University Halle-Wittenberg, 06097 Halle (Salle), Germany

ABSTRACT: **Hereditary adrenal pheochromocytoma is caused by germline mutations in RET, VHL, SDHB, SDHD, and NF1. As these genes differ in function, so may their pheochromocytoma phenotypes, suggesting gene-specific patterns of age-related progression to pheochromocytoma. This possibility was explored for gene carriers with a lifetime risk of pheochromocytoma in excess of 50%. Published age-standardized penetrance rates of VHL-, SDHB-, and SDHD-associated pheochromocytoma were gauged against age-standardized penetrance rates of MEN2-associated pheochromocytoma in 219 institutional carriers of RET mutations conferring highest (codon 918), high (codons 609, 611, 618, 620, 630, and 634) and least high risk (codons 768, 790, 791, 804, and 891). The highest-risk category included SDHB, SDHD, and the highest-risk RET genotype; the high-risk category VHL missense mutations and the high-risk RET genotypes; and the least-high risk category VHL truncating mutations and least-high risk RET genotypes. Detailed information on recurrence rates and intervals was available only for the RET carriers (19–31% and means of 4.3–5.5 years; all RET risk categories combined). Ipsilateral recurrences in adrenal remnants, and contralateral recurrences in virgin adrenals were comparable in incidence (27% and 39%, $P = 0.69$; high-risk RET category) and time to recurrence (means of 4.3 vs. 5.4 year; $P > 0.99$; high-risk RET category), discounting a major effect of tumor spillage at primary subtotal adrenalectomy on pheochromocytoma recurrence. The risk of malignancy usually is low, except for SDHB (38%). For most hereditary pheochromocytomas, endoscopic subtotal adrenalectomy is the procedure of choice. Grouping hereditary pheochromocytoma into preliminary risk categories may improve the management of gene carriers at risk of developing pheochromocytomas.**

KEYWORDS: **multiple endocrine neoplasia type 2; RET proto-oncogene; Von Hippel–Lindau disease; succinate dehydrogenase B and D; neurofibromatosis; age-related penetrance of pheochromocytoma**

Address for correspondence: Henning Dralle, M.D., Department of General, Visceral and Vascular Surgery, Martin-Luther-University Halle-Wittenberg, Ernst-Grube-Straße 40, D-06097 Halle/Saale, Germany. Voice: +49-345-557-2314; fax: +49-345-557-2551.
e-mail: henning.dralle@medizin.uni-halle.de

Ann. N.Y. Acad. Sci. 1073: 417–428 (2006). © 2006 New York Academy of Sciences.
doi: 10.1196/annals.1353.045

INTRODUCTION

Arising from neural crest-derived adrenomedullary chromaffin cells, adrenal pheochromocytomas are heterogeneous neuroendocrine tumors that can display diverse phenotypes. Hereditary pheochromocytomas occur in isolation or in conjunction with other syndromic endocrine tumors. Acting on a single common pathway responsible for culling precursor cells during development,[1] a variety of germline mutations are known to predispose gene carriers to pheochromocytoma: mutations in exons 10, 11, 13, 14, 15, and 16 of the RET proto-oncogene, the susceptibility gene of multiple endocrine neoplasia (MEN) type 2 that encodes the RET receptor tyrosine kinase;[2] mutations in exons 1, 2, and 3 of the von Hippel–Lindau (VHL) tumor suppressor gene;[3–6] mutations in the succinate dehydrogenase (SDH) B and D genes, the susceptibility genes of paraganglioma syndromes 4 and 1 that encode Krebs cycle proteins;[7–12] and mutations in the neurofibromatosis (NF) 1 gene that encodes for neurofibromin, a downregulator of the ras oncogene.[13]

Although hereditary pheochromocytomas are largely similar in appearance, subtle differences in morphology do exist, reflecting separate mechanisms of causation with distinct genotype–phenotype relationships. VHL-, SDHB-, and presumably also SDHD-associated pheochromocytomas are composed of tumor cells intermixed with numerous irregular vessels due to disruption of hypoxia-responsive regulation,[9,14] whereas MEN2-associated pheochromocytomas consist of polygonal cells with admixture of small stromal vessels since only the terminal differentiation of neuroepithelial cells is impaired.[12,14] Because of an earlier arrest or defect in development, VHL-associated pheochromocytomas, unlike their MEN2-associated counterparts, fail to produce adrenergic phenotypes due to lack of phenylethanolamine-*N*-methyltransferase, the enzyme required for conversion of norepinephrine to epinephrine.[15] The MEN2-associated adrenergic phenotype is characterized more by paroxysmal than sustained hypertension, which is more typical of the VHL-associated noradrenergic phenotype.[16]

Germline mutations in different genes may not only account for this phenotypic heterogeneity, but could also translate into different patterns of age-related penetrance of hereditary pheochromocytoma. Such distinct patterns of age-related penetrance of MEN2-associated pheochromocytoma were confirmed for the three different categories of RET receptor tyrosine kinase activation in MEN type 2: alteration of the intracellular substrate recognition pocket of the catalytic core, extracellular ligand-independent dimerization and cross-phosphorylation, and interference with intracellular ATP binding.[2] The current study was devised to explore the patterns of age-related pheochromocytoma penetrance by gauging published age-standardized penetrance rates of VHL-, SDHB-, and SDHD-associated pheochromocytoma against those for MEN2-associated pheochromocytoma from 219 institutional carriers of RET mutations conferring highest, high, and least high risks. Ipsilateral recurrence rates of pheochromocytoma in adrenal remnants then were compared with contralateral recurrence rates in virgin adrenal glands.

METHODS

Age-Related Penetrance of MEN2-Associated Pheochromocytoma (Institutional Reference Population)

The reference population of 219 RET carriers was recruited between November 1994 and April 2005 at this institution, which serves as a tertiary surgical center with referrals of RET carriers from all over Germany. A more detailed analysis of codon-specific progression from adrenomedullary hyperplasia to pheochromocytoma based on 206 of the 219 RET carriers has recently been published, encompassing the most extensive experience on the subject to date.[2] Before genetic analysis and surgery, informed consent was obtained from all patients or their respective guardians. All surgical interventions represented standard practice of care. A diagnosis of adrenal pheochromocytoma always required histopathologic confirmation. For each RET risk category of highest (codon 918), high (codons 609, 611, 618, 620, 630, and 634), and least high risk (codon 768, 790, 791, 804, and 891), age-related, cumulative penetrance rates of MEN2-associated pheochromocytoma were calculated according to Kaplan–Meier.[17] These estimates served as an internal reference standard for subsequent comparisons with VHL, SDHB-, SDHD-, and NF1-associated pheochromocytomas.

Age-Related Penetrance of VHL-, SDHB-, SDHD-, and NF1-Associated Pheochromocytomas (Published Gene Carrier Populations)

To enable valid comparisons between different hereditary pheochromocytomas, standardization of the published heterogeneous populations of gene carriers was required. In a first step, comparative analyses were restricted to gene carriers who developed adrenal pheochromocytomas only, eliminating gene carriers with extra-adrenal pheochromocytomas or paragangliomas. Because gene carriers tend to develop pheochromocytomas more frequently as they age, all comparisons between different germline mutations were based on age-standardized, cumulative penetrance rates, as far as pertinent data were available from the international literature.

RESULTS

Classification of Hereditary Pheochromocytoma

TABLE 1 summarizes the characteristics of RET, VHL, SDHB, SDHD, and NF1 germline mutations. Located on different chromosomes, all five germline

TABLE 1. Classification of hereditary pheochromocytoma

	Multiple endocrine neoplasia type 2	Von Hippel-Lindau disease	Paraganglioma 4	Paraganglioma 1	Neurofibromatosis 1
Gene	RET	VHL	SDHB	SDHD	NF1
Locus	10q11.2	3p25–26	1p23–25	11q23	17q11
Exons	21	3	8	4	60
Hot spots (exons)	10, 11, 13, 14, 15, 16	None	Unknown	None	Unknown
Mode of inheritance	Autosomal-dominant	Autosomal-dominant	Autosomal-dominant	Autosomal-dominant	Autosomal-dominant
Associated tumors	Medullary thyroid cancer, parathyroid hyperplasia/ adenoma	Hemangioma, hemangioblastoma clear-cell renal carcinoma	None	None	Neurofibroma, optic pathway tumors, iris hamartomas
Extra-adrenal (%)	0	13	50	36	6
Lifetime risk of pheochromocytoma (%)	50	59	80	58	0.1—5.5

RET (*RE*arranged during *T*ransfection), VHL (*V*on *H*ippel–*L*indau), SDH (*S*uccinate *D*e*H*ydrogenase), NF (*N*euro*F*ibromatosis).

mutations are inherited as an autosomal-dominant trait that can be associated with various syndromic tumors. At the molecular level, however, all hereditary disorders are autosomal-recessive as additional, deleterious "second hit" mutations are required for tumorigenesis. Unlike most other mutations, RET mutations cluster at hot spots on exons 10, 11, 13, 14, 15, and 16, facilitating DNA-based analysis appreciably. The NF1 gene is not always fully sequenced because of its considerable length (60 exons). It entails a lifetime risk of pheochromocytoma of just 0.1–5.5%, as opposed to the 50–80% pheochromocytoma lifetime risk inherent in the other germline mutations (TABLE 1). Consequently, data on age-related penetrance of NF1-associated pheochromocytoma were unavailable from the literature, precluding further comparisons with the other germline mutations. Because of the high prevalence rates of extra-adrenal tumors, the exclusion of extra-adrenal pheochromocytomas and paragangliomas for standardization purposes affected mainly SDHB and SDHD gene carriers, reducing markedly the amount of pertinent literature data for subsequent comparative analyses.

Age-Standardized Penetrance of Hereditary Adrenal Pheochromocytoma

Apart from the previously mentioned limitations of literature data for SDHB, SDHD, and NF1 germline mutations, most publications presented information on pheochromocytoma penetrance overall unadjusted for patient age, and if so, they chose different time points, for example, by the age of 30, 35, 50, and 70 years. Considering institutional and published data, preliminary groupings of RET categories, VHL missense, VHL truncating, SDHB, and SDHD germline mutations were devised on the basis of age-standardized penetrance rates, mean age at first diagnosis, and multifocality of pheochromocytoma (TABLE 2):[2,3,10,19] The highest-risk category for hereditary adrenal pheochromocytoma included SDHB and SDHD in addition to the highest-risk RET genotype; the high-risk category included VHL missense mutations in addition to the high-risk RET genotypes; and the least-high risk category included VHL truncating mutations in addition to least-high risk RET genotypes. In the highest-risk category, the penetrance of pheochromocytoma obviously is so profound that asymptomatic gene carriers rarely have been reported. The risk of malignancy usually was low in hereditary adrenal pheochromocytoma, except for SDHB carriers (38%), where the impossibility of excluding extra-adrenal tumors may have inflated the actual risk of SDHB-associated adrenal malignancy.

Recurrent Pheochromocytoma after Adrenalectomy for Primary Pheochromocytoma

No systematic investigations of the risk of recurrent hereditary pheochromocytoma have appeared in the literature, except for MEN2-associated

TABLE 2. Age-related penetrance of hereditary adrenal pheochromocytoma*

	Highest risk			High risk			Least high risk	
Gene Codon /Mutation (n)**	RET[a] 918 5***	SDHB[b] 8	SDHD[b] 9***	RET[a] 609–634 27	VHL[c] 98 118	VHL[d] missense 29	RET[a] 768–891 2	VHL[d] truncation 60
Penetrance at age 30 years	43		~50	8		40	0	6
35 years	100	50		18	31		0	
50 years	100	77	86	54		59	4	9
70 years	100			73	60		9	
Age at first diagnosis, yr mean (range)	26.4 (22–31)	31.4 (12–48)	24.9 (5–59)	35.1 (18–53)			46.5 (39–54)	
Multifocal**** (%)	25	28*****	37*****	21		12	3	
Malignant (%)	0	38	0	4			0	

* Discounting NF1 due to low penetrance rates of pheochromocytoma and lack of data.
**: Numbers denote gene carriers, unless in *italics, where they denote families.*
***: Only affected gene carriers.
****: Including bilateral tumors.
*****: Including extra-adrenal tumors.
RET (*RE*arranged during *T*ransfection), VHL (*V*on Hippel-*L*indau), SDH (*S*uccinate *D*e*H*ydrogenase).
[a]: Updated from Machens *et al.* (2005).[2]
[b]: Adapted from Neumann *et al.* (2004).[10]
[c]: Bender *et al.* (2001).[19]
[d]: Maher *et al.* (1996).[3]

pheochromocytoma.[2] TABLE 3 provides our updated experience with the recurrence of MEN2-associated pheochromocytoma, which now also considers the risk of recurrence in adrenal remnants after subtotal adrenalectomy for primary pheochromocytoma. With just three (highest risk RET category) and two (least-high RET risk category) ipsilateral adrenal remnants and contralateral virgin adrenals at risk each, information on recurrence of pheochromocytoma was limited, and no recurrent pheochromocytoma was encountered in the highest and least-high risk RET categories. More data were available for the high-risk RET category, where 11 ipsilateral adrenal remnants and 18 contralateral virgin adrenals were at risk. Ipsilateral recurrences of pheochromocytoma in adrenal remnants, and contralateral recurrences in virgin adrenals were comparable in incidence (27% and 39%, $P = 0.69$; high-risk RET category) and time to recurrence (means of 4.3 years vs. 5.4 years; $P > 0.99$; high-risk RET category). These data discounted a major effect of tumor spillage at primary subtotal adrenalectomy on recurrence of pheochromocytoma in our RET population.

DISCUSSION

The recent fundamental advances in DNA technology have uncovered genotype–phenotype correlations for many forms of hereditary cancer. DNA-based information can be used for the timing of preemptive interventions and biochemical surveillance adapted to the genetic risk. The preliminary grouping of different germline mutations into separate risk categories based on the gene carriers' age-related risk of developing pheochromocytoma may permit a risk-oriented approach to hereditary adrenal pheochromocytoma. Because of the unsatisfactory amount of pertinent data on hereditary pheochromocytoma, and the unpredictability of somatic "second hit" mutations required for tumorigenesis, some limitations nevertheless apply, requiring further research.

Limitations of the Preliminary Risk Categories for Hereditary Pheochromocytoma

Although the risk of MEN2-associated pheochromocytoma is quite well established for the high risk RET category, more data are needed for the highest and least-high RET risk categories, and similarly for the rare SDHB, SDHD, and NF1 germline mutations. However, even within the high risk RET category, for which more data are available, the risk of pheochromocytoma may not be the same for all genotypes, ranging from 13–14% for codon 618 and 620 mutations to 29% for codon 634 mutations in younger RET carriers.[2] VHL germline mutations broadly fall into missense mutations, which carry a high risk of pheochromocytoma, and truncating mutations, which rarely give rise to pheochromocytoma.[3,4] VHL missense mutations, however, may not be a

TABLE 3. Time to recurrent pheochromocytoma after adrenalectomy* for MEN 2-associated pheochromocytoma (University of Halle, 1994–2005)

RET risk category (codons)	Carriers with PCC *n* (%)	Site	Recurrence *n* (%)	Adrenals at risk *n*	Time to recurrence, yr mean	range	Observation period yr since birth mean [95% CI]
Highest (918)	5 (25)	Ipsilateral[a]	0 (0)	3			15.8 [11.3; 20.3]
		Contralateral[b]	0 (0)	3			
High (609–634)	27 (21)	Ipsilateral[a]	3 (27)**$	11	4.3***	3–6	24.9 [21.8; 27.9]
		Contralateral[b]	7 (39)**	18	5.4***	1–14	
		Contralateral[c]	1 (33)	3	6		
Least high (768–891)	2 (3)	Ipsilateral[a]	0 (0)	2			32.9 [27.8; 38.0]
		Contralateral[b]	0 (0)	2			
Total	34 (16)	Ipsilateral[a]	3 (19)$	16	4.3	3–6	27.1 [24.6; 29.6]
		Contralateral[b,c]	8 (31)	26	5.5	1–14	

*:Discounting synchronous bilateral pheochromocytomas.
**: $P = 0.69$ (two-tailed Fisher exact test) for the difference in recurrence between ipsilateral (adrenal remnant) and contralateral (virgin) adrenals.
***: $P > 1.00$ (two-tailed exact Mann–Whitney–Wilcoxon rank sum test) for the difference in time-to-recurrence between ipsilateral (adrenal remnant) and contralateral virgin adrenals.
$:Including a patient with stated bilateral "total" adrenalectomy performed elsewhere for benign bilateral pheochromocytoma.
[a]:Ipsilateral adrenal remnants left *in situ* after ipsilateral subtotal adrenalectomy.
[b]:Contralateral virgin adrenals.
[c]: Contralateral adrenal remnants left *in situ* after contralateral subtotal adrenalectomy.
PCC: Pheochromocytoma.

homogeneous group as the presumed gain of function may not be identical for all VHL missense mutations.[18] Further investigations of this issue have been hampered by the comparative lack of hot spot mutations in the VHL gene so that the few carriers harboring the same VHL missense mutations usually are insufficient to base genotype-specific penetrance rates of pheochromocytoma on.[4] More subject to chance occurrence and ascertainment bias, small numbers can yield higher penetrance rates by chance alone. Codon 167 VHL missense mutations, for which the penetrance of pheochromocytoma is estimated at 53% at the age of 30 years and 82% at the age of 50 years,[3] may have a higher risk of pheochromocytoma than most VHL missense mutations, such as the Y98H VHL genotype.[19] The precision of these risk estimates is unknown, as the number of carriers harboring the codon 167 VHL missense mutation was unspecified.

Surgical Intervention for Primary and Recurrent Hereditary Adrenal Pheochromocytoma

With improved control of concurrent, formerly lethal syndromic tumors, namely, medullary thyroid cancer in MEN type 2 and clear-cell renal cell cancer in VHL, more and more pheochromocytomas keep emerging in an aging population of gene carriers. From a surgical point of view, the benefits of "cortical sparing" subtotal adrenalectomy, lifelong steroid independence and protection from addisonian crisis need to be balanced against the risks of organ preservation, recurrence of pheochromocytoma and malignancy. The risks of ipsilateral recurrence in adrenal remnants and contralateral recurrence in virgin adrenals during the observation period were 19% and 31%, respectively, for all RET carriers combined (and 27% and 39%, respectively, for codon 634 RET carriers only), with mean recurrence intervals of 4.3–5.5 years (TABLE 3). Altogether, one-third of MEN2-associated pheochromocytomas start out as synchronous bilateral tumors, another third develop bilateral tumors one at a time, whereas the last third remain unilateral.[20] In keeping with our data, Lee and associates[21] encountered recurrent pheochromocytomas in three (25%) of their twelve MEN 2 patients after a median follow-up of 138 months. Yip and colleagues[22] found three (33%) contralateral recurrences in ten MEN 2 patients within the first 3 years of follow-up, whereas Brunt and co-workers[23] saw four (33%) contralateral recurrences in twelve MEN 2 patients during a mean follow-up of 57 months, an average of 13 years after the initial procedure. The lack of evidence for clinically relevant tumor spillage during subtotal adrenalectomy in this series, the generally small risk of malignancy, and the lower surgical morbidity render endoscopic subtotal adrenalectomy, coupled with intraoperative ultrasonography, the therapy of choice for most hereditary adrenal pheochromocytomas. The results of adrenal autotransplantation have been disappointing,[24] reaching steroid independence at best in one-third of cases. To maintain steroid independence for prolonged periods, a minimum of 15–30% of adrenal tissue must be preserved.[25] Leaving a small layer of uninvolved adrenal tissue, care should be taken to protect the remnant's segmental arterial tributary and dual venous drainage, the venae comitantes-emissary veins and, where possible, the main adrenal vein.[25,26] When these principles are heeded, repeat subtotal adrenalectomy is feasible for pheochromocytomas recurring in adrenal remnants, with preservation of postoperative adrenocortical function.[27] To keep the option of repeat subtotal adrenalectomy in the event of recurrence, annual biochemical screening will be required for most gene carriers to identify recurrent pheochromocytomas early while they are still small.

CONCLUSION

In face of the substantial progress made during the past decade, our understanding of the mechanisms governing genotype–phenotype correlations has remained somewhat rudimentary. Many hereditary pheochromocytomas are not just part of a constellation of associated tumors that make up the respective hereditary syndrome, but also feature distinct genetic patterns of age-related penetrance. To accommodate the effect of age that can confound genotype–phenotype correlations, provision of age-standardized penetrance rates of hereditary pheochromocytoma is pivotal to enable comparisons between carriers of RET-, VHL-, SDHB-, SDHD-, and NF1-associated pheochromocytoma. As new information is forthcoming, the preliminary risk categories will need to be adjusted to refine the risk-oriented approach to hereditary adrenal pheochromocytoma. More work is wanted to distinguish between hereditary adrenal pheochromocytoma and extra-adrenal or combined adrenal–extra-adrenal pheochromocytomas since these tumors may behave differently, requiring a modified risk-oriented approach.

REFERENCES

1. MAXWELL, P.H. 2005. A common pathway for genetic events leading to pheochromocytoma. Cancer Cell **8:** 91–93.
2. MACHENS, A., M. BRAUCKHOFF, H.-J. HOLZHAUSEN, *et al.* 2005. Codon-specific development of pheochromocytoma in multiple endocrine neoplasia type 2. J. Clin. Endocrinol. Metab. **90:** 3999–4003.
3. MAHER, E.R., A.R. WEBSTER, F.M. RICHARDS, *et al.* 1996. Phenotypic expression in von Hippel-Lindau disease: correlations with germline VHL gene mutations. J. Med. Genet. **33:** 328–332.
4. ZBAR, B., T. KISHIDA, F. CHEN, *et al.* 1996. Germline mutations in the Von Hippel-Lindau disease (VHL) gene in families from North America, Europe, and Japan. Hum. Mutat. **8:** 348–357.
5. NEUMANN, H.P.H., B. BAUSCH, S.R. MCWHINNEY, *et al.* 2002. Germ-line mutations in nonsyndromic pheochromocytoma. N. Engl. J. Med. **346:** 1459–1466.

6. LONSER, R.R., G.M. GLENN, M. WALTHER, *et al.* 2003. Von Hippel-Lindau disease. Lancet **361:** 2059–2067.
7. GIMM, O., M. ARMANIOS, H. DZIEMA, *et al.* 2000. Somatic and occult germ-line mutations in SDHD, a mitochondrial complex II gene, in nonfamilial pheochromocytoma. Cancer Res. **60:** 6822–6825.
8. ASTUTI, D., F. LATIF, A. DALLOL, *et al.* 2001. Gene mutations in the succinate dehydrogenase subunit SDHB cause susceptibility to familial pheochromocytoma and to familial paraganglioma. Am. J. Hum. Genet. **69:** 49–54.
9. GIMENEZ-ROQUEPLO, A.-P., J. FAVIER, P. RUSTIN, *et al.* 2003. Mutations in the SDHB gene are associated with extra-adrenal and/or malignant phaeochromocytomas. Cancer Res. **63:** 5615–5621.
10. NEUMANN, H.P.H., C. PAWLU, M. PECZKOWSKA, *et al.* 2004. Distinct clinical features of paraganglioma syndromes associated with SDHB and SDHD gene mutations. JAMA **292:** 943–951.
11. DANNENBERG, H., F.H. VAN NEDERVEEN, M. ABBOU, *et al.* 2005. Clinical characteristics of pheochromocytoma patients with germline mutations in SDHD. J. Clin. Oncol. **23:** 1894–1901.
12. POLLARD, P.J., J.J. BRIERE, N.A. ALAM, *et al.* 2005. Accumulation of Krebs cycle intermediates and over-expression of HIF1α in tumours which result from germline FH and SDH mutations. Hum. Mol. Genet. **14:** 2231–2239.
13. RASMUSSEN, S.A. & J.M. FRIEDMAN. 2000. NF1 gene and neurofibromatosis 1. Am. J. Epidemiol. **151:** 33–40.
14. VOGEL, T.W.A., F.M. BROUWERS, I.A. LUBENSKY, *et al.* 2005. Differential expression of erythropoietin and its receptor in von Hippel-Lindau-associated and multiple endocrine neoplasia type 2-associated pheochromocytomas. J. Clin. Endocrinol. Metab. **90:** 3747–3751.
15. EISENHOFER, G., J.W. LENDERS, W.M. LINEHAN, *et al.* 1999. Plasma normetanephrine and metanephrine for detecting pheochromocytoma in von Hippel-Lindau disease and multiple endocrine neoplasia type 2. N. Engl. J. Med. **340:** 1872–1879.
16. EISENHOFER, G., M.M. WALTHER, T.T. HUYNH, *et al.* 2001. Pheochromocytomas in von Hippel-Lindau syndrome and multiple endocrine neoplasia type 2 display distinct biochemical and clinical phenotypes. J. Clin. Endocrinol. Metab. **86:** 1999–2008.
17. KAPLAN, E.L. & P. MEIER. 1958. Nonparametric estimation from incomplete observations. J. Am. Stat. Assoc. **53:** 457–481.
18. RATHMELL, W.K., M.M. HICKEY, N.A. BEZMAN, *et al.* 2004. In vitro and in vivo models analyzing von Hippel-Lindau disease-specific mutations. Cancer Res. **64:** 8595–8603.
19. BENDER, B.U., C. ENG, M. OLSCHEWSKI, *et al.* 2001. VHL c.505 T>C mutation confers a high age related penetrance but no increased overall mortality. J. Med. Genet. **38:** 508–514.
20. DRALLE, H., G.F.W. SCHEUMANN, J. KOTZERKE, *et al.* 1992. Surgical management of MEN 2: recent results. Cancer Res. **125:** 167–195.
21. LEE, J.E., S.A. CURLEY, R.F. GAGEL, *et al.* 1996. Cortical-sparing adrenalectomy for patients with bilateral pheochromocytoma. Surgery **120:** 1064–1071.
22. YIP, L., G.J. COTE, S.E. SHAPIRO, *et al.* 2003. Multiple endocrine neoplasia type 2. Evaluation of the genotype-phenotype relationship. Arch. Surg. **138:** 409–416.
23. BRUNT, L.M., T.C. LAIRMORE, G.M. DOHERTY, *et al.* 2002. Adrenalectomy for familial pheochromocytoma in the laparoscopic era. Ann. Surg. **235:** 713–721.

24. DRALLE, H., M. IPTA, E. HENSCHEL, *et al.* 1988. Surgical treatment of sporadic and familial pheochromocytoma. Acta Med. Austriaca **15:** 108.
25. BRAUCKHOFF, M., O. GIMM, P.N. THANH, *et al.* 2003. Critical size of residual adrenal tissue and recovery from impaired early postoperative adrenocortical function after subtotal bilateral adrenalectomy. Surgery **134:** 1020–1028.
26. BAGHAI, M., G.B. THOMPSON, W. YOUNG, *et al.* 2002. Pheochromocytomas and paragangliomas in von Hippel-Lindau disease. A role for laparoscopic and cortical-sparing surgery. Arch. Surg. **137:** 682–689.
27. BRAUCKHOFF, M., O. GIMM, K. BRAUCKHOFF, *et al.* 2004. Repeat adrenocortical-sparing adrenalectomy for recurrent hereditary pheochromocytoma. Surg. Today **34:** 251–255.

Treatment of Bilateral Pheochromocytoma and Adrenal Medullary Hyperplasia

SVANTE JANSSON,[a] AMIR KHORRAM-MANESH,[a] OLA NILSSON,[b] LARS KÖLBY,[a] LARS-ERIK TISELL,[a] BO WÄNGBERG,[a] AND HÅKAN AHLMAN[a]

[a]*Department of Surgery and Transplantation, Sahlgrenska University Hospital, and The Lundberg Laboratory for Cancer Research, Göteborg University, Göteborg, Sweden*

[b]*Department of Pathology, Sahlgrenska University Hospital, and The Lundberg Laboratory for Cancer Research, Göteborg University, Göteborg, Sweden*

ABSTRACT: **The risk for bilateral tumors and long-term outcome after conservative cortical-sparing adrenal surgery was studied in a consecutive single-center series. One hundred fifty-four patients were operated on (1950–2004) for pheochromocytoma (PC = 137), or abdominal paraganglioma (PG = 17). Twenty had MEN 2 (16 MEN 2A; 4 MEN 2B), 15 von Recklinghausen's disease (VRD), and 1 von Hippel–Lindau (VHL) disease. Twelve patients had, or developed, bilateral adrenal medullary tumors; four with MEN 2A, four with MEN 2B, three with VRD, and one with probably hereditary PC associated with brain tumors/meningioma. Two patients with MEN 2B and one with MEN 2A with had bilateral adrenalectomy (adx). Three VRD patients, two MEN 2B and one MEN 2A patients had cortical-sparing surgery. Two patients were operated on unilaterally, but developed small contralateral tumors; one of these (MEN 2A) had a second asymptomatic PC diagnosed at an older age, so surgery was withheld; the other patient (hereditary PC syndrome) had a small contralateral PC diagnosed at autopsy 9 years later. Only three of nine patients with bilateral operations needed corticosteroid replacement after surgery. Four of six patients died of associated tumors (MTC and meningioma). The mean follow-up was 13 (1–25) years. Twelve MEN 2A patients with unilateral adx have been followed up for 20 (4–36) years without developing a second PC. Cortical-sparing adrenal surgery can safely be performed in the majority of patients with bilateral PC. On the basis of our long-term experience of MEN 2A we perform contralateral adrenal resection only if a second PC is confirmed. Five patients underwent adrenal exploration because of clinical and biochemical findings compatible with PC. Four had**

Address for correspondence: Svante Jansson, M.D., Ph.D., Department of Surgery and Transplantation, Sahlgrenska University Hospital, S-413 45 Göteborg, Sweden. Voice: +46313421798; fax: +46313424600.
e-mail: svante.jansson@surgery.gu.se

Ann. N.Y. Acad. Sci. 1073: 429–435 (2006).
doi: 10.1196/annals.1353.046

asymmetrical positive MIBG scans. They all underwent unilateral adx and diffuse medullary hyperplasia was confirmed (medullary weight estimated morphometrically to 1.0–3.4 g vs. normal weight 0.3–0.5 g in matched controls). These patients have been followed for 19 (5–27) years with normal clinical and biochemical findings. In this rare condition removal of the largest adrenal seems adequate.

KEYWORDS: hereditary pheochromocytoma; adrenal medullary hyperplasia; cortex-sparing adrenal surgery

INTRODUCTION

As a consequence of screening/genetic testing the proportion of hereditary pheochromocytoma (PC) has increased from the classical 10% to about 30%.[1] The syndromes most often associated with the development of PC are MEN 2A and B (activating mutations of *RET*), von Hippel–Lindau disease (inactivation of *VHL*), von Recklinghausen's disease (inactivation of *NF1*), and mutations of *SDHB* and *D* resulting in familial paraganglioma syndromes. Also, MEN 1 and Carney's triad can be associated with PC. Underlying germline mutations are expressed in the medulla of both adrenals, which can lead to bilateral PC; for example, after unilateral adx in MEN 2 there is 30–50% risk to develop contralateral tumors within 10 years.[2] There is a gradual development of manifest tumors via diffuse and nodular adrenal medullary hyperplasia (AMH), which has led to recommendations of early surgical intervention to reduce diseased medullary tissue. Nonhereditary AMH is a very rare condition that may cause catecholaminergic symptoms.[3] The surgical strategy for hereditary PC has over time varied from total adx for gene mutation carriers to unilateral adx with surveillance of the least diseased side, and most recently bilateral subtotal adx with preservation of cortical tissue.[4–6] Prophylactic bilateral adx has been abandoned, since addisonian crisis occurred in one-quarter of the patients over 10 years despite adequate corticosteroid replacement.[2] For unilateral PC one can choose between conservative unilateral adx and surveillance (adequate corticosteroid secretion, but most likely need for additional adrenal surgery), or bilateral subtotal adx (a certain risk for inadequate corticosteroid secretion, but less risk for additional adrenal surgery). In bilateral PC cortical-sparing surgery can be performed, saving at least 30% of residual cortex, (i.e., unilateral adx + contralateral subtotal adx or bilateral subtotal adx). The cortisol secretion must be carefully controlled in these patients as well their response to ACTH. The results of autotransplantation of cortical tissue are not convincing and adequate function will most likely require a phase of stimulation with ACTH analogues.[7]

The aim of this study was to review the long-term outcome of individually tailored surgical treatment of bilateral PC at one center.

PATIENTS AND METHODS

A total of 154 consecutive patients with PC (n = 137) or abdominal PG (n = 17) were treated at our unit (the only referral center for western Sweden; population 1.6 million) between 1950 and 2004 (85 females and 69 males, mean age 51 years). One hundred eighteen patients were considered to have sporadic tumors. Twenty had MEN 2 (16 MEN 2A; 4 MEN 2B), 15 VRD, and 1 VHL, that is, 30% were hereditary tumors. Twelve MEN 2A patients underwent unilateral adx and have not yet developed a second PC. These patients belong to seven kindreds; three with codon 634 mutations, one with codon 618 mutation, one with codon 804, and two with yet not identified mutations. Screening for MEN 2 has been performed biochemically (basal and stimulated S-calcitonin) since 1984. All patients with hereditary tumors were followed annually by biochemical screening and, when tests were positive, imaging procedures were performed. Metastatic PC/PG, was diagnosed in 12 patients, but no patient with hereditary tumor was diagnosed so far.

RESULTS

Twelve patients in this series presented with, or developed, bilateral PC (TABLE 1). All four patients with MEN 2B presented with bilateral PC. Four of the 16 MEN 2A patients have developed a contralateral PC 10–19 years after unilateral adx. Three of the 15 VRD patients presented with bilateral PC. The remaining one patient with bilateral tumors was a male with PC and a familial history of brain tumors/meningioma.

Surgical Procedures

MEN 2B: All four MEN 2B patients underwent bilateral adrenal surgery. Two underwent bilateral adx (one 5 years after bilateral resection) and one had unilateral adx with contralateral cortical-sparing resection and lived for 7 years without steroid replacement. These three patients died from widespread medullary thyroid carcinoma (MTC). One female MEN 2B patient underwent bilateral adrenal resection that left 30–40% of cortical tissue. She has been observed for 10 years with no signs of recurrence and has no steroid replacement.

MEN 2A: All four MEN 2A patients that developed bilateral PC had a *RET* mutation at codon 634. One presented with bilateral tumors and underwent bilateral resection; 17 years later completion adx was performed. One female patient underwent unilateral adx at the age of 57; control CT 14 years later revealed a 1-cm tumor in the contralateral adrenal. She was asymptomatic and not willing to undergo surgery, so she was followed for another 12 years until she died from coronary insufficiency. A male patient underwent unilateral adx at the age of 25 years for a small PC. Eighteen years later he developed

TABLE 1. Clinical characteristics of patients with bilateral adrenal medullary tumors

Sex/age	Syndrome/ genotype (site of mutation)	Surgery	Present steroid substitution	Observation time	Outcome
F/28	MEN 2B/n.a.	1bil. res. 2 bil. adx.	Yes	19 years (14 years after adx.)	Died of MTC
M/25	MEN 2B /918	adx. sin + res. dx.	No	7 years	Died of MTC
M/35	MEN 2B/n.a.	bil. adx.	Yes	18 years	Died of MTC
F/20	MEN 2B /918	bil. res.	No	10 years	NED
F/26	MEN 2A /634	1 bil. res. 2 bil. adx.	Yes	42 years (25 years after adx.)	NED
F/57	MEN 2A /634	adx. dx.	No	26 years (12 years with an asympt. PC)	Died from unrelated cause
M/25	MEN 2A /634	1 adx. dx. 2 res. sin	No (normal testing)	20 years (1 year after op 2.)	NED
F/26	MEN 2A /634	adx.dx. (res. sin planned)	No	17 years	New contralat. PC
M/52	VRD/n.a.	adx.sin + res. dx	No	3 years	NED (concomitant GIST)
M/72	VRD/n.a.	adx. dx + res. sin	No	2 years	NED
F/61	VRD/n.a.	adx. sin + res. dx	No	1.5 years	Died from nonrelated cause
M/59	Hereditary PC + brain tumors/n.a.	adx. left	No	9 years	Died of meningioma

Legends: adx = adrenalectomy; res. = resection; bil. = bilateral; contralat. = contralateral; dx = right; NED = no evidence of disease; n.a. = not available; GIST = gastrointestinal stromal tumor; sin = left.

a small PC contralaterally, which led to subtotal resection. He had normal urinary cortisol and serum ACTH and normal response to ACTH. The fourth patient underwent unilateral adx at the age of 26 years. Since then she had two uncomplicated pregnancies and deliveries. Seventeen years later she developed a small PC in the residual adrenal and is now being considered for contralateral resection. The other 12 MEN 2A patients in our series have been followed for a mean of 20 (4–36) years after unilateral adx without developing demonstrable PC.

VRD: Three of 15 VRD patients presented with bilateral PC; all underwent unilateral adx (largest tumor side) and cortical-sparing resection contralaterally and have been observed 1.5–3 years without steroid replacement. In one, the histopathological examination revealed a typical PC in the excised adrenal and a ganglioneuroma contralaterally, and another had concomitant gastrointestinal stromal tumors. The last patient belonged to a family with PC and brain tumors/meningioma and presented with unilateral PC. Nine years later he died from malignant meningioma. At autopsy a small PC was found in the residual adrenal.

In this series of 12 patients with hereditary bilateral PC, 9 underwent bilateral adrenal surgery, 1 had bilateral adx, and 2 underwent completion adx after initial bilateral resections. The latter two patients needed no steroid replacement during 5 and 17 years, respectively. The remaining six patients had cortical-sparing surgery (five unilateral adx + contralateral resection and one bilateral resection) and were observed for 2.5 (1–18) years after primary surgery without steroids.

AMH: Five patients were clinically diagnosed with unilateral PC with moderately elevated urinary catecholamines/metanephrines and one enlarged adrenal on CT (4 MIBG-positive). All patients underwent unilateral adx and exploration of the contralateral adrenal, which in each case was judged to be normal. The histopathological examination of the specimens showed diffuse AMH. Morphometric analyses of the serial sectioned gland were performed in order to assess adrenal medullary weight and volume. The medullary weights were thus estimated at 1–3.4 g versus 0.3–0.5 g in age- and sex-matched controls. After adx these patients have been followed for a mean of 19 (range 5–27) years and have remained asymptomatic with normal biochemical findings.

DISCUSSION

Our long-term study over 54 years demonstrated that all four MEN 2B patients developed bilateral PC. We performed bilateral adx in one patient with large tumors and had to proceed with completion adx in another patient after 5 years, which may reflect different tumor biology in MEN 2B versus MEN 2A. On the other hand, subtotal procedures were adequate treatment of the other two MEN 2B patients observed over 7 and 10 years, respectively, without need for steroid replacement. Three of 15 VRD patients and one of 20 MEN 2A patients presented with bilateral PC. For the VRD patients and most MEN 2A patients we used cortical sparing procedures, most commonly unilateral adx followed by contralateral resection, when a second PC was confirmed. By this conservative strategy only 25% of the MEN 2A patients have undergone additional adrenal surgery 10–19 years after the primary operation; the others were observed for a mean of 20 (range 4–36) years after the initial unilateral adx with no new tumor. With this conservative strategy the majority of our MEN 2A patients could avoid steroid replacement for a considerable period of their lives. Only one MEN 2A patient with previous bilateral resection underwent completion adx. The VRD patients presented with bilateral tumors and were all subjected to unilateral adx + contralateral resection. The predisposition for malignant PC in MEN 2 patients is very low.[8] This risk is somewhat higher for VRD patients (11%). All three VRD patients in this series were subjected to subtotal adx leaving a 30–40% adrenal cortical residue. They have only been observed between 1.5 and 3 years with no demonstrable new tumor.

Nonhereditary AMH-simulating PC has previously been reported and was found in five patients in our series. In hereditary cases AMH is a preneoplastic state of the adrenal medulla, but underlying events for this condition in sporadic cases are not known. Our five patients have been observed for a mean of 19 years after unilateral adx without clinical signs of recurrence in the residual adrenal, which indicates a nonaggressive disorder with no need for bilateral interventions. Similar good results with conservative surgery in nonhereditary AMH have been reported by others as well.[3]

ACKNOWLEDGMENT

This study was supported by grants from the Swedish MRC (5220) and the Swedish Cancer Society (3911).

REFERENCES

1. NEUMANN, H.P.H., B. BAUSCH, S.R. MCWHINNEY, *et al.* 2002. Germ-line mutations in nonsyndromic pheochromocytoma. N. Engl. J. Med. **346:** 1459–1466.
2. LAIRMORE, T.C., D.W. BALL, S.B. BAYLIN, *et al.* 1993. Management of pheochromocytomas in patients with multiple endocrine neoplasia type 2 syndromes. Ann. Surg. **217:** 595–601.
3. DRALLE, H., S. SCHRODER, K.F. GRATZ, *et al.* 1990. Sporadic unilateral adrenomedullary hyperplasia with hypertension cured by adrenalectomy. World J. Surg. **14:** 308–315.
4. VAN HEERDEN, J.A., G.W. SIZEMORE, J.A. CARNEY, *et al.* 1984. Surgical management of the adrenal glands in multiple endocrine neoplasia type II syndrome. World J. Surg. **8:** 612–621.

5. JANSSON, S., L.E. TISELL, M. FJALLING, *et al.* 1988. Early diagnosis of and surgical strategy for adrenal medullary disease in MEN II gene carriers. Surgery **103:** 11–18.
6. YIP, L., J.E. LEE, S.E. SHAPIRO, *et al.* 2004. Surgical management of hereditary pheochromocytoma. J. Am. Coll. Surg. **198:** 525–534.
7. BRAUCKHOFF, M., O. GIMM, P.N. THANH, *et al.* 2003. Critical size of residual adrenal tissue and recovery from impaired early postoperative adrenocortical function after subtotal bilateral adrenalectomy. Surgery **134:** 1020–1027.
8. LENDERS, J.W., G. EISENHOFER, M. MANELLI, *et al.* 2005. Phaeochromocytoma. Lancet **366:** 665–675.

AT_2 Receptor Stimulation May Halt Progression of Pheochromocytoma

MORRIS J. BROWN,[a] ISLA S. MACKENZIE,[a] MICHAEL J. ASHBY,[a] KOTTEKKATTU K. BALAN,[b] AND DEREK S. APPLETON[b]

[a]*Clinical Pharmacology Unit, University of Cambridge, Cambridge CB2 2QQ, United Kingdom*

[b]*Department of Radiology, Addenbrookes Hospital, Cambridge CB2 2QQ, United Kingdom*

ABSTRACT: Two patients with pheochromocytoma are described in whom treatment with a high dose of an angiotensin receptor blocker was associated with cessation of tumor growth as assessed by serial CT scanning and plasma norepinephrine estimation. If the association with drug treatment is causal, the mechanism may be through stimulation of the AT_2 receptor consequent upon the elevation of plasma angiotensin II levels induced by AT_1 receptor blockade. Similar observations in further patients should lead to a placebo-controlled study in patients with malignant or familial pheochromocytoma, or other tumors found to express the AT_2 receptor.

KEYWORDS: pheochromocytoma; angiotensin receptor blocker; treatment; malignant; F-DOPA scan

BACKGROUND

Stimulation of the angiotensin type 2 (AT_2) receptor promotes apoptosis in a number of cell types, including cultured pheochromocytoma (pheo) PC12 cells.[1,2] We therefore wished to observe the possible benefit of AT_2 receptor simulation in a small number of patients in whom curative surgery was either impossible or delayed. Since there is no AT_2 receptor agonist available for clinical use, we used the strategy of blocking the AT_1 receptor with an angiotensin receptor blocker (ARB) in order to increase circulating angiotensin II levels. This occurs because of blockade of negative feedback of angiotensin II upon secretion of renin.

Address for correspondence: Prof. Morris J. Brown, Department of Medicine, Addenbrookes Hospital, Box 110, Cambridge CB2 2QQ, UK. Voice: 44-1223-336743; 44-1223-762576.
e-mail: m.j.brown@cai.cam.ac.uk

Ann. N.Y. Acad. Sci. 1073: 436–443 (2006). © 2006 New York Academy of Sciences.
doi: 10.1196/annals.1353.047

CASE 1

In 1984, a 32-year-old man presented with headaches, sweating, and hypertension. Twenty-four-hour urine VMA excretion was elevated, but equivocal CT scan led to referral for selective venous sampling. This showed reversed epinephrine-to-norepinephrine ratio in the left adrenal vein, and the patient proceeded to surgical adrenalectomy with successful cure of his symptoms and hypertension.

In 1997, he re-presented with hypertension and history of recent pheochromocytoma in a niece. His plasma norepinephrine was elevated less than twofold (1.5 ng/mL), but was not suppressed over 20 min following i.v. injection of pentolinium 2.5 mg.[3] A CT scan showed a 1.5 cm mass in the right adrenal, but plasma epinephrine was normal (26 pg/mL). No hot spots were found on ^{123}I-mIBG scan or selective venous sampling. The patient was therefore managed medically. Blood pressure was controlled by phenoxybenzamine, but there was a progressive increase in plasma norepinephrine to 3.3 ng/L. Additional therapy with an ARB, irbesartan 150 mg, was started in 1999. In view of the rising plasma norepinephrine levels, the dose of irbesartan was increased to 300 mg daily in 2001. Plasma norepinephrine peaked at 4000 ng/mL and then appeared to decline (FIG. 1).

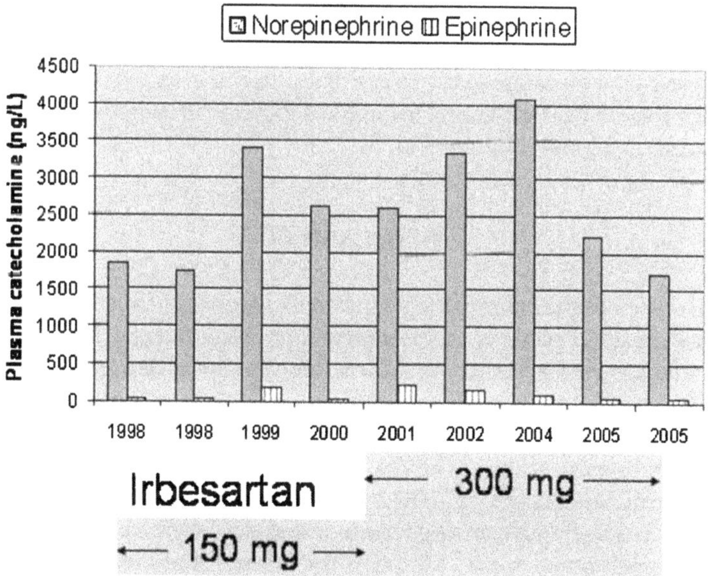

FIGURE 1. Serial plasma catecholamines in Case 1. The results for plasma norepinephrine (*solid columns*) and epinephrine (*hatched columns*) are shown relative to the dose of irbesartan, which was 150 mg daily between 1998 and 2001, and 300 mg daily thereafter.

Over 4 years from 1998 to 2002, the adrenal mass grew approximately 50% in diameter (FIG. 2), but remained negative on mIBG and octreotide scans. From 2002, the size of tumor remained static (FIG. 2). In 2004, two PET scans were performed, with ^{18}F-FDG and ^{18}F-FDOPA. The first of these was negative; the second showed an isolated hot spot in the area of the adrenal mass (FIG. 3). The patient awaits laparoscopic right adrenalectomy.

CASE 2

A 63-year-old man presented in 2000 with sweating, weight loss, and hypertension. Plasma norepinephrine was elevated at 12.0 ng/mL, but plasma epinephrine was normal (28 pg/mL). A large left adrenal phaeochromocytoma was seen on MRI scan and surgically removed. At follow-up over the next year, the patient remained well and normotensive, and in June 2001 plasma norepinephrine was only 3.8 ng/mL. However, in August 2004 the patient re-presented with a recurrence of weight loss, night sweats, fevers, and hypertension. Plasma norepinephrine was once again elevated at 8.4 ng/mL, but epinephrine was normal. CT scanning showed local recurrence in the left adrenal bed. mIBG scanning was negative, but ^{18}F-FDG scanning revealed both local and distal metastases. Surgical exploration revealed multiple peritoneal seedlings and no tumor was excised except for histological confirmation.

The patient was therefore managed medically. Phenoxybenzamine was changed to doxazosin, which was better tolerated in this patient, and ARB therapy started with candesartan 16 mg daily. Over the next year, plasma norepinephrine declined (FIG. 4), and the mass of tumor in the adrenal bed appeared unchanged or slightly reduced (FIG. 5).

DISCUSSION

In this type of observational report, there is no control for what would have happened in these patients in the absence of ARB therapy. However, such observations are the necessary prelude to any attempt at designing and undertaking a controlled study of therapy. This is particularly true of conditions like pheochromocytoma, whose rarity has discouraged recruitment of sufficient patients for therapeutic studies. The first patient provided an unusual opportunity for long-term observation of ARB therapy in a patient with a presumed benign pheochromocytoma, arising contra-lateral to a long-time previous benign adrenal pheochromocytoma. Although the adrenal mass on CT was always likely to be the elusive pheochromocytoma, we considered the benefit of its removal outweighed by the risk of wrongly removing a normal gland from a patient with no other adrenal tissue. This concern was finally removed by the availability of the ^{18}F-DOPA PET scan.[4] Ironically, the patient's course on

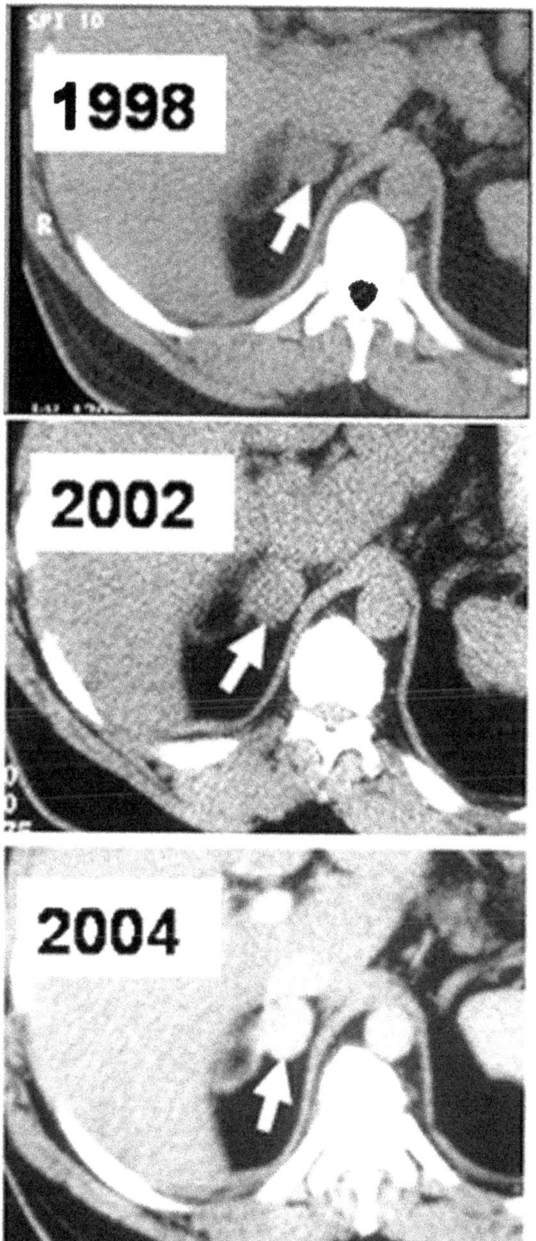

FIGURE 2. Serial CT scans in Case 1. In 1998, the diameter of the right adrenal pheochromocytoma (*arrow*) is smaller than the length of the attached medial limb of normal adrenal, and than the diameter of the aorta. In 2002, the tumor is a similar size to these adjacent tissues, but there is no further increase in 2004.

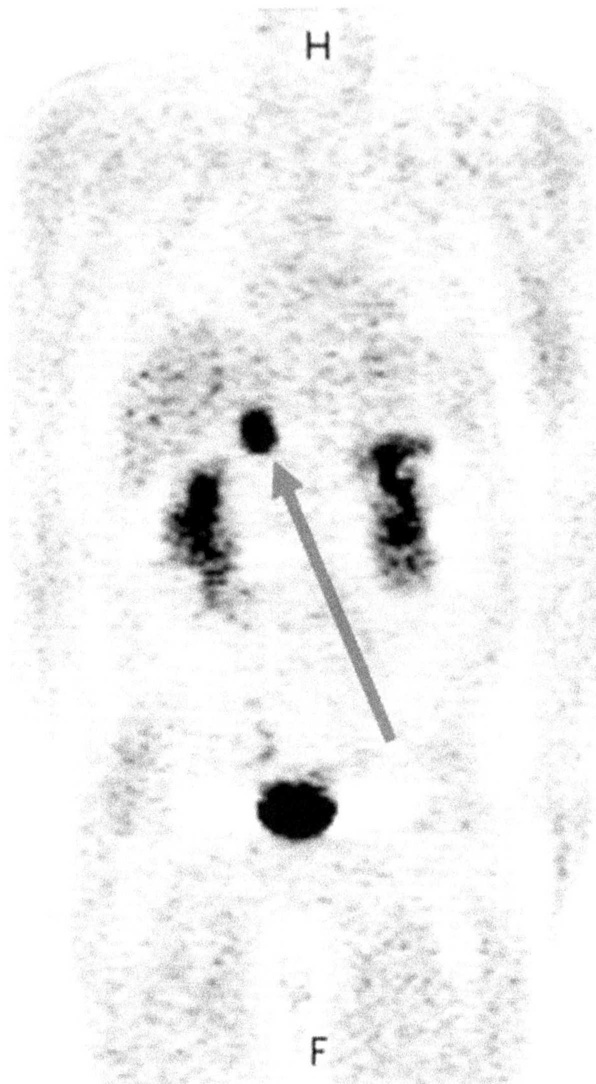

FIGURE 3. ^{18}F-DOPA PET scan in Case 1. The right adrenal pheochromocytoma is shown by *arrow*. DOPA is converted to dopamine in the kidneys, which together with bladder also show as hot spots in F-DOPA scans.

medical treatment has been so benign that the question now is whether there is an absolute indication for surgery with its consequent requirement to swap the phenoxybenzamine and irbesartan for adrenal replacement therapy.

The use of ARB in this patient appears, at the most conservative, to be associated with no change in plasma norepinephrine over 7 years, and a less

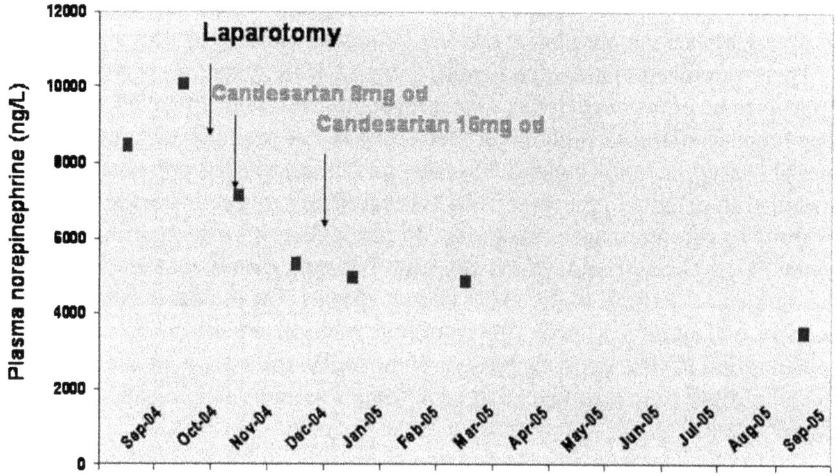

FIGURE 4. Serial plasma norepinephrine in Case 2. Introduction of candesartan is associated with a decline in plasma norepinephrine levels over the subsequent year.

than doubling of tumor diameter of this time. More speculatively, the sequence in FIGURES 1 and 2 may suggest a dose-related effect with high-dose irbesartan, which was required to reduce tumor secretion. The second patient had a sub-acute presentation at recurrence, with a picture of aggressive spread at laparotomy. We therefore feared rapid further clinical deterioration and spread

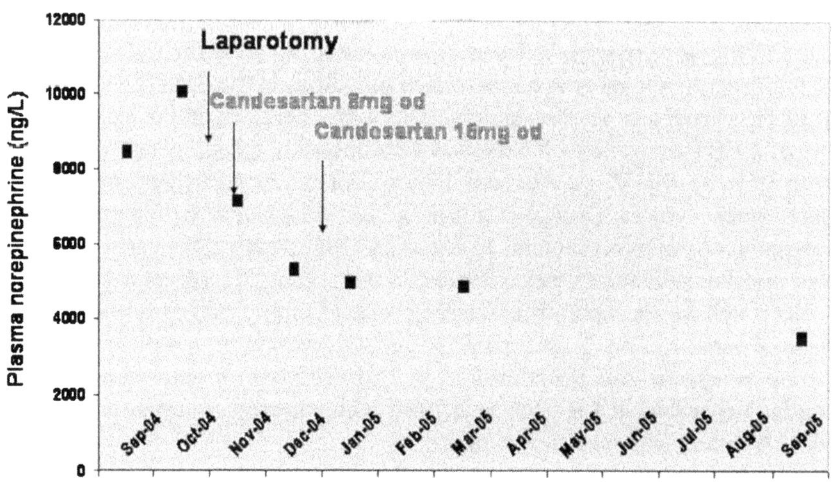

FIGURE 5. Serial CT scans in Case 2. The local spread and adjacent lymph node deposits are arrowed. These show no apparent change over 1 year between 2004 and 2005, when the patient received candesartan 8–16 mg daily.

of tumor. This expectation is the only control against which the actual course to date suggests the possibility of a drug-induced slowing of tumor growth.

The mechanism of potential benefit from ARB treatment is speculative, but appears to be of two main types. One is through stimulation of the AT_2 receptor. The function of this G-protein-coupled receptor has been less clear than that of the AT_1 receptor, but in general AT_2 receptor stimulation has opposite effects to stimulation of the AT_1 receptor.[5] In a number of cultured cell types, stimulation of the AT_2 receptor causes apoptosis. In particular, this effect has been noted in the PC12 pheochromocytoma cell line. The concentration of angiotensin II has tended to be high in the cultured cell studies. On the other hand, *in vivo* induction of apoptosis needs affect a minute fraction of cells in order to oppose proliferation of slow-growing tumors. If the higher rates of apoptosis described in cell culture were reproduced *in vivo,* tissues would totally disappear within days!

The main alternative mechanism would be through blockade of angiotensin II's behavior as a tumor growth factor, acting through the AT_1 receptor. Interestingly, a 16-year retrospective survey of 5,000 patients by the Glasgow hypertension clinic showed a 30% lower incidence of all cancers in patients receiving ACE inhibitors compared to patients on other antihypertensive drugs.[6] The many prospective studies of ACE inhibitors and ARBs are not suitable for detecting a benefit in patients with existing tumors, who would be excluded from such trials. They are probably also underpowered to detect influences on tumor manifestation, especially if the benefit were limited to specific tumor types.

The purpose of the present, anecdotal report is to encourage other physicians to consider high-dose ARB therapy, which is well tolerated and has no apparent downside to its use. Target patients would be any patient with pheochromocytoma in whom surgery is delayed or impossible. In addition, the recognition of high recurrence rates in patients with mutations in the SDHB gene, and of multiple pheochromocytomata in patients with SDHD mutations, may prompt use of ARB therapy in such patients after removal of the index tumor. Patients with VHL or MEN2 may be candidates after removal of their first adrenal pheochromocytoma. Design of a prospective, formal trial is likely to require extension of the target patients to include asymptomatic gene carriers. A further possibility is recruitment of patients with other AT_2 receptor-expressing tumors, and we are currently examining expression in a range of neural crest–derived tumors. This is prompted by our observation, in a patient with carcinoid syndrome and hypertension, that introduction of candesartan 16–32 mg for hypertension has been associated with an arrest of tumor growth and 5HIAA excretion over a 3-year period.

In summary, we present two patients with pheochromocytoma in whom high-dose ARB therapy has been associated temporally with cessation of tumor growth. Further anecdotal experience is encouraged as a prelude to design of a prospective, comparative trial.

REFERENCES

1. STOLL, M., U.M. STECKELINGS, M. PAUL, *et al.* 1995. The angiotensin AT2-receptor mediates inhibition of cell proliferation in coronary endothelial cells. J. Clin. Invest. **95:** 651–657.
2. YAMADA, T., M. HORIUCHI & V.J. DZAU. 1996. Angiotensin II type 2 receptor mediates programmed cell death. Proc. Natl. Acad. Sci. USA **93:** 156–160.
3. BROWN, M.J., D.J. ALLISON, D.A. JENNER, *et al.* 1981. Increased sensitivity and accuracy of phaeochromocytoma diagnosis achieved by plasma adrenaline estimations and a pentolinium suppression test. Lancet **II:** 174–177.
4. BRINK, I., S. HOEGERLE, J. KLISCH & T.A. BLEY. 2005. Imaging of pheochromocytoma and paraganglioma. Familial Cancer **4:** 61–68.
5. HEIN, L., G.S. BARSH, R.E. PRATT, *et al.* 1995. Behavioural and cardiovascular effects of disrupting the angiotensin II type-2 receptor gene in mice. **377:** 744–747.
6. LEVER, A.F., D.J. HOLE, C.R. GILLIS, *et al.* 1998. Do inhibitors of angiotensin-I-converting enzyme protect against risk of cancer? Lancet **352:** 179–184.

Mortality Associated with Pheochromocytoma

Increased Risk for Additional Tumors

AMIR KHORRAM-MANESH,[a] SVANTE JANSSON,[a] BO WÄNGBERG,[a] OLA NILSSON,[b] LARS-ERIK TISELL,[a] AND HÅKAN AHLMAN[a]

[a]*Department of Surgery, The Lundberg Laboratory for Cancer Research, Göteborg University, Sahlgrenska University Hospital, Göteborg, Sweden*

[b]*Department of Pathology, The Lundberg Laboratory for Cancer Research, Göteborg University, Sahlgrenska University Hospital, Göteborg, Sweden*

ABSTRACT: A consecutive series of patients (68 females and 53 males) with pheochromocytoma (PC, $n = 110$) or paraganglioma (PG, $n = 11$) were treated at the Sahlgrenska University Hospital (1950–1997). During the observation period (15 ± 6 years) 42 patients died versus 23.6 expected in the general population ($P < 0.001$). There was no surgical mortality. Twenty patients died of cardiovascular disease, 11 of other tumors, and 7 of other diseases, but only 4 of PC/PG. The main causes of death in this regional series were cardiovascular diseases and tumor in a ratio of 1.3 versus 2.0 in the general Swedish population. Analysis of the mortality in all patients with clinically diagnosed PC ($n = 481$, 259 women and 222 men) based on the National Cancer Registry (1957–1997) showed that the number of deaths in this cohort was 196 versus 153.4 expected ($P < 0.001$). These patients had almost four times higher risk of dying of a tumor than did the general population (similar risk for females and males). There was no increased risk for cardiovascular death; in fact, the risk was lower than expected for men (22 vs. 38 expected). A second tumor diagnosed subsequent to PC occurred in 68 versus 31 expected. In men tumors of the liver and biliary tract and central nervous system and in women malignant melanoma and cervix carcinoma were most frequent. The results from the national series thus confirm an increased risk of a second tumor and increased tumor-related mortality in patients with PC.

KEYWORDS: tumor mortality; pheochromocytoma/paraganglioma; regional/national series

Address for correspondence: Amir Khorram-Manesh, M.D., Ph.D., Department of Surgery, Sahlgrenska University Hospital, S-413 45 Göteborg, Sweden. Voice: +46-31-3421129; fax: +46-31-417364. e-mail: amir.khorram-manesh@surgery.gu.se

Ann. N.Y. Acad. Sci. 1073: 444–448 (2006).
doi: 10.1196/annals.1353.048

INTRODUCTION

Pheochromocytoma/paraganglioma (PC/PG) is a rare disease with a potentially lethal outcome if not diagnosed.[1,2] On account of the high secretion of catecholamines, immediate cardiovascular complications (e.g., myocardial infarction, stroke) can cause death.[2,3] With early tumor diagnosis and adequate treatment, patients with PC/PG are reported to have normal life expectancy.[2,4,5] The main causes of death in the general population are cardiovascular diseases and tumor.[6] However, the causes of death in patients treated for PC/PG with long observation have been less well studied. In some reports, cardiovascular diseases and metastatic PC/PG were found to be the major causes of death.[1–4]

Patients with rare endocrine disorders, (e.g., PC/PG) in the western region of Sweden (1.6 million inhabitants), are referred to the Sahlgrenska University Hospital. The aim of this study was therefore to identify the causes of death in patients treated for PC/PG (1950–1997) in a consecutive series from our center with a long follow-up period. Furthermore, we compared our regional results with a larger series from the same time period, consisting of all cases of clinically diagnosed PC, based on the Swedish National Cancer Registry (NCR).[6] In this national cohort, we also analyzed causes of death and occurrence of a second tumor after the diagnosis of PC.

PATIENTS AND METHODS

In our regional series (1950–1997), 121 consecutive patients (68 women and 53 men) with PC (n = 110), or PG (n = 10) were surgically treated at our hospital. The median age at surgery in this series was 47 years for both women (range 15–82 years) and men (range 23–77 years). In the national series, 481 patients with clinically diagnosed PC in Sweden between 1957 and 1997 were identified (259 women and 222 men, mean age 50 ± 17 years) in NCR. Autopsy-based diagnoses (n = 179) were not included. The inclusion date of a patient was the date the tumor diagnosis was established; diagnoses were classified according to ICD-7.[7] The causes of death in the regional series were obtained from medical records, death certificates, or autopsy results (n = 42).

The observed numbers and causes of death in both series were compared with the expected numbers and causes of death in the control population (entire Swedish population: 8.2 million) by using a Poisson distribution. Additional tumor diagnoses, occurring after diagnosis of PC, were recorded in both series and the occurrence of a second tumor (metastases not included) was compared with that of the control population. It is mandatory for all clinicians, cytologists, and pathologists in Sweden to report all malignant and several benign tumors (including PC/PG) to NCR separately.[6,8] The registry contains no information on stage of disease or treatment given. Its completeness is approximately 98% and it has valid incidence figures.[8] The patients in NCR are coded identically as those registered in the National Registry of Deaths and Main Causes of Death,[6] that is, no patient can be included in a study more than once and the data in these registries can be cross-matched. Confidence intervals (CI) for risk ratios (RR) were calculated exactly. Analyses were performed for men and women separately. Two-tailed tests were used.

RESULTS

During an observation period of 15 ± 6 years after resection for PC/PG in the regional series ($n = 121$), eight patients had, or developed, malignant PC ($n = 6$) or PG ($n = 2$); a total of 42 patients died. The expected number of deaths was 23.6 ($P < 0.001$). Only four patients died of PC/PG. The remaining 38 patients died from other causes; 20 of cardiovascular disease (53%), 11 of tumors (29%), and 7 of other causes, such as trauma, intoxication, gastric bleeding, and uremia (two of the accidentally deceased had brain tumors at autopsy). Three MEN 2B patients died of MTC, three others of intracranial tumors, four of nonrelated carcinoma, and one of leukemia.[9] In the national series, the number of deaths was 196 versus 153.4 expected ($P < 0.001$). The total mortality for men after treatment for PC was not significantly increased, while it was elevated twofold for women. Analyses of causes of death showed that patients with PC had almost four times higher risk of dying of a tumor than expected in the general population. Similar risks were observed both for men and women (RR = 3.4 and 3.9, respectively). There was no increased risk for cardiovascular death (RR 0.73; CI = 0.53–0.98); in men there were only 22 such deaths versus 38 expected, while women had a similar risk as the control population (TABLE 1).

In the national cohort, a second tumor diagnosed subsequent to PC occurred in 68 patients versus 31 expected (RR = 2.20; CI =1.7–2.8). In men a second

TABLE 1. Comparison between causes of death in the normal population versus patients with pheochromocytoma in Sweden (1958–1997)

Cause of death	Sex	Observed	Expected	Risk ratio	95 % CI
All	Total	196	153.4	1.28	1.10–1.47
	Men	102	108.8	0.94	0.76–1.14
	Women	94	44.6	2.11	1.70–2.60
Tumors	Total	95	26.2	3.63	2.94–4.44
	Men	48	14.1	3.41	2.51–4.52
	Women	47	12.1	3.90	2.86–5.18
Cardiovascular	Total	44	60.5	0.73	0.53–0.98
	Men	22	38.0	0.58	0.36–0.88
	Women	22	22.5	0.98	0.61–1.48

tumor was reported in 28 patients versus 13.6 expected (RR = 2.05; CI = 1.4–2.9) and in women 40 versus 17.5 (RR = 2.29; CI = 1.6–3.1). In men tumors of the liver/biliary tract (RR = 8.62; CI = 1.8–25.2) and central nervous system tumors (RR = 13.08; CI = 4.8–28.5) were most frequent. Among women malignant melanomas (RR = 6.61; CI = 1.8–16.9) and carcinomas of the uterine cervix (RR = 7.69; CI = 2.5–17.9) were overrepresented. In the general population breast cancer is common among women with the expected incidence of 5.2. Only four were reported in patients treated for PC (RR = 0.75; CI = 0.2–2.0). In men prostate cancer was expected in 3.6 versus 2 found in patients treated for PC (RR = 0.55; CI = 0.1–2.0).

DISCUSSION

By analyzing our regional consecutive series with long follow-up and without surgical mortality, we found that patients treated for PC/PG had an increased mortality risk compared with the matched control population ($P < 0.001$). These patients had cardiovascular disease as the main cause of death, but had also an increased risk for death of other malignancies. The most common cause of death among patients who had PC, as well as the general population, was cardiovascular diseases and tumor in a ratio of 1.3 and 2.0, respectively.[6,9] In our regional series, only 4 patients died from malignant PC/PG, while 11 died of other malignancies; certain unusual tumor types such as MTC and brain tumors, seemed to be overrepresented. All patients who died from MTC had MEN 2B, while one associated with brain tumors may represent a yet-undescribed syndrome. Neumann *et al.*[10] reported that about 25% of patients with presumably sporadic tumors had genetic causes and were thus susceptible to develop specific tumor types in addition to adrenal PC.

For a rare disease like PC, the NCR[6,8] allows a unique analysis of certain parameters in a large cohort (gender, age, and time after diagnosis) as possible determinants of the risk for a second tumor. The national registries also allow evaluation of the cause of death in a selected population versus the general population.[6,8] Using the entire Swedish population as control group, we could not only show an increased risk of developing certain second tumor in patients with PC, but also a fourfold increased tumor mortality risk versus that of the control population, which may indicate genetic mechanisms in addition to the recognized hereditary syndromes. The large size of the control group reduces the possible statistical error and eliminates the risk of selection errors. In this large cohort we found no excess mortality risk for cardiovascular diseases; in fact the risk for death in cardiovascular diseases was lower than expected for men. Surveillance for additional tumor therefore seems as important as detection of cardiovascular diseases in the lifelong follow-up of patients with PC.

ACKNOWLEDGMENTS

This study was supported by grants from the Swedish MRC (5220) and the Swedish Cancer Society (3911).

REFERENCES

1. Lo, C.Y., K.Y. Lam, *et al.* 2000. Adrenal pheochromocytoma remains a frequently overlooked diagnosis. Am. J. Surg. **179:** 212–215.
2. Kebebew, E. & Q.Y. Duh. 1998. Benign and malignant pheochromocytoma: diagnosis, treatment, and follow-up. Surg. Oncol. Clin. N. Am. **7:** 765–789.
3. Lenders, J.W., G. Eisenhofer, *et al.* 2005. Phaeochromocytoma. Lancet **366:** 665–675.
4. Edström, E., A.L. Hjelm Skog, *et al.* 2003. The management of benign and malignant pheochromocytoma and abdominal paraganglioma. Eur. J. Surg. Oncol. **29:** 278–283
5. O'Halloran, T., G. McGreal, *et al.* 2001. 47 years of phaeochromocytomas. Ir. Med. J. **94:** 200–203.
6. The National Board of Health and Welfare. Centre for Epidemiology. The Cancer Registry. 1999 Cancer incidence in Sweden 97. Article No. 1999–42-008.(ISBN: 91-7201-386-9).
7. World Health Organization. 1957. Manual of International Statistical Classification of Diseases, Injuries and Causes of Death, seventh revision: 1–393. WHO. Geneva.
8. Hansson, L.E., P. Sparen, *et al.* 1999. Survival in stomach cancer is improving: results of a nationwide population-based Swedish study. Ann. Surg. **230:** 162–169.
9. Khorram-Manesh A., H. Ahlman, *et al.* 2005. Long-term outcome of a large series of patients surgically treated for pheochromocytoma. J. Intern. Med. **258:** 55–66.
10. Neumann, H.P.H., B. Bausch, *et al.* 2002. Germ-line mutations in nonsyndromic pheochromocytoma. N. Engl. J. Med. **346:** 1459–1466.

Malignant Pheochromocytoma

State of the Field with Future Projections

HÅKAN AHLMAN

Department of Surgery and the Lundberg Laboratory for Cancer Research, Sahlgrenska Academy, University of Göteborg, Sweden

ABSTRACT: **The prevalence of malignant pheochromocytoma is about 10%, and is somewhat higher for paraganglioma. A problem for clinical follow-up is that patients with "benign" histopathologic findings may develop metastatic disease. At the first international symposium on pheochromocytoma in Bethesda (2005) experts from different disciplines and patients shared their experiences, and the present knowledge of this rare disease was updated. The discussion related to future strategies for better clinical/histopathologic diagnosis and understanding of different geno- and phenotypes. Curative surgery can only seldom be performed because of multiple metastases. The main therapeutic goal is therefore often tumor reduction and control of hypertension. To date the best adjunct to surgery is radionuclide therapy using ^{131}I-MIBG, but the background information for optimal treatment is still incomplete. Certain patients may benefit from ^{131}I-MIBG combined with radiotherapy via somatostatin receptors expressed by the tumor, or the combination with chemotherapy. The need for future multicenter studies was emphasized. In experimental models the work on enhanced expression of amine transporters critical for radiotherapy is continued. Ongoing microarray studies will reveal novel intracellular pathways of importance for proliferation/cell cycle control, which can be inhibited by pharmacologic tools.**

KEYWORDS: **pheochromocytoma; tumor markers; radionuclide therapy; chemotherapy**

INTRODUCTION

Aminergic neurons and neuroendocrine cells synthesize, store, and release amines. Amines are synthesized from precursor amino acids in the cytoplasm before transport into storage vesicles by specific membrane-bound transporters, VMATs. Once released from the cells amines can be subject to active

Address for correspondence: Prof. Håkan Ahlman, Department of Surgery, Sahlgrenska University Hospital, 413 45 Göteborg, Sweden. Voice: +46 31 3421778; fax: +46 31 822104.
e-mail: hakan.ahlman@surgery.gu.se

Ann. N.Y. Acad. Sci. 1073: 449–464 (2006). © 2006 New York Academy of Sciences.
doi: 10.1196/annals.1353.049

reuptake by other transporters at the plasma membrane.[1,2] Two subtypes of vesicular transporters, VMAT 1 and 2, have been characterized with structural similarity but different substrate specificity and tissue distribution;[3,4] serotonin-producing midgut carcinoids mainly express VMAT 1, histamine-producing foregut carcinoids almost exclusively VMAT 2. Pheochromocytoma (PC) and paraganglioma (PG) are neuroendocrine tumors derived from chromaffin cells located in the adrenal medulla and sympathetic paraganglia. PC and mainly abdominal PG can synthesize, store, and secrete catecholamines (CA) and express high levels of VMAT 1 and 2.[5,6] Parasympathetic head and neck PGs are exceptions, with only occasional CA secretion and expression of acetylcholine transporters.[7]

PROGNOSTIC MARKERS

Histopathology

One clinical problem in the follow-up of patients is that no single histopathologic feature of resected PC/PG can predict future metastatic disease. Malignancy has therefore been defined as presence of metastases at sites where chromaffin tissue should not be present, for example, skeleton, lungs, liver, and lymph nodes.[8] Recently, Thompson[9] proposed a scaled score (PASS) for better assessment of malignancy; this score considered not only local invasiveness, but also several other parameters as growth pattern (Zellballen), presence of necrosis, cellularity, spindled morphology, cytological features (nuclear pleomorphism and hyperchromasia), mitotic activity, and atypical mitoses. However, the weighting process was subjective and the diagnostic performance of PASS is not optimal. A total score of ≥ 4 indicates high risk for malignancy, but there are patients with very high scores who have not developed malignant disease. Prospective studies to validate current scoring systems are clearly needed. For other types of neuroendocrine tumors, proliferation rates (Ki-67 index) higher than 5–10% indicate malignancy (carcinoids and endocrine pancreatic tumors of the WHO class 2 type: well-differentiated endocrine carcinomas).[10,11] This figure seems to be lower for PC (> 2.5%).[12] The latter study also observed a reduced number of sustentacular cells (immunoreactive with S100) in tumors with higher proliferation.

Extensive research in fields related to angiogenesis, adhesion molecules, DNA ploidy, new molecular markers, and gene expression abnormalities has indicated possible new associations with malignant PC/PG. Potential markers of malignancy include increased microvessel density and differential expression of VEGF and VEGFR 2,[13–15] p53 and bcl2,[16] Hif2-α,[13] NCAD,[17] tenascin C,[18] COX 2,[19] and secretogranin II and its processing, for example, peptide EM66[20,21] and endoproteases of the prohormone convertase family.[22] However, the apoptosis inhibitor survivin was present in the cytoplasm of both benign and malignant tumors.[23] Expression of TGF-β-related growth factors, the β-subunits of inhibin and activin, their receptors and binding proteins, could not discriminate between benign and malignant tumors,[24] nor could other putative markers for malignant PC, for example, the gap junction protein connexin or galectin 3.[25,26]

Overexpression of HSP 90 (heat-shock protein) may have future therapeutic implications; HSP 90 is a molecular chaperone that maintains the conformation of proteins, which control intracellular oncogenic pathways, including cyclin binding and activation of Cdk4.[27] HSP 90 is also part of the human telomerase complex, which also includes the telomerase RNA component (hTR), its associated protein (TP1), and catalytic subunit (hTERT); hTERT and HSP 90 had high expression in malignant PC, but high telomerase activity was only seen in hTERT-expressing tumors.[28] Overexpression of HSP 90 could thus activate telomerase via hTERT and inhibitors of HSP 90 would then be antiproliferative. From ongoing microarray studies several novel molecular markers will appear in the near future.

Clinical and Biochemical Parameters

Metastases are usually present within 5 years after primary surgery, but may also occur after a very long time in individual patients.[29,30] Well-recognized risk factors for malignant disease are large tumor size (>5 cm) and tumors with extra-adrenal location.[31–33] Malignant PCs/PGs have a defective expression of the CA-synthesizing enzymes, especially downregulation of PNMT, which converts norepinephrine (NE) to epinephrine (E). This means that the noradrenergic phenotype dominates in malignant PC/PG;[34,35] malignant tumors can also have other defects in their synthesis of CA precursors, which may result in elevated levels of DOPA/dopamine in plasma and urine.[35–38] These biochemical markers indicate dedifferentiation, but do not reliably distinguish between benign and malignant tumors. Purely dopamine-secreting tumors are very rare and patients can be normotensive and asymptomatic. An association with inflammatory syndromes has been described.[39] The granular storage protein chromogranin A (CgA) is co-released together with amines/peptides from neuroendocrine tumor cells and is therefore a general tumor marker in plasma. It correlates both with secretory activity and tumor volume.[40] The sum of the two free metanephrines in plasma can also be helpful in predicting tumor size, and the relative profile of normetanephrine versus metanephrine indicates phenotype and, indirectly, location of tumor.[41] Rao *et al.*[42] demonstrated that patients with malignant tumors had higher CgA levels than those with benign tumors, which in turn were different from controls. During chemotherapy CgA levels followed CA markers and reflected the therapeutic response. Plouin *et al.*[43] recently showed that urinary metanephrines very well reflected the growth of malignant tumors and their response to treatment. Novel plasma markers derived from proteomics are needed with potential to distinguish between benign and malignant tumors.

The prevalence of malignant PC is about 10% (5–26%); higher rates (up to 46%) have been reported for extra-adrenal tumors.[32,44] The high figures should be interpreted with some caution, since they may relate to other definitions of malignancy or emanate from studies that are not population-based, with overrepresentation of certain mutations, or from screening studies on imaging.[30,33,44,45]

Genetics

Hereditary factors responsible for development of PC/PG and also for malignant transformation have been underscored. Neumann *et al.*[46] and Bryant *et al.*[47] found that 20–24% of apparently sporadic tumors had underlying germline mutations, most frequently VHL (10%), followed by RET and SDHB and D (5% each). Malignant transformation is most variable for the different hereditary tumor types. The predisposition for malignancy is low for VHL, RET, and SDHD (<5%), relatively low for NF1 (11%), and high for SDHB (50%).[7] In patients with metastatic PC/PG, gene testing for SDHB is most appropriate, since these mutations have high prevalence in these patients (22–37%) and are not associated with specific clinical features.[48] It is notable that extra-adrenal tumors may occur in both VHL and SDHD, but still these patients have low risk for malignant disease in contrast to patients with sporadic extra-adrenal tumors. Another intriguing observation comes from gene expression studies of VHL-PCs and malignant PCs, both showing hypoxia-driven angiogenesis with increased expression of an endothelial nuclear receptor translocator (Hif-2α), in contrast to benign hereditary and sporadic tumors.[49] VHL-PCs and malignant PCs further share the noradrenergic phenotype with main production of NE, despite the fact that VHL tumors only rarely are malignant. PGs also express the noradrenergic phenotype and are usually more aggressive than adrenal tumors with predominant secretion of E.[35,38,50]

Genome-wide studies by comparative genomic hybridization (CGH) have indicated certain regions of loss (6q and 17p) and gain (5p, 7p, and 12q) in malignant PC.[51] Ongoing studies with gene expression profiling of benign versus malignant PCs will generate data with high resolution. After correction for phenotypic influence these studies will address not only malignant characteristics, but also differences between primary and metastases, hereditary and sporadic tumors, and adrenal and extra-adrenal tumors.[52]

IMAGING

The identification of metastases requires imaging studies. Computed tomography and magnetic resonance imaging have high sensitivity (95%) in detecting the primary tumor (somewhat lower for extra-adrenal lesions), but suffer from restricted specificity (50%).[53,54] Therefore, functional imaging of the whole body is usually performed by means of tumor-specific techniques, for example, uptake of the CA analogue metaiodobenzylguanidine (MIBG) via the NE transporter (type I uptake process) at the cell membrane and concentration within secretory granules via VMATs, labeled with either ^{131}I (half-life 8.2 day; 364 keV) or ^{123}I (half-life 13 h; 159 keV). Imaging using ^{123}I and single-photon emission computed tomography has higher sensitivity, better imaging quality, and less radiation, but is more expensive than ^{131}I. PC/PG can be imaged by MIBG with a sensitivity of 77–90% (even higher for ^{123}I) and a specificity of 95%.[55] However, recent studies indicate that ^{131}I-MIBG has much lower detection rate (56%) for malignant tumors, and individual patients can have both MIBG-positive and negative lesions.[56] PCs/PGs can also express somatostatin receptors (SSTRs) on their cell membrane. However, there are relatively few studies on SSTR-expression in PC/PG using immunohistochemistry, real-time polymerase chain reaction, or autoradiography;[57–60] some report expression of all five SSTR subtypes; others show high incidence of SSTR 2 (with high affinity for the somatostatin analogues octreotide/octreotate). Our own studies indicate relatively low numbers of SSTR 2 in accordance with much lower detection rate of benign PC by octreotide scintigraphy than by the MIBG techniques.[61] Higher detection rate by octreotide scintigraphy has been reported for parasympathetic head and neck PG.[62] In the case of malignant tumors it is important to realize that octreotide scintigraphy can serve as a complement to visualizing MIBG-negative lesions,[56,61] even though ^{123}I-MIBG is considered to have better overall detection rate than octreotide scintigraphy.[63]

In pilot studies high scintigraphic ^{123}I-uptake was found in two malignant PGs with high VMAT expression (500–730 copies of VMAT 1 and 1,500–1,700 copies of VMAT 2/1,000 β-actin) in comparison with a third malignant PG with negative imaging and low VMAT expression (330 copies of VMAT 1 and 350 copies of VMAT 2/1,000 β-actin). *In vitro,* the VMAT antagonist reserpine and membrane pump inhibitors each inhibited the uptake of ^{123}I-MIBG into tumor cells equally well. In our analysis of SSTR expression, SSTR 2 was the most abundant receptor subtype, but with relatively low receptor numbers (40–260 copies versus 9,000 copies/1,000 β-actin in midgut carcinoids).[64] Also, the activity concentration ratio in PC tumors versus blood (T/B ratio) was low in comparison with other types of neuroendocrine tumors.[65]

PET using ^{11}C-labeled CA precursors (DOPA, dopamine), E, or analogues (hydroxyephedrine, HED), all of which target the NE transporter, have been used to identify metastatic tumors.[55,66] These substances not only differ in substrate specificity for the transporter, but also in degree of vesicular sequestration. Most recently, ^{18}F-labeled DOPA, or dopamine, has been used. The most sensitive method seems to be ^{18}F-6-fluorodopamine, which is associated with very high T/B ratios and is to date the superior technique to localize metastatic PC/PG.[56] Compared with MIBG imaging the PET techniques that generate low radiation dose are rapid, and do not require iodine blockade of the thyroid. In the case of undifferentiated tumors, negative imaging with these specific scintigraphic and PET techniques may still occur. In such cases ^{18}F-fluorodeoxyglucose PET can be diagnostic.

Most investigators recommend MIBG imaging prior to surgical resection, especially in patients with large (> 5 cm), extra-adrenal, or multiple tumors. It is also important to repeat biochemical testing after surgery to verify that no remaining functional tumor remains, since micrometastases may remain that have not been removed by resection. Biochemical testing is generally performed on an annual basis, followed by imaging studies when CA hypersecretion is indicated biochemically. It would be of crucial importance to be able to define from histopathologic criteria patients at risk for intensified surveillance. In our own population-based series of 154 patients with PC/PG (1950–2004) only 12 patients had malignant tumors (8 PCs + 4 PGs); 4 presented with distant metastases, 4 with locally advanced disease, and 4 developed metastases despite "benign" histopathology. The first group had severe prognosis, while the tumor progression was very slow in the other two groups; only 5 of 8 patients died of disease after a mean observation of 20 (5–35) years. Despite adequate lymphadenectomy in the second group, all patients developed recurrent disease after long latency, indicating residual micrometastases after intentionally curative surgery. The third group emphasizes the need for risk criteria for intensified surveillance of certain patients.[67]

TUMOR MODELS

Lack of established human PC cell lines has hampered the research on tumorigenesis and novel treatment strategies. The rat PC 12 cell line was established 30 years ago[68] and has generated detailed knowledge about this tumor type (derived from one rodent tumor). More recently several different mouse PC (MPC) cell lines were developed by knockout of the tumor suppressor gene NF 1;[69] they all have a high expression of nonmutated *ret* like human tumors and are thus suitable for studies of *ret*-signaling.[70] In MPC cells glucocorticoids control the expression of PNMT, which can be silenced by neurotrophic factors, that is, transcription studies can reveal mechanisms of sympathoadrenal differentiation.[71] Furthermore, the CA gene expression can be modulated via selective nicotinic receptor stimulation.[72] Recently, a model of MPC metastatic to the liver of nude mice has been developed, which allows tumor studies by micro-CT.[73] MEN 2 transgenic mice also develop PC.[74] Comparative genomic hybridization (CGH) studies of secondary genetic changes revealed large similarities between human and mouse PC.[75] Furthermore, knockout of the gene for phosphatase and tension (*Pten*) homologue also predispose for development of PC.[76]

In rats reserpine (which inhibits VMAT and depletes the granular stores of CA) can induce proliferation and tumor transformation of chromaffin cells. During such treatment the cytoplasm of these cells will contain high concentrations of CA, which leads to enhanced catabolism by oxidative deamination. It has been proposed that this process generates endogenous mutagens, for example, quinones, with potential genotoxic effects. Several therapeutic studies have been performed using human PC tumors, or rat cell lines, xenografted to nude mice: for example, Zielke *et al.*[14] inhibited tumor angiogenesis by treatment with VEGF-antibodies. Gross *et al.*[77] used human VHL tumor xenografts to study the antitumor effects of a collagen synthesis inhibitor, halofuginon. Carcinoid tumor research has also faced similar problems with access to only one very unusual human pancreatic carcinoid cell line.[78] We established and characterized the first human midgut carcinoid cell line GOT 1.[79] Xenograft studies of these tumor cells have been most useful in optimizing SSTR-based radiotherapy[80] and to study the marked antitumor effects by the inhibition of the transcription factor NF-kappa B,[81] as first shown in neuroblastoma.[82]

THERAPY

Interventional Treatment

The 5-year survival for patients with malignant PC/PG and distant metastases is less than 50%, but the individual course of disease is most variable.[29,30,38] Radical surgery can be difficult to perform on account of distant metastases, often localized to the skeleton (70%).[32,44] In exceptional cases with sole liver metastases, not accessible to surgical resection, transplantation has been attempted.[83] To date 150 patients with various neuroendocrine tumors have been treated worldwide with liver transplantation.[84] In the series with best results (selected as well-differentiated endocrine carcinomas with Ki-67 5–10% and liver as the only metastatic organ), the overall and recurrence-free survival rates are 80% and 20%, respectively.[11,85] In metastatic disease of PC/PG the main therapeutic goal is often to obtain *tumor reduction* and *control of hypertension*. In the palliative treatment of neuroendocrine tumors it has been suggested that if the main tumor bulk (80–90%) can be safely excised, this is a recommended therapy.[86] However, there are no randomized trials demonstrating any survival advantage of debulking (cytoreductive surgery), but a reduced tumor volume may facilitate for subsequent radio- or chemotherapy. Prior to surgery it is important to control CA symptoms by α-adrenoceptor blockade, sometimes followed by β-adrenoceptor blockade. Patients with malignant PC/PG can have extremely high NE levels, which has potentially cytotoxic effects on the myocardium. For these patients inhibition of the CA synthesis by α-methyl-paratyrosine may be useful pretreatment, despite the side effects on the central nervous system.[87] Surgery is appropriate treatment for lesions at critical sites also for patients with disseminated disease, for example, spinal cord compression.

Tumor reduction can also be achieved by other interventional techniques. *Selective transcatheter embolization* causes complete, but temporary, ischemia distal to the point of injection of embolization material and deprives neuroendocrine metastases of their main oxygen and blood supply with maintained portal perfusion of the normal liver parenchyma. Tumors that produce histamine or CA have been considered relative contraindications for surgery due to risk for uncontrollable release of these substances. However, the first reports on successful embolization of individual patients with PC/PG under strict pharmacological blockade have now appeared.[43,88] The ischemic strategy can be taken further by the use of *chemoembolization*, that is, embolization combined with intra-arterial administration of chemotherapy using iodized oil, doxorubicin, and Gelfoam particles. For other types of neuroendocrine tumors some centers have used temporary occlusion of the hepatic artery via external vessel loops, or via port-operated tourniquets. A combination of peripheral embolization and temporary proximal occlusion of the hepatic artery may have additive ischemic effects. In patients with a high risk for critical hormone release *hyperthermic perfusion* of the liver with cytotoxic drugs has been attempted. During perfusion the venous efferent from the liver (containing CA) can be shunted from the systemic circulation, thus avoiding adverse effects.[86] Other alternatives to surgical resection, also for metastases outside the liver, include *external beam radiation* (effective for bone pain), *cryoablation,* and *radiofrequency ablation*. The local ablative techniques are valuable complements to liver resection for treatment of localized tumors in the residual liver and for recurrent tumors.

Chemotherapy

Chemotherapy with a combination of cyclophosphamide, vincristine, and dacarbazine (CVD)[89] can provide partial tumor responses and palliation of symptoms in as many as 50% of the patients with malignant PC/PG, but this is of short duration.[90] Addition of anthracyclines (doxorubicin) to this regimen has in individual cases enhanced the therapeutic response.[91] Dr. Tito Fojo, an oncologist at the NIH, had similar experience with CVD (16% complete and 55% partial responses); CVD combined with DTIC did not significantly prolong survival. Patients with nonresectable functional tumors should be kept on chronic α-adrenoceptor blockade, in certain cases combined with α-methylparatyrosine.

The overexpression of HSP 90 and hTERT in malignant PC[28] has been one target for new anticancer drugs.[92] If the chaperone HSP 90 controls signaling pathways of importance for proliferation/cell cycle control–specific inhibitors of this protein, for example, 17-allylamino, 17-demethoxygeldanamycin, may be tailor-made treatment for this disease.[93] When geldanamycin was tested on thyroid cancer cell lines, it decreased proliferation, expression of certain oncoproteins, and EGF-induced invasiveness.[94] These drugs have not yet reached clinical trial.

Radionuclide Therapy

Radionuclide therapy has been used for more than 50 years (^{131}I therapy of thyroid cancer), but its radiobiological effects are much less known than those of external beam irradiation. ^{131}I-MIBG therapy for PC/PG was introduced some 20 years ago,[95] but since malignant PCs/PGs are rare tumors, only small numbers of patients have been treated with different protocols. We still do not have adequate information about absorbed doses/dose rates needed for cure, or tolerance levels for normal tissues. Optimal fractionation schedules are also lacking. It is important to bear in mind that radionuclide therapy is limited by the radiation dose to critical organs, that is, the bone marrow for ^{131}I-MIBG.

In 1997 the world experience with ^{131}I MIBG therapy comprised 116 patients treated at 24 centers worldwide.[96] Thereafter, the largest single-center experiences include a series of 12–33 patients and the activity level per fraction has varied considerably.[65] The majority of patients have been treated with low doses of radioactivity (160–190 mCi), while Safford *et al.*[97] treated 33 patients with medium doses (390 mCi), and Rose *et al.*[98] treated 12 patients with high doses (800 mCi). In general, about three-quarters of the patients had symptomatic responses, half had hormonal responses, and one quarter showed tumor regression, indicating effective palliation by this treatment modality. Objective tumor responses correlated with the given levels of activity. In low-dose studies a minority of patients (4%) showed complete remission versus 25% in the high-dose study, which was the only demonstrated cure of bone metastases.[98] The high-dose study has now been updated and includes 30 patients with PC/PG; all with prior surgery and 16 with no prior radiation or chemotherapy. Only three patients showed complete remission, but 16 had partial remission.[99] The high-dose treatment induced high-grade bone marrow toxicity (neutropenia and thrombocytopenia), which in about 10% required stem cell rescue, that is, for high-dose therapy bone marrow must be harvested prior to treatment. No recommendation for *optimal* ^{131}I MIBG therapy can be given from the present retrospective studies with few patients, different protocols, no dosimetric studies, and different individual follow-up.

Also, other radiopharmaceuticals can be considered for radiotherapy of PC/PG. Since some patients have MIBG-positive and -negative lesions, where some of the negative lesions were visualized via SSTR 2, there is a possibility that combined radiotherapy via NE transporters (MIBG) and SSTR 2 (octreotide/octreotate) might have synergistic effects. In ongoing clinical studies of SSTR-based radiotherapy for other neuroendocrine tumors ^{90}Y-DOTA-octreotide and ^{177}Lu-DOTA-octreotate are used.[100,101]

Somewhat divergent side effects (bone marrow toxicity for ^{131}I and nephrotoxicity followed by bone marrow toxicity for ^{177}Lu) also favor combined radiotherapies. On the other hand, the relatively low expression of SSTR 2 and low T/B ratios hitherto shown are suboptimal.

To achieve cure by radiotherapy all disseminated tumors must be eradicated. One advantage with radionuclides is that adjacent tumor cells without radionuclide binding can be effectively irradiated from tumor cells with radionuclide binding and therefore the range of emitted particles is important for therapeutic effects; too long a range will result in low absorbed doses in small tumors, and therefore dosimetric comparisons between different radionuclides are important. To treat small tumors/micrometastases the short-range α-emitter ^{211}At bound to MIBG (MABG) is of interest. The electron emitters ^{177}Lu and ^{90}Y can be bound to somatostatin analogues with high specific activity and may therefore be complements to ^{131}I MIBG for treatment. ^{177}Lu-DOTA-octreotate is valuable for small PC/PG. For large tumors (often with necroses and nonuniform uptake) ^{90}Y-DOTA-octreotide is the only choice because of the long range of electrons emitted.

For future radionuclide therapy it is important to perform preoperative imaging studies using both ^{123}I-MIBG and ^{111}In-DTPA-D-Phe^{1}-octreotide. The biokinetics of each radiopharmaceutical can be evaluated from scintigraphy. Also, surgical biopsy specimens will allow us to determinate activity concentrations in tumor and normal tissues. In the biopsy specimens the quantitative expression of CA transporters/VMATs and SSTR 1–5 can be determined, but we still need a functional assessment of these transporters. *In vitro* studies of uptake mechanisms may give limited information, not taking into account tumor blood flow, synthesis/degradation of the transporters, and sequestration of the radionuclide. Based on the outlined data, individual dose planning can be performed; optimal dose planning will lead to administration of activities near the tolerance of critical organs and to treatment with iterated fractions based on individual responses. As single agent ^{131}I-MIBG seems to have limited efficacy to cure; medium- or high-dose therapy should be reserved for patients with distant metastases, but medium doses can be considered for completion radiotherapy after so-called curative surgery in high-risk patients with probable micrometastases. More knowledge is needed on synergistic effects of chemotherapy combined with radionuclide therapy, as indicated by current studies on neuroblastoma.[102]

FUTURE PROJECTIONS

To date ^{131}I-MIBG therapy is the single most valuable adjunct to surgical treatment of malignant PC/PG. We still lack sufficient background to design the optimal protocol. Several questions need to be addressed in prospective studies: high-dose versus fractionated medium doses, monotherapy with radionuclides versus combined therapies, for example, ^{131}I-MIBG alone or together with SSTR-based therapies, ^{131}I-MIBG alone or together with chemotherapy. A cross-over design can be difficult to achieve in a radiotherapy trial, since the critical organs may not tolerate a second type of therapy (radio- or chemotherapy) when tumor progression occurs. If the progression probability is 30% for one treatment and 60% for the other treatment, the power 80% is achieved with 50 patients in each group; for 100 patients per group the corresponding figures are 56 versus 52%. Considering that malignant PC/PG is a very rare disease, with about 100 new cases each year in the United States, it is evident that any kind of prospective trial will require a multicenter protocol.

Other lines of research will be to find better substrates for CA transporters/VMATs, to which suitable radionuclides can be bound with high specific activity, and to increase the expression of transporters in the tumor cells. Experimentally, this has been achieved by transporter gene transfer[103] or pretreatment with cytotoxic agents, cytokines, and retinoic acid.[104,105] Transduction of adrenal chromaffin cells has resulted in efficient transgene expression at low virus load, which indicates that tailored recombinant adenoviral vectors may be useful for gene therapy of PC/PG.[106] Naked DNA vaccination has not yet been attempted.

Novel principles for targeted therapy interfering with signaling pathways will follow the microarray studies as outlined for inhibition of HSP 90 by geldanamycin. The high expression of angiogenic factors in PC/PG may imply the use of antiangiogenic principles, receptor antibodies, or profiled tyrosine kinase inhibitors with anti-VEGF activity as recently applied for metastatic thyroid carcinoma.[107] One interesting approach to develop anticancer drugs is induced apoptosis after inhibition of the transcription factor NF-kappa B,[108] which seems to be effective treatment experimentally for neuroblastoma and other types of neuroendocrine tumors.[81,82] However, as pointed out by Dr. Fojo, the tumor biology and therapeutic principles regarding neuroblastoma cannot always be translated to PC/PG. The recent hypothesis that stem cells (resistant to apoptosis), present in neuroblastoma, are responsible for tumor recurrence is plausible.

REFERENCES

1. ROTHMAN, J.E. *et al.* 1992. Molecular dissection of the secretory pathway. Nature **355:** 409–415.
2. CALAKOS, N. *et al.* 1994. Vesicle-associated membrane protein and synaptophysin are associated on the synaptic vesicle. J. Biol. Chem. **269:** 24534–24537.
3. ERICKSON, J.D. *et al.* 1992. Expression cloning of a reserpine-sensitive vesicular monoamine transporter. Proc. Natl. Acad. Sci. USA **89:** 10993–10997.
4. ERICKSON, J.D. *et al.* 1996. Distinct pharmacological properties and distribution in neurons and endocrine cells of two isoforms of the human vesicular monoamine transporter. Proc. Natl. Acad. Sci. USA **93:** 5166–5171.
5. ERICKSON, D. *et al.* 2001. Benign paragangliomas: clinical presentation and treatment outcomes in 236 patients. J. Clin. Endocrinol. Metab. **86:** 5210–5216.
6. JAKOBSEN, A.M. *et al.* 2001. Expression of vesicular monoamine transporter (VMAT) 1 and 2 in gastrointestinal endocrine tumors. J. Pathol. **195:** 463–472.
7. LENDERS, J.W.M. *et al.* 2005. Pheochromocytoma. Lancet **366:** 665–675.

8. LACK, E.E. *et al.* 2003. Recommendations for the reporting of extra-adrenal paragangliomas. The Association of Directors of Anatomic and Surgical Pathology. Hum. Pathol. **34:** 112–113.
9. THOMPSON, L.D. 2002. Pheochromocytoma of the adrenal gland scaled score (PASS) to separate benign from malignant neoplasms: a clinicopathologic and immunophenotypic study of 100 cases. Am. J. Surg. Pathol. **26:** 551–566.
10. PELOSI, G. *et al.* 1996. Endocrine tumors of the pancreas: Ki-67 immunoreactivity on paraffin sections is an independent predictor for malignancy. Hum. Pathol. **27:** 1124–1134.
11. ROSENAU, J. *et al.* 2002. Ki67, ECAD, and p53 as prognostic indicators of long-term outcome after liver transplantation for metastatic neuroendocrine tumors. Transplantation **73:** 386–394.
12. VAN DER HARST, E. *et al.* 2000. Proliferative index of pheochromocytomas: does it predict the occurrence of metastases? J. Pathol. **191:** 175–180.
13. FAVIER, J. *et al.* 2002. Angiogenesis and vascular architecture in pheochromocytomas: distinctive traits in malignant tumors. Am. J. Pathol. **161:** 1235–1246.
14. ZIELKE, A. *et al.* 2002. VEGF-mediated angiogenesis of human pheochromocytomas is associated to malignancy and inhibited by anti-VEGF antibodies in experimental tumors. Surgery **132:** 1056–1063.
15. SALMENKIVI, K. *et al.* 2003. VEGF in 105 pheochromocytomas: enhanced expression correlates with malignant outcome. APMIS **111:** 458–464.
16. DE KRIJGER, R.R. *et al.* 1999. Prognostic value of p53, bcl-2, and c-erb B-2 protein expression in pheochromocytomas. J. Pathol. **188:** 51–55.
17. KHORRAM-MANESH, A. *et al.* 2002. NCAD expression in adrenal tumors: upregulation in malignant pheochromocytoma and down-regulation in adrenocortical carcinoma. Endocr. Pathol. **13:** 99–110.
18. SALMENKIVI, K. *et al.* 2001. Increased expression of tenascin in pheochromocytomas correlates with malignancy. Am. J. Surg. Pathol. **25:** 1419–1423.
19. SALMENKIVI, K. *et al.* 2001. Increased expression of cyclooxygenase-2 in malignant pheochromocytomas. J. Clin. Endocrinol. Metab. **86:** 5615–5619.
20. YON, L. *et al.* 2003. Identification of the secretogranin II-derived peptide EM66 in pheochromocytomas as a potential marker for discriminating benign versus malignant tumors. J. Clin. Endocrinol. Metab. **88:** 2579–2585.
21. ANOUR, Y. *et al.* 2005. Development of novel tools for the diagnosis and prognosis for pheochromocytomas using peptide marker immunoassay and gene expression profiling approaches. [abstract at ISP].
22. GUILLERMOT, J. *et al.* 2005. Expression and processing of the neuroendocrine protein secretogranin II in benign *vs.* malignant pheochromocytomas. [abstract at ISP].
23. KOCH, C.A. *et al.* 2002. Survivin: a novel neuroendocrine marker for pheochromocytoma. Eur. J. Endocrinol. **146:** 381–388.
24. HOFLAND, J. *et al.* 2005. Expression of activin and inhibin subunits, receptors and binding proteins and immunohistochemistry of inhibin β-subunits in human pheochromocytomas. [abstract at ISP].
25. WILLENBERG, H.S. *et al.* 2005. Expression of connexins in chromaffin cells of hormal human adrenals, benign and malignant pheochromocytomas. [abstract at ISP].
26. GIMM, O. *et al.* 2005. Distinct expression of galectin-3 in pheochromocytomas. [abstract at ISP].
27. LAI, E.W. *et al.* 2005. Cell cycle regulation in metastatic pheochromocytoma. [abstract at ISP].

28. Boltze, C. *et al.* 2003. Expression profile of the telomeric complex discriminates between benign and malignant pheochromocytoma. J. Clin. Endocrinol. Metab. **88:** 4280–4286.
29. Lenders, J.W. *et al.* 2002. Biochemical diagnosis of pheochromocytoma: which test is best? JAMA **287:** 1427–1434.
30. Khorram-Manesh, A. *et al.* 2005. Long-term outcome of a large series of patients surgically treated for pheochromocytoma. J. Intern. Med. **258:** 55–66.
31. O'Riordain, D.S. *et al.* 1996. Clinical spectrum and outcome of functional extraadrenal paraganglioma. World J. Surg. **20:** 916–921.
32. Goldstein, R.E. *et al.* 1999. Clinical experience over 48 years with pheochromocytoma. Ann. Surg. **229:** 755–766.
33. Gimenez-Roqueplo, A.P. *et al.* 2003. Mutations in the SDHB gene are associated with extra-adrenal and/or malignant pheochromocytomas. Cancer Res. **63:** 5615–5621.
34. Eisenhofer, G. *et al.* 2001. Pheochromocytomas in VHL syndrome and MEN 2 display distinct biochemical and clinical phenotypes. J. Clin. Endocrinol. Metabol. **86:** 1999–2008.
35. van der Harst, E. *et al.* 2002. The value of plasma markers for the clinical behaviour of pheochromocytomas. Eur. J. Endocrinol. **147:** 85–94.
36. Anton, A.H. *et al.* 1967. Dihydroxyphenylalanine secretion in a malignant pheochromocytoma. Am. J. Med. **42:** 469–475.
37. Goldstein, D.S. *et al.* 1986. Plasma 3, 4-dihydroxyphenylalanine (dopa) and catecholamines in neuroblastoma or pheochromocytoma. Ann. Int. Med. **105:** 887–888.
38. John, H. *et al.* 1999. Pheochromocytomas: can malignant potential be predicted? Urology **53:** 679–683.
39. Proye, C. *et al.* 1986. Dopamine-secreting pheochromocytoma: an unrecognized entity? Classification of pheochromocytoma according to type of secretion. Surgery **100:** 1154–1161.
40. Baudin, E. *et al.* 2001. Impact of chromogranin A measurement in the work up of neuroendocrine tumors. Ann. Oncol. Suppl. **12**: 79–82.
41. Eisenhofer, G. *et al.* 2005. Pheochromocytoma catecholamine phenotypes and prediction of tumor size, location, and germ-line mutation using plasma-free metanephrines. Clin. Chem. **51:** 735–744.
42. Rao, F. *et al.* 2000. Malignant pheochromocytoma: chromaffin granule transmitters and response to treatment. Hypertension **36:** 1045–1052.
43. Plouin, P.-F. *et al.* 2005. The course of urinary metanephrine excretion in recurrent and malignant pheochromocytomas and secreting paragangliomas. [abstract at ISP].
44. Thompson, N.W. 1993. Malignant pheochromocytoma. Acta. Chir. Austriaca **4:** 235–241.
45. Edström-Elder, E. *et al.* 2003. The management of benign and malignant pheochromocytoma and abdominal paraganglioma. Eur. J. Surg. Oncol. **29:** 278–283.
46. Neumann, H.P. *et al.* 2002. Germ-line mutations in nonsyndromic pheochromocytoma. N. Engl. J. Med. **346:** 1459–1466.
47. Bryant, J. *et al.* 2003. Pheochromocytoma: the expanding genetic differential diagnosis. J. Nat. Cancer Inst. **95:** 1196–1204.
48. Brouwers, F.M. *et al.* 2005. Importance of SDHB mutation testing in patients with malignant pheochromocytoma. [abstract at ISP].

49. EISENHOFER, G. *et al.* 2004. Malignant pheochromocytoma: current status and initiatives for future progress. Endocr. Rel. Cancer **11:** 423–436.
50. BROWN, W.J. *et al.* 1972. Ultrastructural and biochemical correlates of adrenal and extra-adrenal pheochromocytoma. Cancer **29:** 744–759.
51. DANNENBERG, H. *et al.* 2000. Losses of chromosomes 1p and 3q are early genetic events in the development of sporadic pheochromocytomas. Am. J. Pathol. **157:** 353–359.
52. BROUWERS, F. *et al.* 2005. Gene expression profiling of benign and malignant pheochromocytoma: new markers for prognosis and targets for treatments. [abstract at ISP].
53. MAUREA, S. *et al.* 1993. ^{131}I-MIBG scintigraphy in preoperative and postoperative evaluation of paragangliomas: comparison with CT and MRI. J. Nucl. Med. **34:** 173–179.
54. FRANCIS, I.R. *et al.* 1996. Pheochromocytoma. Radiol. Clin. N. Am. **34:** 1101–1112.
55. PACAK, K. *et al.* 2004. Diagnostic imaging of pheochromocytoma. *In* Pheochromocytoma: Pathophysiology and Clinical Management. H. Lehnert, Ed. Front. Horm. Res. **31:** 107–120.
56. ILIAS, I. *et al.* 2003. Superiority of 6-[^{18}F]-fluorodopamine positron emission tomography versus [^{131}I]-MIBG scintigraphy in the localization of metastatic pheochromocytoma. J. Clin. Endocrinol. Metab. **88:** 4083–4087.
57. REUBI, J.C. *et al.* 1992. In vitro and in vivo detection of somatostatin receptors in pheochromocytomas and paragangliomas. J. Clin. Endocrinol. Metab. **74:** 1082–1089.
58. KUBOTA, A. *et al.* 1994. Identification of somatostatin receptor subtypes and an implication for the efficacy of SMS 201-995 in treatment of human endocrine tumors. J. Clin. Invest. **93:** 1321–1325.
59. EPELBAUM, J. *et al.* 1995. Molecular and pharmacological characterization of somatostatin receptor subtypes in adrenal, extraadrenal and malignant pheochromocytomas. J. Clin. Endocrinol. Metab. **80:** 1837–1844.
60. KIMURA, N. *et al.* 1999. Immunohistochemical expression of somatostatin type 2A receptor in neuroendocrine tumors. Chir. Cancer Res. **5:** 3483–3487.
61. VAN DER HARST, E. *et al.* 2001. ^{123}I-MIBG and ^{111}In-octreotide uptake in benign and malignant pheochromocytoma. J. Clin. Endocrinol. Metab. **86:** 685–693.
62. GAGLIANO, M.S. *et al.* 2005. Different scintigraphic patterns between parasympathetic and sympathetic paragangliomas in patients with PGL-1. [abstract at ISP].
63. KALTSAS, G. *et al.* 2001. Comparison of somatostatin analog and MIBG radionuclides in the diagnosis and localization of advanced neuroendocrine tumors. J. Clin. Endocrinol. Metab. **86:** 895–902.
64. KÖLBY, L. *et al.* 2005. Can quantification of VMAT and SSTR expression be helpful for planning radionuclide therapy of malignant pheochromocytomas? This volume.
65. FORSSELL-ARONSSON, E. *et al.* 2005. Aspects on radionuclide therapy in malignant pheochromocytomas. [abstract at ISP].
66. HOEGERLE, S. *et al.* 2002. Pheochromocytomas: detection with ^{18}F- DOPA whole body PET: initial results. Radiology **222:** 507–512.
67. WÄNGBERG, B. *et al.* 2005. Malignant pheochromocytoma in a population-based study. [abstract at ISP].

68. GREENE, L.A. *et al.* 1976. Establishment of a noradrenergic clonal line of rat adrenal pheochromocytoma cells which respond to nerve growth factor. Proc. Natl. Acad. Sci. USA **73:** 2424–2428.
69. POWERS, J.F. *et al.* 2000. Pheochromocytoma cell lines from heterozygous neurofibromatosis knockout mice. Cell. Tissue Res. **302:** 309–320.
70. POWERS, J.F. *et al.* 2002. High-level expression of receptor tyrosine kinase Ret and responsiveness to Ret-activating ligands in pheochromocytoma cell lines from neurofibromatosis knockout mice. Mol. Cell. Neurosci. **20:** 382–389.
71. POWERS, J.F. *et al.* 2005. Mouse pheochromocytoma cell line reveal transcriptional silencing of adrenergic phenotype by neurotrophin and cAMP. [abstract at ISP].
72. EVINGER, M.J. *et al.* 2005. Mouse pheochromocytoma cells modulate catecholamine gene expression through selective neuronal nicotinic receptor subtypes. [abstract at ISP].
73. OHTA, S. *et al.* 2005. A hepatic model of metastatic pheochromocytoma. [abstract at ISP].
74. SMITH-HICKS, C.L. *et al.* 2000. C-cell hyperplasia, pheochromocytoma and sympathoadrenal malformation in a mouse model of MEN 2B. EMBO J. **19:** 612–622.
75. YOU, M.J. *et al.* 2002. Genetic analysis of Pten and Ink4a/Arf interactions in the suppression of tumorigenesis in mice. Proc. Natl. Acad. Sci USA **99:** 1455–1460.
76. PODSYPANINA, K. *et al.* 2001. An inhibitor of mTOR reduces neoplasia and normalizes p70/S6 kinase activity in Pten ± mice. Proc. Natl. Acad. Sci. USA **98:** 10320–10325.
77. GROSS, D.J. *et al.* 2003. Treatment with halofuginone results in marked growth inhibition of a VHL pheochromocytoma *in vivo*. Clin. Cancer Res. **9:** 3788–3793.
78. EVERS, B.M. *et al.* 1991. Establishment and characterization of a human carcinoid in nude mice and effect of various agents on tumor growth. Gastroenterology **101:** 303–311.
79. KÖLBY, L. *et al.* 2001. A transplantable human carcinoid as model for somatostatin receptor-mediated and amine-transporter mediated radionuclide uptake. Am. J. Pathol. **158:** 745–755.
80. KÖLBY, L. *et al.* 2005. Successful receptor-mediated radiation therapy of xenografted human midgut tumour. Br. J. Cancer **14:** 1144–1151.
81. JOHANSON, V. *et al.* 2006. Antitumoral effects of CHS 828 on three different types of neuroendocrine tumors xenografted to nude mice. Neuroendocrinology **82:** 171–176.
82. SVENSSON, A. *et al.* 2002. CHS 828 inhibits neuroblastoma growth in mice alone and in combination with antiangiogenic drugs. Pediatr. Res. **51:** 607–611.
83. LEHNERT, T. 1998. Liver transplantation for metastatic neuroendocrine carcinoma. Transplantation **66:** 1307–1312.
84. FLORMAN, S. *et al.* 2004. Liver transplantation for neuroendocrine tumors. J. Gastrointest. Surg. **8:** 208–212.
85. OLAUSSON, M. *et al.* 2002. Indications and results of liver transplantation in patients with neuroendocrine tumours. World J. Surg. **26:** 998–1004.
86. AHLMAN, H. *et al.* 2004. Interventional treatment of the carcinoid syndrome. Neuroendocrinology **80:** 67–73.
87. KINNEY, M.A.O. *et al.* 2002. Perioperative management of pheochromocytoma. J. Cardiothor. Vasc. Anesth. **16:** 359–369.

88. TAKAHASHI, K. *et al.* 1999. Malignant pheochromocytoma with multiple hepatic metastases treated by chemotherapy and transcatheter arterial embolization. J. Int. Med. **38:** 349–354.
89. AVERBUCH, S.D. *et al.* 1988. Malignant pheochromocytoma: effective treatment with a combination of cyclophosphamide, vincristine and dacarbazine. Ann. Intern. Med. **109:** 267–273.
90. SCHLUMBERGER, M. *et al.* 1992. Malignant pheochromocytoma: clinical, biological, histologic and therapeutic data in a series of 20 patients with distant metastases. J. Endocrinol. Invest. **15:** 631–642.
91. NAKANE, M. *et al.* 2003. Successful treatment of malignant pheochromocytoma with combination chemotherapy containing anthracycline. Ann. Oncol. **14:** 1449–1451.
92. MALONEY, A. *et al.* 2002. HSP 90 as a new therapeutic target for cancer therapy: the story unfolds. Expert Opin. Biol. Therap. **2:** 3–24.
93. SAUSVILLE, E.A. *et al.* 2003. Clinical development of 17-allylamino, 17-demethoxygeldanamycin. Curr. Cancer Drug Targets **3:** 377–383.
94. PARK, J.W. *et al.* 2003. The heat shock protein 90-binding geldanamycin inhibits cancer cell proliferation, down-regulates oncoproteins, and inhibits EGF-induced invasion in thyroid cancer cell lines. J. Clin. Endocrinol. Metab. **88:** 3346–3353.
95. SISSON, J.C. *et al.* 1984. Radiopharmaceutical treatment of malignant pheochromocytoma. J. Nucl. Med. **25:** 197–206.
96. LOH, K.C. *et al.* 1997. The treatment of malignant pheochromocytoma with ^{131}I-MIBG: a comprehensive review of 116 reported patients. J. Endocrinol. Invest. **20:** 648–658.
97. SAFFORD, S.D. *et al.* 2003. Iodine-131 MIBG is an effective treatment for malignant pheochromocytoma and paraganglioma. Surgery **134:** 956–962.
98. ROSE, E. *et al.* 2003. High-dose ^{131}I-MIBG therapy for 12 patients with malignant pheochromocytoma. Cancer **98:** 239–248.
99. FITZGERALD, P.A. *et al.* 2005. Phase II study of high dose ^{131}I-MIBG therapy for patients with malignant pheochromocytoma/ paraganglioma. [abstract at ISP].
100. KWEKKEBOOM, D.J. *et al.* 2005. Overview of results of peptide receptor radionuclide therapy with 3 radiolabeled somatostatin analogs. J. Nucl. Med. **46:** 62–66.
101. FORRER, F. *et al.* 2005. Treatment with ^{177}Lu-DOTATOC of patients with relapse of neuroendocrine tumors after treatment with ^{90}Y-DOTATOC. J. Nucl. Med. **46:** 1310–1316.
102. SISSON, J.C. *et al.* 1999. Treatment of malignant pheochromocytomas with ^{131}I-MIBG and chemotherapy. Am. J. Clin. Oncol. **22:** 364–370.
103. CUNNINGHAM, S. *et al.* 2000. A gene therapy approach to enhance the targeted radiotherapy of neuroblastoma. Med. Ped. Oncol. **35:** 708–711.
104. ARMOUR, A. *et al.* 1997. The effect of cisplatin pretreatment on the accumulation of MIBG by neuroblastoma cells *in vitro*. Br. J. Cancer **75:** 470–476.
105. MONTALDO, P.G. *et al.* 1996. Increase of MIBG uptake and intracellular half-life during differentiation of human neuroblastoma cells. Int. J. Cancer **67:** 95–100.
106. PERERA, S. *et al.* 2005. Adenoviral sector transduction of bovine chromaffin cells: effects on cell survival and catecholamine uptake. [abstract at ISP].
107. STROCK, C.J. *et al.* 2006. Activity of irinotecan and the tyrosin kinase inhibitor CEP-751 in medullary thyroid carcinoma. J. Clin. Endocrinol. Metab. **91:** 79–84.
108. KARIN, M. *et al.* 2004. The IKK NF-kappa B system: a treasure trove for drug development. Nat. Rev. Drug Discov. **3:** 17–26.

Malignant Pheochromocytomas and Paragangliomas

A Phase II Study of Therapy with High-Dose ^{131}I-Metaiodobenzylguanidine (^{131}I-MIBG)

PAUL A. FITZGERALD,[a,d] ROBERT E. GOLDSBY,[b,d] JOHN P. HUBERTY,[c] DAVID C. PRICE,[c] RANDALL A. HAWKINS,[c] JANET J. VEATCH,[b] FILEMON DELA CRUZ,[b] THIERRY M. JAHAN,[a,d] CHARLES A. LINKER,[a,d] LLOYD DAMON,[a,d] AND KATHERINE K. MATTHAY[b,d]

[a]*Department of Medicine, University of California, San Francisco, California, USA*

[b]*Department of Pediatrics, University of California, San Francisco, California, USA*

[c]*Department of Nuclear Medicine, University of California, San Francisco, California, USA*

[d]*UCSF Comprehensive Cancer Center, University of California, San Francisco, California, USA*

ABSTRACT: Thirty patients with malignant pheochromocytoma (PHEO) or paraganglioma (PGL) were treated with high-dose ^{131}I-MIBG. Patients were 11–62 (mean 39) years old: 19 patients males and 11 females. Nineteen patients had PGL, three of which were multifocal. Six PGLs were nonsecretory. Eleven patients had PHEO. All 30 patients had prior surgery. Fourteen patients were refractory to prior radiation or chemotherapy before ^{131}I-MIBG. Peripheral blood stem cells (PBSCs) were collected and cryopreserved. ^{131}I-MIBG was synthesized on-site, by exchange-labeling ^{131}I with ^{127}I-MIBG in a solid-phase Cu^{2+}-catalyzed exchange reaction. ^{131}I-MIBG was infused over 2 h via a peripheral IV. Doses ranged from 557 mCi to 1185 mCi (7.4 mCi/kg to 18.75 mCi/kg). Median dose was 833 mCi (12.55 mCi/kg). Marrow hypoplasia commenced 3 weeks after ^{131}I-MIBG therapy. After the first ^{131}I-MIBG therapy, 19 patients required platelet transfusions; 19 received GCSF; 12 received epoeitin or RBCs. Four patients received a PBSC infusion. High-dose ^{131}I-MIBG resulted in the following overall tumor responses in 30 patients: 4 sustained complete remissions (CRs); 15 sustained partial remissions (PRs); 1 sustained stable disease (SD);

Address for correspondence: Dr. Paul A. Fitzgerald, Box 1222, University of California, San Francisco, San Francisco, CA 94143-1222. Voice: 415-665-1136; fax: 415-665-8500.
e-mail: paul.fitzgerald@ucsf.edu

Ann. N.Y. Acad. Sci. 1073: 465–490 (2006). © 2006 New York Academy of Sciences.
doi: 10.1196/annals.1353.050

5 progressive disease (PD); 5 initial PRs or SD but relapsed to PD. Twenty-three of the 30 patients remain alive; deaths were from PD (5), myelodysplasia (1), and unrelated cause (1). Overall predicted survival at 5 years is 75% (Kaplan Meier estimate). For patients with metastatic PHEO or PGL, who have good *I-MIBG uptake on diagnostic scanning, high-dose ^{131}I-MIBG therapy was effective in producing a sustained CR, PR, or SD in 67% of patients, with tolerable toxicity.

KEYWORDS: **malignant; pheochromocytoma; paraganglioma; MIBG**

Pheochromocytomas are particularly deadly and deceptive tumors. Their production of catecholamines can cause hypertensive crisis and sudden death. Patients experience symptoms that are often mistaken for other common conditions, leading to delayed diagnoses. Malignant pheochromocytomas are even more treacherous.

Adrenal pheochromocytoma (PHEO) and extra-adrenal pheochromocytoma (paraganglioma, PGL) are rare tumors and malignant PHEOs and PGLs are extremely rare. Because few clinicians are familiar with treating patients with metastatic PHEO/PGL, a variety of management strategies have been used, with such differences probably affecting survival. This paper provides some background regarding malignant PHEO and non–head-neck PGL. We present our Phase II protocol and results to date, using high-dose ^{131}I-MIBG for treating 30 patients with metastatic PHEO/PGL and we describe our approach to overall management of these patients at the University of California, San Francisco.

BACKGROUND

Incidence of Metastatic or Multicentric Pheochromocytomas and Paragangliomas

The yearly incidence of pheochromocytoma has been reported to be 9.5/million (Minnesota),[1] 2.1/million (Sweden),[2] 1.5/million (Australia),[3] and 1.9/million (Denmark).[4] About 40–45% of these cases were diagnosed at autopsy. Nearly 50% of tumors are discovered incidentally during CT scanning for other reasons.[5] At least 8% of incidentally discovered PHEO/PGL tumors have metastasized by the time of their detection.

Metastases are detected in 11% of patients with PHEOs at the time of diagnosis.[6] PGLs are more likely to have metastasized by the time the primary tumor is discovered. Genetic syndromes, predisposing to bilateral PHEOs or multiple PGLs, commonly present in childhood. In one series of childhood cases of PHEO/PGL, 5 of 16 (31%) children were reported to have regional or distant metastases at diagnosis.[7]

Approximately 20–30% of all patients with PHEO/PGL have been found to harbor germline mutations that gives them a predisposition to develop this tumor in multiple locations, either at the same time (synchronous) or at a later date (metachronous). Patients with genetic pheochromocytomas have been found to have metastatic or locally invasive PHEO at the time of diagnosis at the following rates: MEN 2A 4%; VHL 8%; NF-1 12%. Paragangliomas, including those associated with SDHB and SDHD mutations, are commonly malignant (30–50%). Genetic testing for SDHB mutations has proven useful, particularly for patients with metastatic PGL. When a germline defect is discovered, family members may then be screened for the mutation; carriers can have surveillance that may detect PGLs and PHEOs at earlier stages.

Metastases or additional primary tumors may not be apparent initially, because they are small or because scanning was not performed, was not sensitive for the metastases, or did not include the area of metastases in the scanning field. It is not surprising that metastases or second primary tumors are discovered in an additional 5–10% of patients, sometimes many years after resection of the primary tumor.[8]

Clinical and Histopathological Features of Malignant Pheochromocytomas and Paragangliomas

Lehnert *et al.*[9] reviewed the diagnostic criteria for malignant pheochromocytoma. Unlike the case in most other tumors, histopathology cannot accurately determine whether a given PHEO or PGL is benign or malignant. Even the presence of vascular invasion does not predict metastases.

Efforts have been made to predict the metastatic potential of adrenal PHEOs on the basis of cases histology. The Pheochromocytoma of the Adrenal Gland Scaled Score (PASS) considers multiple factors in assessing a given adrenal pheochromocytoma's likelihood of having metastasized. Pheochromocytomas were found to be more aggressive and likely to metastasize when they had a combination of the following characteristics: vascular or capsular invasion, increased mitotic rate, atypical mitoses, necrosis, high cellularity, hyperchromasia. tumor cell spindling, large nests of diffuse growth, cellular monotony, and profound nuclear pleomorphism.[10] Kimura *et al.*[11] recently reviewed the histology of 146 patients with PHEOs and PGLs, correlating surgical histologic with prognosis. However, no histologic scoring system is reliably accurate for determining the metastatic potential of these tumors, such that all PHEOs and PGLs must be considered potentially malignant.

Other methodologies have been used to determine a given tumor's potential for metastasis. MIB-1 nuclear proliferation marker staining was positive in 3 of 6 malignant pheochromocytomas, but in none of 45 apparently benign PHEOs in one series.[12] In another series of 92 pheochromocytomas, the 8 malignant PHEOs expressed markedly increased cyclooxygenase-2 (COX-2) activity, versus weak COX-2 activity in the 84 apparently benign PHEOs.[13]

Benign and malignant PHEOs and PGLs secrete most of the same secretory products. Serum levels of catecholamines, metanephrines, and chromogranin

A cannot reliably distinguish benign from malignant tumors prior to resection. However, when tumor markers are found to be persistently or recurrently high, months or years after the PHEO/PGL resection, metastases or new primary tumors must be suspected.

Neuron-specific enolase (NSE) is a neuroendocrine glycolytic enzyme. Serum levels of NSE have been reported to be normal in patients with benign PHEO and elevated in about half of the patients with malignant PHEO.[14] However, it is possible that NSE levels are related to tumor burden, rather than malignancy *per se*; therefore, the clinical utility of NSE levels remains unproven.

At this point, only the presence of detectable metastases defines a PHEO or PGL as being malignant. However, even this feature may be misleading, because metastases may not be detected at the time of the primary tumor resection for reasons mentioned previously. Also, patients with familial germline mutations can develop new PGLs or PGLs at a later date in different locations, which may be mistaken for metastases or which may themselves metastasize. Additionally, peritoneal seeding of tumor cells at the time of surgery (pheochromocytomatosis) can cause multiple recurrences that may be mistaken for metastases.

DETECTION OF PHEO/PGL METASTASES

Urine and Blood Tumor Markers

Most patients with recurrent or metastatic PHEO/PGL have elevations in plasma or urinary normetanephrine, but some metastases from adrenal pheochromocytomas secrete mostly epinephrine and metanephrine. Plasma fractionated free metanephrines is probably the most sensitive test for detecting recurrent or metastatic PHEO/PGL, but "false positives" occur frequently. Some patients with "nonsecretory" metastases have normal plasma and urine fractionated metanephrines. Serum chromogranin A (CgA) is usually elevated in patients with both secretory and "nonsecretory" PHEO/PGL. Serum CgA is usually elevated in patients with clinically significant metastases. It is an excellent tumor marker for most patients, reflecting tumor burden.[15] Fractionated urine and plasma metanephrines and serum CgA usually normalize by two weeks after a successful resection of a PHEO/PGL. However, patients with normal postoperative tests may still harbor small or nonsecretory metastases.

Detection of Metastases—Scanning

^{a}I-MIBG and ^{111}In-DTPA-Octreotide Scanning

Benzylguanidine was first developed as a guanethidine derivative for potential use as an adrenergic-blocking antihypertensive agent.[16] ^{131}I-metaiodobenzylguanidine (^{131}I-MIBG) was developed at the University of

Michigan for detecting adrenal pheochromocytomas.[17–19] The usefulness of ^{131}I-MIBG scintigraphy was confirmed at the University of California, San Francisco.[20] Most PHEO/PGL metastases can be detected on whole-body scintigraphy with MIBG, tagged with a radioisotope of iodine.[a] ^{123}I-MIBG scanning with single-photon emission computed tomography (SPECT) is more sensitive than ^{131}I-MIBG planar imaging, particularly for PGLs and metastases.[21] Despite the value of I-MIBG in diagnostic scanning for PHEO/PGL, only about two-thirds of metastases are avid for MIBG. Patients with metastases that are avid for *I-MIBG often harbor concurrent metastases or second primaries that are not avid for *I-MIBG and may remain undetected even on post-therapy whole-body scanning after high-dose ^{131}I-MIBG therapy.

There are other problems with *I-MIBG scanning. Patients may have significant bowel activity that may be mistaken for an abdominal paraganglioma or metastasis. Delayed imaging after a laxative is sometimes required in these patients. Because MIBG is excreted in the urine, bladder paragangliomas may not be visualized or may be mistakenly thought to have *I-MIBG uptake. ^{123}I-MIBG SPECT imaging of the bladder during bladder irrigation is sometimes required to elucidate this situation. Another nuclear imaging technique used to locate metastases is ^{111}In-DTPA-octreotide, which is reported to have a sensitivity of only 44%, but often detects metastases that are not visualized with *I-MIBG.

PET Scanning

Positron emission tomography (PET) is the most sensitive scanning technique for imaging PHEO/PGL metastases. PET scanning dramatically displays metastatic tumor burden and the response to therapy.[22]

PET scanning with ^{18}F-deoxyglucose (^{18}FDG) works on account of the fact that deoxyglucose is absorbed into cells by a glucose transporter and accumulates in the cells because it cannot enter glycolytic pathways. An estimated 90% of PHEO and PGL metastases are avid for ^{18}FDG. However, ^{18}FDG PET is nonspecific and may detect other tumors and has increased uptake in areas of increased glucose absorption, such as the brain, inflammation, muscle activity, or bone marrow after G-CSF stimulation.

^{18}F-dopamine PET scanning is both highly sensitive and specific for primary PHEO/PGL and metastases. Although both ^{18}F-dopamine and *I-MIBG are transported into cells by an amine uptake-1 mechanism, ^{18}F-dopamine is more actively transported into neurosecretory vesicles, where it is stored, whereas *I-MIBG may leave the cell. Therefore, ^{18}F-dopamine PET scanning is more sensitive than even ^{123}I-MIBG SPECT scanning. ^{18}F-dopamine PET scanning is more selective than ^{18}FDG-PET for PHEO/PGL metastases, as well as being about 90% sensitive. However, ^{18}FDG PET scanning may underestimate the

[a]I = either ^{123}I or ^{131}I

number of metastases in patients with advanced metastases and a high tumor burden. Also, false-positives may occur with ^{18}FDG PET, such as gallbladder visualization.[23]

Disadvantages of PET scanning include its high cost and radiation exposure. Both ^{18}FDG and ^{18}F-dopamine PET scanning can be combined with CT scanning to produce extraordinarily accurate anatomic imaging. Combined PET/CT fusion imaging is currently the state-of-the-art for accurately detecting and quantifying PHEO/PGL metastases.

CT Scanning

CT scanning without contrast is helpful in determining the density of adrenal nodules, which is measured in Hounsefeld Units (HUs). Adrenal nodules with densities above 10–25 HUs ordinarily are seen with PHEOs, excluding adrenal adenomas and lipomas, but high HU density is seen with other tumors. A mass with a low density of <10 HU on noncontrast CT is not likely a PHEO/PGL. For CT scanning with intravenous contrast enhancement, nonionic contrast is preferred, because it is unlikely to induce hypertensive crisis.[24]

MRI Scanning

MRI scanning can be helpful, particularly for imaging bone and hepatic metastases, given most PHEO/PGLs display increased signal intensity on T_2-weighted imaging. MRI is also preferred for children and pregnant women, due to lack of radiation exposure.[25]

These different scanning techniques can be considered complementary to each other, with no single imaging modality being 100% sensitive and specific for metastatic PHEO or PGL.

Differential Diagnoses for Metastatic PHEO and PGL

The differential diagnosis for apparent PHEO/PGL metastases includes benign paragangliomas, multicentric paragangliomas, second pheochromocytomas, intraperitoneal seeding (pheochromocytomatosis), false-positive scanning, and other malignancies. Patients with VHL germline mutations may have a concurrent renal cell carcinoma and hemangioblastomas. Patients with MEN-2 may have concurrent medullary thyroid carcinoma. Patients with NF-1 usually have concurrent neurofibromas and may develop gliomas and malignant peripheral nerve sheath tumors (MPNSTs, neurofibromosarcoma). Any suspicious mass lesion that is not demonstrated on *I-MIBG or ^{18}F-dopamine PET scanning should be considered for a CT-guided fine-needle aspiration biopsy for definitive diagnosis.

Historical Prognosis for Patients with Benign and Malignant PHEOs and PGLs

Patients with benign phochromocytomas have an increased mortality rate. Although the perioperative mortality rate for patients undergoing unilateral benign adrenal PHEO resection is now only about 3% with optimal medical preparation, anesthesia, surgical, and postoperative care, these patients experience a long-term mortality rate that is higher than that of age-matched controls. A Swedish series of 121 patients with pheochomocytoma reported no peri-operative mortality, but 50% of patients remained hypertensive postoperatively. Of the 121 patients, 42 died during a period averaging 15 years, versus an expected 23.6 deaths in an age-matched general population, yielding a 78% increase in mortality (RR = 1.78). Of the 42 patients who died, 20 deaths were due to cardiovascular disease, 6 from associated neuroectodermal tumors, 5 from other malignancies, 7 from unrelated causes, and 4 from malignant pheochromocytoma.[26]

Patients with metastatic PHEO/PGL, treated with conventional radiation and chemotherapy, have been reported to have a mean 5-year survival rate of about 44%. However, survival can vary from days to decades. The prognosis is worse for those patients whose metastatic disease is discovered at a late stage and those with diffuse pulmonary metastases. Malignant PHEO/PGLs vary tremendously in their aggressiveness, secretory capacity, and sites of metastases. These variables affect each patient's prognosis.

Treatment—Medical Therapy

Bravo has reviewed antihypertensive therapy for patients with pheochromocytoma.[27] About 50% of patients with PHEO/PGL metastases have persistent hypertension after resection of the primary tumor. Hypertensive patients must be involved with home blood pressure monitoring with an accurate automatic sphygmomanometer (arm cuff). Blood pressures should ideally be determined at home once or twice daily and immediately in the event of acute symptoms of headache, perspiration, palpitations, or other unique symptoms that the patient experiences with hypertensive episodes. While phenoxybenzamine is effective and tolerable for short periods preoperatively, most patients experience side effects from phenoxybenzamine, such as fatigue and nasal congestion, making the drug less suitable for chronic therapy. Phenoxybenzamine accumulates in the fetus more than it does the mother, with a fetal:maternal concentration ration of 1.6:1 and has been associated with neonatal hypotension in the newborn.[28]

Calcium channel blockers are effective and usually tolerated better than alpha blockade. They may be used alone or in combination with tolerated doses of alpha-blockers or other antihypertensives. Calcium channel blockers were used successfully as the sole peri-operative management in a French study involving 105 surgeries for pheochromocytomas and paragangliomas. Both nicardipine and nifedipine have been used extensively.[29,30] Blake *et al.*[31] reported the results of using nifedipine to treat five patients with metastatic PHEOs. In one patient, there was a remarkable and reproducible doubling of the tumor-absorbed dose of ^{131}I-MIBG due to prolonged tumoral retention of the isotope; nifedipine also caused this patient's norepinephrine excretion to decline by two-thirds.

Nifedipine is also useful for treating acute hypertensive events in the hospital (during procedures or ^{131}I-MIBG infusion therapy) or at home. Hypertensive patients with metastatic or unresectable secretory PHEO/PGLs are given a supply of nifedipine-10-mg capsules; if the patient measures a blood pressure that exceeds 170 mm Hg, and immediately verifies it, he is instructed to chew one pierced capsule and monitor his blood pressure carefully.

Other antihypertensive medications may be effective as add-on therapy for hypertensive patients with malignant pheochromocytoma or paraganglioma. Elevated catecholamine levels stimulate renin secretion, which increases angiotensin II production and aggravates hypertension. Adding an angiotensin receptor blocker (ARB) or angiotensin-converting enzyme (ACE) inhibitor is often an effective measure. Besides the usual antihypertensive measures, intravenous magnesium sulfate has proven effective in children and pregnant women.[32]

Beta-blocker therapy is given to patients with sustained tachycardia or intermittent tachyarrhythmias, after initiation of antihypertensive therapy. Sustained-action cardio-selective beta-blockers are preferred, such as metoprolol XL. Labetalol is avoided, since it causes misleading elevations in urinary catecholamine determinations in some assays. Labetalol also interferes with norepinephrine uptake-1, and patients taking labetalol should discontinue the drug for at least one 4–7 days before ^{18}F-dopamine PET, *I-MIBG scintigraphy or ^{131}I-MIBG therapy.[33]

Metyrosine partially inhibits tyrosine kinase and tumoral catecholamine secretion; metyrosine does not inhibit norepinephrine uptake-1 and ^{131}I-MIBG scanning and therapy can be used in patients being treated with metyrosine. However, metyrosine does not inhibit tumor growth and its side effects are considerable, exerting an adverse impact on the patient's well-being such that metyrosine therapy is not generally advisable.[34]

Patients with functioning malignant PHEO/PGLs are advised to observe certain precations. Patients are advised to avoid activities that might put physical pressure on large soft tissue tumors, precipitating catecholamine release, and hypertensive crisis. Patients must be counseled to avoid decongestants, cocaine, diet pills, MAO inhibitors, and other drugs that can provoke a hypertensive crisis. Epinephrine, injected by dentists and emergency physicians to help retain local anesthesia, may also precipitate symptoms in patients with secretory metastases. Intravenous ionic contrast for CT scanning may precipitate hypertensive crisis in patients with secretory tumors; however, nonionic intravenous contrast appears to be relatively safe.[35]

Treatment—Surgery

For patients having what appears to be an isolated adrenal pheochromocytoma, a total adrenalectomy is more likely to prevent recurrence than a selective adrenal-sparing surgical procedure,[36] which is sometimes attempted for patients with bilateral pheochromocytomas or familial disease. For patients who are found to have metastases at the time of diagnosis, it is usually best to resect the primary tumor as well as large metastases. Laparoscopic adrenalectomy has become the procedure of choice for pheochromocytomas up to 5 to 6 cm in diameter.[37,38] Large cranial, abdominal, and pulmonary metastases have been successfully resected. The surgical reduction of tumor burden can reduce symptoms and is presumed to prolong survival. These tumors can be indolent and debulking improves local symptoms, catecholamine levels and hypertension. Lower plasma norepinephrine levels may possibly improve *I-MIBG uptake-1, especially when postoperative plasma norepinephrine levels are below 500 ng/mL.[39]

Some tumors, particularly retroperitoneal paragangliomas in the abdomen or pelvis, can become massive, encasing major blood vessels and other organs. Heroic surgery may require vascular grafts, ureter stenting, nephrectomy, and other procedures. Surgical resection of massive paragangliomas can be extremely difficult and the patients must be rendered nomotensive preoperatively. Perioperative intensive monitoring and treatment by an experienced anesthesiologist and surgical team are mandatory. Even so, surgical complications are common. Postoperative pulmonary embolism from pelvic veins is particularly common in patients with massive abdominal or pelvic tumors. Therefore, women should discontinue oral contraceptives 2 months preoperatively and all such patients should be treated with low-molecular-weight heparin postoperatively.

Large invasive pheochromocytomas and paragangliomas are extremely vascular, causing serious problems with hemostasis and making tumor resection difficult and sometimes impossible. Preoperative arterial embolization has proven feasible for some secretory tumors. However, some large tumors cannot be resected, particularly massive retroperitoneal paragangliomas that have encased major blood vessels and involve other organs. Many patients have metastases that are so massive or numerous that surgical debulking is impossible. In these cases, non-surgical approaches to treatment are of the first order.

Treatment—Chemotherapy

The most commonly used chemotherapy regimen for patients with metastatic PGL or PHEO, reported by Averbuch *et al.*[40] uses a combination of cyclophosphamide, vincristine, and dacarbazine/DTIC (CVD). Cyclophosphamide 750 mg/m^2 and vincristine 1.4 mg/m^2 are given on day 1, and dacarbazine 600 mg/m^2 is given on days 1 and 2. The cycle is repeated every 21 days. This chemotherapy regimen, given every 21 days, was reported to cause complete or partial remissions in 7 of 12 patients (57%).

In a review of chemotherapy for patients with metastatic paraganglioma, 5 of 11 achieved a partial remission after various regimens, including: cyclophosphamide, doxorubicin, and DTIC/dacarbazine (CyADIC; cyclophosphamide, vincristine, doxorubicin, and DTIC/dacarbazine (CyVADIC); doxorubicin and dacarbazine (ADIC).[41]

Despite some success with chemotherapy for patients with malignant pheochromocytoma, continuous cycles must be given on a long-term basis, because tumors usually recur during necessary or patient-requested "breaks" in chemotherapy. Chronic chemotherapy has an adverse impact on quality-of-life, because most patients experience recurrent bouts of malaise, nausea, or other adverse reactions after each cycle. Cyclophosphamide can cause sterility, myelosuppression, nausea, alopecia, hemorrhagic cystitis, cardiomyopathy, stomatitis, darkened skin and nails, and an increased risk for second malignancies. Vincristine neurotoxicity can lead to severe peripheral neuropathy with pain, cranial nerve palsies, severe muscle weakness, intestinal ileus and, rarely, ataxia. Dacarbazine can cause myelosuppression, nausea, myalgias, fever, diarrhea, photosensitivity, hepatic and renal dysfunction, and occasional anaphylaxis. Doxorubicin can cause cardiomyopathy and ventricular arrhythmias, myelosuppression, alopecia, onycholysis, nausea, severe stomatitis, esophagitis, and necrotizing enterocolitis. Side effects related to chemotherapy can reduce compliance with repeated cycles of therapy. Nevertheless, many patients do exhibit partial responses to chronic chemotherapy and some patients appear to tolerate it reasonably well.[42]

Zoledronic acid is a third-generation bisphosphonate. Patients with bone metastases are empirically treated with zoledronic acid (Zometa), 4 mg infused intravenously over 20 min. The frequency of the zoledronic acid infusions has varied, being given every 1 to 12 months, depending upon the extent and aggressiveness of the bone metastases and the patient's tolerance for the treatment. Zoledronic acid inhibits osteoclastic bone resorption and has proven useful for other malignancies that metastasize to bone.[43] Zoledronic acid has been reported to provide effective treatment for bone metastases from a variety of tumors, such as breast cancer, prostate cancer, renal cell carcinoma, multiple myeloma, chronic myeloid leukemia, and Ewing's sarcoma. However, there are no data for the effectiveness of zoledronic acid for osseous metastases from pheochromocytoma. Zoledronic acid therapy is generally well tolerated, with the exception of transient flu-like symptoms (that may be severe) within a week following the infusion; hypocalcemia and thrombotic thrombocytopenic purpura, and jaw osteonecrosis occur rarely.

Treatment—Potential Anti-VEGF/VEGFR and Adjuvant Therapies

Vascular endothelial growth factors (VEGFs) are pro-angiogenesis molecules. VEGFs bind to vascular VEGF receptors (VEGFRs), causing receptor dimerization and activation of receptor tyrosine kinase that induces vascular proliferation, a necessary process for tumorigenesis and metastasis. VEGFs are over-expressed in about 70% PGLs[44] and are also over-expressed in PHEOs.[45–47] Mutations in the gene encoding mitochondrial succinate dehydrogenase subunit B (SDHB) in PGLs activate cellular hypoxia pathways that stimulate the production of VEGFs.[48] Middeke *et al.*[49] have demonstrated the importance of VEGF for PHEO angiogenesis *in vitro*.

Potential anti-VEGF drug therapies include monoclonal antibodies against VEGF. Zielke, *et al.*[50] demonstrated that antibodies to VEGF inhibited PHEO tumor growth, both *in vitro,* and *in vivo.* A VEGF monoclonal antibody, bevacizumab, has been approved by the FDA as a first-line treatment for colorectal cancer.[51]

New cancer therapies are targeting VEGF receptors (VEGFRs). Inhibitors of VEGFR-2 may preferentially target tumor vasculature.[52] The initial clinical trials of VEGFR-2 inhibitors were disappointing. However, the results from ongoing clinical trials of second-generation oral VEGFR-2 inhibitors (e.g., ZD6474), for other solid tumors, have been more encouraging.[53,54]

Cyclooxygenase-2 is over-expressed in PHEO/PGL[13] and Cox-2 inhibitors might be helpful in reversing resistance to chemotherapy.[55] Nifedipine may improve the therapeutic uptake of ^{131}I-MIBG into PHEO/PGL metastases in certain patients.[31] Starikova *et al.*[56] demonstrated that nifedipine reduced the mitotic rate and proliferation of PC-12 cells *in vitro.*

Clinical trials of such potential anti-VEGF/VEGFR and adjuvant therapies are required for patients with metastatic PHEO/PGL.

Treatment—Radiation Therapy

External beam radiation therapy completely abolishes tumoral avidity for MIBG and renders subsequent *I-MIBG scanning insensitive and makes ^{131}I-MIBG ineffective therapy for irradiated metastases. Therefore, if ^{131}I-MIBG therapy is planned, radiation should not be given to metastases displaying *I-MIBG avidity prior to ^{131}I-MIBG therapy. External beam radiation therapy may be given subsequently to osseous metastases, if ^{131}I-MIBG therapy is ineffective. Radiation therapy has proven moderately efficacious for relieving pain and inhibiting the growth of bone metastases.[57] Radiation therapy to large cranial bone metastases can produce neurologic improvement. Large abdominal or pelvic paragangliomas generally should not be irradiated, because such radiation is not particularly effective, causes gastrointestinal disturbance, and makes later surgeries relatively contraindicated due to the risk of wound dehiscence, abscesses, and fistulas. Certain small recurrent tumors may be amenable for treatment with CyberKnife stereotactic radiosurgery. It may be useful for localized spinal metastases and can be used for recurrent growth of bone metastases in a previously irradiated field. Cyberknife also carries the advantage to the patient of being given in a single day, rather than over the 5 weeks typically required for conventional external beam radiation therapy.[58]

^{131}I-MIBG Therapy–History

Metaiodobenzylguanidine bears a structural resemblance to norepinephrine (FIG. 1). From pharmacologic studies, benzylguanidine was found to participate in both uptake pathways by adrenal medullary cells, where it is subsequently stored in neurosecretory granules. Because of the effectiveness of ^{131}I for the treatment of thyroid cancer, higher doses of ^{131}I-MIBG for treatment of patients with malignant pheochromocytoma was first used at the University of Michigan and reported in 1984.[59] Two of five patients achieved partial remissions after total doses of 373-484 mCi ^{131}I-MIBG, fractionated as 3–4 separate treatments. Since then, many other patients with malignant PHEO/PGL have been treated with ^{131}I-MIBG elsewhere.[60–66]

Many nonfunctioning PHEO and PGL metastases continue to exhibit norepinephrine uptake-1, such that treatment with ^{131}I-MIBG can be effective for patients with nonfunctioning tumors, as long as scanning demonstrates that the tumors are avid for MIBG. Following therapy with ^{131}I-MIBG, once background radiation has dissipated, a post-treatment whole-body scan can be obtained that indicates the successfulness of the treatment and may locate the presence of metastases that were not appreciated on diagnostic *I-MIBG scanning.

Competitive inhibition of tumoral uptake of ^{131}I-MIBG may be caused by the large amount of “cold” ^{127}I-MIBG that is also infused, a product of the current

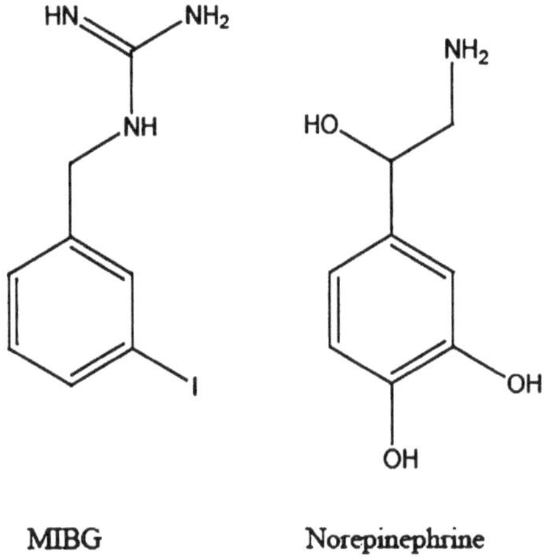

FIGURE 1. Molecular diagrams of metaiodobenzylguanidine and norepinephrine.

exchange labeling method of synthesizing ^{131}I-MIBG. The "no-carrier-added" method of synthesizing ^{131}I-MIBG produces less cold ^{127}I-MIBG. Mairs *et al.*[67] demonstrated that human neuroblastoma xenografts in nude mice had better uptake of no-carrier-added ^{131}I-MIBG than conventional exchange-labeled ^{131}I-MIBG; however, uptake was also increased in the adrenal and heart. No-carrier-added ^{131}I-MIBG is being developed commercially and clinical trials are under way to determine whether it is superior to exchange-labeled ^{131}I-MIBG for treating patients with malignant PHEO/PGL.

Peripheral Blood Stem Cell (PBSC) Leukapheresis and Cryopreservation

PBSC leukapheresis is now widely available and is used for patients with other malignancies before they receive myeloablative chemotherapy. Marrow stimulation with granulocyte colony-stimulating factor (GCSF) allows successful PBSC harvesting in most patients, usually after 1–2 leukapheresis sessions. The reinfusion of the patient's own cryopreserved PBSCs has been extremely effective and engraftment has been successful in over 95% of cases. In 1998, Matthay *et al.*[68] at the University of California, San Francisco, reported a Phase I dose escalation of ^{131}I-MIBG with autologous bone marrow support in refractory neuroblastoma. Sung *et al.*[69] reported the use of autologous stem cell transplantation after high-dose chemotherapy in patients with high-risk neuroblastoma.

Patients with extensive PHEO/PGL bone metastases can have bone marrow involvement with tumor, such that tumor cells could be inadvertantly harvested along with the PBSCs during the leukopheresis procedure. Such marrow involvement is a relative contraindication to PBSC leukapheresis. Advances in purging the harvested PBSCs of tumor cells have been reported.[70]

High-Dose ^{131}I-MIBG Therapy—The UCSF Experience

A Phase I-II dose-escalation protocol for ^{131}I-MIBG therapy for patients with malignant pheochromocytoma and related tumors was begun in 1991 at the University of California, San Francisco (UCSF). A concurrent UCSF Phase I pediatric oncology protocol investigated the use of ^{131}I-MIBG therapy for children with malignant neuroblastoma. In 1997, on the basis of the Phase I toxicity dose escalation studies, the protocol was revised and formally entered Phase II.

In 2003, Rose *et al.*[71] described the experience with the first 12 patients with metastatic pheochromocytoma treated with high-dose ^{131}I-MIBG therapy at the University of California, San Francisco. Of these 12 patients, 5 had received prior external beam radiation and/or chemotherapy. Their median single treatment dose was 800 mCi (37 GBq) or 11.5 mCi/kg (ranges,

386–866 mCi or 6.6–18.3 mCi/kg). Their median cumulative dose was 1015 mCi (range, 386–1690 mCi). Three of the twelve patients had complete responses; two had soft-tissue and skeletal metastases and one had intraperitoneal seeding of tumor, with recurrent disease. Seven patients had a sustained partial response (PR), two had an initial PR with progressive disease (PD) and death at 13 and 11 months, respectively. Two patients did not respond and died with PD. Grade 3 thrombocytopenia followed 79% (15 of 19) of ^{131}I-MIBG treatments. Grade 3 and 4 neutropenia followed 53% and 19% of treatments, respectively.

We have now treated 32 patients for our ongoing Phase II trial. Of these patients, we have post-therapy data to evaluate the responses of 30 patients. All patients had surgery for their primary tumor and had unresectable metastases. These 30 patients met strict eligibility criteria (TABLE 1).

Of these 30 patients, there were 19 males and 11 females. Ages ranged from 10 to 62 years (mean 39 years; seven patients were under age 18 years). Nineteen patients had paragangliomas: 10 juxta-renal, 8 periaortic/aortic bifurcation, 2 pelvis, 1 atrium/mediastinum, 1 lung apex/periverterbal. Four of seven patients with paragangliomas, who have had genetic testing, have been found to harbor germline mutations in the gene encoding succinate dehydrogenase subunit B (SDHB). Eleven patients had pheochromocytomas: seven of the left adrenal, four of the right adrenal. Distant metastases were present in 27 of the 30 patients (90%) (TABLE 2).

High-dose ^{131}I-MIBG resulted in the following overall tumor responses in these 30 patients: 4 sustained complete remissions (CR); 15 sustained partial remissions (PR); 1 sustained stable disease (SD); 5 had initial PR or SD, but relapsed to progressive disease (PD); 5 had PD. Patient follow-up has ranged from 7 to 154 months. The criteria for remission are listed in TABLE 3. Patients with sustained remission were noted to have a gradual response to high-dose ^{131}I-MIBG, with improvements in tumor markers and scans continuing for up to 24 months in some patients (FIG. 2).

Of the 30 treated patients, 23 remain alive. Dating from the time of initial ^{131}I-MIBG therapy, overall survival at 5 years has been 75% by Kaplan-Meier estimate (FIG. 3). Of note, there was a considerable delay between the diagnosis of the primary tumor and the time of ^{131}I-MIBG therapy: median, 68 months; mean, 45 months; range, 2 to 310 months.

Eight patients have died. One patient died from a non-tumor-related cause after a sustained PR. Another patient died after a PR lasting 5 years, at which time she developed PD and myelodysplastic syndrome with monosomy 7, a known potential risk for ^{131}I-MIBG therapy.[72–74] This patient died suddenly and unexpectedly during myeloablative therapy and allogenic marrow transplant. Six of the 30 patients have died from aggressive progressive disease (PD). Five of these six patients had abdominal or pelvic paragangliomas as their primary tumor.

TABLE 1. Eligibility criteria for high-dose ^{131}I-MIBG therapy for patients with metastatic pheochromocytoma or paraganglioma—UCSF Phase II Protocol

Inclusion criteria

- Histological documentation of pheochromocytoma or paraganglioma.
- Tumor not amenable to surgical excision.
- Tumor with *I-MIBG avidity that is at least twice background.
- >3 weeks since chemotherapy.
- >2 weeks since major surgery.
- >4 weeks since completion of prior radiation therapy; no radiation therapy for 4 months after ^{131}I-MIBG, except for progressive disease.
- No treatment with an investigational agent concurrently or within 30 days before therapy.
- Patients who have received previous chemotherapy or radiation therapy must have evidence of persistent disease on *I-MIBG scan and elevated tumor markers or measurable lesions by CT/MRI before receiving high-dose ^{131}I-MIBG.
- ≥ 4 years of age.
- Agreement to use birth control for at least 2 months before (women) and for at least 6 months after (men and women) ^{131}I-MIBG therapy.
- Required initial laboratory data (minimum levels):
  - Neutrophil count $\geq 1{,}000/\mu L$
  - Platelet count $\geq 80{,}000/\mu L$
  - AST (SGOT) $\leq 2.5 \times$ ULN
  - Total bilirubin $\leq 2.5 \times$ ULN
  - Creatinine $\leq 2 \times$ ULN

Measurable tumor

- Lesions that can be accurately measured in at least one dimension (longest diameter to be recorded) as >10 mm as measured with CT/MRI scanning, *OR*
- Lesions <10 mm diameter or bone lesions in the presence of demonstrable uptake of *I-MIBG on diagnostic scanning, plus elevated levels of a tumor marker specific for pheochromocytomas: urine catecholamines or metanephrines or serum CgA.

Exclusion criteria

- Estimated life expectancy <12 weeks.
- Karnofsky performance status $<60\%$.
- Psychiatric illness that precludes informed consent.
- Pregnancy or nursing.
- Brain lesions that are parenchymal and MIBG-avid.
- Uncontrolled intercurrent illness, including but not limited to: ongoing active infections, symptomatic congestive heart failure, unstable angina pectoris, cardiac arrhythmia, or psychiatric illness/social situations that would limit compliance with study requirements.
- Second Malignancies:
  - Patients with a "currently active" second malignancy, other than non-melanoma skin cancers, are not eligible.
  - Patients are not considered to have a "currently active" second malignancy if they have been cancer-free for ≥ 5 years.

TABLE 2. Sites of metastases in 30 patients with metastatic paraganglioma or pheochromocytoma—UCSF Phase II Protocol

- Distant metastases: 27/30 = 90%
  - Bone: 23/30 = 77%
  - Liver: 12/30 = 40%
  - Local nodes (in addition to distant metastases): 11/30 = 37%
  - Distant nodes: 6/30 = 20%
  - Lungs: 4/30 = 13%
  - Muscle: 3/30 = 10%
  - Pituitary: 1/30 = 3%
- Local metastases only: 3/30 = 10%
  - Local nodes: 2/30 = 6%
  - Peritoneal seeding: 1/30 = 3%

UCSF Protocol for ^{131}I-MIBG Therapy

Peripheral Blood Stem Cell (PBSC) Leukapheresis and Cryopreservation

Patients who are candidates for high-dose ^{131}I-MIBG have a PBSC leukapheresis prior to therapy. PBSC leukapheresis is now widely available and is used for patients with other malignancies before they receive myeloablative chemotherapy. Marrow stimulation with granulocyte colony-stimulating factor (GCSF) allows successful PBSC collection in most patients, usually after 1–2 leukapheresis sessions. Cyclophosphamide rebound has not been required for successful PBSC harvesting in patients with metastatic PHEO and PGL. The reinfusion of the patient's own cryopreserved PBSCs has been extremely effective with successful engraftment in over 95% of cases.

Patients with extensive PHEO/PGL bone metastases may have bone marrow involvement with tumor, creating a risk that tumor cells could be inadvertently harvested along with the PBSCs during the leukapheresis procedure. Therefore, patients with significant bone metastases have a bone marrow biopsy prior to PBSC harvest to help determine whether the marrow is involved

TABLE 3. Definitions of tumor responses—UCSF Phase II Protocol

Complete response (CR): Sustained disappearance of all lesions visible on *I-MIBG scan and CT/MRI scan and normal catecholamines, metanephrines, and CgA.

Partial response (PR): Sustained decrease in metastases visible on *I-MIBG scan, and ≥30% reduction in the sum of the longest diameter of soft-tissue metastases, and ≥ 50% decrease in initially-elevated catecholamines, metanephrine, and CgA.

Stable disease (SD): No significant change in *I-MIBG scan, no change in CT/MRI of metastases, no change in tumor markers to qualify for PR or PD.

Progressive disease (PD): New metastases on *I-MIBG scan, or increase of ≥20% increase in maximum diameter of metastases or new metastases on CT/MRI scan, or > 20% increase in initially-elevated catecholamines, metanephrines, or serum CgA levels.

PR/SD → PD: Initial PR or SD relapsing to PD.

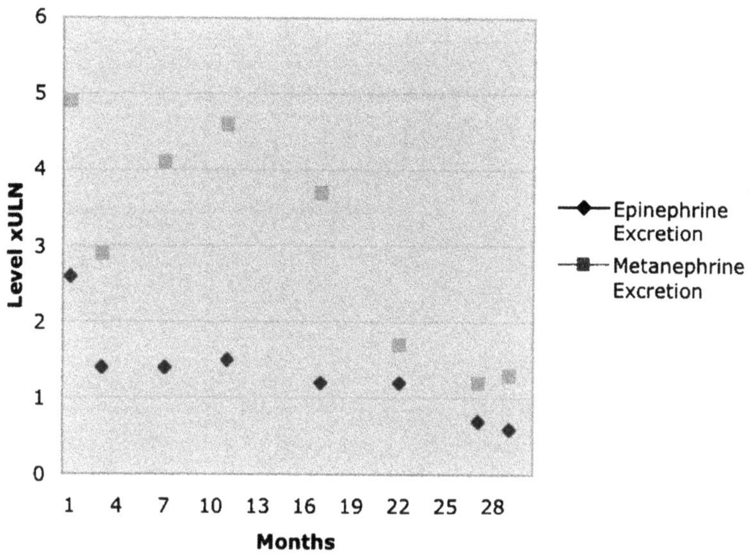

FIGURE 2. Plot of urinary epinephrine and metanephrine excretion in a patient with metastatic adrenal pheochromocytoma, months after a single intravenous dose of ^{131}I-MIBG: 808 mCi (13 mCi/kg). ULN: upper limit of normal.

with tumor. Such marrow involvement is a relative contraindication to PBSC leukapheresis, although exceptions can be made if marrow involvement is limited.

Patient Evaluation and Preparation for High-Dose ^{131}I-MIBG Therapy

Prospective subjects for this Phase II clinical trial were carefully evaluated in preparation for ^{131}I-MIBG therapy, as detailed in TABLE 1. Patients with hypertension are treated with antihypertensive medications as described above. Menstruating women received one intramuscular injection of sustained-release medroxyprogesterone acetate (Depo-Provera) 150 mg before high-dose ^{131}I-MIBG therapies in order to prevent menorrhagia during thrombocytopenia. Patients continue to receive their usual analgesics and other medications. However, all medications known to interfere with MIBG uptake are prohibited, particularly labetalol, tricyclics, phenothiazines, and decongestants.

^{131}I-MIBG Formulation

UCSF Nuclear Medicine obtains ^{131}I from commercial sources as a reactor product. Although a fission ^{131}I product is now available, most exchange labelings of ^{127}I-MIBG for therapy at UCSF have been with MDS Nordion's ^{131}I reactor product. On the morning of therapy, the UCSF nuclear pharmacist (J.P.H.) synthesizes the ^{131}I-MIBG by exchange-labeling 15 mCi (reactor)

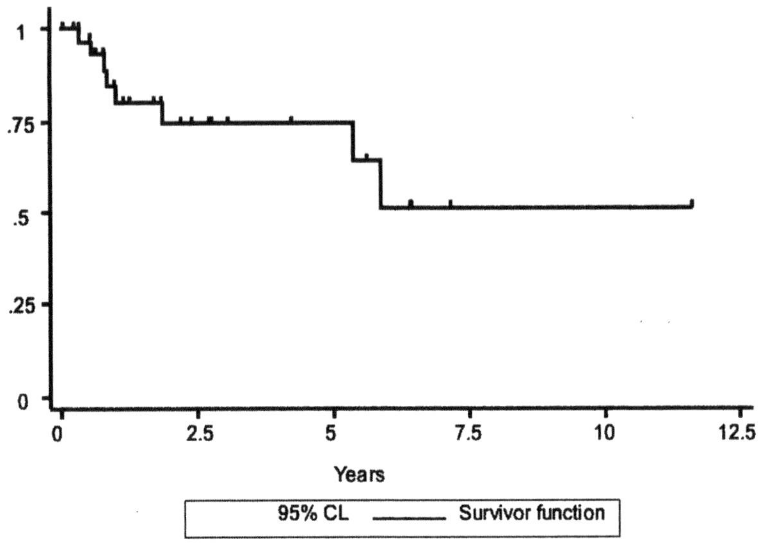

FIGURE 3. Standard Kaplan–Meier overall survival estimate with 95% confidence limits (CL) for 30 patients with metastatic paraganglioma or pheochromocytoma, from the time of ^{131}I-MIBG therapy. The survival estimate includes all-cause mortality, including two patients with non-tumoral mortality.

or 50 mCi (fission) ^{131}I/mmol ^{127}I-MIBG in a solid-phase Cu^{2+}-catalyzed exchange reaction.

All exchange labelings have been conducted using the solid-phase (ammonium sulfate) method with Cu^{2+} catalysis, typically incubating 600–1400 mCi ^{131}I with a much larger amount of ^{127}I-MIBG. (Molar ratio of approximately 1:1000) in a protected hot-cell designed for this purpose. On account of shielding constraints, hot-cell activities are limited to 2 Ci and room activity to 1500 mCi. The nuclear pharmacist delivers the ^{131}I-MIBG to the patient's room in a lead-shielded container.

This exchange-labeling process of synthesizing ^{131}I-MIBG yields a mixture of ^{131}I-MIBG and ^{127}I-MIBG in a molar ratio of about 1:1,000; this is known as "carrier added" ^{131}I-MIBG. About 97–98% of the radioactive isotope ^{131}I is bound to MIBG, leaving only about 2–3% free ^{131}I-MIBG; this is known as having a high "specific activity".

UCSF Hospital Care During ^{131}I-MIBG Therapies

Patients are admitted to the University of California, San Francisco on Thursdays to lead-lined rooms that had been prepared in advance by UCSF Environmental Health and Safety. Adults are admitted to the oncology unit, whereas children are admitted to UCSF Children's Hospital Pediatric Clinical Research Center.

All patients with hypertension were treated with antihypertensives. Nifedipine was used preferentially. Labetalol was not used, on account of its known inhibition of MIBG uptake into tumors.

On the evening of admission, all patients receive a bladder catheter; an intravenous line is established, and intravenous 0.9 normal saline solution is infused for the duration of the hospitalization. A second peripheral intravenous line is established with an angiocatheter, heparin-locked, and lightly taped in preparation for the ^{131}I-MIBG infusions.

For thyroid protection against free ^{131}I, all patients receive potassium iodide (KI) and potassium perchlorate ($KClO_4$). For nausea prophylaxis, patients are administered granisetron 2 mg orally daily for 5 to 7 days, beginning on the morning of the ^{131}I-MIBG infusions. In the event of vomiting, intravenous granisetron or ondansetron is used. For sedation or additional anti-emetic effect, lorazepam 1 mg was administered intravenously or orally every 6 to 8 hours.

For prophylaxis against deep vein thrombosis, all adult patients receive low molecular weight heparin (enoxaparin 40 mg) subcutaneously daily for the first 3 days of their hospitalization, while they have a bladder catheter and are at bed rest. The patients receive their usual medications, as long as they are not known to interfere with ^{131}I-MIBG uptake.

In preparation for the ^{131}I-MIBG infusion, each patient's bladder catheter is drained into a lead-lined container by the bedside, from which it is constantly pumped away into a continuously flushing toilet.

UCSF ^{131}I-MIBG Infusion Protocol and Dosing

Adult patients are gently sedated with lorazepam 1 mg intravenously immediately prior to the isotope infusion. ^{131}I-MIBG is infused intravenously over 120 min via a peripheral intravenous line. The isotope activity is pumped from a shielded vial through micropore tubing past an infrared bubble detector. Blood pressure and pulse are measured remotely every 15 min with an automated monitoring device during the isotope infusion. For systolic hypertension reaching 170 mm Hg, nifedipine 10 mg was administered orally. After the isotope infusion, the intravenous line used for the infusion is removed. A physician, nuclear pharmacist, and radiation safety specialist are present during each infusion of ^{131}I-MIBG.

The individual doses of ^{131}I-MIBG ranged from 557 mCi to 1185 mCi (mean 833 mCi). Expressed as mCi/kg body weight, the doses ranged from a low of 7.4 mCi/kg (large adult) to 18.75 mCi/kg (mean 12.6 mCi/kg).

Three days after the ^{131}I-MIBG infusion, the bladder catheter is typically removed. A laxative is administered to patients who are constipated. Four days after the isotope infusion, a whole-body post-therapy scan is obtained. Most patients are discharged on their fifth to seventh day following the isotope infusion, as long as their γ radiation levels are below 7 mRem/h at 1 m for adults and 2 mRem/h for children. The patients whose γ radiation levels measuring 2–7 mRem/hr at 1 m are discharged with explicit radiation safety precautions.

Patient Evaluation After ^{131}I-MIBG Therapy

Following ^{131}I-MIBG therapy, patients receive a post-therapy scintigraphy scan prior to discharge, and then return home for close hematological surveillance and support. Patients are followed very carefully after high-dose ^{131}I-MIBG therapy as follows: CBC with absolute neutrophil counts twice weekly for at least 6 weeks and then every 3 months; thorough serum biochemistries once weekly for 6 weeks and then every 3 months; *I-MIBG whole-body scanning every 3–4 months; volumetric imaging of metastases with CT or MRI every 3–4 months; serum chromogranin A every 1 to 3 months; 24-h urine fractionated catecholamines and metanephrines every 3–4 months; serum TSH and thyroxine every 3 months. Pulmonary function testing was required for patients with pulmonary metastases. An echocardiogram was required for patients with cardiac avidity for ^{131}I-MIBG. A hematologist–oncologist follows all patients.

Myelosuppression After ^{131}I-MIBG: Patient Care

Aspirin is prohibited following high-dose ^{131}I-MIBG therapies because it inhibits platelet aggregation, an unwanted effect in view of expected thrombocytopenia. Patients developed myelosuppression, generally commencing about 2.5–3 weeks after ^{131}I-MIBG therapies. Thrombocytopenia usually appeared first and was treated with platelet transfusions for platelet counts less than 20,000/μL at the discretion of the hematologist. After 30 initial ^{131}I-MIBG therapies, the grades of thrombocytopenia at nadir were: Grade 1 (> 75,000/μL) 4 patients; Grade 2 (≥ 50,000/μL and ≤ 75,000/μL) 2 patients; Grade 3 (> 10,000/μL and < 50,000/μL) 21 patients; and Grade 4 (≤ 10,000/μL).

GCSF was empirically administered to patients with an absolute neutrophil count (ANC) below 500/μL. Antibiotics (usually levofloxacin) were administered for fever or prophylactically to patients with an ANC below 200/μL. Erythropoietin analogues are empirically given for significant anemia. Red blood cell transfusions were administered as clinically indicated. Infusion of autologous cryopreserved peripheral blood stem cells (PBSCs) were administered to four patients with an ANC <200/μL, Hct <25%, or PLT

<20,000/μL (treatment-dependent for over 2 weeks). No patient developed irreversible myelosuppression after ^{131}I-MIBG therapies.

Non-hematological Adverse Reactions to High-Dose ^{131}I-MIBG

Most patients experienced varying degrees of nausea or anorexia, beginning the evening after the ^{131}I-MIBG infusions. The nausea is believed due to radiation sickness, aggravated by oral administration of KI and $KClO_4$. The nausea was usually mild and transient. Patients with a heavy tumor burden tended to experience more prolonged anorexia and nausea that lasted up to 3–4 weeks, long after the isotope had dissipated by excretion or decay.

Many patients experienced transient thinning of scalp hair after high-dose ^{131}I-MIBG. Sialadenitis occurred in several patients whose parotid tenderness appeared to be subjectively relieved by sour lemon candies. Primary ovarian or testicular failure were documented in three patients who had received repeated doses of 131I-MIBG and had extensive pelvic bone metastases.

Several patients have developed Graves' disease after MIBG therapy. One of these 30 patients developed Graves' disease 26 months after receiving ^{131}I-MIBG. Another patient, recently treated, developed Graves' disease 3 months after ^{131}I-MIBG. A child (treated at UCSF under the concurrent neuroblastoma ^{131}I-MIBG treatment protocol) also developed Graves' disease after ^{131}I-MIBG. Graves' disease may have been triggered by the large doses of KI that were administered for thyroid protection, with a mechanism akin to amiodarone-induced hyperthyroidism.

Many feared toxicities have *not* developed after high-dose ^{131}I-MIBG. The normal liver absorbs a large portion of the administered ^{131}I-MIBG by a cation transporter mechanism, and the liver shows significant uptake of ^{131}I-MIBG on the post therapy scans. Therefore, liver enzymes were monitored weekly in all patients for 6 weeks and then regularly thereafter. No patients developed hepatic toxicity after high-dose ^{131}I-MIBG therapies. Patients with numerous large hepatic metastases did not show any sign of liver toxicity, despite significant uptake of isotope into their hepatic metastases. The normal adrenal medulla takes up ^{131}I-MIBG, but no patients have developed primary adrenal insufficiency. The sympathetic nervous system has robust norepinephrine uptake-1 activity, but we have not observed adrenergic insufficiency in any patient. The heart can have significant uptake of ^{131}I-MIBG, but no therapy-related cardiac toxicity has been observed.

CONCLUSION

For patients with paraganglioma or pheochromocytoma metastases having good *I-MIBG uptake on diagnostic scanning, high-dose ^{131}I-MIBG therapy can be effective therapy. In our experience, 67% of patients had a sustained CR,

PR, or SD. The calculated 5-year survival was 75% from time of treatment. While there is some significant potential toxicity, this therapeutic approach is generally very well tolerated. The results from this ongoing Phase II study demonstrate the efficacy of high-dose ^{131}I-MIBG therapy for selected patients with malignant pheochromocytoma and paraganglioma. However, novel therapies are needed. We may be able to improve such patients' outcomes with refinements in ^{131}I-MIBG synthesis and dosing, and by developing techniques to improve these tumors' sensitivity to ^{131}I-MIBG as well as their uptake and retention of the isotope.

ACKNOWLEDGMENTS

The Pediatric Clinical Research Center, Children's Hospital, University of California, San Francisco is supported in part by Grant 2M01 RR01271 from the National Institutes of Health, Department of Health and Human Services; The Jason Krantz Memorial Fund; Steven H. Fugaro, M.D.; and The Genevieve Woods Trust.

REFERENCES

1. BEARD, C.M. *et al.* 1983. Occurrence of pheochromocytoma in Rochester, Minnesota, 1950 through 1979. Mayo Clin. Proc. **58:** 802–804.
2. STENSTROM, G. & K. SVARDSUDD. 1986. Pheochromocytoma in Sweden 1958-1981. An analysis of the National Cancer Registry Data. Acta Med. Scand. **220:** 225–232.
3. HARTLEY, L. & D. PERRY-KEENE. 1985. Phaeochromocytoma in Queensland: 1970–83. Aust. N. Z. J. Surg. **55:** 471–475.
4. ANDERSEN, G.S. *et al.* 1988. The incidence rate of phaeochromocytoma and Conn's syndrome in Denmark, 1977–1981. J. Hum. Hypertens. **2:** 187–189.
5. BAGUET, J.P. *et al.* 2004. Circumstances of discovery of phaeochromocytoma: a retrospective study of 41 consecutive patients. Eur. J. Endocrinol. **150:** 681–686.
6. SUTTON, M.G. *et al.* 1981. Prevalence of clinically unsuspected pheochromocytoma: review of a 50-year autopsy series. Mayo Clin. Proc. **56:** 354–360.
7. CIFTCI, A.O. *et al.* 2001. Pheochromocytoma in children. J. Pediatr. Surg. **36:** 447–452.
8. TANAKA, S. *et al.* 1993. Malignant pheochromocytoma with hepatic metastasis diagnosed 20 years after resection of the primary adrenal lesion. Intern. Med. **32:** 789–794.
9. LEHNERT, H. *et al.* 2004. Malignant pheochromocytoma. *In* Pheochromocytoma. Pathophysiology and Clinical Management. Frontiers of Hormone Research. Vol. 31, A.B. Grossman, Ed.: 155–162. S. Karger. Basel, Switzerland.
10. THOMPSON, L.D.R. 2002. Pheochromocytoma of the adrenal gland scaled score (PASS) to separate benign from malignant neoplasms. Am. J. Surg. Pathol. **26:** 551–556.

11. KIMURA, N. *et al.* 2005. Histological grading of adrenal and extra-adrenal pheochromocytomas and relationship to prognosis: a clinicopathological analysis of 116 adrenal pheochromocytomas and 30 extra-adrenal sympathetic paragangliomas including 38 malignant tumors. Endocr. Pathol. **16:** 23–32.
12. BROWN, H.M. *et al.* 1999. Predicting metastasis of pheochromocytomas using DNA flow cytometry and immunohistochemical markers of cell proliferation. Cancer **86:** 1583–1589.
13. SALMENKIVI, K. *et al.* 2001. Increased expression of cyclooxygenase-2 in malignant pheochromocytomas. J. Clin. Endocrinol. Metab. **86:** 5615–5619.
14. OISHI, S. & T. SATO. 1988. Elevated serum neuron-specific enolase in patients with malignant pheochromocytoma. Cancer **61:** 1167–1170.
15. RAO, F. *et al.* 2000. Malignant pheochromocytoma: chromaffin granule transmitters and response to treatment. Hypertension **36:** 1045–1052.
16. SHORT, J.H. & T.D. DARBY. 1967. Sympathetic nervous system blocking agents. III. Derivatives of benzylguanidine. J. Med. Chem. **10:** 833–840.
17. SISSON, J.C. *et al.* 1981. Scintigraphic localization of pheochromocytoma. N. Engl. J. Med. **305:** 12–17.
18. SHAPIRO, B. *et al.* 1984. The location of middle mediastinal pheochromocytomas. J. Thoracic Cardiovasc. Surg. **87:** 814–820.
19. SHAPIRO, B. *et al.* 1985. Iodine-131 metaiodobenzylguanidine for the locating of suspected pheochromocytoma: experience in 400 cases. J. Nucl. Med. **26:** 576–585.
20. HATTNER, R.S. *et al.* 1984. Scintigraphic detection of pheochromocytomas using m-iodo (I-131) benzylguanidine. Noninvasive Med. Imaging **1:** 105–109.
21. TSUCHIMOCHI, S. *et al.* 1997. Metastatic pulmonary pheochromocytomas: positive I-123 MIBG imaging with negative I-131 MIBG and equivocal I-123 MIBG planar imaging. Clin. Nucl. Med. **22:** 687–690.
22. ARGIRIS, A. *et al.* 2003. PET scan assessment of chemotherapy response in metastatic paraganglioma. Am. J. Clin. Oncol. **26:** 563–566.
23. PACAK, K. *et al.* 2004. Functional imaging of endocrine tumors: role of positron emission tomography. Endocr. Rev. **25:** 569–580.
24. MUKHERJEE, J.J. *et al.* 1997. Pheochromocytoma: effect of nonionic contrast medium in CT on circulating catecholamine levels. Radiology **202:** 227–231.
25. ILIAS, I. & K. PACAK. 2004. Anatomical and functional imaging of metastatic pheochromocytoma. Ann. N.Y. Acad. Sci. **1018:** 495–504.
26. KHORRAM-MANESH, A. *et al.* 2004. Mortality associated with pheochromocytoma in a large Swedish cohort. Eur. J. Surg. Oncol. **30:** 556–559.
27. BRAVO, E.L. 2002. Pheochromocytoma: an approach to antihypertensive management. Ann. N. Y. Acad. Sci. **970:** 1–10.
28. SANTEIRO, M.L. *et al.* 1996. Phenoxybenzamine placental transfer during the third trimester. Ann. Pharmacother. **30:** 1249–1251.
29. COMBEMALE, F. *et al.* 1998. Exclusive use of calcium channel blockers and cardioselective beta-blockers in the pre- and peri-operative management of pheochromocytomas. 70 cases. Ann. Chir. **52:** 341–345.
30. LEBUFFE, G. *et al.* 2005. The effect of calcium channel blockers on outcome following the surgical treatment of phaeochromocytomas and paragangliomas. Anaesthesia **60:** 439–444.
31. BLAKE, G.M. *et al.* 1988. Modification by nifedipine of ^{131}I-metaiodobenzylguanidine kinetics in malignant phaeochromocytoma. Eur. J. Nucl. Med. **14:** 345–348.

32. MINAMI, T. *et al.* 2002. An effective use of magnesium sulfate for intraoperative management of laparoscopic adrenalectomy for pheochromocytoma in a pediatric patient. Anesth. Analg. **95:** 1243–1244.
33. KHAFAGI, F.A. *et al.* 1989. Labetalol reduces iodine-131 MIBG uptake by pheochromocytoma and normal tissues. J. Nucl. Med. **30:** 481–489.
34. STEINSAPIR, J. *et al.* 1997. Metyrosine and pheochromocytoma. Arch. Intern. Med. **157:** 901–906.
35. MUKHERJEE, J.J. *et al.* 1997. Pheochromocytoma: effect of nonionic contrast medium in CT on circulating catecholamine levels. Radiology **202:** 227–231.
36. DINER, E.K. *et al.* 2005. Partial adrenalectomy: The National Cancer Institute experience. Urology **66:** 19–23.
37. GUERRIERI, M. *et al.* 2005. Laparoscopic adrenalectomy in pheochromocytomas. J. Endocrinol. Invest. **28:** 523–527.
38. DAVIES, M.J. *et al.* 2004. A comparison of open and laparoscopic approaches to adrenalectomy in patients with phaeochromocytoma. Anaesth. Intensive Care **32:** 224–229.
39. ELDADAH, B.A. *et al.* 2004. Cardiac uptake-1 inhibition by high circulating norepinephrine levels in patients with pheochromocytoma. Hypertension **43:** 1227–1234.
40. AVERBUCH, S.D. *et al.* 1988. Malignant pheochromocytoma: effective treatment with a combination of cyclophosphamide, vincristine, and dacarbazine. Ann. Intern. Med. **109:** 267–273.
41. PATEL, S.R. *et al.* 1995. A 15-year experience with chemotherapy of patients with paraganglioma. Cancer **76:** 1476–1480.
42. KOSHIHARA, K. *et al.* 1989. Remarkable regression of malignant paraganglioma in the retroperitoneum and neck after chemotherapy: report of a case and a review of the literature. Jpn. J. Med. **28:** 772–776.
43. MICHAELSON, M.D. & M.R. SMITH. 2005. Bisphosphonates for treatment and prevention of bone metastases. J. Clin. Oncol. **23:** 8219–8224.
44. BRIEGER, J. *et al.* 2005. Vascular endothelial growth factor expression, vascularization and proliferation in paragangliomas. ORL J. Otorhinolaryngol. Relat. Spec. **67:** 119–124.
45. TONG, A.L. *et al.* 2004. [Expression of transforming growth factor alpha, tumor necrosis factor alpha, and vascular endothelial growth factor of human pheochromocytoma tissues]. Zhongguo Yi Xue Ke Xue Yuan Xue Bao. **26:** 426–431.
46. TAKEKOSHI, K. *et al.* 2004. Expression of vascular endothelial growth factor (VEGF) and its cognate receptors in human pheochromocytomas. Life Sci. **74:** 863–871.
47. SALMENKIVI, K. *et al.* 2003. VEGF in 105 pheochromocytomas: enhanced expression correlates with malignant outcome. APMIS. **11:** 458–64.
48. GIMENEZ-ROQUEPLO, A.P. *et al.* 2002. Functional consequences of a SDHB gene mutation in an apparently sporadic pheochromocytoma. J. Clin. Endocrinol. Metab. **87:** 4771–4774.
49. MIDDEKE, M. *et al.* 2002. *In vitro* and *in vivo* angiogenesis in PC12 pheochromocytoma cells is mediated by vascular endothelial growth factor. Exp. Clin. Endocrinol. Diabetes **110:** 386–392.
50. ZIELKE, A. *et al.* 2002. VEGF-mediated angiogenesis of human pheochromocytomas is associated to malignancy and inhibited by anti-VEGF antibodies in experimental tumors. Surgery **132:** 1056–1063.

51. FERRARA, N. *et al.* 2004. Discovery and development of bevacizumab, an anti-VEGF antibody for treating cancer. Nat. Rev. Drug Discovery **3**: 391–400.
52. ZACHARIAH, A. & G. SCOFF. 2005. Update on angiogenesis inhibitors. Curr. Opin. Oncol. **17:** 578–583.
53. RYAN, A.J. & S.R. WEDGE. 2005. ZD6474–a novel inhibitor of VEGFR and EGFR tyrosine kinase activity. Br. J. Cancer **92:** S6–13.
54. HOLDEN, S.N. *et al.* 2005. Clinical evaluation of ZD6474, an orally active inhibitor of VEGF and EGF receptor signaling, in patients with solid, malignant tumors. Ann. Oncol. **16:** 1391–1397.
55. ZATELLI, M.C. *et al.* 2005. Cyclooxygenase-2 inhibitors reverse chemoresistance phenotype in medullary thyroid carcinoma by a permeability glycoprotein-mediated mechanism. J. Clin. Endocrinol. Metab. **90:** 5754–5760.
56. STARIKOVA, A.M. *et al.* 1998. Nifedipine-induced morphological differentiation of rat pheochromocytoma cells. Neuroscience **86:** 611–617.
57. YU, L. *et al.* 1996. Radiation therapy of metastatic pheochromocytoma: case report and review of the literature. Am. J. Clin. Oncol. **19:** 389–393.
58. GERSZTEN, P.C. & W.C. WELCH. 2004. Cyberknife radiosurgery for metastatic spine tumors. Neurosurg. Clin. N. Am. **15:** 491–501.
59. SISSON, J.C. *et al.* 1984. Radiopharmaceutical treatment of malignant pheochromocytoma. J. Nucl. Med. **24:** 197–206.
60. CHARBONNEL, B. *et al.* 1988. Le traitement des pheochromocytomas malins par la 131-I-metaiodobenzylguanidine. Ann. Endocrinol. (Paris) **49:** 344–347.
61. BRENDEL, A. *et al.* 1989. Radionuclide therapy of pheochromocytomas and neuroblastomas using Iodine-131-metaiodobenzylguanidine (MIGB). Clin. Nucl. Med. **14:** 19–21.
62. TRONCOME, L. *et al.* 1990. The diagnostic and therapeutic utility of radioidonated metaiodobenzylguanidine (MIBG): 5 years experience. Europ. J. Nucl. Med. **16:** 325–335.
63. LOH, K.C., P.A. FITZGERALD, *et al.* 1997. The treatment of malignant pheochromocytoma with Iodine-131 metaiodobenzylguanidine (^{131}I-MIBG): a comprehensive review of 116 reported patients. J. Endocrinol. Invest. **20:** 648–658.
64. MUKHERJEE, J.J. *et al.* 2001. Treatment of metastatic carcinoid tumors, phaeochromocytoma, paraganglioma and medullary carcinoma of the thyroid with ^{131}I-meta-iodobenzylguanidine (^{131}I-mIBG). Clin. Endocrinol. **55:** 47–60.
65. SAFFORD, S.D. *et al.* 2003. Iodine-131 metaiodobenzylguanidine is an effective treatment for malignant pheochromocytoma and paraganglioma. Surgery **134:** 956–063.
66. KORAL, K.F. *et al.* 1989. Calculating radiation absorbed dose for pheochromocytoma tumors in 131-I MIBG therapy. Int. J. Radiat. Oncol. Bio. Phys. **17:** 211–218.
67. MAIRS, R.J. *et al.* 1995. Enhanced tumour uptake and *in vitro* radiotoxicity of no-carrier-added ^{131}I-metaiodobenzylguanidine: implications for targeted radiotherapy of neuroblastoma. Eur. J. Cancer **31:** 576–581.
68. MATTHAY, K.K. *et al.* 1998. Phase I dose escalation of ^{131}I-metaiodobenzylguanidine with autologous bone marrow support in refractory neuroblastoma. J. Clin. Oncol. **16:** 229–236.
69. SUNG, K.W. *et al.* 2002. Double high-dose chemotherapy with autologous stem cell transplantation in patients with high-risk neuroblastoma: a pilot study in a single center. J. Kor. Med. Sci. **17:** 537–543.

70. CHOU, T. *et al.* 2005. Isolation and transplantation of highly purified autologous peripheral CD34+progenitor cells: purging efficacy, hematopoietic reconstitution following high dose chemotherapy in patients with breast cancer: results of a feasibility study in Japan. Breast Cancer **12:** 178–188.
71. ROSE, B. *et al.* 2003. High-dose ^{131}I-Metaiodobenzylguanadine therapy for 12 patients with malignant pheochromocytoma. Cancer **98:** 1–10.
72. BENNETT, J.M. & R.S. KOMROKJI. 2005. The myelodysplastic syndromes: diagnosis, molecular biology and risk assessment. Hematology **10:** 258–269.
73. WEISS, B. *et al.* 2003. Secondary myelodysplastic syndrome and leukemia following ^{131}I-metaiodobenzylguanidine therapy for relapsed neuroblastoma. J. Pediatr. Hematol. Oncol. **25:** 543–547.
74. GARAVENTA, A. *et al.* 2003. Second malignancies in children with neuroblastoma after combined treatment with ^{131}I-metaiodobenzylguanidine. Cancer **97:** 1332–1338.

Can Quantification of VMAT and SSTR Expression Be Helpful for Planning Radionuclide Therapy of Malignant Pheochromocytomas?

LARS KÖLBY,[a] PETER BERNHARDT,[b] VIKTOR JOHANSON,[a] BO WÄNGBERG,[a] ANDREAS MUTH,[a] SVANTE JANSSON,[a] EVA FORSSELL-ARONSSON,[b] OLA NILSSON,[c] AND HÅKAN AHLMAN[a]

[a]*Departments of Surgery,* [b]*Radiation Physics, and* [c]*Pathology at the Lundberg Laboratory for Cancer Research, Göteborg University, Sahlgrenska University Hospital, 413 45 Göteborg, Sweden*

ABSTRACT: Tumor-specific uptake of the radio-iodinated norepinephrine analogue meta-iodobenzylguanidine (MIBG) or uptake of radiolabeled somatostatin analogues via somatostatin receptors (SSTRs) are possibilities to diagnose and treat malignant pheochromocytomas/paragangliomas (PCs/PGs). The aims of this study were to investigate the quantitative expression of vesicular monoamine transporters (VMAT 1, 2) and all five SSTRs in malignant pheochromocytoma/paraganglioma (PC/PG) to evaluate the possibilities for tumor-specific radionuclide therapy. High scintigraphic ^{123}I-MIBG uptake was found in two malignant PGs with high VMAT expression (500–730 copies of VMAT 1, 1,500–1,700 copies of VMAT 2 per 1,000 β-actin), while no ^{123}I-MIBG uptake was found in the malignant PG with low VMAT expression (330 copies of VMAT 1, 350 copies of VMAT 2 per 1,000 β-actin). The two patients with high VMAT expression and high ^{123}I-MIBG uptake were treated with ^{131}I-MIBG (2–3 × 8 GBq). *In vitro*, the VMAT antagonist, reserpine, and the membrane pump inhibitor, clomipramine, inhibited the uptake of ^{123}I-MIBG into tumor cells equally well (48% and 53% reduction respectively, $P <$ 0.001). SSTR2 was the most abundant receptor subtype, but in the two malignant PGs its expression was only 110–260 copies/1,000 β-actin. The transporters at the cell membrane and in the vesicular membrane both appear to be of importance for the uptake of ^{123}I-MIBG into malignant PC/PG. Quantitative determination of VMAT expression may be helpful in selecting patients suitable for radionuclide therapy with ^{131}I-MIBG. The present data indicate that SSTR-mediated

Address for correspondence: Lars Kölby, M.D., Ph.D., Lundberg Laboratory for Cancer Research, Institute for Surgical Sciences, Department of Surgery, Göteborg University, Sahlgrenska University Hospital, SE-413 45 Göteborg, Sweden. Voice: 46-31-342-1000; fax: 46-31-41-7364.
e-mail: lars.kolby@surgery.gu.se

**Ann. N.Y. Acad. Sci. 1073: 491–497 (2006). © 2006 New York Academy of Sciences.
doi: 10.1196/annals.1353.051**

radionuclide therapy will not be effective treatment of malignant PC/PG.

KEYWORDS: malignant pheochromocytoma; VMAT; SSTR; radionuclide therapy

INTRODUCTION

Malignant pheochromocytoma/paraganglioma (PC/PG) is a rare disease with a prevalence of 5–26% of all PCs/PGs depending on the cohort of patients examined.[1–4] No single histological feature of resected PC/PG predicts future metastatic disease. Malignancy is often first diagnosed by the presence of metastases to the skeleton, lungs, liver, and lymph nodes. Metastases usually present within 5 years, but can also occur after a very long time. Risk factors for malignant disease are large tumor size (>5 cm) and extra-adrenal tumors. Malignant tumors have a defective expression of CA-synthesizing enzymes, that is, the norepinephrine (NE) phenotype is common. Without treatment the overall 5-year survival of malignant PC/PG is less that 50%.[5] Surgery is the only potential cure of malignant PC/PG. The palliative treatment is directed toward tumor reduction and control of hypertension. Cytotoxic treatment can alleviate symptoms and may induce remission, but only with limited duration.[6]

Tumor-specific radiation therapy is one alternative for palliative treatment of metastatic disease. ^{131}I-MIBG is a synthetic NE analogue that is taken up by the membrane pump and concentrated in tumor cells via vesicular monoamine transporters (VMAT).[7] Patients treated with ^{131}I-MIBG showed lessened symptoms and in some cases objective tumor regression also.[8–10] ^{123}I-MIBG scintigraphy has high sensitivity and specificity in detecting PC/PG, but malignant tumors can be MIBG-negative and individual patients can have both positive and negative lesions.[11]

Somatostatin receptor (SSTR)-mediated radionuclide therapy shows promising results for the treatment of SSTR-positive neuroendocrine tumors such as carcinoids.[12] Some PCs/PGs express SSTRs and can be visualized by octreotide scintigraphy with relatively high sensitivity for malignant tumors. This technique serves as a complement to ^{123}I-MIBG scintigraphy and MIBG-negative lesions can sometimes be visualized by octreotide scintigraphy.[11] SSTR-mediated radionuclide therapy may therefore have a role in the treatment of malignant PC/PG.

The aims of the present study were to investigate the mechanisms behind MIBG uptake in malignant PC/PG, to quantitate the expression of VMAT 1 and 2, and SSTR1–5, and to relate the expression to scintigraphic uptake in patients with benign and malignant PC/PG. Such studies may in the future be helpful to identify patients suitable for MIBG/SSTR-based radionuclide therapy.

MATERIAL AND METHODS

Patient Material

Tumor biopsy specimens from 10 patients with PC/PG (7 benign/3 malignant) were obtained at surgery. All but one of the patients had undergone ^{123}I-MIBG- and/or SSTR scintigraphy prior to surgery. Two patients with malignant PC underwent palliative treatment with ^{131}I-MIBG (2–3 therapies with 8 GBq). Patient 5 had MEN2 and was previously operated on for medullary thyroid carcinoma. Patients 6 and 7 were mother and son in a family with hereditary PC only (affecting at least four individuals in three generations).

^{123}I-MIBG Binding in Cell Cultures

The binding of ^{123}I-MIBG was studied in the primary tumor cell culture established from one of the patients with malignant PG (patient 9). Preparation and characterization of tumor cell cultures have been described previously.[13] Tumor cells were incubated at 37°C for 4 h with 100 μL RPMI 1640 medium containing approximately 500 Bq ^{123}I-MIBG (corresponding to 10 nM of MIBG). For blockade of ^{123}I-MIBG uptake at the vesicular membrane or plasma membrane, the medium was supplemented with reserpine (1 μM) or clomipramine (1 μM) 30 min before the addition of MIBG, respectively. After incubation the medium was removed and the cells were washed rapidly three times with 1 mL Ca- and Mg-free DPBS. The amount of cell-bound ^{123}I was determined in a gamma counter. Correction was made for background and radioactive decay. The binding of ^{123}I-MIBG was expressed as a fraction of activity administered per well.

Quantitative Real-Time PCR

Total RNA was prepared from tumor biopsies, followed by RNA purification, DNase treatment, and cDNA synthesis. A primer pair and a probe were designed for each subtype of the SSTR and VMAT using assays by design for gene service expression (Applied Biosystems, Foster City, CA) and sequence data from GenBank. Primers and probes for the following genes were used: SSTR1, SSTR2, SSTR3, SSTR4, SSTR5, VMAT1, and VMAT2.

The probes were labeled with a fluorescent 5′-reporter dye (FAM; 6-carboxy-fluorescein) and a 3′-quencher dye (TAMRA; 6-carboxy-tetramethyl-rhodamine). Primers and probes for SSTR, VMAT, and β-actin (TaqMan® β-actin Control Reagent, part. no. 401846) were purchased from Applied Biosystems.

Real-Time PCR Assay

The threshold (Ct) for SSTR 1-5, VMAT 1 and 2 and β-actin was determined for each sample and compared to standards.

RESULTS

Result of ^{131}I-MIBG Therapy

Patient 9 received three courses of therapy and had an almost complete remission of symptoms (hormonal and spinal cord compression) accompanied by the reduction of urinary norepinehrine from 16,000 nM to 2,700 nM. Patient 8 received two courses of therapy with no symptom relief or tumor response. After the first therapy the MIBG uptake was much reduced. This patient died within 6 months from an undifferentiated PG.

^{123}I-MIBG Binding in Cell Cultures

In vitro, the VMAT antagonist, reserpine, and the membrane pump inhibitor, clomipramine, inhibited the uptake of ^{123}I-MIBG into tumor cells equally well (48% and 53 % reduction, respectively, $P < 0.001$).

Quantitative Expression of VMAT1 and 2 and SSTR1–5

The results of quantitation of VMAT1 and 2 and SSTR1–5 expression are shown in TABLES 1 and 2.

DISCUSSION

Treatment of disseminated malignant PC/PG is a challenge. Debulking surgery can reduce the tumor burden and hormonal symptoms but a survival advantage has not been proven. Debulking surgery may have a role in facilitating for subsequent radio- or chemotherapy. In disseminated disease, ^{131}I-MIBG radiotherapy seems to be effective for lesions diagnosed by MIBG scintigraphy, while chemotherapy shows more variable results of limited duration.[6] Since malignant PC/PG can be visualized by octreotide scintigraphy, radiation therapy via SSTR may also be an alternative: [14] case 10 in this study had a negative MIBG scintigraphy, but a positive octreotide scintigraphy. The best criteria to select patients for such forms of therapy have been scintigraphic studies of the uptake of either MIBG or somatostatin analogues. In this study we have

TABLE 1. VMAT quantification and result of MIBG scintigraphy

Case No.	VMAT1[a]	VMAT2[a]	^{123}I-MIBG scintigraphy
A. Benign tumors ($n = 5$)			
1. PC	960	1,800	Neg
2. PC	680	1,300	Not performed
3. PC	130	380	Neg
4. PC	430	430	Pos
5. PC, MEN2	270	850	Pos
6. PC, hereditary	770	3,100	Pos
7. PC, hereditary	4,800	9,800	Pos
B. Malignant tumors (n = 3)			
8. PG	500	1,500	Pos
9. PG	730	1,700	Pos
10. PG	330	350	Neg

[a]Per 1,000 β-actin.

investigated whether quantitation of the MIBG transporter VMAT1 and 2 or SSTR1–5 in tumor biopsies can be helpful to select patients for MIBG- or SSTR-mediated radiation therapy. From this limited series it seems as if high expression of VMAT1, or 2, relates to visualization by ^{123}I-MIBG scintigraphy. The cell culture experiments corroborated previous findings in benign PC that the uptake of ^{123}I-MIBG into tumor cells was dependent on transport via both the cell membrane and vesicular membrane; the uptakes were equally well inhibited by clomipramine or reserpine.[7] The SSTR expression in PC/PG seemed considerably lower than in other neuroendocrine tumors. In midgut carcinoid tumors we have found a mean of 9,000 copies of SSTR2 per 1,000 β-actin versus only 40–260 copies of SSTR2 per 1,000 β-actin in PC/PC in the present study. The activity concentrations in tumor tissue versus blood (T/B) after injection of ^{111}In-octreotide can be up to 1,200 in carcinoids versus about 40 for PC/PG in the present study.[15] With such background data successful SSTR-mediated radiation therapy could be predicted for carcinoid tumors but, from the limited material in the present study, it seems less likely that SSTR-based radiotherapy for PC/PG will be successful.

TABLE 2. SSTR quantification, result of octreotide scintigraphy, and tumor-to-blood (T/B) ratios

Case No.	SSTR1[a]	SSTR2[a]	SSTR3[a]	SSTR4[a]	SSTR5[a]	Octreotide scintigraphy	T/B ratio
1. PC	330	110	n.d.	n.d.	2	Neg	40
6. PC	260	40	1.6	n.d	10	Neg	40
8. PG	3	260	n.d.	n.d.	n.d.	Pos	Not performed
9. PG	7	110	n.d.	n.d.	n.d.	Pos	Not performed

[a]Per 1,000 β-actin; n.d. = not detectable.

Today, tumor-specific radiation therapy with ^{131}I-MIBG seems to be the most promising alternative for PC/PG. Selection of suitable patients can be made from scintigraphic studies/dosimetry, or by determining VMAT expression and T/B ratios. Since MIBG uptake is influenced by several mechanisms, a better selection of patients could be performed if these mechanisms were known and were possible to determine for each individual patient. Recent experimental studies have shown that the specific uptake of MIBG can be enhanced by gene therapy, certain cytokines, and retinoic acid.[16,17] In the future it is therefore possible that therapeutic manipulation of malignant PC/PG may be one way to increase tumor responsiveness to ^{131}I-MIBG.

ACKNOWLEDGMENTS

We wish to thank Siv Tuneberg, Ann Wikström, Annki Illerskog, Ellinor Andersson, Gülay Altiparmak, and Malin Bengtsson for expert technical assistance. This study was supported by the Swedish MRC (5220), the Swedish Cancer Society (3427, 4956 and 3911), I.B. & A. Lundberg Research Foundation, Assar Gabrielsson Foundation, the Swedish Society of Medicine, the Swedish Society for Medical Research, the Göteborg Medical Society, the King Gustav V Jubilee Clinic Cancer Fund, Göteborg, Sahlgrenska University Hospital Research Funds, Gunvor & Josef Anérs Stiftelse, Axel Linders Stiftelse, Gunnar, Arvid & Elisabeth Nilssons Stiftelse, B. Uhlanders fond, C. Landgrens Minnesfond, Serena Ehrenströms Foundation and Wilhelm, Martina Lundgrens Vetenskapsfond, and Camilla Landgrens Memorial Fund.

REFERENCES

1. Gimenez-Roqueplo, A.P. *et al.* 2003. Mutations in the SDHB gene are associated with extra-adrenal and/or malignant phaeochromocytomas. Cancer Res. **63:** 5615–5621.
2. Goldstein, R.E. *et al.* 1999. Clinical experience over 48 years with pheochromocytoma. Ann. Surg. **229:** 755–64; discussion 764–766.
3. Mundschenk, J. & H. Lehnert. 1998. Malignant pheochromocytoma. Exp. Clin. Endocrinol. Diabetes **106:** 373–376.
4. Neumann, H.P. *et al.* 2002. Germ-line mutations in nonsyndromic pheochromocytoma. N. Engl. J. Med. **346:** 1459–1466.
5. John, H. *et al.* 1999. Pheochromocytomas: can malignant potential be predicted? Urology **53:** 679–683.
6. Averbuch, S.D. *et al.* 1988. Malignant pheochromocytoma: effective treatment with a combination of cyclophosphamide, vincristine, and dacarbazine. Ann. Intern. Med. **109:** 267–273.
7. Kölby, L. *et al.* 2003. Uptake of meta-iodobenzylguanidine in neuroendocrine tumours is mediated by vesicular monoamine transporters. Br. J. Cancer. **89:** 1383–1388.

8. Safford, S.D. *et al.* 2003. Iodine-131 metaiodobenzylguanidine is an effective treatment for malignant pheochromocytoma and paraganglioma. Surgery **134:** 956–962; discussion 962–963.
9. Rose, B. *et al.* 2003. High-dose ^{131}I-metaiodobenzylguanidine therapy for 12 patients with malignant pheochromocytoma. Cancer **98:** 239–248.
10. Loh, K.C. *et al.* 1997. The treatment of malignant pheochromocytoma with iodine-131 metaiodobenzylguanidine (^{131}I-MIBG): a comprehensive review of 116 reported patients. J. Endocrinol. Invest. **20:** 648–658.
11. Ilias, I., S. Alesci & K. Pacak. 2004. Current views on imaging of adrenal tumors. Horm. Metab. Res. **36:** 430–435.
12. Kwekkeboom, D.J. *et al.* 2003. Treatment of patients with gastro-entero-pancreatic (GEP) tumours with the novel radiolabelled somatostatin analogue [177Lu-DOTA(0),Tyr3]octreotate. Eur. J. Nucl. Med. Mol. Imaging **30:** 417–422.
13. Westberg, G. *et al.* 1997. Secretory patterns of tryptophan metabolites in midgut carcinoid tumor cells. Neurochem. Res. **22:** 977–983.
14. Lehnert, H., J. Mundschenk & K. Hahn. 2004. Malignant pheochromocytoma. Front Horm. Res. **31:** 155–162.
15. Forssell-Aronsson, E. *et al.* 2004. Biodistribution data from 100 patients i.v. injected with ^{111}In-DTPA-D-Phe1-octreotide. Acta Oncol. **43:** 436–442.
16. Boyd, M. *et al.* 2001. Expression in UVW glioma cells of the noradrenaline transporter gene, driven by the telomerase RNA promoter, induces active uptake of [^{131}I]MIBG and clonogenic cell kill. Oncogene **20:** 7804–7808.
17. Cunningham, S. *et al.* 2000. A gene therapy approach to enhance the targeted radiotherapy of neuroblastoma. Med. Pediatr. Oncol. **35:** 708–711.

Aspects on Radionuclide Therapy in Malignant Pheochromocytomas

EVA FORSSELL-ARONSSON,[a] PETER BERNHARDT,[a] BO WÄNGBERG,[b] LARS KÖLBY,[b] OLA NILSSON,[c] AND HÅKAN AHLMAN[b]

[a]*Department of Radiation Physics at the Lundberg Laboratory for Cancer Research, Göteborg University, Sahlgrenska University Hospital, SE-413 45 Göteborg, Sweden*

[b]*Department of Surgery at the Lundberg Laboratory for Cancer Research, Göteborg University, Sahlgrenska University Hospital, SE-413 45 Göteborg, Sweden*

[c]*Department of Pathology at the Lundberg Laboratory for Cancer Research, Göteborg University, Sahlgrenska University Hospital, SE-413 45 Göteborg, Sweden*

ABSTRACT: **Malignant pheochromocytomas/paragangliomas (PCs/PGs) often have distant metastases to the skeleton, liver, and lungs. Radionuclide therapy is valuable for treatment of disseminated tumor disease and could be used as adjuvant therapy after surgery. Patients with local and/or distant metastases of PC/PG should be investigated preoperatively by scintigraphy using both ^{123}I-MIBG and ^{111}In-DTPA-D-Phe^{1}-octreotide, to evaluate the possibilities for radionuclide therapy (i.e., a dosimetric estimation of radiation dose to the tumor tissue versus critical normal tissues). Individual patient dose-planning should be performed. For patients in whom positive therapeutic effects are anticipated radionuclide therapy can be applied. Therapy with both ^{131}I-MIBG and ^{177}Lu-octreotate might be favorable in individual patients with lesions visualized by both metaiodobenzylguanidine (MIBG) and octreotide scintigraphy with enhanced therapeutic effects and reduced side effects.**

KEYWORDS: **malignant pheochromocytoma; radionuclide therapy; MIBG; octreotate; dosimetry**

INTRODUCTION

Surgery can provide cure of malignant pheochromocytoma/paraganglioma (PC/PG), but due to the type of tumor dissemination curative resections can seldom be performed. The aim of further treatment is therefore often directed

Address for correspondence: Prof. Eva Forssell-Aronsson, Ph.D., Department of Radiation Physics, Göteborg University, Sahlgrenska University Hospital, SE-413 45 Göteborg, Sweden. Voice: +46 31 3421000; fax: +46 31 822493.
e-mail: eva.forssell_aronsson@radfys.gu.se

Ann. N.Y. Acad. Sci. 1073: 498–504 (2006).
doi: 10.1196/annals.1353.052

toward tumor reduction and control of hypertension. To obtain tumor reduction and palliation of hormonal symptoms, *individual* treatment can be initiated by surgical debulking, or ablative procedures, followed by radionuclide therapy (mediated via catecholamine transporters or somatostatin receptors [sstr]), and/or chemotherapy (using multiple agents). Since recurrent tumors are common even after resection with curative intent, one should also consider radionuclide therapy in an adjuvant setting in patients with minimal residual disease.

Radionuclide therapy is so far the most valuable treatment for metastatic PC/PG. The ^{131}I-labeled norepinephrine analogue meta-iodobenzylguanidine (MIBG) has been used with some success, working by specific catecholaminergic uptake at the cell membrane and concentrated into secretory granules via vesicular monoamine transporters (VMAT 1 and 2). Radionuclide therapy is limited by the radiation dose to the critical organs, which for ^{131}I-MIBG is the bone marrow.

Although radionuclide therapy has been used for more than 50 years (starting with ^{131}I therapy of differentiated thyroid cancer), there is still very limited radiobiological knowledge about this type of therapy compared to external radiation therapy. There is a lack of knowledge about the absorbed doses and dose rates (1) needed for tumor cure and (2) tolerated by normal tissues. The influence of other factors (e.g., fractionation schedule) must also be known to optimize the therapy. Due to the relatively poor results of ^{131}I-MIBG therapy in most studies on PC/PG patients, optimization of ^{131}I-MIBG therapy must first be done in order to fully utilize the potential of radionuclide therapy.

EXPERIENCE OF MIBG THERAPY IN MALIGNANT PC/PG

A review of the experience of ^{131}I-MIBG therapy in malignant PC/PG was published in 1997 containing data on 116 patients from 24 centers in 10 countries.[1] Thereafter, more results have been published from single centers, and some of the studies with the highest number of patients are given in TABLE 1.[2–4] The activity level per fraction in these studies varied considerably

TABLE 1. Experience of MIBG therapy in malignant PC/PG

Place of study	Reference	No. of patients	Dose/fraction	Total activity
Review "worldwide"	1	116	160 mCi (96–300) Low dose	490 mCi (100–2,300)
London	2	15	190 mCi (100–300) Low dose	590 mCi (200–1,600)
Duke (Durham)	3	33	390 mCi (70–510) Low-medium dose	550 mCi (70–1,220)
San Francisco	4	12	800 mCi (390–870) High dose	1,020 mCi (390–1,700)

(96–870 mCi), so the studies could be divided into low-, medium-, and high-activity dose. The overall results showed a symptomatic response in 76–100%, hormonal response in 45–89%, and tumor response in 30–83%. These studies demonstrate that MIBG can be an effective palliative treatment for many patients. The tumor response seemed to correlate with the activity level given, while the symptomatic and hormonal response did not. In the low-dose studies, complete remission (CR) was obtained in only 4% of the patients versus 25% CR for the high-dose regimen. CR in patients with skeletal metastases was only obtained in the high-dose study, while CR in soft tissue metastases was found in all studies. In contrast to the mild toxicity seen in the low-dose groups, the high-dose regimen induced severe bone marrow toxicity in many patients, that is, 79% had grade 3 thrombocytopenia, 72% had grade 3–4 neutropenia, and one patient required stem cell infusion. These results highlight the importance of bone marrow harvest before using high doses. However, no firm conclusions for optimal ^{131}I-MIBG therapy can be drawn from these studies. All performed studies are retrospective, with few patients per center; no strict study protocols were used; and all patients were treated and followed on individual basis. In none of the studies were dosimetric investigations were performed.

PATIENT SELECTION FOR ^{131}I-MIBG THERAPY

In our long-term consecutive series of 154 patients with PC/PG followed during 1950–2004, we have shown that only 12 patients had malignant tumors (8 PCs and 4 PGs): 4 patients presented with distant metastases; 4 with locally advanced disease; and 4 patients developed metastases despite "benign" diagnosis at primary surgery.[5] This series is population-based and may better reflect the natural history of malignant tumors and it has less selection bias than series from national reference centers. The first group had the worst prognosis, while the tumor progression was very slow in the other two groups; and only 5 of 8 patients died of PC/PG after an observation time of 20 years (5–35 years). Therefore, medium- or high-dose ^{131}I-MIBG therapy should be reserved for patients with distant metastases and progressive disease. The final selection of patients for radionuclide therapy should be based on careful dosimetric analyses.

OTHER RADIOPHARMACEUTICALS FOR THERAPY

Several other radiopharmaceuticals might be used for targeted therapy of PC/PG, such as analogues of somatostatin, vasoactive intestinal peptide, epinephrine, and dopamine. Of these, the radiolabeled somatostatin analogues might have the highest potential for therapy. There are few studies on the sstr expression by PC/PG, either with RT-PCR, and immunohistochemistry or autoradiography of binding sites; some report expression of all 5 sstr subtypes and others a high incidence of sstr2 (with high affinity for octreotide/octreotate).[6–9] Our own pilot studies on the quantitative sstr expression have shown relatively low levels of sstr1 and 2 in PC/PG versus very high levels in midgut carcinoids (<300 versus 9,000 per 1,000 copies of β-actin).[10] In carcinoid and EPT, the tumor-to-blood activity concentration ratio (T/B) is as high as 50–1,500,[11] and promising clinical therapeutic studies with the radiolabeled somatostatin analogues ^{90}Y-DOTA-octreotide and ^{177}Lu-DOTA-octreotate are ongoing.[12–14] The T/B values of radiolabeled somatostatin analogues for PC/PG was limited to values around 40 (in two patients), but more tumor biopsy data are required before any firm conclusion on the uptake can be made.[10]

RADIONUCLIDE SELECTION

In malignant PC/PG, disseminated metastases commonly occur, and to obtain long-lasting cure, all disseminated tumors must be eradicated. One benefit of radionuclide therapy is also that neighboring unlabeled tumor cells will be irradiated from the tumor cells with activity uptake, resulting in an effective therapeutic effect. However, if the range of the particles emitted by the radionuclide is too long, low absorbed dose will be obtained in small tumors, resulting in suboptimal therapeutic effects. FIGURE 1 shows a dosimetric

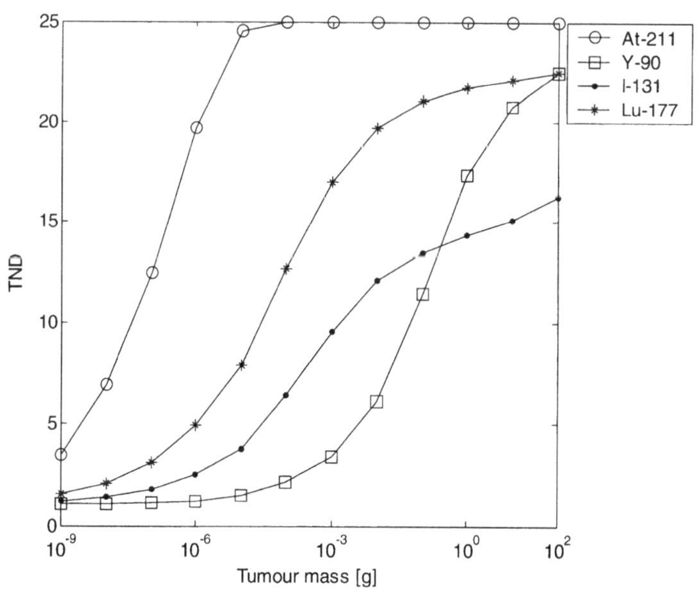

FIGURE 1. The tumor-to-normal-tissue mean absorbed dose rate ratio (TND)[15] for some radionuclides of interest for therapy using MIBG and somatostatin. The estimations assumed a 25-fold higher radionuclide activity in the tumor tissue compared to surrounding normal tissues.

comparison of some radionuclides of interest for MIBG- and sstr-based therapy.[15] ^{131}I had very low absorbed dose values for small tumors and therefore the alpha emitter ^{211}At bound to MIBG (MABG) might be valuable for the treatment of small tumor/micrometastases. The electron-emitting ^{177}Lu and ^{90}Y have been bound to somatostatin analogues in high specific activities. From a dosimetric point, ^{177}Lu-DOTA-octreotate might be a complement to ^{131}I-MIBG for eradication of the smallest PC/PG tumors (FIG. 1). This combination might also give fewer side effects than each radiopharmaceutical alone; the main side effect of MIBG is bone marrow toxicity, but of radiolabeled somatostatin analogues nephrotoxicity followed by bone marrow toxicity. An optimal dose-planning resulting in administration of activities up to the tolerance levels for both bone marrow and kidney will enable administration of higher activities and/or more fractions. ^{90}Y-DOTA-octreotide is only suitable for treatment of large PC/PG tumors with nonuniform uptake on account of the long range of the electrons emitted.

CONCLUSIONS

We propose that patients with local and/or distant metastases of PC/PG should be investigated preoperatively by scintigraphy using both ^{123}I-MIBG and ^{111}In-DTPA-D-Phe^{1}-octreotide to evaluate the possibility for radionuclide therapy. The biokinetics of the radiopharmaceuticals is evaluated from the scintigraphic tissue uptake, and during surgery tumor biopsies can be taken to allow a more accurate determination of the radionuclide concentration in tumor versus normal tissues. High tumor-to-normal-tissue concentration ratios are favorable for tumor therapy. Valuable data can also be obtained by determination of the quantitative expression of VMAT 1 and 2 and of sstr1-5 in individual tumor biopsy. On the basis of these data, individual dose-planning should be performed, and patients in whom positive therapeutic effects are anticipated can have radionuclide therapy. The combination of ^{131}I-MIBG and ^{177}Lu-octreotate might be more favorable in individual patients with enhanced therapeutic effects and reduced side effects than a single high dose ^{131}I-MIBG with severe bone marrow toxicity (requiring stem cell rescue).

FUTURE USE

Further studies are needed to evaluate methods to enhance therapy using ^{131}I-MIBG and ^{177}Lu-octreotate, such as methods to increase the uptake by tumor tissue (by increasing the transport capacity, or receptor expression) and methods to reduce irradiation of the critical organs. Furthermore, the choice of radionuclide depends on the homogeneity of the activity distribution in tissue, and the tumor size. Using the MIBG uptake mechanisms, the alpha emitter

^{211}At bound to MIBG (MABG) needs to be further evaluated for treatment of malignant PC/PG. More knowledge is also needed on the possible synergistic effects of chemotherapy in combination with radionuclide therapy.

ACKNOWLEDGMENTS

The study was supported by grants from the Swedish Research Council (5220), the Swedish Cancer Society (3427, 3911, and 4956), and the King Gustav V Jubilee Clinic Cancer Foundation in Göteborg, Sweden.

REFERENCES

1. LOH, K.-C. *et al.* 1997. The treatment of malignant pheochromocytoma with iodine-131 metaiodobenzylguanidine (^{131}I-MIBG): a comprehensive review of 116 reported patients. J. Endocrinol. Invest. **20:** 648–658.
2. MUKHERJEE, J.J. *et al.* 2001. Treatment of metastatatic carcinoid tumours, phaeochromocytoma, paraganglioma and medullary carcinoma of the thyroid with ^{131}I-meta-iodobenzylguanidine (^{131}I-mIBG). Clin. Endocrinol. **55:** 47–60.
3. SAFFORD, S.D. *et al.* 2003. Iodine-131-metaiodobenzylguanidine is an effective treatment for malignant pheochromocytoma and paraganglioma. Surgery **134:** 956–962.
4. ROSE, B. *et al.* 2003. High-dose ^{131}I-metaiodobenzylguanidine therapy for 12 patients with malignant pheochromocytoma. Cancer **98:** 239–248.
5. WÄNGBERG, B. *et al.* 2006. Malignant pheochromocytoma in a population-based study. Ann. N.Y. Acad. Sci., submitted.
6. REUBI, J.C. *et al.* 1992. In vitro and in vivo detection of somatostatin receptors in pheochromocytomas and paragangliomas. J. Clin. Endocrinol. Metab. **74:** 1082–1089.
7. KUBOTA, A. *et al.* 1994. Identification of somatostatin receptor subtypes and an implication for the efficacy of somatostatin analogue SMS 201-995 in treatment of human endocrine tumors. J. Clin. Invest. **93:** 1321–1325.
8. EPELBAUM, J. *et al.* 1995. Molecular and pharmacological characterization of somatostatin receptor subtypes in adrenal, extraadrenal and malignant pheochromocytomas. J. Clin. Endocrinol. Metab. **80:** 1837–1844.
9. KIMURA, N. *et al.* 1999. Immunohistochemical expression of somatostatin type 2A receptor in neuroendocrine tumors. Clin. Cancer Res. **5:** 3483–3487.
10. KÖLBY, L. *et al.* 2006. Can quantification of VMAT and sstr expression be helpful for planning radionuclide therapy of malignant pheochromcytomas? Ann. N. Y. Acad. Sci. This volume.
11. FORSSELL-ARONSSON, E. *et al.* 2004. Biodistribution data from 100 patients i.v. injected with ^{111}In-DTPA-D-Phe^{1}-octreotide. Acta Oncol. **43:** 436–442.
12. KWEKKEBOOM, D.J. *et al.* 2005. Radiolabeled somatostatin analog [^{177}Lu-DOTA0, Tyr3]octreotate in patients with endocrine gastroenteropancreatic tumors. J. Clin. Oncol. **23:** 2754–2762.

13. FORRER, F. *et al.* 2005. Treatment with ^{177}Lu-DOTATOC of patients with relapse of neuroendocrine tumors after treatment with ^{90}Y-DOTATOC. J. Nucl. Med. **46:** 1310–1316.
14. KWEKKEBOOM, D.J. *et al.* 2005. Overview of results of peptide receptor radionuclide therapy with 3 radiolabeled somatostatin analogs. J. Nucl. Med. **46:** 62S–66S.
15. BERNHARDT, P. *et al.* 2001. Dosimetric comparison of radionuclides for therapy of somatostatin receptor-expressing tumors. Int. J. Radiat. Oncol. Biol. Phys. **51:** 514–524.

Courses of Malignant Pheochromocytoma

Implications for Therapy

JAMES C. SISSON,[a] BARRY L. SHULKIN,[b] AND NAZANENE H. ESFANDIARI[c]

[a]*Division of Nuclear Medicine, Department of Radiology, University of Michigan Health System, Ann Arbor, Michigan 48109, USA*

[b]*Division of Nuclear Medicine, Department of Radiological Sciences, St. Jude Children's Research Hospital, Memphis, Tennessee 38105, USA*

[c]*Division of Endocrinology and Metabolism, Department of Internal Medicine, University of Michigan Health System, Ann Arbor, Michigan 48109, USA*

ABSTRACT: Survival of patients with metastatic pheochromocytoma that have exceeded 30 years without therapy to reduce tumors have been reported. We reviewed the records of 38 patients with malignant pheochromocytoma who had received ^{131}I-metaiodiobenzylguanidine (^{131}I-MIBG) treatments between 1981 and 1996 to evaluate longevity. Survival from diagnosis to last follow-up exceeded 5 years in 21 of 38 (55%) and $\geq$10 years in 50%. In 17 of 21, the interval from diagnosis to ^{131}I-MIBG therapy was greater than 5 years. Survival following ^{131}I-MIBG was $\geq$5 years in 12 of 17 and $\geq$10 years in 7 of 17 patients despite continued evidence of excessive circulating catecholamines. Objective responses to ^{131}I-MIBG therapy were seen in about 30% and were usually of a few years, duration, but one individual exhibited marked reductions in volume and function of tumors that have persisted for 21 years. No feature, including a remission of >5 years following surgical excision, was found to predict prolonged survival. In summary, many patients with malignant pheochromocytoma will follow a course extending over many years. The role of ^{131}I-MIBG therapy in longevity is uncertain, but this radiopharmaceutical reduces evidence of tumors in some patients. Criteria for selecting patients who will benefit from treatment remain to be determined.

KEYWORDS: malignant pheochromocytoma; metaiodobenzylguanidine; patient longevity; long-term survival

Address for correspondence: James C. Sisson, M.D., Division of Nuclear Medicine, UH B1 G505D, University of Michigan Health System, Ann Arbor, MI 48109-0028. Voice: 734-936-5387; fax: 734-936-8182.

e-mail: jsisson@umich.edu

Ann. N.Y. Acad. Sci. 1073: 505–511 (2006).
doi: 10.1196/annals.1353.053

INTRODUCTION

In the strategy of therapy for potentially lethal diseases, prolongation of life is paramount. To appreciate beneficial effects, the probable courses of the disorder without treatment must be taken into account. Survival of patients with malignant pheochromocytoma, even those with distant metastases, has exceeded 10 years.[1–10] Tumor doubling time is then likely to be more than 2 years. These patterns prompted the review of patients with malignant pheochromocytoma initially seen at the University Michigan from 1981 to 1995 for treatments with ^{131}I-metaiodobenzylguanidine (MIBG). The periods of time before and after the therapies were given special attention.

A number of patients who eventually developed malignant pheochromocytoma appeared to have a benign, completely resected, tumor at the outset; more than 5 years between diagnosis and recurrence has not been rare.[5,6,11–13] These observations have led some to recommend that all patients treated for pheochromocytoma should have reevaluations for extended periods of time with the expectation of eventually uncovering malignancy.[11–13] How this manifestation affects survival has not been closely examined. Nine of our patients treated with ^{131}I-MIBG exhibited this phenomenon. For these individuals, the intervals between initial operation and recrudescence are recorded, and these periods are related to their subsequent survival.

MATERIALS AND METHODS

Thirty-eight patients were treated with one to six intravenous infusions of ^{131}I-MIBG for malignant pheochromocytoma between 1981 and 1995 (treatments completed in 1996). Nearly all received multiple infusions, often at intervals of 3 to 4 months but some were extended through a period of 3 years, and one patient received four courses of therapy over 4.5 years. Results have been published for 28 patients treated with ^{131}I-MIBG alone[14] and 6 who received the radiopharmaceutical followed by chemotherapy.[15] Four additional patients were given ^{131}I-MIBG between those two studies. The available records were reviewed, but for three patients too little information was available to assess the intervals in question.

RESULTS

Of the 38 patients, 21 (55%) were known to have survived for >5 years (7–45 years of age), and 50% were alive for ≥10 years following the diagnosis of pheochromocytoma (TABLE 1). Of these 21 patients, the age at diagnosis ranged from 10 to 69 years; only 3 of these patients were females. Information on the remaining 17 patients was sparse: the age at diagnosis ranged from 14 to 66 years; seven were females; and at least three died within 5 years of diagnosis.

Manifestations of excessive catecholamines, symptoms, and hypertension were present in each of the 21 subjects listed in TABLE 1. The pheochromocytoma in patient 11 arose as a component of MEN 2 A. Associated disorders of polycythemia in patients 8 and 18 and a familial hypercoagulation state in patient 12 suggested the possibilities of syndromes, but no genetic tests for germline mutations that result in pheochromocytomas were done. In only patient 11, who manifested MEN 2 A, was there a family history of pheochromocytoma.

The time from diagnosis of pheochromocytoma to treatment with ^{131}I-MIBG ranged from 0.1 years to 20 years (TABLE 1). This interval exceeded 5 years in all but 4 patients, and in 13 it was $\geq$10 years. None of the patients attained a complete remission following treatments (as noted previously).[14,15] In our prior evaluations, about 30% of those treated with ^{131}I-MIBG were shown to have objective decreases in tumor volume and/or hormone metabolite secretions from the tumors. Recent information recorded that patient 1 exhibited a marked reduction in tumor volume and function that has persisted for 21 years after radiopharmaceutical therapy.

From the longevity data available on 17 patients, the interval after ^{131}I-MIBG treatments was at least 5 years for 12 patients, >10 years for 7, and >20 years for 3 (TABLE 1), each with evidence of persisting tumors. However, in the 12 patients surviving for at least 5 years, a relationship was not apparent between the interval spanning diagnosis to ^{131}I-MIBG therapy, ranging from 0.1 years to 20 years, and the subsequent survival of 5–21 years. Nor was the occurrence of partial remissions, seen in patients 1, 2, 4, 9, and 12, associated with a distinct pattern of post-therapy survival, 4–21 years (TABLE 1). Moreover, patients 6, 8, 16, 18, and 21 manifested no objective responses to treatment, but their survivals were among the longest.

Ten patients manifested recurrences more than 5 years after the initial resection of a pheochromocytoma that was thought to be curative (TABLE 1, footnote[a]). These individuals had been cared for by a variety of physicians in multiple institutions, and it is unknown how frequently, and with what laboratory tests, evaluations were carried out in the interlude. These individuals appeared to live longer after initial diagnosis, but, from the incomplete follow-up data, there was no real difference in survival subsequent to ^{131}I-MIBG treatments.

DISCUSSION

Ascertainment bias will afflict studies of any rare tumor. Some malignant pheochromocytomas may cause inanition and death within a few months of diagnosis, and patients with such tumors would have been excluded from our study. Nevertheless, it appears that, in a number of individuals, malignant pheochromocytoma may progress very slowly, even over decades. This concept is supported in 11 reports of $\geq$10-year survival in the presence of metastatic

TABLE 1. Patients with malignant pheochromocytoma: known survival > 5 years

Patient	Age at initial diagnosis (year)	Gender (m/f)	Primary tumor site	Metastasis major site	Initial diagnosis to recurrence[a] (year)	Initial diagnosis to MIBG Rx (year)	MIBG Rx to follow-up (year)	Total survival (year)	Status at follow-up	MIBG treatments No.	MIBG treatments total (mCi/GBq)
1	18	f	extra adr	bone		0.1	21	21	alive[b]	2	400/14.8
2	13	f	extra adr	bone		2	12	14	alive	3	767/28.4
3	40	m	extra adr	bone		2	8	10	alive	3	385/14.2
4	63	m	l adrenal	bone		3	4	7	dead	3	608/22.5
5	39	m	r adrenal	mediastinum		6	5	11	alive	2	507/18.8
6	30	m	l adrenal	lung		7	27	34	alive	2	430/15.9
7	48	m	l adrenal	bone, liver		8		8	unknown[c]	2	312/11.5
8[d]	17	m	extra adr	regional		8	17	25	dead	2	246/ 9.1
9	51	m	l adrenal	regional		10	3	13	dead	6	825/30.5
10	11	m	thorax	bone		11		11	unknown[c]	4	916/33.9
11[e]	25	m	r adrenal	liver	12	12	5	17	alive	2	360/13.3
12[f]	39	f	r adrenal	liver	10	12	5	17	dead	3	854/31.6
13	48	m	r adrenal	bone	12	13		13	unknown[c]	1	325/12.0
14	42	m	r adrenal	regional	12	14	4	18	alive	1	200/ 7.4
15	56	m	r adrenal	bone	11	14	1	15	dead	2	429/15.9
16	23	m	r adrenal	liver	6	14	22	36	alive	3	587/21.7
17	33	m	r adrenal	mediastinum	8	15		15	unknown[c]	1	240/ 8.9
18[d]	10	m	extra adr	bone		16	16	32	dead	4	605/22.4
19	36	m	l adrenal	lung	8	16	1	17	alive	2	544/20.1
20	69	m	extra adr	liver	10	19	6	16	alive	2	419/15.5
21	15	m	r adrenal	bone	15	20	25	45	alive	3	480/17.7

[a]Patients whose recurrence was more than 5 years after diagnosis. In others, there was persistence or early recurrence.
[b]Persisting marked reduction in tumor.
[c]No information after last treatment with ^{131}I-MIBG.
[d]Polycythemia.
[e]MEN2A.
[f]Familial hypercoagulability.

disease: one patient dying at 20 years[1]; three reaching ≥20 years[2]; one living for 25 years[3]; one alive at 21 years[4]; two living longer than 20 years[5]; two of 14 patients, longest 22 years[6]; one surviving 26 years[7]; one alive for more than 30 years[8]; one alive at 16 years;[9] one dead after 11 years.[10]

In our 38 patients, survivals from time of diagnosis were greater than 5 years in at least 55% and greater than 10 years in 50%. The role of ^{131}I-MIBG treatment in longevity remains uncertain. An interval of ≥10 years from diagnosis to treatment was present in 13 patients and already gave evidence of slow progression of disease. Some patients had objective improvements following ^{131}I-MIBG treatments, but the benefits were incomplete, and, except in two patients, sustained for only a few years. A pattern of infrequent, partial, and temporary responses to ^{131}I-MIBG is similar to that reported by others, as noted in reviews of the literature.[16,17] In recent reports, rates of objective improvements have been similar in six[10] and 33 patients.[18] However, 3 of 12 individuals treated with high-dose ^{131}I-MIBG exhibited complete remissions; 2 of the remitted pheochromocytomas were nonsecretory, but the disappearance of scintigraphic and CT evidence of disease has endured for 8.5 years in one.[19] In addition, two patients had marked partial responses to multiple ^{131}I-MIBG therapies, and, in one, diminutions of tumor have persisted for 16 years.[10] And one of our patients enjoyed substantial reductions in tumor volume and hormonal markers that have been sustained for 21 years. These latest observations give hope of long-term effects from ^{131}I-MIBG therapy, but enhanced survival will require study of numerous patients over decades.

When considering therapy for a patient with malignant pheochromocytoma, is there any way to predict the course of disease? Observations for a period of many months may be insufficient to predict accurately the long-term course a patient will take; for example, two of our patients (patients 18 and 21) appeared to have developed extensive metastases during the few years following diagnosis and then manifested stable patterns of disease for a prolonged period before ^{131}I-MIBG treatment. It is possible that growth-inhibiting substances, released by paracrine or autocrine mechanisms from the tumors, and/or activation of autoimmune forces brought about this pattern of malignant growth. Identification of such inhibiting factors could not only predict the course of disease but also lay a basis for new therapeutics.

Research into tumor-suppressor genes,[20] angiogenetic forces,[21] and proteomics[22] may lead to accurate predictions of which tumors will progress rapidly. Other types of analyses have shown that plasma methoxytyramine and dopamine levels have been associated with multiple deposits of tumor;[23] these, and possibly other, catecholamine-related products may be portents of aggressive malignancy.

Without predictors of the course of malignant pheochromocytoma, it will be difficult to withhold treatment in a symptomatic patient while awaiting a pattern of progression to appear. Objective responses observed in indices of tumor function and volume over a year or two following treatments may be the best guides of success.

Why some malignant pheochromocytomas recur years after apparently complete resection is unknown. The reappearance of tumor more than 5 years after surgical excision was seen in 10 of our patients. This early delay in tumor progression was not associated with a greater overall longevity than that seen in the patients whose residual malignancy was observed sooner. In the literature, 3–8% of patients who were originally thought to harbor benign disease have developed recurrences after 5 years: one patient (cohort not described)[5]; two of 14 patients[6]; three of 98[11]; 14 of 176[12]; and five of 121.[13] In at least one series, urinary catecholamines and metabolites were found to be normal after the operation.[11] For patients with apparently benign pheochromocytoma, prediction of events will be difficult, but proteomics offers some hope,[22] and, if measured at regular intervals, the plasma-free metanephrines, which offer high sensitivities,[24,25] may provide an early clue.

In summary, patients with malignant pheochromocytoma may exhibit a slow progression of disease extending over decades. Years of observation are necessary to project the ultimate course. However, without early prognosticators, therapy that is found to help at least some patients cannot be withheld. Still, success must include accurate measurements of survival. For the few patients who will have delayed recurrence after initial excision, methods must be devised to detect these resurgent tumors at the earliest time to give the best opportunity for cure through reoperation.

ACKNOWLEDGMENTS

Evaluations and treatments of patients were supported by the General Clinical Research Center at the University of Michigan, Grant No. M01-RR00042. Carol Kruise was especially helpful in preparing this manuscript. This research was approved by the IRB for Medicine at the University of Michigan Health System.

REFERENCES

1. TRAUB, Y.M. & J.B. ROSENFELD. 1970. Malignant pheochromocytoma with pleural metastasis of unusually long duration. Chest **58:** 546–550.
2. REMINE, R.H. *et al.* 1974. Current management of pheochromocytoma. Ann. Surg. **179:** 740–747.
3. VAN DEN BROEK, P.J. & J. DE GRAEFF. 1978. Prolonged survival in a patient with pulmonary metastases of malignant pheochromocytoma. Neth. J. Med. **21:** 245–247.
4. ABEMAYOR, E. *et al.* 1980. Multiple sequential pulmonary resections for metastatic pheochromocytoma with long-term survival. Am. J. Surg. **140:** 696–697.
5. BRENNAN, M.F. & H.R. KEISER. 1982. Persistent and recurrent pheochromocytoma: the role of surgery. World J. Surg. **6:** 397–402.
6. MORNEX, R *et al.* 1992. Malignant pheochromocytoma: a series of 14 cases observed between 1966 and 1990. J. Endocrinol. Invest. **15:** 643–649.

7. YOSHIDA, S.M. *et al.* 2001. Twenty-six-years' survival with multiple bone metastasis of malignant pheochromocytoma. Arch. Orthop. Trauma. Surg. **121:** 598–600.
8. YOUNG, A.L. *et al.* 2002. Familial malignant catecholamine-secreting paraganglioma with prolonged survival associated with mutation in the succinate dehydrogenase B gene. J. Clin. Endocrinol. Metab. **87:** 4101–4105.
9. MARNIX, G.E.H. *et al.* 2005. Repeated [^{131}I]metaiodobenzylguanidine therapy in two patients with malignant pheochromocytoma. J. Clin. Endocrinol. Metab. **90:** 5888–5895.
10. BOMANJI, J.B. *et al.* 2003. Treatment of neuroendocrine tumours in adults with ^{131}I-MIBG therapy. Clin. Oncol. **15:** 193–198.
11. VAN HEERDEN, J.A. *et al.* 1990. Long-term evaluation following resection of apparently benign pheochromocytoma(s)/paraganglioma(s). World J. Surg. **14:** 325–329.
12. AMAR, L. *et al.* 2005. Year of diagnosis, features at presentation, and risk of recurrence in patients with pheochromocytoma or secreting paraganglioma. J. Clin. Endocrinol. Metab. **90:** 2110–2116.
13. KHORAM-MANESH, A. *et al.* 2005. Long-term outcome of a large series of patients surgically treated for pheochromocytoma. J. Intern. Med. **258:** 55–66.
14. SHAPIRO, B. *et al.* 1991. Radiopharmaceutical therapy of malignant pheochromocytoma with [^{131}I]metaiodobenzylguanidine: results from ten years of experience. J. Nucl. Med. Biol. Med. **35:** 269–276.
15. SISSON, J.C. *et al.* 1999. Treatment of malignant pheochromocytomas with 131-I metaiodiobenzylguanidine and chemotherapy. Am. J. Clin. Oncol. **22:** 364–370.
16. KOH, K-C. *et al.* 1997. The treatment of malignant pheochromocytoma with iodine-131 metaiodobenzylguanidine (^{131}I-MIBG): a comprehensive review of 116 reported patients. J. Endocrinol. Invest. **20:** 648–658.
17. SISSON, J.C. 2002. Radiopharmaceutical treatment of pheochromocytoma. Ann. N.Y. Acad. Sci. **970:** 54–60.
18. SAFFORD, S.D. *et al.* 2003. Iodine-131 metaiodobenzylguanidine is an effective treatment for malignant pheochromocytoma and paraganglioma. Surgery **134:** 956–963.
19. ROSE, B. *et al.* 2003. High-dose ^{131}I-metaiodobenzylguanidine therapy for 12 patients with malignant pheochomocytoma. Cancer **98:** 239–248.
20. OHTA, S. *et al.* 2005. Downregulation of metastasis suppressor genes in malignant pheochromocytoma. Int. J. Cancer **114:** 139–143.
21. ROOIJENS, P.P. *et al.* 2004. The significance of angiogenesis in malignant pheochromocytoma. Endocr. Path. **15:** 39–45.
22. BROUWERS, F.M. *et al.* 2005. Low molecular weight proteomic information distinguishes metastatic from benign pheochromocytoma. Endocr. Relat. Cancer **12:** 263–272.
23. EISENHOFER, G. *et al.* 2005. Biochemical and clinical manifestations of dopamine-producing paragangliomas: utility of plasma methoxytyramine. J. Clin. Endocrinol. Metab. **90:** 2068–2075.
24. SAWKA, A.M. *et al.* 2003. A comparison of biochemical tests for pheochromocytoma: measurement of fractionated plasma metanephrines compared with the combination of 24-hour urinary metanephrines and catecholamines. J. Clin. Endocrinol. Metab. **88:** 553–558.
25. EISENHOFER, G. *et al.* 2003. Biochemical diagnosis of pheochromocytoma: how to distinguish true- from false-positive test results. J. Clin. Endocrinol. Metab. **88:** 2656–2666.

Malignant Pheochromocytoma in a Population-Based Study

Survival and Clinical Results

BO WÄNGBERG,[a] ANDREAS MUTH,[a] AMIR KHORRAM-MANESH,[a] SVANTE JANSSON,[a] OLA NILSSON,[b] EVA FORSSELL-ARONSSON,[c] LARSERIK TISELL,[a] AND HÅKAN AHLMAN[a]

[a]*Department of Surgery,* [b]*Department of Pathology, and* [c]*Department of Radiophysics, The Lundberg Laboratory for Cancer Research, Göteborg University, Sahlgrenska University Hospital, SE 41345 Göteborg, Sweden*

ABSTRACT: One hundred fifty-four consecutive patients with pheochromocytoma (PC, $n = 137$) or paraganglioma (PG, $n = 17$) were treated at our unit. Twenty patients had MEN 2, 15 VRD, and 1 VHL tumors. Twelve had malignant tumors and were classified according to mode of presentation: (1) Distant metastases ($n = 4$); three underwent surgical debulking (with chemotherapy in one); and three had ^{131}I-MIBG therapy. Within 4 years two patients died of tumor progression. (2) Locally advanced disease ($n = 4$), all resected for cure. (3) Malignancy disclosed during follow-up after adrenalectomy with "benign" histopathology ($n = 4$). All patients in groups 2 and 3 developed recurrence 9 (1–17) years after primary surgery; four underwent resection, one remains tumor-free. The others were treated chronically with phenoxybenzamine, combined with ^{131}I-MIBG in one. These eight patients were observed 20 (5–35) years after primary surgery and 11 (1–19) years after recurrence. This series is population-based and may better reflect the natural history of malignant PC/PG than the series from national referral centers. Active surgical treatment and phenoxybenzamine resulted in low tumor-related mortality in groups 2 and 3; five patients died 8–30 years after diagnosis, four of PC/PG (three from group 2 and one from group 3) and one of other causes. We propose tumor uptake studies (MIBG- and octreotide scintigraphy) in patients with nonresectable metastases; to select individual radionuclide therapy data on the expression of CA-transporters/somatostatin receptors may be helpful. To diagnose PC/PG early, screening of adrenal incidentalomas has been suggested. In a regional population-based prospective study, 503 incidentalomas were reported during 18 months, but only one patient with PG was identified.

Address for correspondence: Bo Wängberg, Department of Surgery, Sahlgrenska University Hospital, SE 41345 Göteborg, Sweden. Voice: +46313421000; fax: +4631417364.
e-mail: bo.wangberg@surgery.gu.se

Ann. N.Y. Acad. Sci. 1073: 512–516 (2006). © 2006 New York Academy of Sciences.
doi: 10.1196/annals.1353.054

KEYWORDS: **malignant pheochromocytoma; paraganglioma; prognosis; treatment**

INTRODUCTION

Pheochromocytomas (PCs) are rare tumors originating from chromaffin cells of the adrenal medulla (80–85%) or extra-adrenal paraganglia (15–20%), the so-called paraganglioma (PG). Abdominal PCs/PGs usually produce catecholamines (CA). Specific germline mutations account for up to 24% of patients with apparent sporadic PC.[1,2] So far, five genes associated with familial PC/PG have been identified: von Hippel–Lindau (*VHL*), MEN 2 (*RET*), neurofibromatosis type 1 (*NF 1*), and the paraganglioma syndromes (*SDHB* and *D*). Malignant PC/PG in familial disease is uncommon, except for mutations of the *SDHB* with a malignancy rate of 50%.[3] The only absolute proof of malignancy is the presence of chromaffin metastases at sites not normally containing chromaffin tissue. Several studies use the classic definition, that is, the presence of metastases and/or extensive local invasion.[4] The frequency of malignant PC/PG is estimated to be 5–26%, depending on the definition used and on the population studied; it is even higher for PG.[1,3,5,6,7] With modern imaging techniques, an increasing number of adrenal tumors is found in patients undergoing abdominal examination without a suspicion of adrenal disease; that is, adrenal incidentalomas are detected in 2–4% of examinations. PC and subclinical Cushing's syndrome are the most common hormone-producing conditions in these patients, and screening for adrenomedullary hyperfunction is recommended for early diagnosis of PC.[8]

MATERIALS AND METHODS

Patients Treated for Pheochromocytoma or Paraganglioma

One hundred fifty-four consecutive patients with PC/PG were treated at our unit (referral center for western Sweden; population 1.6 million) during the period 1950–2004. One hundred thirty-seven patients had a PC and 17 PG; the mean age was 51 years and the female/male ratio was 85/69.

Pheochromocytoma in a Prospective Study of Adrenal Incidentaloma

During 18 months, all adrenal incidentalomas were reported directly from the radiology departments in our region to a central database. Patients reported underwent clinical evaluation, biochemical testing for medullary (urinary catecholamines + fractionated metanephrines and plasma chromogranin A) and cortical hyperfunction, and computed tomography scans.

RESULTS

Patients Treated for Pheochromocytoma and Paraganglioma

Familial disease was documented in 36 patients (20 MEN 2, 15 VRD, and 1 VHL), but no genetic screening of apparently sporadic cases was performed during the study period. No malignant PCs/PGs were identified among these patients.

Twelve patients had clinically and histologically proven malignant tumors (eight PC and four abdominal PG) that were detected as follows: (1) presentation with distant metastases ($n = 4$); (2) presentation with locally advanced disease ($n = 4$); and (3) late presentation of metastatic disease despite "benign" PC at prior adrenalectomy ($n = 4$).

Group 1: Three patients were first treated with surgical debulking and two received fractionated ^{131}I-MIBG radiotherapy (2–3 × 8 Gbq). The third patient (PG with no uptake of ^{123}MIBG) was treated with chemotherapy (cyclophosphamide, vincristine, and dacarbazine) followed by spine surgery and external radiation therapy due to severe compression of the spinal cord. The fourth patient had ^{131}MIBG therapy (1 × 8 Gbq) without prior tumor reduction. Within 4 years after diagnosis, two patients treated with radiotherapy died of tumor progression and the third patient died of a fatal accident; ^{131}I-MIBG-therapy had caused marked tumor regression. This patient had similar uptake sites at octreotide scintigraphy and ^{123}MIBG at initial workup. The ^{123}MIBG-negative patient, treated with surgery, chemotherapy, and external radiotherapy, is still symptom-free with normal biochemistry 4 years after diagnosis. The tumor lesions of this patient that showed initial high uptakes at octreotide scintigraphy are now barely visible after treatment.

Group 2: Four patients presented with locally advanced disease (3 PC/1 PG) and underwent resection for cure. All these patients developed recurrent disease after a mean observation of 4.5 years (range 1–7 years) and were then treated with surgery and phenoxybenzamine ($n = 3$) or ^{131}I-MIBG therapy ($n = 1$). Three of the patients died of metastasizing disease after a mean of 15.6 years (range: 8–30 years). One patient is still treated with phenoxybenzamine for palliation, 19 years after primary surgery and 18 years after repeat surgery.

Group 3: Four patients were initially operated upon for tumors without histological or clinical signs of malignancy (3 PC/1 PG), but tumor recurrence was observed after a mean of 12.8 years (range 4–17 years). One patient with PG had a local recurrence that could be resected; there is no evidence of disease 33 years after primary surgery (17 years after repeat surgery). Three patients had distal metastases of PC that were treated with phenoxybenzamine for palliation. At the latest follow-up, one patient is alive with minimal symptoms 26 years after adrenalectomy (12 years after repeat surgery) and one patient died of unrelated causes 5 years after adrenalectomy (1 year after repeat surgery).

The third patient died of disseminated disease 23 years after adrenalectomy (6 years after repeat surgery).

Pheochromocytoma in a Prospective Study of Adrenal Incidentaloma

In our population-based study, 503 accidentally found adrenal tumors were reported in 489 patients during 18 months. The screening for PC/PG only resulted in the finding of one patient with PG. The tumor was situated close to the adrenal and was excised without complications with biochemical normalization.

DISCUSSION

Our large prospective study of adrenal incidentaloma in our region indicates a much lower incidence of PC/PG than previously reported.[8] The series of 154 consecutive patients treated for PC/PG with long follow-up is also population based. It therefore has a lesser selection bias than the series from national referral centers and may better reflect the natural history of malignant PC/PG. Clinical presentation with distant metastases (1) was associated with the worst prognosis; tumor-related death in 2 of 4 patients within 4 years. Active surgical treatment combined with symptomatic medical therapy resulted in low tumor-related mortality for patients with locally advanced disease (2) and clinically proven malignancy during observation (3). All eight patients in the latter two groups developed recurrence 9 (1–17) years after primary surgery; four patients with localized disease underwent resection but only one has remained tumor-free. The other four patients were treated with chronic α-adrenoceptor blockade, combined with ^{131}MIBG in one. These eight patients were observed for 20 (5 35) years after primary surgery and 11 (1–19) years after their first recurrence. Micrometastases seem to be present in the patients in groups 2 and 3 since recurrent tumors developed in all during the long observation time. Completion radiotherapy following surgical resection can be one attempt to eradicate residual minute lesions and prolong the recurrence-free period (since effective chemotherapy is lacking). We propose that patients with nonresectable metastases should be investigated by tumor uptake (MIBG- and octreotide scintigraphy) prior to surgery in order to select the best individual radiotherapy (or a combination thereof). By studies of activity concentrations in tumor biopsy specimens and normal tissue/blood (taken during surgery), the responsiveness to radionuclide therapy can be assessed from, for example, tumor/blood (T/B) ratios but probably also from quantitative studies on CA transporters and somatostatin receptors (SSTR). Successful radiotherapy with somatostatin analogues relates to high T/B values, shown to be up to 1,200 for carcinoids and endocrine pancreatic tumors compared to 40 for PC/PG in pilot studies.[9,10] It also relates to high expression of SSTR2 (9,000 copies/1,000 β-actin for carcinoids; less than 300 for PC/PG in pilot studies). On the other hand, the expression of VMAT 1 and 2 seems to be relatively high in MIBG-positive PC/PG. In patients with negative uptake studies (most likely reflecting dedifferentiated tumors), chemotherapy remains a therapeutic option.

High-dose radionuclide therapy is associated with bone marrow toxicity (^{131}I MIBG) and nephrotoxicity (^{177}Lu octreotate) and the complete remission rate is low.[11] It is therefore important to initiate this type of treatment first at signs of progressive disease, for example, mainly in patients presenting with distal metastases. In these cases debulking surgery may facilitate the distribution of radionuclide to multiple small lesions in several organs. Novel treatment strategies with less toxicity are clearly needed, such as inhibitors of angiogenesis and of tumor-specific signal transduction.

REFERENCES

1. NEUMANN, H.P. *et al.* 2002. Germ-line mutations in nonsyndromic pheochromocytoma. N. Engl. J. Med. **346:** 1459–1466.
2. BRYANT, J. *et al.* 2003. Pheochromocytoma: the expanding genetic differential diagnosis. J. Natl. Cancer Inst. **95:** 1196–1204.
3. GIMENEZ-ROQUEPLO, A.P. *et al.* 2003. Mutations in the SDHB gene are associated with extra-adrenal and/or malignant phaeochromocytomas. Cancer Res. **63:** 5615–5621.
4. LACK, E.E. 1997. Tumors of the Adrenal Gland and Extra-Adrenal Paraganglia. Armed Forces Institute of Pathology. Washington, DC.
5. GOLDSTEIN, R.E. *et al.* 1999. Clinical experience over 48 years with pheochromocytoma. Ann. Surg. **229:** 755–764.
6. EDSTROM-ELDER, E. *et al.* 2003. The management of benign and malignant pheochromocytoma and abdominal paraganglioma. Eur. J. Surg. Oncol. **29:** 278–283.
7. LENDERS, J.W. *et al.* 2005. Phaeochromocytoma. Lancet **366:** 665–675.
8. MANTERO, F. *et al.* 2000. A survey on adrenal incidentaloma in Italy. J. Clin. Endocrinol. Metab. **85:** 637–644.
9. FORSSELL-ARONSSON, E. *et al.* 2004. Biodistribution data from 100 patients i.v. injected with ^{111}In-DTPA-D-Phe-octreotide. Acta Oncol. **43:** 436–442.
10. KÖLBY, L. *et al.* Can quantification of VMAT and SSTR expression be helpful for planning radionuclide therapy of malignant pheochromocytomas? Ann. N. Y. Acad. Sci. This volume.
11. ROSE, B. *et al.* 2003. High-dose ^{131}I-metaiodobenzylguanidine therapy for 12 patients with malignant pheochromocytoma. Cancer **98:** 239–248.

Does the Expression of *c-kit* (CD117) in Neuroendocrine Tumors Represent a Target for Therapy?

CHRISTIAN A. KOCH,[a] OLIVER GIMM,[b] ALEXANDER O. VORTMEYER,[c] HAIFA K. AL-ALI,[d] PETER LAMESCH,[e] RUDOLF OTT,[f] REGINE KLUGE,[g] UTA BIERBACH,[h] AND ANDREA TANNAPFEL[i]

[a]*Division of Endocrinology and Nephrology, University of Leipzig, Germany*

[b]*Department of Surgery, University of Halle, Germany*

[c]*National Institutes of Health, NINDS, Bethesda, Maryland, USA*

[d]*Division of Hematology and Oncology, University of Leipzig, Germany*

[e]*Department of Surgery, Sankt Georg Hospital, Leipzig, Germany*

[f]*Department of Surgery II, University of Leipzig, Germany*

[g]*Department of Nuclear Medicine, University of Leipzig, Germany*

[h]*Division of Pediatric Hematology and Oncology, University of Leipzig, Germany*

[i]*Ruhr University of Bochum, Bochum, Germany*

ABSTRACT: Neuroendocrine tumors are very heterogeneous, develop from a variety of tissues, and can be difficult to diagnose. Without the clinical manifestation of metastases, it is often difficult to characterize them as malignant. Even so-called completely (R0) resected tumors can spread clinically visible metastases within a few months after initial surgery. Treatment options for neuroendocrine tumors including pheochromocytoma are limited. Molecular targeted therapies using tyrosine kinase inhibitors might prove to be helpful in patients with these tumors. In an immunohistochemical study, we examined KIT in 26 pheochromocytomas, 8 of which were malignant (3 adrenal pheochromocytomas, 5 paragangliomas). KIT expression was found in one of these 8 malignant tumors. This 2.5-cm-large adrenal pheochromocytoma originated from a woman with neurofibromatosis type 1 and spread into spine, skull, and lung. KIT expression could be demonstrated in 5% of tumor cells. On the basis of KIT expression immunohistochemically, we treated patients with neuroendocrine (i.e., medullary thyroid cancer) and other tumors with imatinib 400 mg per day, but without efficacy after 2 months of therapy. Similar results were shown by other investigators. Therefore,

Address for correspondence: Christian A. Koch, M.D., F.A.C.P., F.A.C.E., Professor and Director, Division of Endocrinology, University of Mississippi, 2500 North State Street, Jackson, MS 39216. USA. Voice: 601-984-5525; fax: 601-984-5769.
e-mail: ckoch@medicine.umsmed.edu

Ann. N.Y. Acad. Sci. 1073: 517–526 (2006). © 2006 New York Academy of Sciences.
doi: 10.1196/annals.1353.055

monotherapy with imatinib may not be efficacious in patients with neuroendocrine tumors that express KIT. Tyrosine kinase inhibitors such as sorafenib that targets several receptors in addition to KIT may be more efficacious in treating patients with neuroendocrine tumors.

Keywords: neuroendocrine; tumor; pheochromocytoma; imatinib; neurofibromatosis type 1

Neuroendocrine tumors can develop from a variety of tissue types, such as the thyroid gland, lung, breast, pancreas, gut, adrenal gland, kidney, uterine cervix, prostate, skin, and others.[1–11] Often these tumors are under- or misdiagnosed, which underscores the difficulties in classifying them.[12] Except for surgery, treatment options for neuroendocrine tumors are usually limited. Somatostatin analoga commonly do not stop tumor growth, neither do chemotherapeutic regimens including 5-Fluorouracil and streptotozocin. If a neuroendocrine tumor is completely resected and no metastases are visible and detectable by various imaging modalities/methods, the question arises whether an adjunctive therapy (for instance with 5-FU and streptotozocin) should be initiated.[13] To assist in making this decision, factors such as the MIB-1 proliferation index and other parameters have been used but remain controversial. If metastases are present in a patient with a neuroendocrine tumor, surgical debulking (especially of liver metastases) has been regarded as effective therapy in some tumor types, such as medullary thyroid carcinoma.[14] Chemotherapeutic regimens usually do not show much effect in patients with metastatic neuroendocrine tumors.

With the discovery of *c-kit*, a receptor tyrosine kinase encoded by a gene located on chromosome 4q12, new hopes in molecular targeted tumor therapy have been raised.[15,16] *c-kit* is usually expressed in hematopoietic cells (myeloblasts), mast cells, the interstitial cells of Cajal (important for the gastrointestinal system), germ cells, and melanocytes.

Many nonendocrine tumors are associated with *c-kit* expression. Most gastrointestinal stromal tumors (GIST) have activating mutations of *c-kit*. Mutations in *c-kit* are also found in mastocytosis and germ cell tumors, such as dysgerminomas and seminomas. KIT can also be overexpressed or amplified in acute myeloblastic and chronic myeloic leukemia. The prevalence of KIT expression in human tumors has been reported in several studies.[17–31] Such studies have to be critically viewed, because false-positive KIT expression may occur. Interpretation of KIT expression depends not only on the antibody directed to KIT, but also on the expression pattern.[18] Went *et al.*[20] acknowledged this problem by testing different antibodies (polyclonal rabbit DAKO A4502, Novocastra NCL-CD117, NeoMarkers MS-271, MBL code no. 566, Santa Cruz sc-1494, Santa Cruz sc-13508, and Santa Cruz sc-168), and by considering staining as true-positive if the reaction product was localized to the cell membrane alone or to the cell membrane and cytoplasm simultaneously, because in these cases the preabsorption controls (negative controls) were negative. Tumors showing purely cytoplasmic staining were shown to be false-positive. Truly KIT-positive tumors included GISTs (100%), seminomas (84%), adenoid-cystic carcinomas (65%), malignant melanomas (35%), large-cell carcinomas of the lung (17%), neural tumors such as oligodendrogliomas (12%), primitive neuroectodermal tumors (17%), glomus tumors (11%), breast carcinomas, female genital tumors, adenocarcinomas of the lung (18%), small-cell carcinomas of the lung (6%), adenocarcinomas of the gastrointestinal tract (9%), paragangliomas (14%), adrenal pheochromocytomas (3%), thyroid carcinomas, and urinary tract tumors (kidney and bladder). However, mutations in *c-kit* in immunohistochemically KIT-positive tumors were rare, with the exception of GISTs. KIT positivity by immunohistochemistry may be associated with the presence of multiple copies of the wild-type KIT gene in tumor cells.[19] In addition to *c-kit*, the platelet-derived growth factor receptor (PDGFR) is also located on chromosome 4. Medullary carcinoma of the thyroid, Merkel cell carcinoma of the skin, esthesioneuroblastoma, carcinoma of the adrenal gland, neurofibroma, and many other tumors were KIT-negative in the study of Went *et al.*[20]

Positive KIT expression in tumors often encourages investigators to initiate a therapeutic trial with the tyrosine kinase inhibitor imatinib mesylate (Gleevec), a drug that targets KIT and PDGF. Newer tyrosine kinase inhibitors, such as gefitinib (Iressa), erlotinib (Tarceva), PTK 787/PZ 222584, SU11248 (Sutent), AG-013736, and sorafenib (BAY 43-9006) aim to target several receptors simultaneously including KIT, PDGF, EGF-R, VEGF, and Raf.[15,16] Some investigators suggest using KIT expression as a prognostic marker.[23,30,32]

In vitro studies suggest that imatinib can inhibit tumor growth in the most aggressive neuroblastic tumors and in neuroendocrine tumors.[22,33] Lankat-Buttgereit *et al.*[33] looked at neuroendocrine tumor cells from insulinomas, gastrinomas, and "carcinoids" and found that imatinib inhibits neuroendocrine tumor cell growth independently of KIT expression. Interestingly, KIT is expressed in mature beta-cells and in the pancreas in development.[34]

For patients with neuroendocrine tumors, the response rates to Gleevec therapy are highly variable.[25,35–38] In a phase II trial of imatinib mesylate in patients with advanced carcinoid tumor, Carr *et al.*[35] found only a modest effect on tumor growth. In up to 70% of cases of small cell lung cancer, KIT overexpression is found. Dy *et al.*[38] treated 29 patients with recurrent and refractory KIT-positive small cell lung cancer with imatinib mesylate (Gleevec) 400 mg twice a day for 28 days and could not demonstrate an objective response or confirmed stable disease. Similar results were obtained in a phase II clinical trial by Krug *et al.*[25] In a phase II trial, Ugurel *et al.*[36] found lack of efficacy of imatinib mesylate in patients with advanced metastatic melanoma.

Therefore, initial clinical studies should discourage investigators from using imatinib mesylate as an adjuvant therapy for patients with neuroendocrine tumors that are completely (R0) resected. In contrast, Gronchi *et al.*[39] recently showed that in patients with GISTs, adjuvant treatment with imatinib mesylate can slow the progression of disease. In addition, Blackstein *et al.*[40] demonstrated that the response rate and progression-free survival in patients with GISTs that are KIT-negative does not differ from those with KIT-positive GISTs, implying that a therapeutic trial of imatinib mesylate may be helpful for all patients with GISTs regardless of CD117 expression.

Pheochromocytomas are neuroendocrine tumors that are usually benign, but metastatic lesions have been reported in up to 36% of patients.[41,42] Patients with

(A)

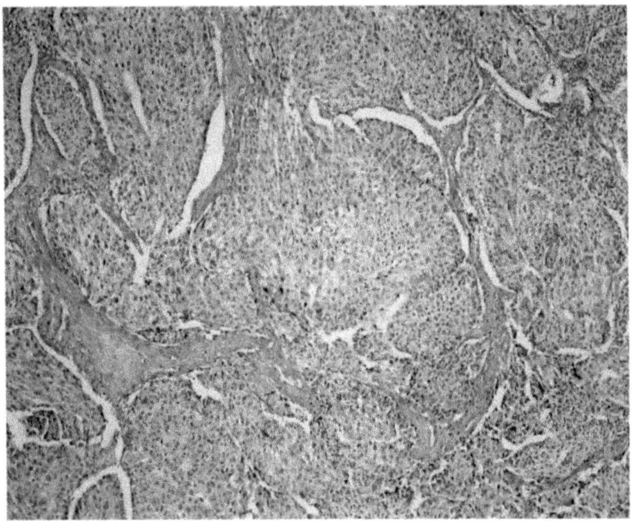

(B)

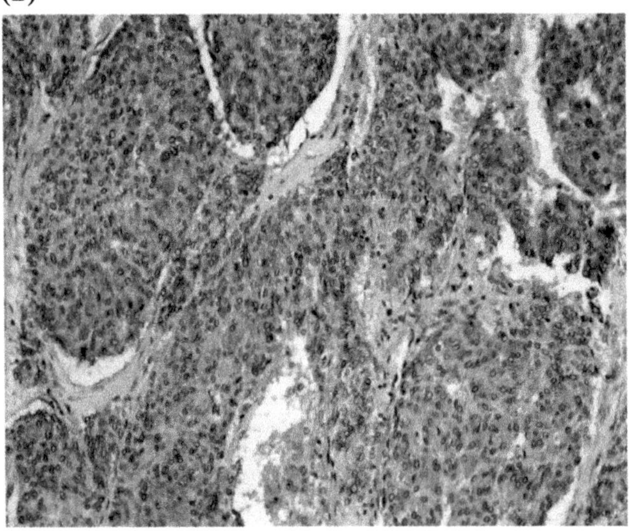

FIGURE 1. (Clinically) metastatic adrenal pheochromocytoma associated with NF1. (**A**) Hematoxylin and eosin. (**B**) Cytoplasmic KIT immunreactivity (5% of tumor cells). (**C**) MIB-1 proliferation index immunreactivity (<2%).

(C)

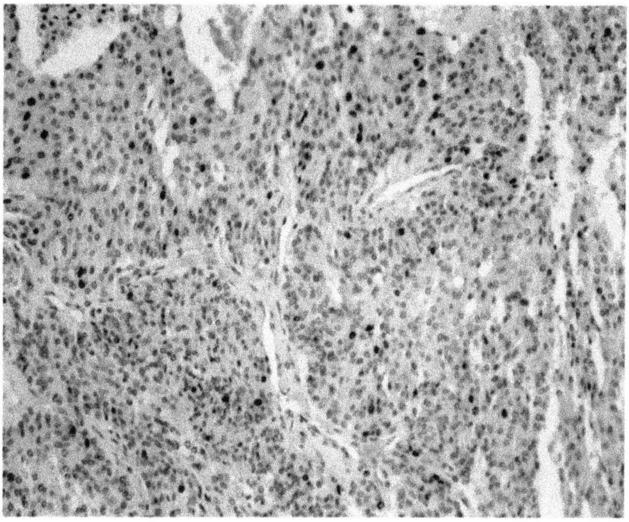

FIGURE 1. *Continued.*

malignant pheochromocytomas are difficult to treat and have a 5-year survival rate of approximately 44%. Distinguishing benign from malignant pheochromocytomas is hard and is only clear cut when metastases are present.[41,43] Went *et al.*[20] found KIT expression in about 14% of pheochromocytomas. In an immunohistochemical analysis using a polyclonal rabbit antibody directed to KIT/CD117, we aimed to assess KIT expression in 26 pheochromocytomas. Twelve tumors were MEN2-associated with known germline mutations in *RET*, 2 were metastatic from patients with NF1, 7 were sporadic (1 with metastasis to the heart at 2-year follow-up), and 5 were metastatic paragangliomas with several recurrences. The objective was to explore whether KIT could serve as a potential marker to distinguish benign from malignant lesions and as a potential target for therapy with imatinib mesylate (Gleevec). Moderate cytoplasmic staining of KIT was found in one of the eight metastatic tumors (FIG. 1). This metastatic (to skull, spine, lung) 2.5-cm adrenal pheochromocytoma originated in a woman with NF1 at the age of 17 (FIG. 2).

On the basis of positive KIT expression immunohistochemically, we (H.K.A.A.) treated patients with tumors refractory to standard therapy (i.e., advanced sporadic medullary thyroid cancer; olfactory neuroblastoma) with Gleevec 400 mg per day which did not show efficacy after 2 months of therapy.

In conclusion, a variety of neuroendocrine tumors including pheochromocytomas show KIT expression to variable degrees. Whether this serves as a prognostic marker or potential target for tyrosine kinase inhibitor therapy remains to be shown.[44]

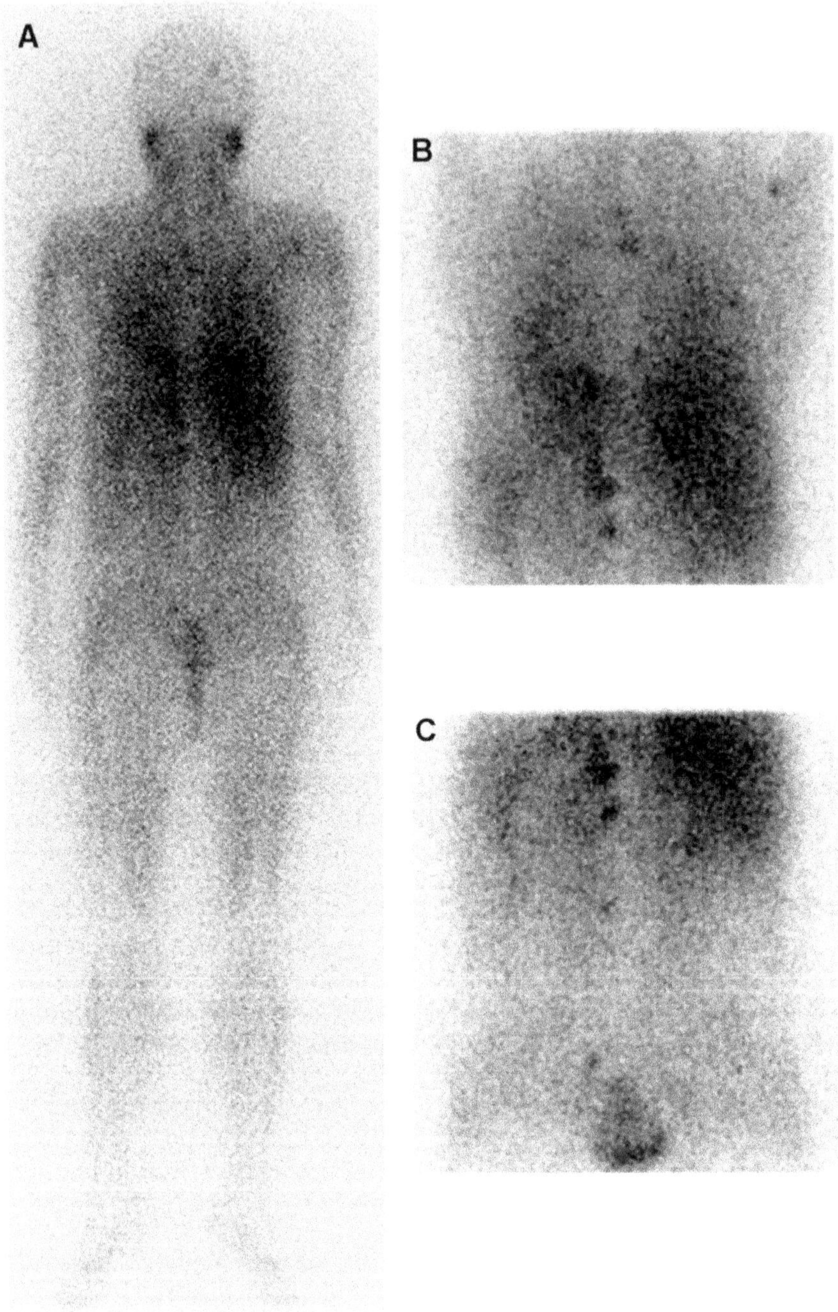

FIGURE 2. **(A–C)** 193 MBq I-123-MIBG scan. **(D, E)** Scintigram 5 days after application of 7.8 GBq I-131-MIBG.

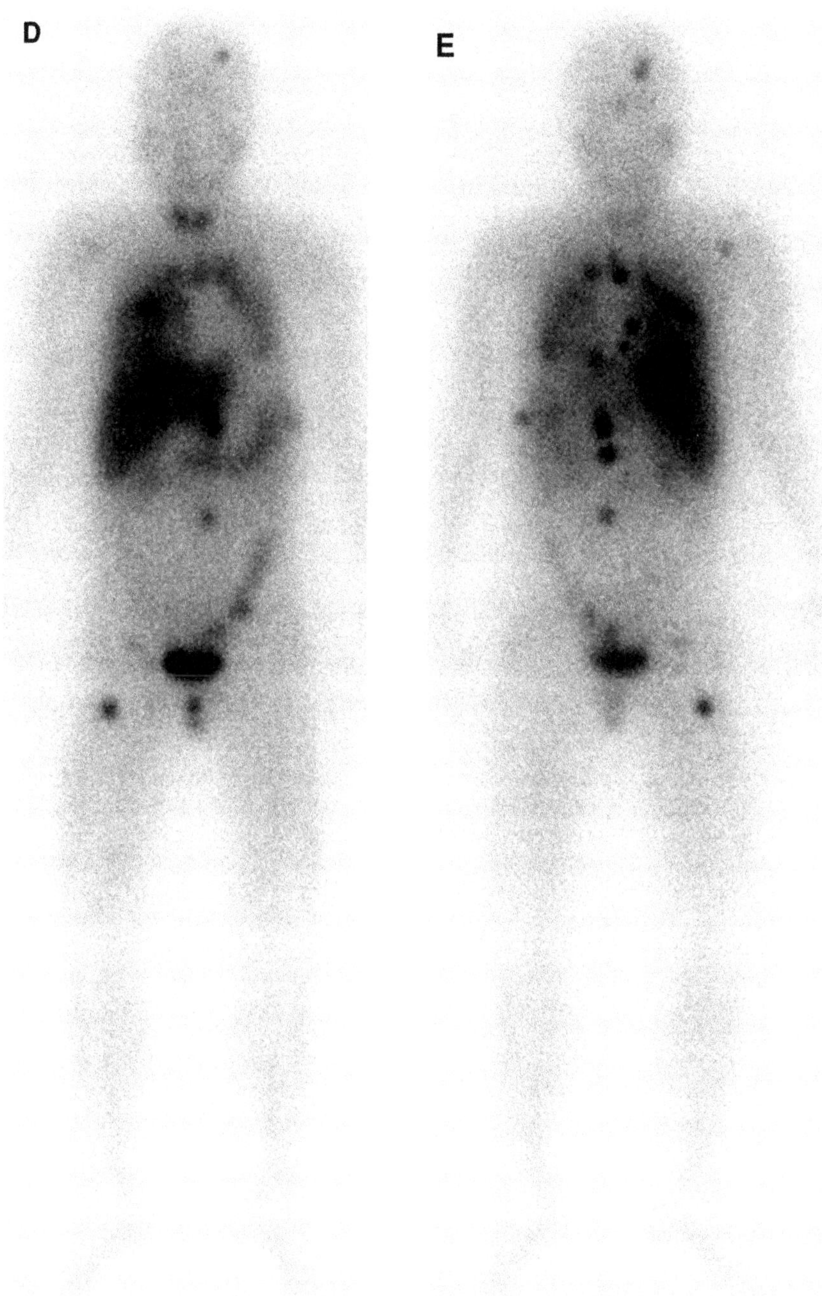

FIGURE 2. *Continued.*

REFERENCES

1. ILIAS, I. *et al.* 2005. Cushing's syndrome due to ectopic corticotropin secretion: twenty years' experience at the National Institutes of Health. J. Clin. Endocrinol. Metab. **90:** 4955–4962.
2. MIEHLE, K. *et al.* 2004. Pancreatic neuroendocrine tumor with ectopic adrenocorticotropin production upon second recurrence. J. Clin. Endocrinol. Metab. **89:** 3731–3736.
3. KOCH, C.A. *et al.* 2003. Adrenal ganglioneuroma in a patient presenting with severe hypertension and diarrhea. Endocr. Rel. Cancer **10:** 99–107.
4. KOCH, C.A. *et al.* 2003. Hypotension in a woman with metastatic dopamine-secreting carotid body tumor. Endocr. Pract. **9:** 310–314.
5. KOCH, C.A. *et al.* 2002. New insights into the genetics of familial chromaffin cell tumors. Ann. N.Y. Acad. Sci. **970:** 11–28.
6. KOCH, C.A. *et al.* 1999. Carcinoid syndrome caused by an atypical carcinoid of the uterine cervix. J. Clin. Endocrinol. Metab. **84:** 4209–4213.
7. YU, J. *et al.* 2004. Ectopic Cushing's syndrome caused by an esthesioneuroblastoma. Endocr. Pract. **10:** 119–124.
8. ARIOGLU, E. *et al.* 2000. Natural history of a proinsulin-secreting insulinom: from symptomatic hypoglycemia to clinical diabetes. J. Clin. Endocrinol. Metab. **85:** 3628–3630.
9. GRANBERG, D. & K. OBERG. 2005. Neuroendocrine tumours. Cancer Chemother. Biol. Response. Modif. **22:** 471–483.
10. PLOCKINGER, U. *et al.* 2004. Guidelines for the diagnosis and treatment of neuroendocrine gastointestinal tumours. A consensus statement on behalf of the European Neuroendocrine Tumour Society (ENETS). Neuroendocrinology **80:** 394–424.
11. KOCH, C.A., K. PACAK, G.P. CHROUSOS. 2005. Endocrine tumors. *In* Principles and Practice of Pediatric oncology, 5th edition. P. Pizzo & D.G. Poplack, Eds. Lippincott Williams & Wilkins. Philadelphia, PA.
12. SOLCIA, E., G. KLOPPEL & L.H. SOBIN. 2000. Histological typing of endocrine tumours, 2nd edition. Springer. Berlin, Heidelberg, New York.
13. OBERG, K. 2001. Chemotherapy and biotherapy in the treatment of neuroendocrine tumours. Ann. Oncol. **12:** S111–S114.
14. CHEN, H. *et al.* 1998. Effective long-term palliation of symptomatic, incurable metastatic medullary thyroid cancer by operative resection. Ann. Surg. **227:** 887–895.
15. ADJEI, A.A. 2005. Targeting multiple signal transduction pathways in lung cancer. Clin. Lung. Cancer **7:** S39–S44.
16. FAVARO, J.P. & D.J. GEORGE. 2005. Targeted therapy in renal cell carcinoma. Expert Opin. Investig. Drugs **14:** 1251–1258.
17. MATSUDA, R. *et al.* 1993. Expression of the c-kit protein in human solid tumors and in corresponding fetal and adult normal tissues. Am. J. Pathol. **142:** 339–346.
18. KOSTOULA, V. *et al.* 2005. Expression of c-kit (CD117) in neuroendocrine tumours-a target for therapy? Oncol. Rep. **13:** 643–647.
19. SHITO, H. *et al.* 2005. Kit and platelet-derived growth factor receptor alpha tyrosine kinase gene mutations and KIT amplifications in human solid tumors. J. Clin. Oncol. **23:** 49–57.
20. WENT, P.T. *et al.* 2004. Prevalence of KIT expression in human tumors. J. Clin. Oncol. **22:** 4514–4522.

21. ZHANG, P.J. *et al.* 2003. The role of calretinin, inhibin, melan-A, BCL-2, and c-kit in differentiating adrenal cortical and medullary tumors: an immunohistochemical study. Mod. Pathol. **16:** 591–597.
22. VITALI, R. *et al.* 2005. c-kit is preferentially expressed in MYCN-amplified neuroblastoma and its effect on cell proliferation is inhibited in vitro by STI-571. Int. J. Cancer **106:** 147–152.
23. UCCINI, S. *et al.* 2005. Clinical and molecular evidence for c-kit receptor as a therapeutic target in neuroblastic tumors. Clin. Cancer. Res. **11:** 380–389.
24. WILCZYNSKI, S.P. *et al.* 2005. Expression and mutational analysis of tyrosine kinase receptors c-kit, PDGFRalpha, and PDGFRbeta in ovarian cancers. Hum. Pathol. **36:** 242–249.
25. KRUG, L.M. *et al.* 2005. Imatinib mesylate lacks activity in small cell lung carcinoma expressing c-kit protein: a phase II clinical trial. Cancer **103:** 2128–2131.
26. LEE, E.S. *et al.* 2005. Occurrence of c-kit positive tumor cells in hepatitis B virus-associated hepatocellular carcinoma. Am. J. Clin. Pathol. **124:** 31–36.
27. KORJA, M. *et al.* 2005. No GIST-type c-kit gain of function mutations in neuroblastic tumours. J. Clin. Pathol. **58:** 762–765.
28. MIETTINEN, M. & J. LASOTA. 2005. KIT (CD117): a review on expression in normal and neoplastic tissues, and mutations and their clinicopathologic correlation. Appl. Immunohistochem. Mol. Morphol. **13:** 205–220.
29. CETIN, N. *et al.* 2005. CD117 expression in glial tumors. J. Neurooncol **75:** 195–202.
30. ZHAO, P. *et al.* 2005. Clinicopathological significance of expression of c-kit protein in neuroendocrine lung carcinoma. Zhonghua. Yi. Xue. Zha. Zhi. **85:** 1526–1529.
31. FJALLSKOG, M.L. *et al.* 2003. Expression of molecular targets for tyrosine kinase receptor antagonists in malignant endocrine pancreatic tumors. Clin. Cancer Res. **9:** 1469–1473.
32. OCHEL, H.J. *et al.* 2005. Effects of imatinib mesylate on adenoid cystic carcinomas. Anticancer Res. **25:** 3659–3664.
33. LANKAT-BUTTGEREIT, B. *et al.* 2005. Effects of the tyrosine kinase inhibitor imatinib on neuroendocrine tumor cell growth. Digestion **71:** 131–140.
34. RACHDI, L. *et al.* 2001. Expression of the receptor tyrosine kinase KIT in mature beta-cells and in the pancreas in development. Diabetes **50:** 2021–2028.
35. CARR, K. *et al.* 2004. A phase II trial of imatinib in patients with advanced carcinoid tumor. J. Clin. Oncol. **22:** 344–348.
36. UGUREL, S. *et al.* 2005. Lack of clinical efficacy of imatinib in metastatic melanoma. Br. J. Cancer **92:** 1398–1405.
37. MODI, S. *et al.* 2005. A phase II trial of imatinib mesylate monotherapy in patients with metastatic breast cancer. Breast Cancer Res. Treat. **90:** 157–163.
38. DY, G.K. *et al.* 2005. A phase II NCCTG/CALGB trial of imatinib in patients with c-kit expressing relapsed small cell lung cancer. Abstract No. 7048. ASCO. Orlando, FL.
39. GRONCHI, A. *et al.* 2005. Surgery of residual disease following imatinib mesylate in advanced gastrointestinal stromal tumors. Abstract No. 9038. American Society of Clinical Oncology. Orlando, FL.
40. BLACKSTEIN, M.E. *et al.* 2005. Clinical benefit of imatinib in patients with metastatic gastrointestinal stromal tumors negative for the expression of CD117 in the S0033 trial. Abstract No. 9010. American Society of Clinical Oncology. Orlando, FL.

41. BROUWERS, F.M. *et al.* 2005. Low molecular weight proteomic information distinguishes metastatic from benign pheochromocytoma. Endocr. Rel. Cancer **12:** 263–272.
42. EISENHOFER, G. *et al.* 2004. Malignant pheochromocytoma: current status and initiatives for future progress. Endocr. Rel. Cancer **11:** 423–436.
43. KOCH, C.A. *et al.* 2002. Survivin: a novel neuroendocrine marker for pheochromocytoma. Eur. J. Endocrinol. **146:** 381–388.
44. VON MEHREN, M. 2005. Targeted therapy with imatinib: hits and misses? J. Clin. Oncol. **23:** 8–10.

Expression and Processing of the Neuroendocrine Protein Secretogranin II in Benign and Malignant Pheochromocytomas

JOHANN GUILLEMOT,[a] LAURE BARBIER,[a] ERWAN THOUENNON,[a] VIRGINIE VALLET-ERDTMANN,[b] MAITE MONTERO-HADJADJE,[a] HERVE LEFEBVRE,[a] MARC KLEIN,[c] MIHAELA MURESAN,[c] PIERRE-FRANÇOIS PLOUIN,[d] NABIL SEIDAH,[e] HUBERT VAUDRY,[a] YOUSSEF ANOUAR,[a] AND LAURENT YON[a]

[a]*INSERM U413, Laboratory of Cellular and Molecular Neuroendocrinology, European Institute for Peptide Research (IFRMP 23), University of Rouen, 76821 Mont-Saint-Aignan, France*

[b]*INSERM U625, University of Rennes I, Rennes, France*

[c]*Department of Endocrinology, Hôpital de Brabois, University of Nancy, Nancy, France*

[d]*Department of Hypertension, Hôpital Européen Georges Pompidou, Paris, France*

[e]*Laboratory of Biochemical Neuroendocrinology, Clinical Research Institute of Montreal, Montreal, Quebec, Canada*

ABSTRACT: The aim of the present study was to compare the expression levels of secretogranin II (SgII), prohormone convertases (PC)1 and PC2, and the proteolytic processing of SgII in benign versus malignant pheochromocytomas. Quantitative (Q)-PCR experiments indicated that SgII, PC1, and PC2 mRNAs were overexpressed in pheochromocytoma compared to non-tumoral chromaffin cells ($P < 0.001$) and in benign compared to malignant tumors ($P < 0.01$). Western blot analysis using a human SgII antiserum revealed the occurrence of a 97-kDa band corresponding to the expected size of SgII, with significantly higher quantities in benign than in malignant tumors ($P < 0.05$). Using antisera directed against sequential regions of SgII (N-terminal, secretoneurin [SN], EM66, internal, and C-terminal sequences), we observed distinct processing profiles between benign and malignant pheochromocytomas. In contrast, using PC1 and PC2 antisera no differences between the two types of tumors were found. RIA measurement showed that EM66

Address for correspondence: Laurent Yon, INSERM U413, Laboratory of Cellular and Molecular Neuroendocrinology, European Institute for Peptide Research (IFRMP23), University of Rouen, 76821 Mont-Saint-Aignan, France. Voice: 33-235-14-6945; fax: 33-235-14-6946.
e-mail: laurent.yon@univ-rouen.fr

Ann. N.Y. Acad. Sci. 1073: 527–532 (2006). © 2006 New York Academy of Sciences.
doi: 10.1196/annals.1353.056

median values between benign and malignant chromaffin cell tumors were significantly different (128.5 vs. 6.3 ng/mg protein, respectively; $P < 0.001$). Taken together, these results indicate that, in pheochromocytoma, malignancy is associated with reduced PC1, PC2, and SgII mRNA expression and decreased levels of processing products of SgII, in line with the low concentrations of EM66 that occur in malignant tumors. These data support the notion that SgII-processing products, such as EM66, could represent prognostic markers of pheochromocytomas.

KEYWORDS: **EM66; pheochromocytoma; proteolytic processing; secretogranin II; malignancy; neuroendocrine tumor**

INTRODUCTION

Chromogranins (Cgs) are a family of soluble proteins present in dense core vesicles of adrenal medullary cells, where they are co-stored and co-released with catecholamines. The major members of this family are chromogranin A, chromogranin B, and SgII.[1] Their primary amino acid sequences are characterized by a high abundance of acidic residues and by the occurrence of multiple pairs of basic residues, which constitute consensus cleavage sites for endoproteases. In fact, as large precursor proteins, Cgs undergo proteolytic processing by prohormone convertases (PCs) to generate bioactive peptides.[2] Although the function of SgII is not yet established, two SgII-derived peptides, that is, secretoneurin (SN) and EM66, have been implicated in the modulation of the inflammatory response[3] and the control of feeding behavior, respectively.[4] The ubiquitous distribution of Cgs in nervous, endocrine, and neuroendocrine tissues makes granins useful markers of normal and tumoral neuroendocrine cells. In particular, measurement of Cg levels can be used to diagnose or monitor the progression of neuroendocrine tumors.[1] Using polyclonal antibodies against SgII and derived fragments of the protein, Vallet *et al.*[5] have shown that SgII represents a valuable marker for nonfunctioning pituitary adenomas and we have demonstrated that low tissue concentrations of the SgII-derived peptide EM66 are associated with malignant differentiation of pheochromocytomas.[6]

The aim of the present study was to compare the mRNA expression levels of SgII, PC1, and PC2 in benign versus malignant pheochromocytomas. We have also investigated the proteolytic processing of SgII using a series of polyclonal antisera directed against different regions of the protein.

MATERIALS AND METHODS

Normal adrenal glands and pheochromocytoma tissue were kept frozen at –80°C until Q-PCR, Western blot analysis, or radioimmunoassay (RIA).[6] After extraction and purification, SgII, PC1, and PC2 mRNA levels relative to glyceraldehyde-3-phosphate dehydrogenase (GAPDH) mRNA level,

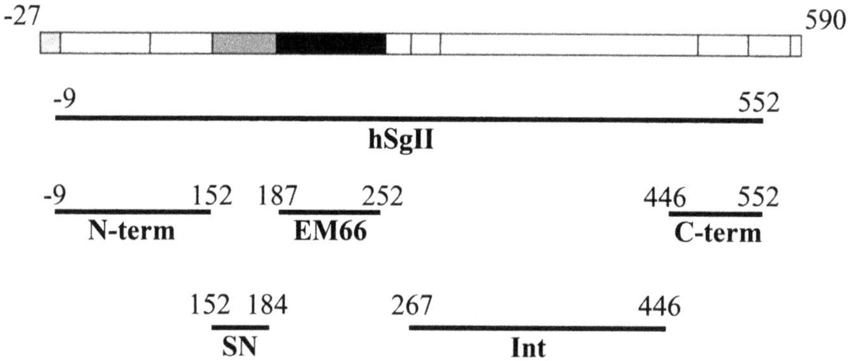

FIGURE 1. Schematic representation of the structure of hSgII. The regions of the protein (with the position of the N- and C-terminal amino acids) against which polyclonal antisera have been produced are indicated. The light gray zone represents the signal peptide; the gray zone, SN, and the black zone, EM66. hSgII, human SgII; N-term, N-terminal region; Int, internal region; C-term, C-terminal region.

were determined by Q-PCR as previously described.[7] Western blot analysis was performed on protein extracts from normal adrenal glands and pheochromocytomas using six different antibodies directed against human SgII (hSgII) (VV493-P), SN (733–145), EM66 (736–1806), N-terminal (N161-S), C-terminal (C107-B), and internal sequences (I180-C) of SgII (FIG. 1).[5,6] EM66 concentrations in benign and malignant tumors were determined by RIA as previously described.[6] Antibodies against PC1 and PC2 were raised in rabbit.[8]

RESULTS AND DISCUSSION

Q-PCR analysis showed that the levels of SgII, PC1, and PC2 mRNAs were significantly lower in normal adrenal glands than in benign ($P < 0.001$) and malignant pheochromocytomas ($P < 0.01$) (FIG. 2). In addition, mRNA expression of SgII, PC1, and PC2 was 3 to 4.5 times higher in benign than in malignant tumors. These results indicate that tumorigenesis of adrenochromaffin cells is associated with increased expression of SgII and PC1/2 mRNAs. In agreement, we have previously shown that SgII mRNA levels are higher in PC12 cells, a rat pheochromocytoma cell line, than in rat adrenomedullary chromaffin cells.[9] The fact that SgII mRNA levels correlate with the differentiation status of tumoral cells (benign vs. malignant) suggests that measurement of the SgII transcript is a potential prognostic tool.

Western blot analysis using the anti-hSgII antiserum revealed the presence of a 97-kDa band corresponding to the size of SgII in normal adrenal glands and pheochromocytomas although the intensity of the band was different (FIG. 3). Indeed, consistent with the observed differences in SgII mRNA levels,

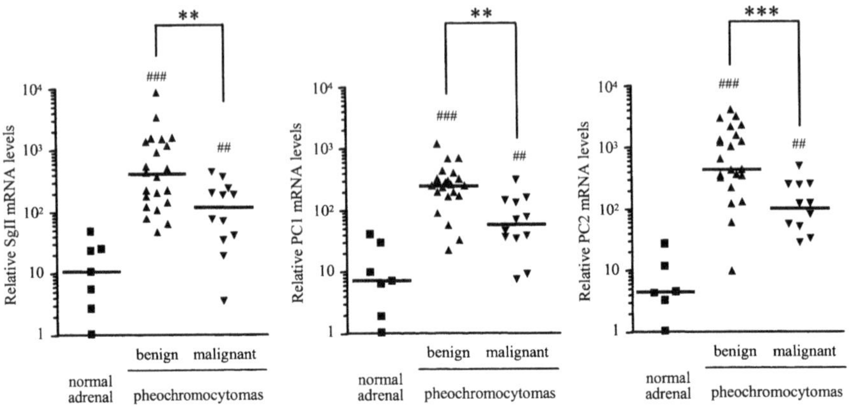

FIGURE 2. Relative SgII, PC1, and PC2 mRNA levels in normal adrenal gland and pheochromocytoma extracts. The *bars* represent the median value for each group. ##, $P < 0.01$; ###, $P < 0.001$ pheochromocytomas versus normal adrenal glands; **, $P < 0.01$; ***, $P < 0.001$ benign versus malignant pheochromocytomas.

significantly higher concentrations of SgII were detected in benign compared to malignant tumors ($P < 0.05$). Several additional immunoreactive bands of lower molecular mass (64, 46, and 31 kDa) were observed, mainly in benign pheochromocytomas (FIG. 3). The 97-kDa band of adrenal glands and chromaffin tumors was recognized by various antisera directed against sequential regions of SgII, except for the C-terminal antiserum. While the 64-kDa band systematically occurred, the 46-kDa band was only revealed by the anti-EM66 and anti-Int antisera and the 31-kDa band by the anti-Int antiserum. These patterns could provide insight into the processing mechanisms of SgII in normal and tumoral chromaffin cells. Whatever the antiserum used, benign and malignant pheochromocytomas exhibited distinct processing profiles, the latter showing fewer immunoreactive bands. Western blot experiments using antisera against PC1 and PC2 showed no significant differences in protein levels between normal adrenal glands, and benign and malignant tumors. In all samples, the antisera detected a 66-kDa band corresponding to the mature form of the enzymes. However, in benign pheochromocytomas, the PC2 antibodies detected an additional band of 75 kDa corresponding to the precursor form of the protein. Taken together, these results indicate that SgII undergoes differential processing in normal versus tumoral, and in benign versus malignant chromaffin cell tumors.

RIA experiments revealed that patients bearing a benign pheochromocytoma ($n = 22$) had EM66 concentrations in the range of 3.2–1221 ng/mg protein with a median value of 117.8 ng/mg protein. The EM66 levels in malignant chromaffin neoplasms ($n = 7$) ranged from 2.9 to 9.7 ng/mg protein with a median value of 6.3 ng/mg protein. Statistical analysis using the nonparametric Mann–Whitney test indicated that the concentration of EM66 in benign tumors

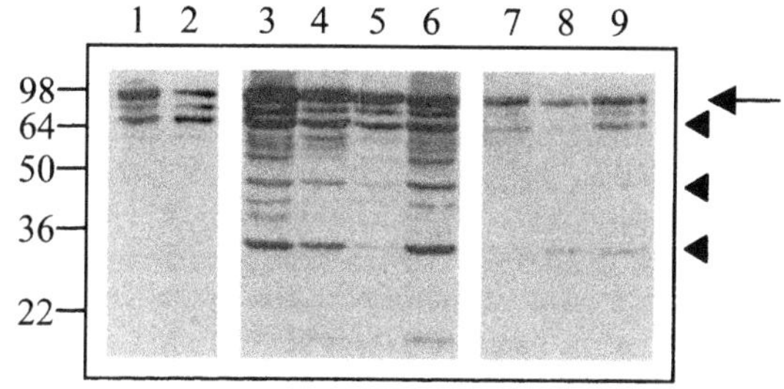

FIGURE 3. Western blot immunodetection of normal adrenal gland (lanes 1–2), and benign (lanes 3–6), and malignant (lanes 7–9) pheochromocytoma extracts using antisera directed against hSgII. The *arrow* indicates the position of hSgII and the *arrowheads* the position of the immunologically related peptides of 64 kDa, 46 kDa, and 31 kDa. Molecular mass markers (in kilodaltons) are indicated on the *left*.

was significantly higher than in malignant tumors ($P < 0.001$). This result is in agreement with the higher SgII mRNA and protein levels and the higher concentrations of processing products of SgII observed in benign compared to malignant pheochromocytomas. These data strengthen our hypothesis that measurement of EM66 concentrations in pheochromocytomas may help to discriminate between benign and malignant tumors.[6]

Taken together, our results indicate that SgII, PC1, and PC2 mRNAs are overexpressed in pheochromocytomas compared to normal chromaffin tissues but with lower expression levels in malignant than in benign tumors. Moreover, malignancy is associated with reduced levels of processing products of SgII, in line with the low concentrations of EM66 measured in malignant pheochromocytomas, thus emphasizing the notion that SgII-derived peptides, notably EM66, may represent valuable prognostic markers of pheochromocytomas.

ACKNOWLEDGMENTS

This work was supported by INSERM (U 413), the European Institute for Peptide Research (IFRMP 23), the COMETE-2 network (Programme Hospitalier de Recherche Clinique AOM-02068), and the Conseil Régional de Haute-Normandie. J.G. is recipient of a fellowship from the Conseil Régional de Haute-Normandie. E.T. is recipient of a fellowship from the Ministry of Research.

REFERENCES

1. TAUPENOT, L., K.L. HARPER & D.T. O'CONNOR. 2003. The chromogranin-secretogranin family. N. Engl. J. Med. **348:** 1134–1149.
2. LASLOP, A., C. WEISS, D. SAVARIA, *et al.* 1998. Proteolytic processing of chromogranin B and secretogranin II by prohormone convertases. J. Neurochem. **70:** 374–383.

3. Wiedermann, C.J. 2000. Secretoneurin: a functional neuropeptide in health and disease. Peptides **21:** 1289–1298.
4. Boutahricht, M., J. Guillemot, M. Montero-Hadjadje, *et al.* 2005. Biochemical characterisation and immunohistochemical localisation of the secretogranin II-derived peptide EM66 in the hypothalamus of the jerboa (*Jaculus orientalis*): modulation by food deprivation. J. Neuroendocrinol. **17:** 372–378.
5. Vallet, V.S., J.Y. Li & J. Duval. 1997. Secretogranin II (SgII) distribution and processing studies in human normal and adenomatous anterior pituitaries using new polyclonal antibodies. Regul. Peptides **86:** 155–163.
6. Yon, L., J. Guillemot, M. Montero, *et al.* 2003. Characterization and localization of the secretogranin II-derived peptide EM66 in pheochromocytomas. EM66 may be a valuable marker for discriminating benign versus malignant tumors. J. Clin. Endocrinol. Metab. **88:** 2579–2585.
7. Falluel-Morel, A., N. Aubert, D. Vaudry, *et al.* 2004. Opposite regulation of the mitochondrial apoptotic pathway by C2-ceramide and PACAP through a MAP-kinase-dependent mechanism in cerebellar granule cells. J. Neurochem. **91:** 1231–1243.
8. Seidah, N.G., M. Marcinkiewicz, S. Benjannet, *et al.* 1991. Cloning and primary sequence of a mouse candidate prohormone convertase PC1 homologous to PC2, Furin, and Kex2: distinct chromosomal localization and messenger RNA distribution in brain and pituitary compared to PC2. Mol. Endocrinol. **5:** 111–122.
9. Grumolato, L., E. Louiset, D. Alexandre, *et al.* 2003. PACAP and NGF regulate common and distinct traits of the sympathoadrenal lineage: effects on electrical properties, gene markers and transcription factors in differentiating PC12 cells. Eur. J. Neurosci. **17:** 71–82.

Development of Novel Tools for the Diagnosis and Prognosis of Pheochromocytoma Using Peptide Marker Immunoassay and Gene Expression Profiling Approaches

YOUSSEF ANOUAR,[a] LAURENT YON,[a] JOHANN GUILLEMOT,[a] ERWAN THOUENNON,[a] LAURE BARBIER,[a] ANNE-PAULE GIMENEZ-ROQUEPLO,[b] JEROME BERTHERAT,[c] HERVE LEFEBVRE,[a] MARC KLEIN,[d] MIHAELA MURESAN,[d] ERIC GROUZMANN,[e] PIERRE-FRANÇOIS PLOUIN,[f] HUBERT VAUDRY,[a] AND ABDEL G. ELKAHLOUN[g]

[a]*INSERM U413, Laboratory of Cellular and Molecular Neuroendocrinology, European Institute for Peptide Research (IFRMP 23), University of Rouen, Mont-Saint-Aignan, France*

[b]*Department of Genetics, Hôpital Européen Georges Pompidou, Paris, France*

[c]*Department of Endocrinology, INSERM U567, Institut Cochin, Paris, France*

[d]*Department of Endocrinology, Hôpital de Brabois, Nancy, France*

[e]*Division of Clinical Pharmacology and Toxicology, CHU Vaudois, Lausanne, Switzerland*

[f]*Hypertension Unit, Hôpital Européen Georges Pompidou, Paris, France*

[g]*Genome Technology Branch, NHGRI, NIH, Bethesda, USA*

ABSTRACT: Pheochromocytomas (PHEOs) are rare catecholamine-producing neoplasias that arise from chromaffin cells of the adrenal medulla or from extra-adrenal locations. These neuroendocrine tumors are usually benign, but may also present as or develop into a malignancy. There are currently no means to predict or to cure malignant tumors which have a poor prognosis. We have recently validated several assays for the measurement of peptides derived from chromogranin A (CgA) and secretogranin II (SgII) in order to determine whether these secreted neuroendocrine products could provide useful, complementary markers for the diagnosis and prognosis of PHEOs. Both the CgA-derived peptide WE14 and the SgII-derived peptide EM66 proved to be sensitive

Address for correspondence: Youssef Anouar, INSERM U413, Laboratory of Cellular and Molecular Neuroendocrinology, European Institute for Peptide Research (IFRMP23), University of Rouen, 76821 Mont-Saint-Aignan, France. Voice: 33-235-14-6661; fax: 33-235-14-6946.
e-mail: youssef.anouar@univ-rouen.fr

**Ann. N.Y. Acad. Sci. 1073: 533–540 (2006). © 2006 New York Academy of Sciences.
doi: 10.1196/annals.1353.057**

circulating markers for the diagnosis of PHEO. In addition, much higher EM66 levels were measured in benign than in malignant tumoral tissues, suggesting that this peptide could represent a valuable tool for the prognosis of PHEO. We have also initiated a comparative microarray study of benign and malignant PHEOs, which allowed the identification of a set of about 100 genes that were differentially expressed and best discriminated the two types of tumors. A large majority of these genes were expressed at lower levels in the malignant disease and were associated with various characteristics of chromaffin cells, such as hormone secretion signaling and machinery, peptide maturation, and cellular morphology. Altogether, these studies provide novel tools for the management of PHEO, and new insights for the understanding of tumorigenesis in chromaffin cells, which may offer potential therapeutic strategies.

Keywords: chromogranin A; expression profiling; markers; peptide; secretogranin II; pheochromocytoma

INTRODUCTION

Pheochromocytomas (PHEOs) are chromaffin cell tumors characterized by excessive production and release of catecholamines that generally provoke paroxysmal or sustained hypertension with potentially lethal cardiovascular effects. These tumors usually occur in the adrenal gland but may also arise from diffuse chromaffin tissue with a more aggressive phenotype.[1] Although most PHEOs are sporadic, familial tumors due to mutations of oncogenes and oncosuppressors including RET, VHL, NF1, and succinate dehydrogenase (SDH) genes are increasingly recognized.[2]

The diagnosis of PHEO has significantly improved during the last years with the introduction of sensitive and specific biochemical tests, such as measurements of the concentrations of plasma and urinary catecholamines (epinephrine and norepinephrine) and catecholamine metabolites (metanephrine and normetanephrine) produced by the tumor.[3] It is now well established that determination of plasma or urinary metanephrines provides better diagnostic results than catecholamines and represents the test of choice for the diagnosis of PHEO.[2,3] Although these tests are highly accurate for the diagnosis of a tumor, false-positive and false-negative results are still observed and remain a problem since PHEO is a life-threatening disease if left untreated. Besides, malignancy of PHEO is another major problem because malignant tumors can be diagnosed only after metastasis. There is no histological or biochemical means to predict or to evidence malignant disease that has a poor clinical outcome.

Using two different approaches based on peptide immunoassay and gene expression profiling, the present studies were designed with the aim of characterizing novel molecular markers of benign and malignant PHEO, and to provide clinicians with useful and reliable tools to improve the diagnosis and evaluate the prognosis of these tumors. In addition, such studies may also uncover targets for therapeutic treatment of PHEO.

MATERIALS AND METHODS

Sample Collection

Blood samples from healthy volunteers (HV) and PHEO patients were collected, and tumoral tissues were provided by a French network for collection of adrenal tumors (COMETE-2 network, PHRC AOM-02068) and by the Rouen, Nancy, and Lausanne University Hospital centers. After collection, samples were kept frozen at –80°C.

Radioimmunoassays

The concentrations of EM66 and WE14 in serum and tissues were measured by RIA as previously described.[4–6] EM66 and WE14 antisera, raised in rabbits and used at a final dilution of 1:48,000 and 1:280,000, respectively, were incubated with 7,000 cpm of tracer/tube in the presence of graded concentrations of standards (EM66 and WE14), serum or tissue samples. After a 2-day incubation at 4°C, the antibody-bound fraction was immunoprecipitated by addition of 200 μL goat anti-rabbit γ-globulins (1:30), 200 μL normal rabbit serum (1:150), and 1 mL of 5% polyethyleneglycol 8000. After centrifugation, the pellets were counted.

Microarray Analysis

Total RNA was extracted from each tumor using the Tri-reagent (Sigma-Aldrich, Saint-Quentin Fallavier, France) and further purified on RNeasy mini-columns (Qiagen, Courtaboeuf, France). RNA was labeled by reverse transcription in the presence of Cy3 or Cy5 fluor-dUTP (Amersham Pharmacia Biotech, Les Ulis, France). The labeled cDNAs were hybridized to a microarray containing oligonucleotides (Qiagen) that correspond to approximately 24,400 nonredundant human genes.[7] Each microarray slide was hybridized with labeled cDNAs made from a tumor and reference cDNAs prepared from human normal adrenal medulla. Hybridized microarrays were scanned and the resulting images of fluorescence were filtered, analyzed, and quantitated using the DeArray algorithm (Scanalytics, Fairfax, USA). Statistical analysis was performed using the JMPδ statistical package (SAS, Inc. http://affylims.cit.nih.gov). Hierarchical clustering of the data was carried out using the Cluster and Tree View software. Functional distribution of the genes differentially expressed between benign and malignant PHEO was based on gene annotations provided by Gene Ontology (http://www.geneontology.org).

RESULTS AND DISCUSSION

In addition to producing catecholamines, PHEOs are known to produce and release various peptides and proteins. Among these, chromogranins (Cgs) are a family of acidic proteins whose major members are chromogranin A (CgA), chromogranin B, and secretogranin II (SgII).[8] These proteins are co-stored and co-secreted with catecholamines in normal and tumoral chromaffin cells, and have been therefore proposed as potential markers for the diagnosis of PHEO.[8] We have recently characterized several novel peptides derived from the intravesicular proteolytic processing of Cgs that also occur in PHEO.[4–6,9] Using polyclonal antibodies raised against EM66 and WE14, two peptides derived from SgII and CgA, respectively, we found that circulating levels of these peptides were significantly higher in PHEO patients compared to HVs (FIG. 1). Thus, preoperative plasma EM66 concentration was 5-fold higher than the concentration measured in the group of HVs ((11.8 [5.8–27.4]) vs. 2.6 [1.9–3.7] ng/mL, $P < 0.001$) (FIG. 1A). Similarly, the median preoperative value of WE14 was about 4-fold higher than the median value determined in HVs (3.7 ng/mL vs. 1 ng/mL, $P < 0.001$) (FIG. 1B). It is noteworthy that measurement of metanephrines in PHEO patients included in the present study, who all had higher EM66 levels relative to control values, yielded one false-negative result.[10] Although the sensitivity of chromogranin peptide measurement remains to be determined in larger cohorts, these data show that determination of the concentrations of peptides, such as EM66 or WE14, based on simple and highly sensitive immunologic assays, may represent a valuable supplementary tool for the diagnosis of PHEO.

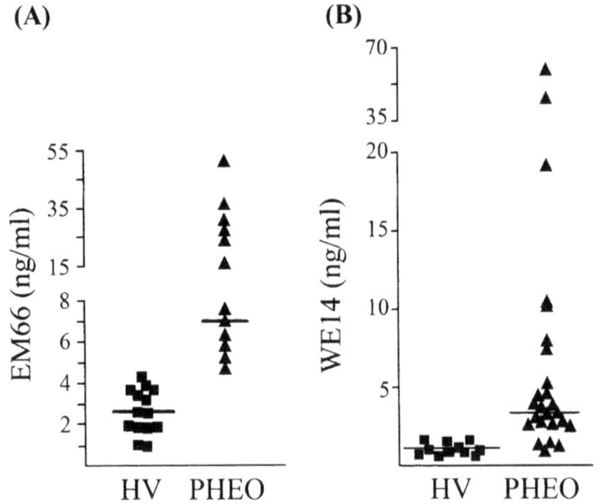

FIGURE 1. Scattergrams of EM66 (**A**) and WE14 (**B**) concentrations in plasma of healthy volunteers (HV) and patients with pheochromocytoma (PHEO). The *bars* represent the median value for each group.

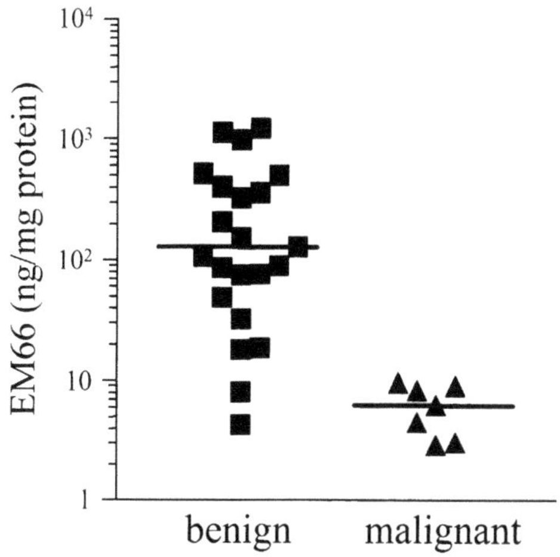

FIGURE 2. Scattergram of EM66 concentrations in tissue extracts from benign and malignant PHEO. The *bars* represent the median value for each group.

We have also measured the concentrations of EM66 in 22 benign and 7 malignant PHEO tissues and found that the concentrations of this marker are several-fold higher in benign than in malignant tumors (118 ng/mg protein vs. 6.3 ng/mg protein, $P < 0.001$) (FIG. 2), suggesting that EM66 measurement may allow discrimination between benign and malignant PHEO, and thus may also serve as a prognostic tool. Together, these results confirm our previous observations,[6] and highlight the relevance of the examination of chromogranin-derived peptides, notably EM66, as a means for the detection of PHEO and for prediction of malignancy.

The other approach that we have undertaken for a more general appreciation of the genetic programs underlying tumoral progression in PHEO is the analysis of the transcriptome of benign and malignant tumors. The ability to define different cancer states, recurrence of disease, and response to therapies using microarray-based gene expression profiling has been demonstrated in multiple studies.[11] Transcriptome analysis using a microarray containing about 34,000 human gene probes allowed identification of a set of about 100 genes that were differentially expressed ($P < 0.001$, Student's *t*-test) and that could blindly discriminate between nine benign and nine malignant PHEOs. A vast majority of these genes is overexpressed in benign PHEO and about a third of them had no known function (FIG. 3). Among the genes whose expression was repressed in malignant tumors are those implicated in vesicular trafficking, peptide maturation, or catecholamine metabolism, suggesting that malignancy is associated with a loss or a reduction in the expression of various traits of the neuroendocrine phenotype. This finding implies that neuroendocrine features are probably maintained in benign tumors, and indicates that transformation of chromaffin cells is accompanied by a dedifferentiation process.

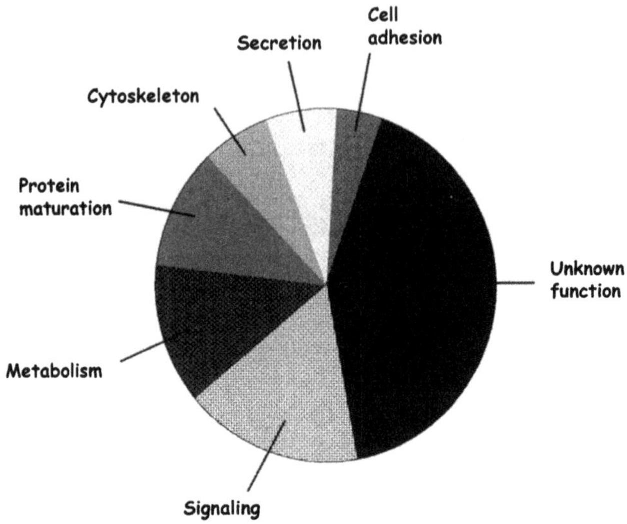

FIGURE 3. Functional classification of the genes differentially expressed between malignant and benign PHEO based on Gene Ontology database.

Conversely, among the few genes whose expression is enhanced in malignant PHEO is that encoding the cytoskeleton protein γ tubulin, a constituent of centrosomes that is overexpressed in different cancers. Enhanced expression of γ tubulin was associated with aberrant organization of the mitotic spindle and abnormal chromosomal distribution in tumoral cells.[12] The genes encoding the cytokine granulocyte-macrophage colony-stimulating factor 2 (GM-CSF2) and the interleukin 2 receptor γ subunit were also overexpressed in malignant tumors. Interestingly, GM-CSF2 and IL2, which enhance the anti-tumoral immune response, have been used in immunotherapy for the treatment of different metastatic tumors including colorectal carcinoma, melanoma, and renal cell carcinoma.[13] Collectively, these data indicate that gene expression profiling of benign and malignant PHEO could provide insights into the mechanisms of tumorigenesis in chromaffin cells which may lead to the discovery of highly discriminating markers of PHEO subtypes, and ultimately offer perspectives on possible therapeutic interventions to combat this cancer.

In conclusion, our studies using peptide marker immunoassays and transcriptome analysis in benign and malignant PHEO have uncovered novel peptide and gene markers that could be useful for the diagnosis and prognosis of this tumor. In addition, the characterization of the molecular signature of PHEO subtypes may provide unsuspected clues to better understand the course of malignancy and, consequently, to devise new therapeutic strategies that may attenuate or cure this disease.

ACKNOWLEDGMENTS

This work was supported by INSERM (U 413), the European Institute for Peptide Research (IFRMP 23), the COMETE-2 network (Programme Hospitalier de Recherche Clinique AOM-02068), the Conseil Régional de Haute-Normandie, and the Fédération des Maladies Orphelines. J.G. is recipient of a fellowship from the Conseil Régional de Haute-Normandie. E.T. is recipient of a fellowship from the Ministry of Research.

REFERENCES

1. Amar, L., A. Servais, A.P. Gimenez-Roqueplo, *et al.* 2005. Year of diagnosis, features at presentation, and risk of recurrence in patients with pheochromocytoma or secreting paraganglioma. J. Clin. Endocrinol. Metab. **90:** 2110–2116.
2. Bertherat, J. & A.P. Gimenez-Roqueplo. 2005. New insights in the genetics of adrenocortical tumors, pheochromocytomas and paragangliomas. Horm. Metab. Res. **37:** 384–390.
3. Lenders, J.W., G. Eisenhofer, M. Mannelli & K. Pacak. 2005. Pheochromocytoma. Lancet **366:** 665–675.
4. Anouar, Y., C. Desmoucelles, L. Yon, *et al.* 1998. Identification of a novel secretogranin II-derived peptide [SgII(187- 252)] in adult and fetal human adrenal glands using antibodies raised against the human recombinant peptide. J. Clin. Endocrinol. Metab. **83:** 2944–2951.
5. Montero-Hadjadje, M., H. Vaudry, V. Turquier, *et al.* 2002. Localization and characterization of evolutionarily conserved chromogranin A-derived peptides in the rat and human pituitary and adrenal glands. Cell Tiss. Res. **310:** 223–236.
6. Yon, L., J. Guillemot, M. Montero-Hadjadje, *et al.* 2003. Characterization and localization of the secretogranin II-derived peptide EM66 in pheochromocytomas. EM66 may be a valuable marker for discriminating benign versus malignant tumors. J. Clin. Endocrinol. Metab. **88:** 2579–2585.
7. Grumolato, L., A.G. Elkahloun, H. Ghzili, *et al.* 2003. Microarray and suppression subtractive hybridization analyses of gene expression in pheochromocytoma cells reveal pleiotropic effects of pituitary adenylate cyclase-activating polypeptide on cell proliferation, survival, and adhesion. Endocrinology **144:** 2368–2379.
8. Taupenot, L., K.L. Harper & D.T. O'Connor. 2003. The chromogranin-secretogranin family. N. Engl. J. Med. **348:** 1134–1149.
9. Turquier, V., H. Vaudry, S. Jegou & Y. Anouar. 1999. Frog chromogranin A messenger ribonucleic acid encodes three highly conserved peptides. Coordinate regulation of proopiomelanocortin and chromogranin A gene expression in the pars intermedia of the pituitary during background color adaptation. Endocrinology **140:** 4104–4112.
10. Guillemot, J., Y. Anouar, M. Montero-Hadjadje, *et al.* 2005. Circulating EM66 is a highly sensitive marker for the diagnosis and follow-up of pheochromocytoma. Int. J. Cancer **118:** 2003–2012.

11. Ramaswamy, S. & T.R. Golub. 2002. DNA microarrays in clinical oncology. J. Clin. Oncol. **20:** 1932–1941.
12. Kronenwett, U., S. Huwendiek, J. Castro, *et al.* 2005. Characterisation of breast fine-needle aspiration biopsies by centrosome aberrations and genomic instability. Br. J. Cancer **92:** 389–395.
13. Eklund, J.W. & K.M. Kuzel. 2004. A review of recent findings involving interleukin-2-based cancer therapy. Curr. Opin. Oncol. **16:** 542–546.

Gene Expression Profiling of Benign and Malignant Pheochromocytoma

FREDERIEKE M. BROUWERS,[a] ABDEL G. ELKAHLOUN,[b] PETER J. MUNSON,[c] GRAEME EISENHOFER,[d] JENNIFER BARB,[c] W. MARSTON LINEHAN,[e] JACQUES W.M. LENDERS,[f] RONALD DE KRIJGER,[g] MASSIMO MANNELLI,[h] ROBERT UDELSMAN,[i] IDRIS T. OCAL,[i] BARRY L. SHULKIN,[j] STEFAN R. BORNSTEIN,[k] JAN BREZA,[l] LUCIA KSINANTOVA,[l] AND KAREL PACAK[a]

[a]*Reproductive Biology and Medicine Branch, National Institute of Child Health and Human Development, National Institutes of Health, Bethesda, Maryland 20892, USA*

[b]*Genome Technology Branch, National Human Genome Research Institute, National Institutes of Health, Bethesda, Maryland 20892, USA*

[c]*Mathematical and Statistical Computing Laboratory, Center for Information Technology, National Institutes of Health, Bethesda, Maryland 20892, USA*

[d]*Clinical Neurocardiology Section, National Institute of Neurological Disorders and Stroke, National Institutes of Health, Bethesda, Maryland 20892, USA*

[e]*Urologic Oncology Branch, Center for Cancer Research, National Cancer Institute, National Institutes of Health, Bethesda, Maryland 20892, USA*

[f]*Department of Internal Medicine, St. Radboud University Hospital, Nijmegen, the Netherlands*

[g]*Department of Pathology, Josephine Nefkens Institute, Erasmus MC–University Medical Center, 3000 DR Rotterdam, the Netherlands*

[h]*Department of Clinical Pathophysiology, University of Florence, Florence, Italy*

[i]*Departments of Surgery and Pathology, Yale University, New Haven, Connecticut 06520, USA*

[j]*Department of Radiological Sciences, St. Jude Children's Research Hospital, Memphis, Tennessee 38105, USA*

[k]*Department of Medicine, University of Dresden, Dresden, Germany*

[l]*Department of Urology, Comenius University and PET Center, BIONT, Bratislava, Slovak Republic for the Pheochromocytoma Research Support Organization (PRESSOR), Slovak Republic*

Address for correspondence: Karel Pacak, M.D., Ph.D., D.Sc., Reproductive Biology and Medicine Branch, National Institute of Child Health and Human Development, National Institutes of Health, Building 10, CRC, Room 1E-1-3140, 10 Center Drive, MSC-1109, Bethesda, MD 20892-1109, USA. Voice: 301-402-4594; fax: 301-402-4712.
e-mail: karel@mail.nih.gov

Ann. N.Y. Acad. Sci. 1073: 541–556 (2006). © 2006 New York Academy of Sciences.
doi: 10.1196/annals.1353.058

ABSTRACT: There are currently no reliable diagnostic and prognostic markers or effective treatments for malignant pheochromocytoma. This study used oligonucleotide microarrays to examine gene expression profiles in pheochromocytomas from 90 patients, including 20 with malignant tumors, the latter including metastases and primary tumors from which metastases developed. Other subgroups of tumors included those defined by tissue norepinephrine compared to epinephrine contents (i.e., noradrenergic versus adrenergic phenotypes), adrenal versus extra-adrenal locations, and presence of germline mutations of genes predisposing to the tumor. Correcting for the confounding influence of noradrenergic versus adrenergic catecholamine phenotype by the analysis of variance revealed a larger and more accurate number of genes that discriminated benign from malignant pheochromocytomas than when the confounding influence of catecholamine phenotype was not considered. Seventy percent of these genes were underexpressed in malignant compared to benign tumors. Similarly, 89% of genes were underexpressed in malignant primary tumors compared to benign tumors, suggesting that malignant potential is largely characterized by a less-differentiated pattern of gene expression. The present database of differentially expressed genes provides a unique resource for mapping the pathways leading to malignancy and for establishing new targets for treatment and diagnostic and prognostic markers of malignant disease. The database may also be useful for examining mechanisms of tumorigenesis and genotype–phenotype relationships. Further progress on the basis of this database can be made from follow-up confirmatory studies, application of bioinformatics approaches for data mining and pathway analyses, testing in pheochromocytoma cell culture and animal model systems, and retrospective and prospective studies of diagnostic markers.

KEYWORDS: pheochromocytoma; paraganglioma; gene expression; microarray; metastases; catecholamines

INTRODUCTION

Pheochromocytomas are rare catecholamine-producing neuroendocrine tumors with diverse clinical presentations and phenotypes depending on the interplay of numerous factors, including genetics, tumor location, and type of catecholamine produced.[1] Most are benign solitary tumors arising from adrenal medullary chromaffin tissue or more occasionally from extra-adrenal chromaffin tissue, where they are defined as paragangliomas. For these, treatment by surgical resection is relatively straightforward and usually curative. An important proportion of tumors, however, presents as or develops into metastatic disease. For these there is invariably no cure. There are also no pathological markers to reliably distinguish malignant from benign disease or to predict malignant tendency of a resected primary mass. Definitive diagnosis of malignant pheochromocytoma continues to rely on identification of metastases at non-chromaffin sites (e.g., liver, bones, and lungs) distant from that of the primary tumor.[1]

Although there remains a lack of pathological markers for malignant disease, several interdependent factors are now identified to be associated with increased risk for malignancy. Most malignant tumors produce predominantly norepinephrine (noradrenergic biochemical phenotype), in contrast to 50% of solitary adrenal tumors that produce a mixture of both norepinephrine and epinephrine (adrenergic biochemical phenotype).[2] Extra-adrenal tumors are almost always characterized by a noradrenergic phenotype and have a relatively high risk of malignancy.[3,4] More recently, germline mutations of the succinate dehydrogenase subunit B (SDHB) gene were identified to be associated with both high rates of extra-adrenal tumor locations and malignant disease.[5,6] This contrasts with other hereditary syndromes, such as multiple endocrine neoplasia type 2 (MEN 2) and von Hippel–Lindau (VHL) syndrome, both associated with low rates of malignancy, the former characterized by an adrenergic phenotype and predominantly adrenal tumors and the latter by a noradrenergic phenotype with both adrenal and extra-adrenal paragangliomas.[7]

In the present study we used oligonucleotide microarray analysis to examine gene expression profiles in a large series of benign and malignant pheochromocytomas with carefully characterized locations, hereditary or sporadic backgrounds, and catecholamine phenotypes. The study used sophisticated statistical approaches involving multiple comparisons—taking into account catecholamine biochemical phenotypes, hereditary factors, and tumor location—to establish differences in gene expression between benign and malignant pheochromocytoma. The ultimate goals of these comparisons are to establish the molecular pathways involved in malignant transformation, identify targets for new treatments, and develop new diagnostic markers for predicting malignant potential. This initial report, rather than addressing the aforementional goals, provides a description of the methods and design of the analyses, with reporting of results restricted to a general overview of global differences in gene expression for each of the numerous comparisons of the study.

MATERIALS AND METHODS

Tumor Procurement

Tumor specimens were collected from patients who underwent surgery at several centers: National Institutes of Health, Bethesda, MD; Yale University, New Haven, CT; University of Michigan, Ann Arbor, MI; and at several European university hospitals (Dresden, Germany; Florence, Italy; Nijmegen and Rotterdam, the Netherlands; and Bratislava, Slovak Republic). Specimens were procured under Institutional Review Board–approved protocols compliant with international guidelines with informed consent from patients.

Tumor samples were frozen and stored at –80°C shortly after surgical resection. Total RNA was extracted from tumors using a standard Trizol preparation protocol (Life Technologies, Inc. Rockville, MD). Quality and quantity of RNA were sufficient for gene expression profiling in 103 tumors from 93 patients. Five tumors (seven slides, as two tumors were done in duplicate) were excluded on account of poor array spot quality ($n = 4$) or inability to classify a tumor as metastatic or recurrent ($n = 1$). Consequently, the final analysis was on the basis of 98 tumors collected from 90 patients (46 female, 42 male, and 2 unknown), including 20 patients with metastatic disease and 70 patients with benign disease. The majority of tumors came from patients with apparently sporadic pheochromocytoma, but the study set also includes tumors from 12 VHL, 12 MEN 2A (one with metastatic disease), 5 SDHB (three with metastatic disease), 4 SDHD patients, and 1 neurofibromato type 1 patient. Multiple tumors were included from three patients, including two with two separate extra-adrenal tumors each, and one patient with seven abdominal metastatic lesions.

Tumor Catecholamines

Tumor tissue concentrations of catecholamines (norepinephrine, epinephrine, and dopamine) were quantified by liquid chromatography with electrochemical detection.[8] Samples of tumor tissue were weighed frozen and homogenized in 5 to 10 volumes of 0.4 M perchloric acid containing 0.5 mM EDTA. Homogenates were centrifuged and supernatants collected for catecholamine determinations.

Oligonucleotide Microarrays

Microarray slides were generated from 34,580 longmer oligonucleotide probes obtained from the Human Genome Oligonucleotide Set Version 3.0 from Qiagen Inc. (Valencia, CA, USA). Each 70 basepair oligomer was sequence-optimized to represent a specific gene using BLAST (Basic Local Alignment Search Tool) for nucleotide sequence to minimize cross-hybridization with other genes. The set represented over 26,121 unique Refseq genes, over 24,048 unique Ensembl genes, and over 25,416 unique Unigene genes. The set also contained 12 unique positive controls (housekeeping genes) and 12 unique negative controls (random sequence) provided in 16 replicates. The gene description and annotation of these oligonucleotides were based on the Ensembl database dated from February 2005.

Dried oligonucleotides were resuspended in $3 \times$ SSC solution and spotted on epoxy-coated slides. The slides were then cleaned by vigorous shaking in a 0.5% SDS solution for 2 min and incubated for 20 min in water at 50°C. The slides were finally air-dried by centrifugation and ready for hybridization.

Probe Labeling and Hybridization

The detailed protocols for probe labeling and hybridization are available through the website: http://research.nhgri.nih.gov/nhgri_cores/microarray.html. In brief: 5 μg of each total RNA sample or 150 ng of human normal adrenal medulla polyA reference (Cat. 637451, BD Biosciences Clontech, Palo Alto, CA, USA) was reverse-transcribed with random hexamers in the presence of 5-(3-aminoallyl)-dUTP. After purification, the cDNAs are coupled with either Cy3 or Cy5 for 1 h and then purified using the PCR cleaning kit from Qiagen. Labeled cDNAs were then hybridized to the slides in a 1 × final *in situ* hybridization buffer from Agilent Technologies (Agilent Technologies, Palo Alto, CA, USA). The hybridization was performed overnight at 60°C in a rotisserie oven. The slides are then washed in a series of SSC/SDS buffers and dried by centrifugation.

Scanning and Image Analysis

A laser confocal scanner from Agilent Technologies was used to scan the hybridized Cy3 and Cy5 probes on the chips. The fluorescent intensities at the spot and nearby background locations on the array were measured using the DEARRAY software (http://www.scanalytics.com). For each spot, a quality indicator (was greater than 100 fluorescent units, spot size greater than 50 units) was recorded.

Clinical Characteristics for Data Analysis

Data were analyzed according to a series of comparisons on the basis of the hypothesis that gene expression profiles would differ according to multiple variables, including benign versus malignant potential, location of primary tumors and metastases, catecholamine biochemical phenotype, and presence of any underlying germline mutation.

Malignant disease was defined on the basis of the occurrence of metastases at sites where chromaffin cells are normally absent (e.g., liver, lungs, and bones). Tumor samples in patients with malignant disease included metastases and primary tumors from which metastases developed, the latter with both adrenal and extra-adrenal locations. Tumors were classified as benign if there was no evidence of metastases at resection, care being taken to distinguish multifocal paragangliomas from true metastatic lesions at nonchromaffin locations. Tumors were classified as having a noradrenergic versus an adrenergic catecholamine phenotype according to the relative tissue concentrations of norepinephrine and epinephrine, as described elsewhere.[9] The presence of a relevant disease-causing germline mutation was confirmed by analysis of genomic DNA for mutations of the SDHB, SDHD, VHL, and RET genes.

TABLE 1. Study comparisons

	Tumors (n)	Patients (n)
Series 1—Focus on malignant disease		
1. Metastatic versus benign tumors		
Metastatic	20	20
Benign	71	69
Total	91	89
2. Metastatic versus benign tumors with consideration of biochemical profile		
Metastatic	16	16
Noradrenergic	12	12
Adrenergic	4	4
Benign	61	60
Noradrenergic	33	32
Adrenergic	28	28
Total	77	76
3. Metastatic versus benign tumors with consideration of SDHB mutation status		
Metastatic	10	8
SDHB+	5	3
SDHB –	5	5
Benign	17	16
SDHB+	3	2
SDHB –	14	14
Total	27	24
4. Metastatic primary versus benign tumors		
Metastatic	8	8
Benign	24	23
Total	32	31
5. Metastases versus metastatic primary tumors		
Metastases	8	8
Primary	10	10
Total	18	18
6. Metastatic adrenal-derived versus metastatic PGG-derived tumors		
PGG	7	7
Adrenal	9	9
Total	16	16
Series 2—Focus on influences of hereditary factors and biochemical profiles		
A. MEN 2A versus VHL tumors		
MEN 2A	10	10
VHL	12	12
Total	22	22
B. Sporadic adrenergic versus noradrenergic tumors		
Adrenergic	16	16
Noradrenergic	17	17
Total	33	33
C. Relationships of gene expression with tumor epinephrine content	87	80
D. VHL versus SDHB tumors		
VHL	12	12
SDHB	6	5
Total	18	17

PGG-paraganglioma.

Study Comparisons

Study comparisons were divided into two series, with numbers of samples in each comparison dependent on the availability of clinical data required for defining the various groups of that comparison (TABLE 1). The first and major series of comparisons was directed at defining sets of genes involved in malignant transformation. This series comprised six comparisons: (1) metastatic versus benign tumors (all tumors included with no consideration of biochemical profile, underlying mutation, tumor location, or nature of malignancy as a primary malignant tumor or a metastatic lesion); (2) metastatic versus benign tumors with additional consideration of adrenergic versus noradrenergic biochemical profile by two-way analysis of variance (ANOVA) [but no consideration of underlying mutation, tumor location, or nature of malignancy as a metastatic lesion or a primary malignant tumor]; (3) metastatic versus benign tumors with additional consideration of SDHB mutation status by two-way ANOVA (confined to noradrenergic tumors from patients tested positive or negative for SDHB mutations and without VHL, RET, or SDHD mutations); (4) metastatic primary versus benign tumors (confined to malignant primary and benign noradrenergic tumors from patients without VHL, RET, or SDHD mutations); (5) metastatic primary tumors versus distant metastatic lesions (all involving different patients); and (6) metastatic paraganglioma-derived versus metastatic adrenal-derived tumors.

The second series of analyses was directed at defining sets of genes critical to the adrenergic versus noradrenergic phenotype or differentially expressed according to underlying mutations of VHL, RET, and SDHB genes. This series also served as a positive control, building on a similar series of comparisons carried out in a previous cDNA microarray study.[10] The series comprised three comparisons and one analysis by linear regression: (A) MEN 2A versus VHL tumors (excluding malignant tumors); (B) sporadic adrenergic versus sporadic noradrenergic tumors (excluding malignant tumors); (C) relationships of gene expression with tumor epinephrine content by linear regression analysis; and (D) VHL versus SDHB tumors.

Statistical Analysis

Image data for each chip were reduced to intensity values for the test and reference channels and quality indicators for each spot, as described above. Data were then normalized between chips. Only spots achieving the highest quality score (1.0) for all chips were included in the subsequent analysis. Quantile normalization was applied separately to intensities from each channel to adjust for chip-to-chip variation in responsivity. An adaptive, variance-stabilizing transform was then applied to each channel to establish a measurement scale in which the variance was uniform. This transformation (denoted as the "symmetric adaptive transform") has been extensively and successfully used with single-channel oligonucleotide microarray data as an effective alternative to median-adjusted-log10-transform, to control for variation between chip responsiveness. We here extend it in a novel application to two-channel microarray data. Differences between transformed intensities for each channel were then computed for each spot and chip, yielding the relative intensity index used in subsequent analysis.

Quality Control, Printing Batch, and Lot Effects

Transformed intensity data from the two channels on each chip were found to be highly correlated ($R > 0.9$), as expected. Six chips with unusually low correlation values (R between 0.83 and 0.89), indicating possible problems with mRNA quality in one or the other channel, image registration, or scanning, were marked as outliers and dropped from the study. Transformed intensities were also subjected to a principal-components analysis (PCA), to further scan for potential outliers and other data artifacts. The six chips identified with low R values also appeared as outliers on the first principal component. Chips were printed in two separate batches, and reference RNA was obtained in six distinct lots. Plots of the first 10 principal components versus the sequence number of each chip revealed a clear batch and lot effect, necessitating the use of batch-corrected analysis subsequently.

ANOVA with Batch Correction

Data were analyzed in reference to each of the study comparisons using a one- or two-way ANOVA, with blocking. Two-way ANOVA is valuable when a confounding factor is known to influence the outcome variable, such as the greater incidence of noradrenergic tumors among malignancies. Both the confounding factor (noradrenergic status) and the factor of interest (malignant vs. benign) can be accounted for by entering both into a two-way ANOVA. Variation due to the six identified print batch or reagent lots (block effect) was removed before the study comparison was addressed using a blocked ANOVA. In some cases, a patient sample was hybridized to multiple chips. Rather than simply averaging the chip intensities, which would have confounded the batch correction, each replicate chip was given a fractional weight, inversely proportional to the number of replicate chips used. Thus, identical, unit statistical weight was applied to each unique sample. Significance values, direction, and magnitude of differential expression were computed for each gene (spot), for each comparison, and genes with $P < 0.001$ were reported in separate gene lists. False-discovery rate values (estimated number of false detection divided by total genes detected) were calculated for each comparison.

Gene Ontology Analysis

The functional distribution of the differentially expressed genes was established on the basis of the annotation provided by the gene ontology (GO) database (http://www.geneontology.org). Numbers of genes per GO term category were analyzed to detect disproportionate numbers of genes using the following formula for a hypergeometric distribution: $P = \Pr(X \geq x \mid N, K, n)$, where x is the number of genes with the GO term per comparison, N is the total number of genes in the database with any GO annotation, K is the total number of genes in database with the specific GO term, and n is the number of genes with any GO annotation per comparison. Statistical significance was defined by a P value less than 0.05 using Fisher's exact test.

RESULTS

Series 1: Malignant Pheochromocytoma

Comparison of the data for all benign and malignant pheochromocytomas (comparison 1) yielded a total of 636 genes that discriminated benign from malignant disease at a significance level of $P < 0.001$ (TABLE 2). Consideration of the influence of catecholamine biochemical phenotype in comparison 2 indicated a considerably larger number of 2,246 genes that discriminated adrenergic from noradrenergic tumors. Additional consideration of the confounding influence of catecholamine biochemical phenotype, by two-way ANOVA, yielded a 53% larger number of 976 genes that discriminated ($P < 0.001$) malignant from benign tumors in comparison 2 than in comparison 1. Among these 976 differentially expressed genes in comparison 2, 516 were also differentially expressed in comparison 1. Most (70%) differentially expressed genes showed lower expression in metastatic than benign tumors (TABLE 2).

Comparison of SDHB-positive with SDHB-negative tumors (comparison 3) yielded a total of 613 genes that differentiated ($P < 0.001$) these two groups of tumors, with 59% of differentially expressed genes more highly expressed in SDHB-positive than SDHB-negative tumors (TABLE 2). Additional consideration of the confounding influence of SDHB mutation status by two-way ANOVA, however, revealed only 19 genes that distinguished benign from malignant pheochromocytoma. This negligible yield did not exceed the number of genes expected to show a difference ($P < 0.001$) by chance alone (i.e., calculated from the expected false-discovery rate).

Excluding adrenergic tumors and metastases at sites distant from the primary source of the malignancy in comparison 4 indicated a total of 383 genes that differentiated ($P < 0.001$) benign from primary malignant tumors (TABLE 2). Eighty-nine percent of these differentially expressed genes were more highly expressed in benign than in malignant primary tumors.

TABLE 2. Numbers of differentially expressed genes at $P < 0.001$

Study comparison	Number (FDR)	Number of genes with higher expression in:	
	Series 1		
1. Metastatic versus benign tumors	636 (4.3%)	Metastatic tumors	134
		Benign tumors	502
2. Metastatic versus benign tumors with consideration of biochemical profile	2,246 (1.2%)	Noradrenergic tumors	1,354
		Adrenergic tumors	892
	976 (2.8%)	Metastatic tumors	293
		Benign tumors	683
3. Metastatic versus benign tumors with consideration of SDHB mutation status	613 (4.4%)	SDHB positive tumors	364
		SDHB negative tumors	249
	19 (100%)	Metastatic tumors	7
		Benign tumors	12
4. Metastatic primary versus benign tumors	383 (7.1%)	Metastatic primary tumors	44
		Benign tumors	339
5. Metastases versus metastatic primary tumors	2,836 (1.0%)	Metastases	1,372
		Metastatic primary tumors	1464
6. PGG-derived versus adrenal-derived metastatic tumors	619 (4.4%)	Metastatic PGG-derived	290
		Metastatic adrenal-derived	329
	Series 2		
A. MEN 2A versus VHL tumors	887 (3.0%)	MEN 2A tumors	259
		VHL tumors	628
B. Sporadic adrenergic versus noradrenergic tumors	179 (15.1%)	Adrenergic tumors	108
		Noradrenergic tumors	71
C. Relationships of gene expression with tumor epinephrine content	1,725 (1.6%)	Positive relationships	602
		Negative relationships	1,123
D. VHL versus SDHB tumors	1,165 (2.3%)	VHL tumors	355
		SDHB tumors	810

Abbreviation: FDR, false discovery rate (percent of genes expected to show differential expression at $P < 0.001$ by chance); PGG, paraganglioma.

Comparison of primary tumors from patients with malignant disease with metastatic lesions of other patients (comparison 5) yielded 2,836 genes that discriminated ($P < 0.001$) between these two groups of tumors (TABLE 2). Among these genes, there were near equal proportions showing higher (48%) and lower (52%) expression in metastatic lesions than in primary malignant tumors.

Among all malignant primary tumors and metastases, comparison of adrenal-derived with paraganglioma-derived malignancies yielded 619 differentially expressed genes that discriminated between ($P < 0.001$) tumors on the basis of the adrenal versus extra-adrenal location of the primary tumor (TABLE 2). Among these differentially expressed genes, 47% showed higher expression in paraganglioma-derived malignancies and 53% in adrenal-derived malignancies.

Series 2: Influences of Hereditary Factors and Biochemical Profiles

Comparison of benign adrenal pheochromocytomas from patients with MEN 2A and VHL syndrome (comparison A) yielded 887 differentially

($P < 0.001$) expressed genes that discriminated between these two groups of hereditary adrenergic and noradrenergic tumors (TABLE 2). Most (72%) of these genes showed higher expression in tumors from VHL than MEN 2A patients. Among benign sporadic pheochromocytomas there were 179 genes that discriminated ($P < 0.001$) adrenergic from noradrenergic tumors (comparison B). Sixty percent of these differentially expressed genes showed higher levels of expression in adrenergic than in noradrenergic tumors.

Linear regression analysis using all data from benign and malignant tumors (comparison C) indicated 1,725 genes showing significant ($P < 0.001$) positive or negative relationships with percentage of epinephrine contents of tumors (TABLE 2). Thirty-five percent of these genes showed positive relationships and 65% negative relationships with increasing epinephrine content. As might be expected, expression of the gene for phenylethanolamine-*N*-methyltransferase showed a positive relationship with tumor epinephrine content and, among all 1,725 genes, represented the single gene with the strongest relationship to epinephrine content.

Comparison of tumors from VHL patients with those from patients with SDHB mutations (comparison D) yielded 1,165 genes that discriminated ($P < 0.001$) between these two groups of tumors (TABLE 2). Seventy percent of these genes showed higher expression in SDHB than in VHL tumors.

GO Analysis

GO analysis of differentially expressed genes ($P < 0.001$ level of significance) for comparisons of benign with malignant primary tumors and metastases (comparisons 1 and 2) indicated disproportionate numbers of differentially expressed genes related to angiogenesis or translation (TABLE 3). The comparison of malignant primary with benign tumors (4) indicated a disproportionate number of differentially expressed genes associated with signal transduction, while the comparison of malignant primary tumors with metastases (5) indicated an importance of genes related to cell proliferation, cytoskeletal function, and regulation of transcription. The comparison of VHL with MEN 2A (A) tumors showed disproportionate numbers of differentially expressed genes associated with cell motility, cytoskeletal function, extracellular matrix, and nucleotide metabolism, while the comparison of VHL with SDHB tumors (D) showed an importance of genes related to ATP binding, nucleotide metabolism, and protein transport.

DISCUSSION

The global differences in gene expression among the multiple comparisons of this study illustrate the importance of a carefully collected comprehensive clinical dataset for analysis and interpretation of microarray-generated

TABLE 3. Selected gene ontology (GO) summaries

GO term (total of genes listed in database with this GO term)	Comparison							
	1	2	4	5	6	A	B	D
Genes $P < 0.001$ (n)	636	976	383	2,836	619	887	179	1,165
Genes with GO listings (%)	41	41	38	47	52	50	56	52
Angiogenesis (56)	4*	4*		1		3	2*	4
Apoptosis/antiapoptosis (556)	8	9	8	51	9	13	1	22
ATP binding (1,731)	23	33	9	131	30	37	11	75*
Cell cycle (575)	9	9		45	14	17	3	15
Cell motility (157)	1	2	1	9	3	9*	2	7
Cell proliferation (611)	8	12	7	59*	11	22	11*	21
Cytoskeleton (665)	11	11	8	64*	14	25*	5	24
Electron transport (583)	7	12	4	46	11	14	10*	19
Extracellular matrix (295)	2	5	5	23	7	22*	4	8
Glucose metabolism (32)				1	2	3		1
Ion transport (721)	12	22	3	54	10	20	3	32
Neurotransmitter (110)	4	4	2	10	1	4		5
Nucleotide (545)	7	17	3	43	15	21*	1	27*
Lipid metabolism (201)	4	6	3	16	2	5	1	3
Protein transport (258)	2	8	3	19	4	7	2	15*
Regulation of transcription (1,962)	24	34	16	174*	29	48	10	57
Signal transduction (1,003)	16	25	13*	77	16	22	6	27
Transcription factor (789)	12	16	4	70	8	18	3	28
Translation (151)	5	13*	2	7	2	1		7

*$P < 0.05$ indicates disproportionate number of genes with a particular GO annotation by Fisher's exact test.

Data for comparison 2 are restricted to genes differentially expressed between benign and malignant tumors. Data for comparison 3 are not shown. The total number of genes in the database with any GO annotation is 17,052.

gene expression profiles in human tumor samples. Consideration of germline mutations and variations in catecholamine biochemical phenotypes and tumor locations are several factors shown here to be associated with differences in gene expression that can assist in comparisons of benign with malignant pheochromocytoma.

The major strengths of our study are the large sample set and the detailed clinical information available for most tumors. The large sample set is extraordinary given the rarity of the tumor, and even more remarkable considering the inclusion of 20 malignant tumors, an even more infrequent entity than benign tumors, which, when diagnosed, are often not resected.

The detailed clinical information available to us allowed identification of confounding variables influencing comparisons of malignant with benign tumors. Use of ANOVA to correct for the influence of tumor catecholamine phenotype in comparisons of malignant versus benign tumors (comparison 2) exemplifies how such information can be applied to enrich a database of differentially expressed genes. This comparison yielded 50% more genes than when the major influence of catecholamine biochemical phenotype was not considered (comparison 1). Moreover, the overlap of differentially expressed genes for both comparisons indicated that differential expression of almost one out of five genes in comparison 1 most likely reflected confounding influences (e.g., catecholamine phenotype) not directly related to malignancy. Thus, the overall yield of correctly identified differentially expressed genes in comparison 2 was nearly twice that of comparison 1. The foregoing differences in yields are explained by major differences in gene expression between adrenergic and noradrenergic tumors,[10] and the predominant noradrenergic phenotype of malignant tumors and adrenergic phenotype of many benign adrenal tumors.[2,9]

Separate identification and analysis of subgroups of malignant primary tumors and distant metastases arising from these primary tumors, SDHB mutation-positive and -negative malignancies, and malignancies arising from adrenal versus extra-adrenal locations, provide other information useful for identifying differences in gene expression crucial for determining malignant potential and pathways of malignant transformation. The distinction of malignant primary tumors from subsequent metastases is not often considered in other studies of malignant pheochromocytoma, but has several important implications. The genes distinguishing benign from malignant primary tumors (comparison 4) may be particularly important for identifying prognostic markers of malignancy. In contrast, the more than sevenfold-higher number of genes differentially expressed between malignant primary tumors and metastatic lesions (comparison 5) may reflect the malignant transformation process or adaptation to a new environment to facilitate survival.

A limitation accompanying the abundance of clinical information is that the necessary subgrouping requires a large dataset of tumors for the various comparisons. Although reasonably large, the sample size was not adequate enough to assess the contributions of all considered variables to the malignant process. The relatively small numbers of malignant and benign tumors identified as arising from SDHB mutations is one example where insufficient sample size limited interpretation. Although the comparison of SDHB-positive versus SDHB-negative benign and malignant tumors yielded a large number of differentially expressed genes, additional consideration of these two variables by ANOVA indicated little difference between SDHB-dependent benign and malignant tumors (comparison 3). Whether this reflects lack of difference between the two groups of SDHB-positive tumors or limited sample size and statistical power of the comparison is unclear.

Another limitation to this and any other study of malignant and benign pheochromocytoma is that there is currently no method other than lifelong follow-up to establish that a pheochromocytoma is not malignant (i.e., truly benign). Since malignant disease can occur 17 or more years after diagnosis of the initial tumor, with patients asymptomatic during this interval,[11,12] it is realistic to assume that some tumors classified as benign in this study may later turn out to metastasize. Such misclassification may lead to a diminished yield of differentially expressed genes, but would not be expected to result in any increase in false-positive rates of gene detection.

What are the future directions for use of the database of differentially expressed genes? This database, available on request as a Filemaker Pro file (Santa Clara, CA), provides a valuable resource from which hypotheses may be generated and tested in further studies on pheochromocytoma. Identification of subsets of genes involved in the malignant process can benefit from application of data mining and pathway analysis tools, but will require validation studies—preferably in different tumor sample sets—before hypotheses about specific pathways of malignancy, targets for treatment, and diagnostic or prognostic markers of malignancy can be tested. Development of tissue arrays for detection of panels of differentially expressed proteins is one approach that might be used in retrospective studies involving archival paraffin-embedded tissues or prospective studies required to validate hypotheses about diagnostic and prognostic markers of malignancy.

Although primarily directed at benign versus malignant pheochromocytoma, the various comparisons in the database are also useful for generating other testable hypotheses about mechanisms of tumorigenesis and genotype–phenotype relationships, including insight into the key genes determining catecholamine biochemical phenotypes. Epinephrine-producing pheochromocytomas in MEN 2A and predominantly norepinephrine-producing tumors in VHL syndrome have highly distinct gene expression profiles, suggesting development from different populations of noradrenergic and adrenergic chromaffin cells.[10] Dahia and colleagues[13] have reported similar highly distinct expression profiles falling into two broad groups of pheochromocytomas, one group including tumors in MEN 2A patients, and the other tumors due to mutations of VHL, SDHD, and SDHB genes. These findings fit with others indicating that familial pheochromocytomas develop by a single pathway linking mutations in disease-causing genes to failure of apoptosis after withdrawal of growth factors during chromaffin cell development.[14] As advanced elsewhere in this volume by Huynh *et al.*,[15] epinephrine-producing tumors in MEN 2A are hypothesized to develop due to susceptibility of more fully developed PNMT-expressing chromaffin cells to the effects of activating RET mutations, whereas norepinephrine-producing pheochromocytomas in VHL syndrome develop from neural crest progenitors before their final development into differentiated epinephrine-producing adrenal chromaffin cells.

The findings presented here that close to 90% of differentially expressed genes in benign and malignant primary pheochromocytomas are underexpressed in malignant compared to benign tumors fits with other observations of a less differentiated biochemical phenotype in malignant tumors, as characterized by lack of production of epinephrine and relatively high production of dopamine compared to norepinephrine.[16,17] This may reflect predominant development of malignant pheochromocytomas from neural crest progenitors arrested in an early stage of development with a malignancy-prone lineage able to populate both adrenal and extra-adrenal sites of chromaffin tissue. The matching of gene expression profiles in neural crest progenitors with those in different groups of pheochromocytomas and mechanistic studies linking these progenitors to effects of specific genes provides possible approaches to test the foregoing hypotheses.

In summary, the present gene expression profiling study in a large sample set, combined with use of advanced statistical approaches to analyze influences of multiple variables, provides a valuable database of differentially expressed genes to help address outstanding questions about genotype–phenotype relationships, tumorigenesis, and malignant potential and transformation pathways in pheochromocytoma.

ACKNOWLEDGMENTS

We thank Edwin Lai and Thanh-Truc Huynh for their technical assistance. This work was supported by the intramural program of the National Institute of Child Health and Human Development, the National Institute of Neurological Disorders and Stroke, the National Human Genome Research Institute, the National Cancer Institute, and the Center for Information Technology, National Institutes of Health.

REFERENCES

1. EISENHOFER, G. *et al.* 2004. Malignant pheochromocytoma: current status and initiatives for future progress. Endocr. Relat. Cancer **11:** 423–436.
2. RAO, F., H. R. KEISER & D. T. O'CONNOR. 2000. Malignant pheochromocytoma: chromaffin granule transmitters and response to treatment. Hypertension **36:** 1045–1052.
3. O'RIORDAIN, D.S. *et al.* 1996. Clinical spectrum and outcome of functional extraadrenal paraganglioma. World J. Surg. **20:** 916–921; discussion 922.
4. WHALEN, R.K., A. F. ALTHAUSEN & G. H. DANIELS. 1992. Extra-adrenal pheochromocytoma. J. Urol. **147:** 1–10.
5. ASTUTI, D. *et al.* 2001. Gene mutations in the succinate dehydrogenase subunit SDHB cause susceptibility to familial pheochromocytoma and to familial paraganglioma. Am. J. Hum. Genet. **69:** 49–54.
6. GIMENEZ-ROQUEPLO, A. P. *et al.* 2003. Mutations in the SDHB gene are associated with extra-adrenal and/or malignant phaeochromocytomas. Cancer Res. **63:** 5615–5621.
7. LENDERS, J.W. *et al.* 2005. Phaeochromocytoma. Lancet **366:** 665–675.
8. EISENHOFER, G. *et al.* 1986. Simultaneous liquid-chromatographic determination of 3,4-dihydroxyphenylglycol, catecholamines, and 3,4-dihydroxyphenylalanine in plasma, and their responses to inhibition of monoamine oxidase. Clin. Chem. **32:** 2030–2033.

9. EISENHOFER, G. *et al.* 2005. Pheochromocytoma catecholamine phenotypes and prediction of tumor size and location by use of plasma free metanephrines. Clin. Chem. **51:** 735–744.
10. EISENHOFER, G. *et al.* 2004. Distinct gene expression profiles in norepinephrine- and epinephrine-producing hereditary and sporadic pheochromocytomas: activation of hypoxia-driven angiogenic pathways in von Hippel-Lindau syndrome. Endocr. Relat. Cancer **11:** 897–911.
11. TANAKA, S. *et al.* 1993. Malignant pheochromocytoma with hepatic metastasis diagnosed 20 years after resection of the primary adrenal lesion. Intern. Med. **32:** 789–794.
12. BABA, T. *et al.* 1985. A malignant pheochromocytoma with ileus, polyuria and hypercalcemia: a case of recurrence 17 years after the initial operation. Endocrinol. Jpn. **32:** 337–345.
13. DAHIA, P.L. *et al.* 2005. A HIF1alpha regulatory loop links hypoxia and mitochondrial signals in pheochromocytomas. PLoS Genet. **1:** 72–80.
14. LEE, S. *et al.* 2005. Neuronal apoptosis linked to EglN3 prolyl hydroxylase and familial pheochromocytoma genes: developmental culling and cancer. Cancer Cell. **8:** 155–167.
15. HUYNH, T.T. *et al.* 2006. Transcriptional regulation of phenylethanolamine *N*-methyltransferase in pheochromocytomas from patients with von Hippel-Lindau syndrome and multiple endocrine neoplasia type 2. Ann. N.Y. Acad. Sci. This volume.
16. JANUSZEWICZ, W. *et al.* 2001. Dopamine and dopa urinary excretion in patients with pheochromocytoma–diagnostic implications. Blood Press. **10:** 212–216.
17. van der HARST, E. *et al.* 2002. The value of plasma markers for the clinical behaviour of phaeochromocytomas. Eur. J. Endocrinol. **147:** 85–94.

Pathology of Pheochromocytoma and Extra-adrenal Paraganglioma

ARTHUR S. TISCHLER,[a] NORIKO KIMURA,[b] AND ANNE MARIE MCNICOL[c]

[a]*Department of Pathology, Tufts University School of Medicine, Boston, Massachusetts 02111 USA*

[b]*Department of Pathology, Tohoku Rosai Hospital, Sendai, 981-8563 Japan*

[c]*Department of Pathology, University of Glasgow, Glasgow G4 0SF, United Kingdom*

ABSTRACT: The 2004 WHO classification of endocrine tumors defines pheochromocytoma as a tumor arising from chromaffin cells in the adrenal medulla. Closely related tumors in extra-adrenal sympathetic and parasympathetic paraganglia are classified as extra-adrenal paragangliomas. A pheochromocytoma is an intra-adrenal sympathetic paraganglioma. While arbitrary, this nomenclature serves to emphasize important distinctive properties of intra-adrenal tumors that must be taken into account in clinical practice and research. Those include an often adrenergic phenotype, a relatively low rate of malignancy, and a predilection to occur in particular hereditary syndromes. Current roles of pathology are limited to distinguishing primary or metastatic pheochromocytomas/paragangliomas from other endocrine or nonendocrine tumors, and flagging tumors that show features suggestive of malignant potential or syndromic disease. Future roles may involve more definitive assessment of malignancy, genotype–phenotype correlation, and identification of targets for therapy. Pathology practice currently rests mostly on interpretation of conventional histological sections stained with hematoxylin and eosin, with variable ancillary application of immunohistochemical staining. Malignancy is currently defined by the presence of metastases, not local invasion. Local invasion alone is a poor predictor of metastases, and the absence of apparent invasion does not preclude development of metastases. The two types of aggressive behavior might therefore have different biological underpinnings, and those will be resolved most effectively if consistent terminology is employed. In order to be optimally informative, pathology reports must employ consistent nomenclature and incorporate standard elements. Templates or checklists for minimal standard reporting are recommended by several pathology associations, but identification of some recommended and optional elements is currently subjective or inconsistent.

Address for correspondence: Arthur S. Tischler, Department of Pathology, Tufts University School of Medicine, Tufts New England Medical Center, Box 802, 750 Washington Street, Boston, MA 02111 USA. Voice: 617-636-1038; fax: 617-636-8302.
e-mail: atischler@tufts-nemc.org

Ann. N.Y. Acad. Sci. 1073: 557–570 (2006).
doi: 10.1196/annals.1353.059

KEYWORDS: **pheochromocytoma; paraganglioma; pathology; histology; malignancy; reporting**

INTRODUCTION

According to the WHO classification of tumors, updated in 2004, "Pheochromocytomas... arise in the adrenal medulla and are derived from chromaffin cells of neural crest origin," "extra-adrenal paragangliomas arise from chromaffin cells in sympathoadrenal and parasympathetic paraganglia," and "a pheochromocytoma is an intra-adrenal sympathetic paraganglioma."[1] Nomenclature limiting use of the term *pheochomocytoma* to tumors of the adrenal medulla was inculcated in U. S. pathologists in 1950 by H.T. Karsner, who wrote the fascicle entitled "Tumors of the Adrenal" in the first series of the Armed Forces Institute of Pathology *Atlas of Tumor Pathology*. Noting the previous application of the term by other authors to various tumors in extra-adrenal locations, including head and neck paragangliomas and even appendiceal carcinoid tumors, Karsner commented that "[t]he confusion in terminology encumbers the exchange of experience which can be so constructive in fields where no one pathologist's experience is enough," adding that "[a]n agreement in nomenclature, even on an arbitrary basis, is helpful."[2] Karsner's original definition, which encompassed tumors "in or near the adrenal," was refined in the second series fascicle of 1985 to include only intra-adrenal neoplasms. By then, the AFIP fascicles had become the definitive *vade mecum* for pathologists in the United States, and for them the arbitrary nomenclature became the norm. Pathologists in other countries were slower to adopt the same conventions but gradually, accommodated them.

Although the current nomenclature has its origin in an arbitrary convention, "special" treatment of intra-adrenal tumors can in fact be justified on the basis of several distinctive characteristics. Those include a lower rate of malignancy (~5% overall versus ~20% for extra-adrenal paragangliomas associated with the sympathetic nervous system[3]), an often adrenergic phenotype (extra-adrenal paragangliomas are almost always noradrenergic[4]), and a proclivity to occur in association with particular genetic disorders (particularly MEN2).[5]

On the other hand, it can be reasonably argued that this classification may detract from efforts to understand the pathobiology of tumors that, overall, are more similar than different. Pheochromocytomas and extra-adrenal paragangliomas often have similar or identical morphology (FIG. 1), share a mostly identical neuroendocrine phenotype, and sometimes have the same genetic predisposition. Nonetheless, most pathologists agree in principle with the need for consistency and accept the idea that the WHO nomenclature, while imperfect, should be adhered to. At the same time, it is recognized that the biological basis for differences in genotype, phenotype, and malignancy based on anatomic site must be resolved.

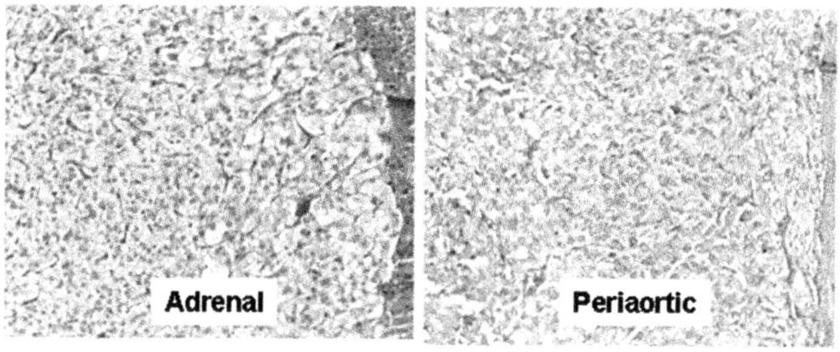

FIGURE 1. Pheochromocytomas and extra-adrenal paragangliomas may have similar or identical histological appearances.

Unfortunately, even in recent publications precise and consistent nomenclature has been difficult to attain, especially in papers written by clinicians and especially for clinically functional tumors producing signs and symptoms of catecholamine secretion. Contributing factors include both lack of familiarity with the WHO nomenclature and resistance to its arbitrary distinctions. The situation is improving as a result of cooperation between pathologists and clinicians with a shared interest in pathobiology.

CURRENT AND FUTURE ROLES OF PATHOLOGY IN MANAGEMENT OF PHEOCHROMOCYTOMAS AND PARAGANGLIOMAS

The current roles of pathology in management of pheochromocytomas and extra-adrenal paragangliomas are limited to diagnosis, documentation of malignant behavior, and recording of findings that may be clues to malignant potential or occult syndromic disease. It is anticipated that future roles will involve more definitive assessment of malignancy, genotype–phenotype correlation, and identification of targets for therapy.

Pheochromocytomas and other paragangliomas show enormous variability in cytology and histological pattern and must be distinguished from a variety of endocrine and nonendocrine tumors. In the adrenal gland, the principal differential diagnosis is adrenal cortical adenoma or carcinoma. Elsewhere, the possibilities include hepatic and hepatoid tumors, alveolar soft part sarcoma, and primary or metastatic carcinomas with endocrine or nonendocrine phenotype. Immunohistochemical staining procedures routinely available in most pathology laboratories can now reliably make the necessary distinctions, provided they are applied judiciously and with appreciation of potential artifacts. The latter include technical artifacts, such as enhancement of endogenous biotin staining by heat-based antigen retrieval methods,[6] nonspecific staining of some neuroendocrine cell types by serum,[7] and cross-reactivities of commercially touted antibodies that are often of dubious quality. The

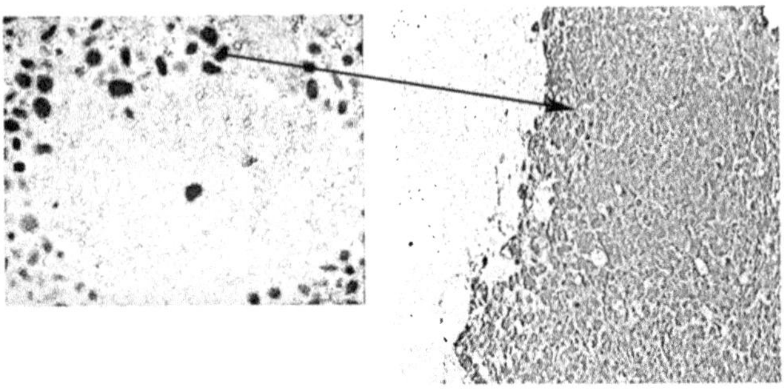

FIGURE 2. Intense immunoreactivity for CgA discriminates pheochromocytoma (right side of right panel) from normal or neoplastic adrenal cortex (left side of right panel). CgA is one of many markers localized to the matrix of membrane-bound secretory granules. Other neuroendocrine markers, for example, synaptophysin, are localized to the granule membranes and may be enriched in the membranes of small agranular "synaptic-like" vesicles. Both types of secretory organelle are shown on left.

single most specific and reliable generic neuroendocrine marker currently used in pathology practice is chromogranin A (CgA), a major constituent of the matrix of catecholamine-containing secretory granules. Immunoreactivity for CgA will readily distinguish pheochromocytomas and other paragangliomas from nonendocrine tumors or tumors of the adrenal cortex (FIG. 2). Staining of pheochromocytomas for CgA is usually extensive, and the diagnosis should be made with caution for tumors that show little or no staining. Distinction of pheochromocytomas and paragangliomas from other neuroendocrine tumors that also express CgA is a process of deduction that often involves panels of antibodies, for example, demonstration of immunoreactive tyrosine hydroxylase (TH, the rate-limiting enzyme in catecholamine biosynthesis) and exclusion of staining for cytoskeletal filament proteins that are often expressed in pulmonary and gastrointestinal neuroendocrine tumors. Staining for CgA and TH may be weaker and more variable in parasympathetic paragangliomas than in their sympathoadrenal counterparts.

Malignancy of pheochromocytomas and paragangliomas is currently defined by the presence of metastases.[1] Despite its potential lethality, local invasion alone, even when extensive, is a poor predictor of metastases, and the absence of apparent invasion does not preclude development of metastases. Some pathologists challenge this convention as "unnecessary mysticism," noting that other locally invasive tumors that have minimal metastatic potential are nonetheless classified as malignant (e.g., basal cell carcinomas of the skin). However, as for tumor nomenclature, most pathologists agree that a consistent definition of malignancy is critical for assessing criteria that in the future will more precisely define risk from either metastases or local growth. There is currently little information correlating extent of local invasion with propensity for local recurrence.

An important obstacle to determining criteria for malignancy is the fact that pheochromocytomas/paragangliomas metastasize infrequently and often late. Consequently, it has been difficult to validate proposed criteria in large studies with adequate follow-up. Most existing analyses are therefore retrospective. In addition, the clustering of gene expression profiles in tumors with different underlying genetic predispositions[8,9] suggests that any particular finding may carry different weights in different patient cohorts. For example, extensive local invasion might pose essentially no risk in an adequately excised tumor from a patient with MEN2A, while even minimal invasion might be ominous in a tumor with mutated SDHB. Because the prevalence of syndromic mutations varies geographically, studies reported from different countries or regions might offer very different conclusions. A further confounding factor is that it may be difficult to distinguish a metastatic pheochromocytoma/paraganglioma from an independent second primary tumor, particularly if the latter is associated with normal or reactive lymphoid tissue that could be mistaken for a lymph node containing metastatic tumor. Some studies therefore limit the definition of tumor metastasis to tumor deposits in locations where paraganglia are not present, such as liver, lung, or bone. While often unavoidable, this policy of exclusion need not be employed arbitrarily because lymph node metastases can often be recognized as such, for example, as irregular tumor deposits in the subcapsular sinus of a lymph node.

Although pathologists generally agree that malignancy can be ascertained only by development of metastases and not by histological features, some evidence suggests that it may in fact be possible to histopathologically differentiate tumors that pose a significant risk of metastasis from those that do not. No single histological feature is alone able to identify metastatic potential, including capsular or vascular invasion, extreme cytological atypia, or areas resembling pediatric neuroblastoma (FIG. 3). However, multifactorial scoring systems may be informative. A seminal study by Linnoila *et al.* in 1990[3] examined multiple histological and nonhistological parameters of 120 sympathoadrenal paragangliomas and developed a statistical model according to which >70% of the tumors could be classified correctly with >95% probability on the basis of four factors: extra-adrenal location, coarse nodularity, confluent necrosis, and absence of hyaline globules. Most malignant tumors had 2 or 3 of those features, while 89% of benign tumors had one or none. Unfortunately, a number of subsequent papers that deal with assessment of markers for malignancy blur the distinction between intra-adrenal and extra-adrenal tumors, so that the powerful independent predictive value of anatomic site is obscured.

In 2002 Thompson proposed the PASS system (pheochromocytoma of adrenal scaled score), specific to the adrenal gland, which scores multiple microscopic findings, including dependent and independent variables identified by Linnoila *et al.*, to arrive at a total score predictive of metastatic potential (TABLE 1).[10] All tumors that metastasized had a score > 4, but 17 of 50 with a score > 4 had not metastasized in a follow-up period of ~5 years, and one

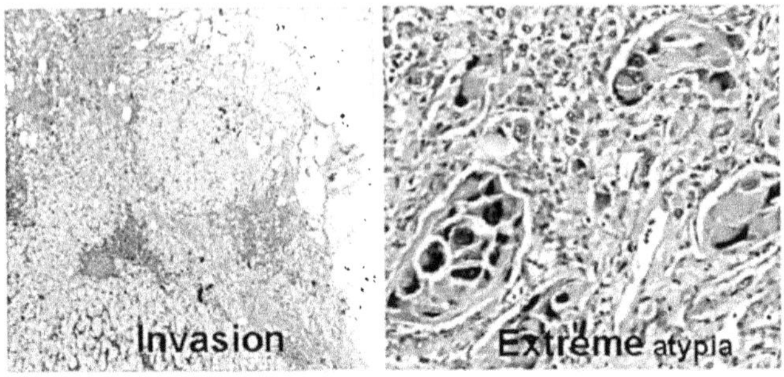

FIGURE 3. No single histological feature, including invasion or extreme cytological atypia, is sufficient to diagnose a pheochromocytoma as malignant. Invasion of periadrenal fat is shown at top right of left panel.

with a score >15 had not metastasized in ~28 years. In his paper Thompson notes that the PASS score provides a threshold for risk but does not quantitate the risk above that threshold, and he further notes that a score ≤ 3 does not guarantee that a patient will not at some point develop metastases.

In the United Kingdom, the Royal College of Pathologists has recently adapted a synoptic reporting template based on Linnoila *et al.*[3] (TABLE 2). The PASS system is referenced but not formally adopted because it requires validation and appears to have a high-false positive rate. The template advises that a diagnosis of "benign" tumor cannot be made.

Immunohistochemistry has been used as an ancillary technique for assessment of malignant potential, with mixed results. The marker most consistently correlated with malignancy is the labeling index of tumor cells stained for the proliferation marker Ki-67, which is performed on paraffin sections using monoclonal antibody MIB-1.[11–13] However, some studies do not show a

TABLE 1. Proposed pheochromocytoma of the adrenal gland scoring scale (PASS score)[a]

Feature	Assigned score
Large nests of cells or diffuse growth (>10%) of tumor volume	2
Necrosis (confluent or central in large cell nests)	2
High cellularity	2
Cellular monotony	2
Presence of spindle-shaped tumor cells (even if focal)	2
Mitotic figures (>3 per 10 high power fields)	2
Extension of tumor into adjacent fat	2
Vascular invasion	1
Capsular invasion	1
Profound nuclear pleomorphism	1
Nuclear hyperchromasia	1
Total possible score	20

All tumors that metastasized were reported to have scores ≥ 4[10].
[a]From Thompson.[10]

TABLE 2. Summary of recommended reporting template for pheochromocytomas by the Royal College of Pathologists, 2005[a]

Gross description

Nature of specimen: Right adrenalectomy □ Left adrenalectomy □ Other (define) □
Nature of surgery: Open □ Laparoscopic □ Not known □
Weight of specimen: g
Dimensions of specimen:___×___×___ mm.
Coarse nodularity: Yes □ No □
Adrenal capsule: Intact □ Breached □
Excision complete: Yes □ No □
Uninvolved adrenal: Identified □ Not identified □ Not applicable □
Other tissues included (define)

Microscopic description

Predominant cell type: Large □ Small □
Hyaline globules: Yes □ No □
Mitotic count: (30 HPF × 400)
Confluent necrosis: Yes □ No □
Vascular invasion: Yes □ No □
Capsular invasion: Yes □ No □
Infiltration into surrounding tissues: Yes □ No □
Sustentacular cells: Yes □ No □ Not assessed □
Other components:
Ganglioneuroma □ Neuroblastoma □ Ganglioneuroblastoma □
Uninvolved adrenal identified: Yes □ No □ Not applicable □
Medullary hyperplasia: Yes □ No □ Not assessed □

[a]Provided by Dr. Anne M. McNicol.

correlation of MIB-1 labeling with malignancy. Studies of MIB-1 labeling show a striking lack of methodological consistency, and many papers do not provide sufficient methodological details to permit replication. Sampling methods that have been used include counts of random fields or "hot spots," results have been expressed as a percentage of cells labeled, labeled cells per field or optical density units, and varying numbers of cells or fields have been scored. Although many pathologists now include an assessment of MIB-1 labeling in diagnostic reporting of pheochromocytomas/paragangliomas, there is currently no prospect of standardization. From a practical perspective, cell counting is a tedious and time-consuming task. In order to gain acceptance, any method ultimately advocated for standardized reporting should be based on comparative data balancing optimal efficacy and minimal effort. Scoring of labeled cells per medium power field has been used in Japan (TABLE 3), where immunohistochemical staining of Ki67 is almost routinely done for every malignancy and is not considered a special task. Although the originally reported method was averaging based on counts of 20 fields of highest labeling,[12] continuing experience suggests that counts of far fewer fields may have equivalent predictive value (N. Kimura, unpublished material).

TABLE 3. Proposed scoring scale for pheochromocytmas and extra-adrenal sympathetic paragangliomas by Kimura *et al.*[a]

Feature	Assigned score
Histological pattern	
Uniform cell nests	0
Large and irregular cell nests	1
Pseudo-rosettes (even if focal)	1
Cellularity	
Low (<150 cells/mm^2)	0
Moderate (150–250 cells/mm^2)	1
High (more than 250 cells/mm^2)	2
Necrosis (confluent or central in large cell nests)	2
Vascular or capsular invasion	1
Ki -67 immunoreactivity	
> 1% or 20 cells per medium power field	1
(avg. count per 200 × field, based on 20 fields with highest labeling)	
> 3% or 50 cells per medium power field	2
Catecholamine phenotype	
Adrenergic	0
Noradrenergic or "nonfunctional"	1
Total possible score	10

NOTE: Metastases were reported in 13% of tumors with scores 1–2, 63% with 3–6, and 100% with 7–10. In addition, 5-year survivals of patients in the three groups were reported to be 92%, 69%, and 0, respectively.[12]

[a]Excerpted from Kimura *et al.*[12]

An expanding list of other immunohistochemical markers reported to correlate with malignancy[14] includes telomerase reverse transcriptase, heat-shock protein 90, vascular endothelial growth factor (VEGF), hypoxia-inducible transcription factor 1α (HIF1α), cyclooxygenase-2, N-cadherin, tenascin C, and specific cleavage products of chromogranin and secretogranin proteins.[15] Absence of labeling for cell adhesion molecule CD44-S has also been reported to correlate with malignancy.[11] As is the case for morphological characteristics, it has not been ruled out that different immunohistochemical marker profiles carry different weights in tumors with different genetic backgrounds. For example, hypoxia-sensitive markers reported to be associated with malignancy, such as VEGF and HIF1α also characterize pheochromocytomas/paragangliomas in patients with von Hippel–Lindau disease,[8,9] and those tumors are usually benign.[14] For sporadic pheochromocytomas, the assessment of chromosomal gains and losses by comparative genomic hybridization (CGH) in combination with PASS score and immunohistochemical staining for MIB-1 and CD44-S has been reported to predict metastatic potential more accurately than PASS score alone.[11] However, it must be borne in mind that specific patterns of secondary genetic changes detected by CGH segregate with specific syndromic mutations,[16] and that a substantial number of apparently sporadic tumors are in fact syndromic.[17]

A 2005 scoring system proposed by Kimura for both pheochromocytomas and extra-adrenal paragangliomas combines histological, immunohistochemical, and biochemical characteristics to arrive at a score reported to predict both the metastatic potential of tumors and the prognosis for patients with tumors that metastasize (TABLE 3).[12] An important element of the system is notation of whether a tumor is adrenergic or noradrenergic. Anatomic site is therefore indirectly weighted because extra-adrenal paragangliomas are almost invariably noradrenergic.

Most pathologists do not currently employ any formal scoring system in routine practice for reasons including the lack of prospective validation and uncertainty as to how to recognize some of the scored parameters. However, major features of the scoring systems are incorporated into reporting templates that are endorsed by pathology associations (TABLES 2, 4, and 5). The listing of potentially unfavorable findings will presumably flag a tumor for some type of follow-up, but the nature of the required follow-up remains unclear.

An exciting prospect is that pathologists in the near future might play a role in management of malignant pheochromocytomas/paragangliomas by immunohistochemically identifying overexpression of proteins that are drug targets, as is already routine for a number of other malignancies. One immediate possibility is drugs targeting heat-shock proteins, which are already in clinical trials.[18]

Pathology presently plays an important role in identifying clues that may lead to identification of patients with previously undetected familial pheochromocytoma/paraganglioma syndromes. In general, a finding of multicentric tumors is suggestive of familial disease. In the adrenal gland, familial disease may be manifest as multiple pheochromocytomas and/or diffuse and nodular hyperplasia, usually detected by gross examination of the specimen. These changes should be carefully searched for and their presence or absence should be documented. They are most likely to occur in MEN2 (but are not always present in MEN2) and are usually not present in other syndromes.

Some evidence suggests that microscopic findings may also provide clues to underlying genotypes. Pheochromocytomas that occur in patients with VHL disease have been reported to exhibit distinctive features consisting of a thick vascular capsule, myxoid and hyalinized stroma, small cells with clear or amphophilic cytoplasm, intermixed small vessels, and absence of hyaline globules.[19] These changes are not always present and it is not known whether they correlate with specific VHL mutations. They may also overlap with findings in other familial or sporadic pheochromocytomas or may be partially mimicked by unrelated findings. For example, the collapsed vascular scaffold of residual normal adrenal medulla adjacent to a pheochromocytoma may resemble a thick vascular capsule. Immunohistochemical staining for phenylethanolamine N-methyltransferase (PNMT), the enzyme that synthesizes epinephrine from norepinephrine, may be a useful ancillary technique because pheochromocytomas in VHL disease are usually noradrenergic,[9] and therefore

TABLE 4. Summary of recommended final anatomic diagnostic checklist for pheochromocytoma[a]

Organ (adrenal gland)	Required
Site (right or left)	"
Surgical procedure	"
Pathologic diagnosis (pheochromocytoma)	"
A. Size of tumor (__cm × __cm × __cm)	"
B. Weight of tumor (__gm)	"
C. Extent of tumor (confined to adrenal, beyond adrenal but not into adjacent organs, or into adjacent organs)	"
Margins of resection (free of tumor, or tumor present at margins)	"
Lymph nodes	"
A. Number examined	
B. Number positive	
C. Comment	
Additional tumor features	"
A. Blood vessel invasion (not identified, or identified, specify intratumoral, or peritumoral)	"
B. Lymph vessel invasion (not identified, or identified, specify intratumoral, or peritumoral)	"
C. Mitotic activity (specify mitotic rate per 50-high power fields)	"
D. Nuclear atypia (mild, moderate, or marked)	"
E. Necrosis (present or absent)	"
F. Comment	
Additional findings and comments (adrenal medullary hyperplasia, cortical lesions, etc.)	Optional
Ancillary studies	"
Special stains are performed, the results are as follows (list stains and results)	
Interpretation	
Immunohistochemical studies are performed, the results are as follows (list studies and results)	
Interpretation	

[a]Excerpted from the Association of Directors of Anatomic and Surgical Pathology checklist for adrenal cortical carcinoma and pheochromocytoma, Ver 1.1,11–03, http://www.adasp.org/

PNMT-negative (FIG. 4). A caveat, however, is that high-quality monoclonal antibodies, such as those long used for CgA or TH, are not widely available for PNMT.

Minimal standards of care for processing and reporting of pathology specimens are recommended by pathology organizations in the United States and United Kingdom (TABLES 2, 4, and 5). Nonetheless, the quality of reports is substantially affected by experience, starting with the approach to the gross specimen. Gross description and tissue sampling are often performed by pathology residents, who are the least experienced members of the pathology team. Education and oversight must emphasize the importance of judgment, particularly with respect to tissue sampling. Most experienced pathologists agree that sampling should be "liberal," and emphasize that samples should represent all morphologically variant areas of a tumor, the tumor capsule, and the interface with adjacent soft tissue. A suggested general guideline of at least one section

TABLE 5. Summary of recommended final anatomic diagnosis checklist for extra-adrenal paragangliomas[a]

Anatomic site of tumor
Surgical procedure
Pathologic diagnosis (terminology based on anatomic site, e.g., "urinary bladder paraganglioma")
Tumor size (__cm × __cm × __cm) and weight (__gm)
Gross description (external and cut surfaces)
Microscopic description (including presence and quantitation of mitotic figures)
Margins of resection (free of tumor, or tumor present at margins)
Presence and approximate extent of necrosis
Presence or absence of invasion (vessels, adjacent tissues, or organs)
Unusual pathologic features
Special studies

[a]Excerpted from the Association of Directors of Anatomic and Surgical Pathology (http://www.adasp.org/) and from Lack *et al.*[21]

per cm of tumor is a minimum applied to many types of tumor. However, there is presently little agreement, and little discussion, of how sections should be used for ancillary studies. If the appearance of a tumor varies from slide to slide, as is often the case, should all of the slides be stained for each marker

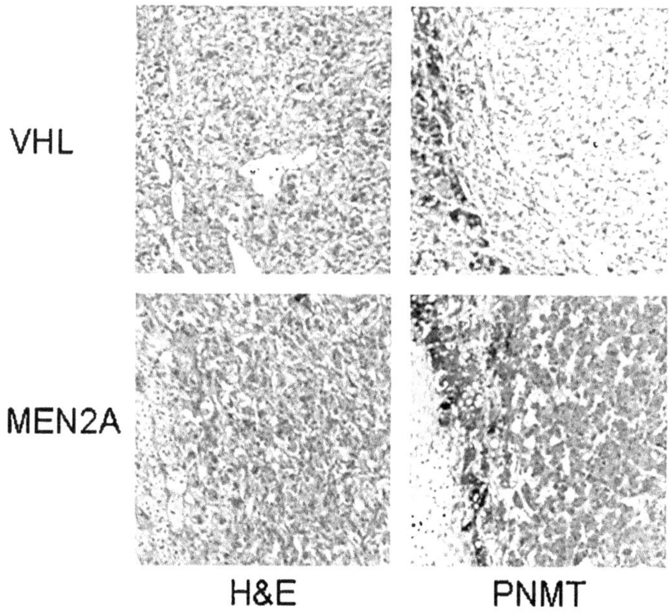

FIGURE 4. Immunohistochemical staining for PNMT confirms an adrenergic phenotype and may aid in genotype–phenotype correlation. Each panel shows pheochromocytomas (right) separated from normal cortex (lower left) by a thin rim of residual normal adrenal medulla that serves as a positive control for PNMT-staining. Pheochromocytomas in VHL disease are typically PNMT-negative, while those in MEN2 are typically positive.

studied? If a tumor is large, should staining be performed on sections representing both the center and the periphery? Although the logical answer to both questions is yes, that approach may be precluded by constraints of cost and time. These issues remain to be resolved both in the design of protocols for clinical studies and in clinical practice.

In the United States, the project of standardizing pathology reporting is one of the tasks undertaken by the Association of Directors of Anatomic and Surgical Pathology (ADASP), an organization founded in 1989 to promote effective education, administration, and practice of anatomic pathology. ADASP issues recommendations for reporting of major tumor types, and those recommendations are available in pathology journals and textbooks, as well as on the organization's website (www.adasp.org). In preparing its recommendations, ADASP initially chose pathologists expert in each field to assemble groups to write specific cancer protocols. The protocols, including those for adrenal gland[20] and extra-adrenal paragangliomas[21] were subsequently updated to generate checklists that comply with requirements adopted in 2004 by the American College of Surgery (ACS) Commission on Cancer (COC) for accreditation of cancer centers in the USA. As described on the ADASP website, "these revised ADASP diagnostic checklists have been divided into required and optional. The term *required* in this context only signifies compliance with the COC guidelines. ADASP realizes that specimens and practices vary and it will not be possible to report these elements in every case." Relevant portions of the current checklists for adrenal gland tumors and extra-adrenal paragangliomas are excerpted in TABLES 4 and 5.

It should be noted that a number of items listed in the ADASP checklists are generic descriptors required in all tumor reporting but not necessarily highly correlated with the behavior of pheochromocytomas or extra-adrenal paragangliomas. For example, tumor size and weight may show some correlation with metastatic potential but not as independent variables.[11] In addition, pheochromocytoma currently receives relatively short shrift as part of a combined ADASP checklist/reporting template for adrenal cortical carcinoma and pheochromocytoma. However, the checklists already incorporate major elements of the various proposed scoring systems and leave flexibility to add additional elements. A more detailed checklist was recently adopted for use in the United Kingdom (TABLE 2).

ACKNOWLEDGMENTS

This review represents a distillation of discussions at the Pathology Breakout Session at the First International Symposium on Pheochromocytoma, Bethesda, MD, October 22, 2005. We thank Dr. Ernest Lack for comments on the manuscript.

REFERENCES

1. DeLellis, R.A., R.V. Lloyd, P.U. Heitz & C. Eng, Eds. 2004. Tumours of Endocrine Organs. IARC Press. Lyon.
2. Karsner, H.T. 1950. Tumors of the Adrenal. Atlas of Tumor Pathology, Section VIII, fascicle 29. Armed Forces Institute of Pathology. Washington, DC.
3. Linnoila, R.I., H.R. Keiser, S.M. Steinberg & E.E. Lack. 1990. Histopathology of benign versus malignant sympathoadrenal paragangliomas: clinicopathologic study of 120 cases including unusual histologic features. Hum. Pathol. **21:** 1168–1180.
4. Lloyd, R.V., J.C. Sisson, B. Shapiro & A.A. Verhofstad. 1986. Immunohistochemical localization of epinephrine, norepinephrine, catecholamine-synthesizing enzymes, and chromogranin in neuroendocrine cells and tumors. Am. J. Pathol. **125:** 45–54.
5. Bryant, J., J. Farmer, L.J. Kessler, *et al.* 2003. Pheochromocytoma: the expanding genetic differential diagnosis. J. Natl. Cancer Inst. **95:** 1196–1204.
6. Srivastava, A., A.S. Tischler & R.A. Delellis. 2004. Endogenous biotin staining as an artifact of antigen retrieval with automated immunostaining. Endocr. Pathol. **15:** 175–178.
7. Tischler, A.S., P. Tsokas, M. Shahsavari & J.F. Powers. 1998. Immunoreactivity of normal rabbit serum with epinephrine (E) cells of the rat adrenal medulla after microwave antigen retrieval. Cell Tissue Res. **293:** 563–566.
8. Dahia, P.L., K.N. Ross, M.E. Wright, *et al.* 2005. A HIF1alpha regulatory loop links hypoxia and mitochondrial signals in pheochromocytomas. PLoS Genet. **1:** 72–80.
9. Eisenhofer, G., T.T. Huynh, K. Pacak, *et al.* 2004. Distinct gene expression profiles in norepinephrine- and epinephrine-producing hereditary and sporadic pheochromocytomas: activation of hypoxia-driven angiogenic pathways in von Hippel-Lindau syndrome. Endocr. Relat. Cancer **11:** 897–911.
10. Thompson, L.D. 2002. Pheochromocytoma of the adrenal gland scaled score (PASS) to separate benign from malignant neoplasms: a clinicopathologic and immunophenotypic study of 100 cases. Am. J. Surg. Pathol. **26:** 551 566.
11. August, C., K. August, S. Schroeder, *et al.* 2004. CGH and CD 44/MIB-1 immunohistochemistry are helpful to distinguish metastasized from nonmetastasized sporadic pheochromocytomas. Mod. Pathol. **17:** 1119–1128.
12. Kimura, N., T. Watanabe, T. Noshiro, *et al.* 2005. Histological grading of adrenal and extra-adrenal pheochromocytomas and relationship to prognosis: a clinicopathological analysis of 116 adrenal pheochromocytomas and 30 extra-adrenal sympathetic paragangliomas including 38 malignant tumors. Endocr. Pathol. **16:** 23–32.
13. Liu, T.H., Y.J. Chen, S.F. Wu, *et al.* 2004. Distinction between benign and malignant pheochromocytomas. Zhonghua Bing Li Xue Za Zhi **33:** 198–202.
14. Eisenhofer, G., S.R. Bornstein, F.M. Brouwers, *et al.* 2004. Malignant pheochromocytoma: current status and initiatives for future progress. Endocr. Rel. Cancer **11:** 423–436.
15. Portela-Gomes, G.M., M. Stridsberg, L. Grimelius, *et al.* 2004. Expression of chromogranins A, B, and C (secretogranin II) in human adrenal medulla and in benign and malignant pheochromocytomas: an immunohistochemical study with region-specific antibodies. APMIS **112:** 663–673.

16. DANNENBERG, H., P. KOMMINOTH, W.N. DINJENS, *et al.* 2003. Molecular genetic alterations in adrenal and extra-adrenal pheochromocytomas and paragangliomas. Endocr. Pathol. **14:** 329–350.
17. LENDERS, J.W., G. EISENHOFER, M. MANNELLI & K. PACAK. 2005. Phaeochromocytoma. Lancet **366:** 665–675.
18. DYMOCK, B.W., X. BARRIL, P.A. BROUGH, *et al.* 2005. Novel, potent small-molecule inhibitors of the molecular chaperone Hsp90 discovered through structure-based design. J. Med. Chem. **48:** 4212–4215.
19. KOCH, C.A., D. MAURO, M.M. WALTHER, *et al.* 2002. Pheochromocytoma in von Hippel–Lindau disease: distinct histopathologic phenotype compared to pheochromocytoma in multiple endocrine neoplasia type 2. Endocr. Pathol. **13:** 17–27.
20. LACK, E.E. 1999. Recommendations for the reporting of tumors of the adrenal cortex and medulla. Association of Directors of Anatomic and Surgical Pathology. Virchows. Arch. **435:** 87–91.
21. LACK, E.E., R.V. LLOYD, J.A. CARNEY & J.W. WOODRUFF. 2003. Recommendations for the reporting of extra-adrenal paragangliomas. The Association of Directors of Anatomic and Surgical Pathology. Hum. Pathol. **34:** 112–113.

Distinct Expression of Galectin-3 in Pheochromocytomas

OLIVER GIMM,[a] ULF KRAUSE,[b] MICHAEL BRAUCKHOFF,[a] CUONG HOANG-VU,[a] AND HENNING DRALLE[a]

[a]*Department of General, Visceral and Vascular Surgery, Martin-Luther-University Halle-Wittenberg, 06097 Halle/Saale, Germany*

[b]*Institute of Pathology, Martin-Luther-University Halle-Wittenberg, 06097 Halle/Saale, Germany*

ABSTRACT: Unless distant metastases or local invasion are present, the diagnosis of malignant pheochromocytoma is challenging. Hence, biological markers are sought after and we thought to examine galectin-3 in such a role. Four malignant and 24 benign (10 sporadic, 14 hereditary) pheochromocytomas were analyzed for the expression of galectin-3. One malignant pheochromocytoma with distant metastases showed strong and one malignant undifferentiated pheochromocytoma with local invasion showed partly strong cytoplasmic staining. Nine of 10 sporadic and all hereditary benign pheochromocytomas had absent/weak staining. One benign sporadic pheochromocytoma had moderate cytoplasmic staining. The distinct expression in various types of pheochromocytomas is intriguing and requires further investigation.

KEYWORDS: pheochromocytoma; malignancy; galectin-3

INTRODUCTION

Pheochromocytomas are rare, catecholamine-producing endocrine tumors, most often deriving from the adrenal medulla. Overall, about 10% are thought to be malignant. Recent research has shown that percentages of malignancy vary between the various types of hereditary as well as sporadic pheochromocytomas. Concerning multiple endocrine neoplasia type 2 (MEN 2) and von Hippel–Lindau (VHL)–associated pheochromocytomas, fewer than 5% are considered malignant (reviewed in Refs. 1 and 2). In contrast, the malignancy of sporadic and neurofibromatosis Type 1 (NF1)–associated pheochromocytoma

Address for correspondence: Oliver Gimm, M.D., Department of General, Visceral and Vascular Surgery, Martin-Luther-University Halle-Wittenberg, Ernst-Grube-Str. 40, 06097 Halle/Saale, Germany. Voice: +49-345-557-2314; fax: +49-345-557-2551.
e-mail: oliver.gimm@medizin.uni-halle.de

**Ann. N.Y. Acad. Sci. 1073: 571–577 (2006). © 2006 New York Academy of Sciences.
doi: 10.1196/annals.1353.028**

TABLE 1. Markers of malignancy in pheochromocytoma (PCC)

		Benign PCC (%)	Malignant PCC (%)	*P*	Reference
Ki-67/MIB-1					
Mean (range) scores		1 (0.5–3)	5 (1–18)	<0.001	7
Mean scores		0.21	3	<0.0005	6
Scores > 2.5%		0	50		
Mean scores		1	5	<0.001	10
Mean scores	non-metastasized		3.5		27
	metastasized		12.8		
hTERT					
mRNA detection		7	100	<0.01	8
mRNA detection		9	100	<0.01	9
S100					
No staining		6	42	0.001	6

is higher than 10% (reviewed in Ref. 1). The highest percentage (>30%) of malignancy has been reported in patients with pheochromcytoma–paraganglioma syndrome and *SDHB* germline mutations.[3,4]

In contrast to other tumors, malignancy in pheochromocytoma can generally not be proven on histopathological examination. Hence, biological markers that enable differentiation between benign and malignant pheochromocytomas are sought after. In this regard, Ki-67/MIB-1 [5–7] and hTERT [8,9] are among the most promising markers (TABLE 1). In addition, depletion of S100-positive sustentacular cells has been shown to be a negative marker of malignancy[6] (TABLE 1). However, S100 is not an independent marker of malignancy and dependent on tumor weight.[10]

Galectin-3 is a member of the galectin family and belongs to a group of soluble β-galactoside-binding lectins. So far, at least 10 different galectins have been identified. Overall, their function still remains largely obscure.[11] Concerning galectin-3, a complex expression pattern has been demonstrated that depends on the cell type and the activation state of the cell. Galectin-3 appears in the nucleus and cytoplasm, on the plasma membrane, and in the extracellular space,[12] but is mainly found in the cytoplasm.[13] It has been identified as an inhibitor of apoptosis (reviewed in Ref. 13) and also appears to be involved in cell growth, adhesion, differentiation, angiogenesis, and metastasis (reviewed in Ref. 14). Concerning endocrine tumors, galectin-3 has been shown to be a marker of malignancy of thyroid tumors. Overexpression of galectin-3 has been demonstrated in thyroid carcinoma, while its expression in normal tissue and adenoma was either absent or weak.[15,16] In addition, overexpression of galectin-3 in transfected galectin-3 cDNA normal thyroid follicular cells led to acquisition of the malignant phenotype.[17] We thought to determine the role of galectin-3 in pheochromocytomas.

MATERIAL AND METHODS

Patient Selection

A total of 28 pheochromocytomas from 28 patients were analyzed. Four of the pheochromocytomas were considered malignant for the following reasons: the presence of distant metastases ($n = 1$), undifferentiated appearance and extensive local infiltration ($n = 1$), and lymph node metastases ($n = 2$). All malignant pheochromocytomas were sporadic. Of the 24 benign pheochromocytomas, 10 were considered sporadic and 14 were hereditary. Of the 14 patients with hereditary pheochromocytoma, 12 had germline *RET* mutations (MEN 2A: $n = 10$, MEN 2B: $n = 2$), 1 had germline *VHL* mutation, and 1 had germline *SDHB* mutation.

Pathological Analysis

Immunohistochemical studies were performed following standard protocols as described before.[18] A commercially available antibody against galectin-3 (Santa Cruz Biotechnology, Santa Cruz, CA) was used at a dilution of 1:100. The antibody against CD95 (Santa Cruz Biotechnology) was used at a dilution of 1:500. Strong galectin-3 expression was found in endothelial cells (see FIG. 1A, B, G, H, M), and as has been described before.[19] This served as an internal control.

RESULTS

One malignant pheochromocytoma with distant metastases showed strong cytoplasmic staining (FIG. 1I) and one malignant undifferentiated pheochromocytoma with local invasion showed partly strong cytoplasmic staining (FIG. 1K). In contrast, those two pheochromocytomas, which were considered malignant because of the presence of lymph node metastases, stained negative/weak (FIG. 1L, M). Only one of 10 benign sporadic pheochromocytomas showed moderate cytoplasmic staining (FIG. 1D), while the remaining ones had absent/weak staining (FIG. 1A–C). All hereditary pheochromocytomas were benign and stained negative/weak (FIG. 1E–H).

Interestingly, staining patterns of CD 95 were very similar to galectin-3 staining patterns (FIG. 2A–F).

DISCUSSION

In this study, we show for the first time that galectin-3 is differentially expressed in pheochromocytomas. Those two pheochromocytomas that were

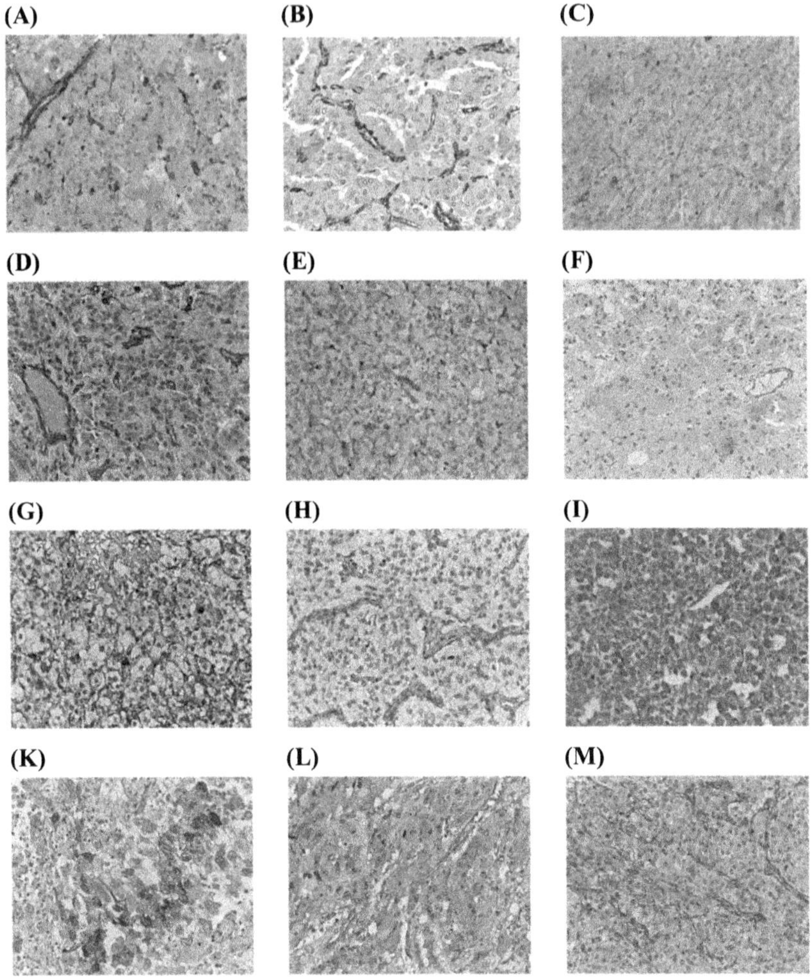

FIGURE 1. Immunohistochemical analysis of pheochromocytoma using the anti-galectin-3 antibody from Santa Cruz Biotechnology (magnification, ×20). (**A–C**): Benign sporadic pheochromocytoma (no staining). (**D**) Benign sporadic pheochromocytoma (strong cytoplasmic staining). (**E**) Benign hereditary (MEN 2A) pheochromocytoma. (**F**) Benign hereditary (MEN 2B) pheochromocytoma. (**G**) Benign hereditary (VHL) pheochromocytoma. (**H**) Benign hereditary (SDHB) pheochromocytoma. (**I–K**) Malignant sporadic pheochromocytoma (strong cytoplasmic staining). (**L–M**) Malignant sporadic pheochromocytoma (absent cytoplasmic staining).

clearly malignant because of the presence of distant metastases or extensive local infiltration showed (partly) strong cytoplasmic staining. In contrast, those two pheochromocytomas that were thought to be malignant because of the presence of lymph node metastases showed absent/weak galectin-3 staining. This is intriguing since some investigators question whether lymph node metastases

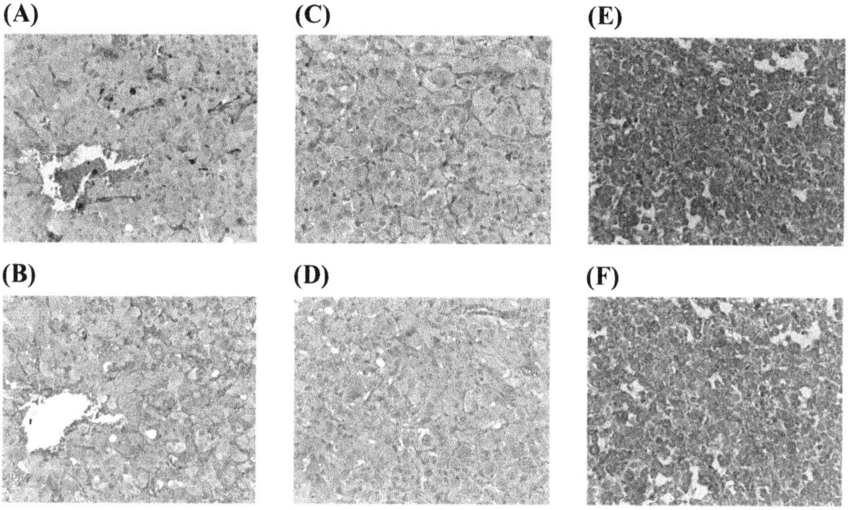

FIGURE 2. Immunohistochemical analysis of pheochromocytoma using the antibodies against galectin-3 (**A, C, E**) and CD95 (**B, D, F**) from Santa Cruz (magnification, × 20). (**A–B**) Benign sporadic pheochromocytoma (absent/weak staining). (**C–D**) Benign hereditary pheochromocytoma (absent/weak staining). (**E–F**) Malignant sporadic pheochromocytoma (strong cytoplasmic staining).

are an unambiguous sign of malignancy in the case of pheochromocytoma. Only one benign sporadic pheochromocytoma showed moderate staining intensity. Unfortunately, this is the only patient for whom no follow-up data are available. The pheochromocytoma of this patient stained negative for Ki-67/MIB-1 and S100 (data not shown). The absence of S100 staining argues for a malignant pheochromocytoma, while the negative Ki-67/MIB-1 staining does not.[10] Also of note, all hereditary benign pheochromocytomas showed absent/weak galectin-3 staining.

In prostate cancer, nuclear expression of galectin-3 has been shown to be associated with tumor suppression whereas cytoplasmic galectin-3 promoted tumor progression.[20] A similar observation has been made in other carcinomas (reviewed in Ref. 21). Summarizing the published data, it appears that cytoplasmic galectin-3 is associated with an aggressive phenotype as opposed to nuclear galectin-3. Regarding pheochromocytomas, it is intriguing that we only observed cytoplasmic galectin-3.

Recently, galectin-3 has been identified as a new binding partner of β-catenin.[22] It has also been shown that the pheochromocytoma cell line PC12 is capable of responding to WNT7A, a member of the Wingless family, by increase in β-catenin stability.[23] Still, the precise role of β-catenin in pheochromocytoma is not known.

Concerning T cells, galectin-3 expression conferred resistance to apoptosis induced by anti-CD95 antibody.[24] More recently, galectin-3 has been shown to be a novel binding partner of CD95/APO-1/Fas.[25] Thus, endogenous galectin-3 appears to determine the routing of CD95 apoptotic pathways. The role of CD95 in pheochromocytoma, however, is unclear. Soluble Fas antigen has been reported to be highest in patients with pheochromocytoma (3.0 ± 1.2 ng/mL) as compared to aldosterone-producing adrenal adenomas (2.2 ± 1.2 ng/mL) and healthy donors (0.8 ± 0.3 ng/mL).[26] In our study, staining for CD95 and galectin-3 appeared to be very similar, thus supporting the hypothesis that these two substances interact in pheochromocytoma.

In summary, our data show distinct galectin-3 staining patterns in various types of pheochromocytomas. If the results are confirmed in larger series, the precise role of galectin-3 in the pathogenesis of pheochromocytomas should be further investigated.

ACKNOWLEDGMENT

The authors thank Kathrin Hammje for superb lab assistance.

REFERENCES

1. Bryant, J., J. Farmer, L.J. Kessler, *et al.* 2003. Pheochromocytoma: the expanding genetic differential diagnosis. J. Natl. Cancer Inst. **95:** 1196–1204.
2. Brauckhoff, M., O. Gimm & H. Dralle. 2004. Preoperative and surgical therapy in sporadic and familial pheochromocytoma. Front. Horm. Res. **31:** 121–144.
3. Gimenez-Roqueplo, A.P., J. Favier, P. Rustin, *et al.* 2003. Mutations in the SDHB gene are associated with extra-adrenal and/or malignant pheochromocytomas. Cancer Res. **63:** 5615–5621.
4. Neumann, H.P., C. Pawlu, M. Peczkowska, *et al.* 2004. Distinct clinical features of paraganglioma syndromes associated with SDHB and SDHD gene mutations. JAMA **292:** 943–951.
5. Brown, H.M., R.A. Komorowski, S.D. Wilson, *et al.* 1999. Predicting metastasis of pheochromocytomas using DNA flow cytometry and immunohistochemical markers of cell proliferation: a positive correlation between MIB-1 staining and malignant tumor behavior. Cancer **86:** 1583–1589.
6. van der Harst, E., H.A. Bruining, H. Jaap Bonjer, *et al.* 2000. Proliferative index in pheochromocytomas: does it predict the occurrence of metastases? J. Pathol. **191:** 175–180.
7. Ohji, H., I. Sasagawa, O. Iciyanagi, *et al.* 2001. Tumour angiogenesis and Ki-67 expression in phaeochromocytoma. BJU Int. **87:** 381–385.
8. Boltze, C., J. Mundschenk, N. Unger, *et al.* 2003. Expression profile of the telomeric complex discriminates between benign and malignant pheochromocytoma. J. Clin. Endocrinol. Metab. **88:** 4280–4286.
9. Isobe, K., T. Yashiro, S. Omura, *et al.* 2004. Expression of the human telomerase reverse transcriptase in pheochromocytoma and neuroblastoma tissues. Endocr. J. **51:** 47–52.

10. CLARKE, M.R., R.J. WEYANT, C.G. WATSON, *et al.* 1998. Prognostic markers in pheochromocytoma. Hum. Pathol. **29:** 522–526.
11. PESHEVA, P., S. KUKLINSKI, B. SCHMITZ, *et al.* 1998. Galectin-3 promotes neural cell adhesion and neurite growth. J. Neurosci. Res. **54:** 639–654.
12. WANG, J.L., J.G. LAING & R.L. ANDERSON. 1991. Lectins in the cell nucleus. Glycobiology **1:** 243–252.
13. KRZESLAK, A. & A. LIPINSKA. 2004. Galectin-3 as a multifunctional protein. Cell Mol. Biol. Lett. **9:** 305–328.
14. TAKENAKA, Y., T. FUKUMORI & A. RAZ. 2004. Galectin-3 and metastasis. Glycoconj. J. **19:** 543–549.
15. NASCIMENTO, M.C., H. BISI, V.A. ALVES, *et al.* 2001. Differential reactivity for galectin-3 in Hurthle cell adenomas and carcinomas. Endocr. Pathol. **12:** 275–279.
16. GASBARRI, A., C. MARCHETTI, G. IERVASI, *et al.* 2004. From the bench to the bedside: galectin-3 immunodetection for improving the preoperative diagnosis of the follicular thyroid nodules. Biomed. Pharmacother. **58:** 356–359.
17. TAKENAKA, Y., H. INOHARA, T. YOSHII, *et al.* 2003. Malignant transformation of thyroid follicular cells by galectin-3. Cancer Lett. **195:** 111–119.
18. GIMM, O., A. PERREN, L.P. WENG, *et al.* 2000. Differential nuclear and cytoplasmic expression of PTEN in normal thyroid tissue, and benign and malignant epithelial thyroid tumors. Am. J. Pathol. **156:** 1693–1700.
19. STRIK, H.M., M.H. DEININGER, B. FRANK, *et al.* 2001. Galectin-3: cellular distribution and correlation with WHO-grade in human gliomas. J. Neurooncol. **53:** 13–20.
20. CALIFICE, S., V. CASTRONOVO, M. BRACKE, *et al.* 2004. Dual activities of galectin-3 in human prostate cancer: tumor suppression of nuclear galectin-3 vs tumor promotion of cytoplasmic galectin-3. Oncogene **23:** 7527–7536.
21. CALIFICE, S., V. CASTRONOVO & F. VAN DEN BRULE. 2004. Galectin-3 and cancer [review]. Int. J. Oncol. **25:** 983–992.
22. SHIMURA, T., Y. TAKENAKA, S. TSUTSUMI, *et al.* 2004. Galectin-3, a novel binding partner of beta-catenin. Cancer Res. **64:** 6363–6367.
23. CARICASOLE, A., T. FERRARO, L. IACOVELLI, *et al.* 2003. Functional characterization of WNT7A signaling in PC12 cells: interaction with A FZD5 × LRP6 receptor complex and modulation by Dickkopf proteins. J. Biol. Chem. **278:** 37024–37031.
24. YANG, R.Y., D.K. HSU, F.T. LIU. 1996. Expression of galectin-3 modulates T-cell growth and apoptosis. Proc. Natl. Acad. Sci. USA **93:** 6737–6742.
25. FUKUMORI, T., Y. TAKENAKA, N. OKA, *et al.* 2004. Endogenous galectin-3 determines the routing of CD95 apoptotic signaling pathways. Cancer Res. **64:** 3376–3379.
26. KUSHLINSKII, N.E., T.A. BRITVIN, G.A. POLYAKOVA, *et al.* 2002. Plasma content of soluble fas antigen in patients with adrenal tumors and tumor-like pathologies. Bull. Exp. Biol. Med. **134:** 171–174.
27. AUGUST, C., K. AUGUST, S. SCHROEDER, *et al.* 2004. CGH and CD 44/MIB-1 immunohistochemistry are helpful to distinguish metastasized from nonmetastasized sporadic pheochromocytomas. Mod. Pathol. **17:** 1119–1128.

Expression of Connexins in Chromaffin Cells of Normal Human Adrenals and in Benign and Malignant Pheochromocytomas

HOLGER S. WILLENBERG,[a] MATTHIAS SCHOTT,[a] WOLFGANG SAEGER,[b] ANNETTE TRIES,[a] WERNER A. SCHERBAUM,[a] AND STEFAN R. BORNSTEIN[c]

[a]*Department of Endocrinology, Diabetes and Rheumatology, University Hospital Duesseldorf, Germany*

[b]*Institute of Pathology of the Marienkrankenhaus Hamburg, Germany*

[c]*Department of Medicine, University of Dresden, Dresden, Germany*

ABSTRACT: Decrease in connexin (Cx) expression and loss of gap junctional intercellular communication (GJIC) have been associated with aberrant cell growth and enhanced neoplastic phenotype. We studied the expression of Cx26, Cx32, Cx43, and Cx50 in chromaffin cells of 10 normal human adrenal glands, 10 benign, and 13 malignant pheochromocytomas. Immunohistochemistry showed that Cx50 expression seemed to be the predominant form of Cx expressed in human chromaffin cells, whereas Cx43 immunoreactivity was the most prominent form found in the adrenal cortex. However, Western blotting revealed that nonphosphorylated and singly and doubly phosphorylated forms of Cx43 were present within the malignant adrenomedullary cells at the same time. Cx26 and Cx32 were distributed inhomogeneously with no emphasis of expression in the types of tissues studied. Cx50 expression was diminished in malignant pheochromocytomas. We conclude that there is a differential expression of Cx in human adrenals. Immunohistological testing for Cx expression does not however allow differentiation of benign from malignant pheochromocytomas.

KEYWORDS: adrenal tumor; chromaffin cell; pheochromocytoma; connexins; human

INTRODUCTION

Gap junctions are small intercellular membrane channels, allowing the direct exchange of ions and small molecules <1,000 Dalton. Two hemi-channels

Address for correspondence: Stefan R. Bornstein, M.D., Department of Medicine, University of Dresden, Fetscherstr. 74, D-01307 Dresden, Germany. Voice: +490351 458-3100; fax: +490351 458-4303.

e-mail: Stefan.Bornstein@uniklinikum-dresden.de

Ann. N.Y. Acad. Sci. 1073: 578–583 (2006). © **2006 New York Academy of Sciences.**
doi: 10.1196/annals.1353.060

from each neighboring cell form a membrane pore, composed of six protein subunits, named connexins (Cx). To date, at least 21 different Cx have been discovered.[1] Gap junctions are hypothesized to play an important role for cell homeostasis, embryogenesis, and growth control. Loss of gap junctional intercellular communication (GJIC) has been associated with carcinogenesis and most tumors, including adrenocortical tumors[2] have dysfunctional GJIC.

Though the majority of pheochromocytomas are benign lesions, rates between 5% and 26% of all pheochromocytomas are estimated to be malignant, although in numerous studies malignant lesions account for 36% to 46% of cases.[3,4] Histological studies of removed tumors do not allow a safe characterization of the chromaffin tissue as benign or malignant.[5] Therefore, malignancy is defined by the presence of metastases in tissues of nonchromaffin origin (e.g., lymph nodes, bone, liver, lung, and brain) or by tumor invasion into surrounding structures.

To test the hypothesis that a diminished expression of Cx may be associated with malignancy in pheochromocytomas, we studied the expression of Cx26, Cx32, Cx43, and Cx50 in chromaffin cells of normal human adrenal glands and in benign and malignant pheochromocytomas by means of immunohistochemistry analysis. Tissues from two different malignant pheochromocytomas were employed to derive primary cultures. Cultured cells have been subjected to Western blotting.

MATERIALS AND METHODS

Tissue from normal human adrenal glands (n = 10, mean patient age: 50 ± 23 years), benign (n = 10, mean patient age: 50 ± 15 years) and malignant (n = 13; mean patient age: 58 ± 6 years) pheochromocytomas were embedded in paraffin. While normal adrenal glands were harvested from patients undergoing surgical treatment of renal carcinoma, adrenomedullary tumors have been removed because of underlying catecholamine excess. Only those tumors have been classified as malignant whose patients had developed metastases to tissues of nonchromaffin origin. In addition, human malignant pheochromocytoma cells were obtained from a metastatic tumor of the liver and a large adrenomedullary tumor in two different patients. Purified human malignant pheochromocytoma cell cultures were established according to a protocol of the group led by P. Hornsby.[6]

Immunostaining was performed as described previously.[7] Tumor specimen were reviewed during the diagnostic procedure by at least two independent investigators. We employed the following affinity isolated antibodies for immunohistological studies: polyclonal rabbit anti-Cx26 (71-0500, ZYMED Laboratories, San Francisco, CA, USA; 1:500), polyclonal rabbit anti-Cx32 (71-0600, ZYMED; 1:1000), rabbit anti-Cx43 (C6219, Sigma-Aldrich St. Louis, MO; 1:10000), and monoclonal mouse anti-Cx50 (33-4300, ZYMED;

TABLE 1. Staining scores obtained from the immunohistological studies

	Normal cortex	Normal medulla	Benign pheo	Malignant pheo
Cx26 (1:100)	**2.0**	0.0	**1.8**	**1.7**
Cx32 (1:100)	**1.5**	0.0	0.3	1.0
Cx43 (1:100)	**2.2**	0.2	0.8	0.3
Cx50 (1:100)	**1.5**	**1.5**	**2.0**	0.5

NOTE: Bold numbers reflect the observation that staining was specific and positive. The table reflects that expression of immunoreactive proteins for Cx32 and Cx43 was actually reserved for adrenocortical cells. Though normal adrenal medulla did not stain with the antibody to Cx26, pheochromocytomas did, independently of their biological behavior. A difference could be noted between benign and malignant pheochromocytomas when investigated for Cx50. However, some malignant pheochromocytomas showed a slight reaction when stained with an antibody to Cx50.

1:1000). For characterization of chromaffin cells, a mouse monoclonal antibody directed to human chromogranin A (DakoCytomation, Hamburg, Germany) was used in dilutions of 1:200. All sections were counterstained with hematoxylin. The staining score is expressed in arbitrary units: no staining was rated 0, staining of less than 25% of cells was rated 1, staining of 25% to 50% was rated 2, and clear staining of more than 50% of cells was rated 3. The mean ratings are presented in TABLE 1.

For Western blotting, cells were grown in six-well plates until they reached ~ 90% confluence. Cells were lysed in 2 × SDS-Page buffer (125 mM Tris-HCL, 4% (w/v) SDS, 20% (w/v) glycerol, 100 mM DTT, 0.2% (w/v) bromphenol blue; pH 6.8) followed by brief sonification. Samples were applied to SDS-polyacrylamide gels of 10% (w/v) acryamide, followed by electrophoresis and blotting. Immunodetection was performed using as primary antibody a 1:1000 dilution of rabbit polyclonal anti-Cx43 (Sigma-Aldrich) and a 1:5000 dilution of antirabbit secondary antibody conjugated to HRP (DakoCytomation). Antigen/antibody complexes were visualized by enhanced chemiluminescence (ECL) and exposed to Hyperfilm-ECL (Amersham Biosciences, GE Healthcare Biosciences AB, Uppsala, Sweden). β-actin was used as gel-loading control.

RESULTS

The results of the immunohistological studies are given in TABLE 1. We found immunoreactive Cx26 in normal adrenal cortex but not in normal chromaffin cells. However, in pheochromocytomas, Cx26 was expressed at a level comparable to that of the normal adrenal cortex. No difference between benign and malignant tissue could be noted. There was little expression of Cx32 in normal adrenal cortex and in malignant pheochromocytomas. However, there was no staining in normal adrenal medulla and benign pheochromocytomas. As expected, Cx43 was expressed in normal adrenal cortex (FIG. 1). However,

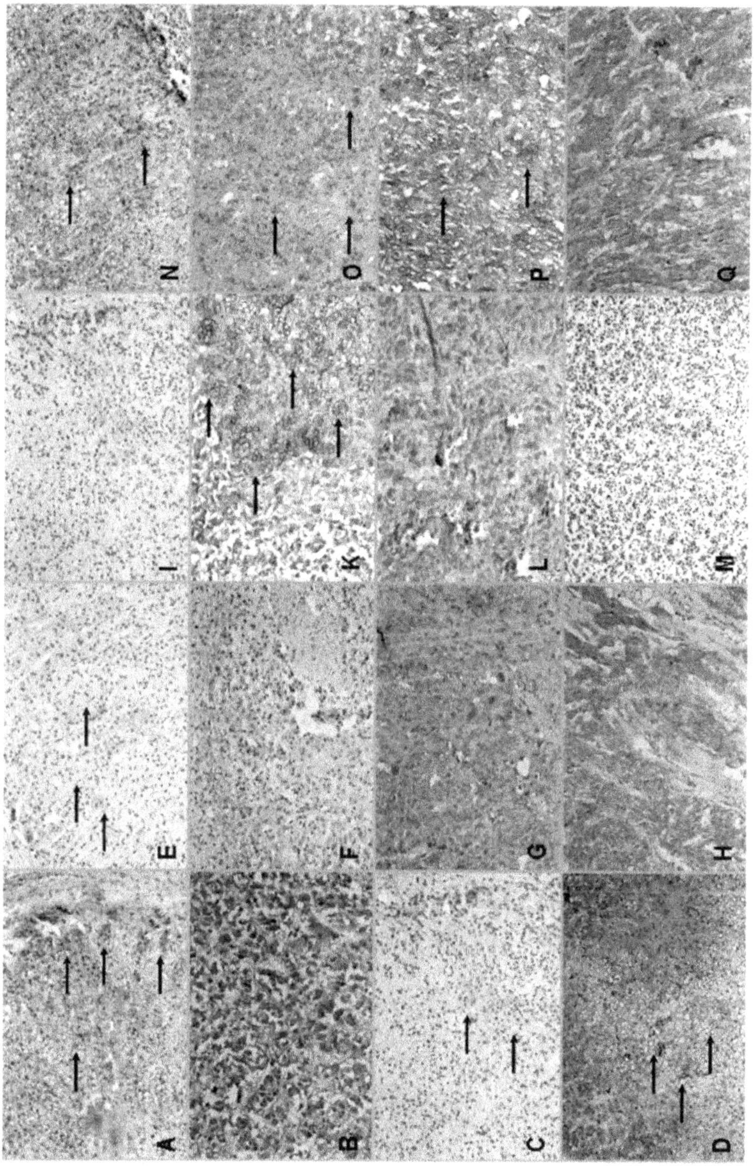

FIGURE 1. Representative histological sections of normal adrenal cortex (Panels A, E, I, K—right part, and N), normal adrenal medulla (Panels B, F, K—left part, and O), benign pheochromocytomas (Panels C, G, L, and P), and malignant pheochromocytomas (Panels D, H, M, and Q) (magnification 20×). Tissue was stained with specific antibodies to Cx26 (Panels, A–D), Cx32 (Panels E–H), Cx43 (Panels K–M), or Cx50 (Panels N–Q). Panel I shows a typical negative control in the staining procedure when tissue was not exposed to primary antibody. *Arrows* point to stained cells, which in the great majority of cases showed a typical reactivity in the membranes.

we found almost no immunoreactivity for Cx43 in all chromaffin tissues studied. On the other hand, Cx43 is found in numerous endocrine-neuroendocrine tissues. Cx43 transcripts have been demonstrated in rat adrenal medulla via RT-PCR.[8] Therefore, we investigated phosphorylation of Cx43 in the cell line. Three Cx bands can be detected in unstimulated human malignant pheochromocytoma cells: the nonphosphorylated (P0), singly (P1) and doubly (P2) phosphorylated forms (data not shown).

Cx50 expression did not vary between adrenal medulla and adrenal cortex. However, we saw a difference in the staining rates between expression in chromaffin cells of benign and malignant pheochromocytomas.

DISCUSSION

Gap junctions have been implicated in important physiological processes, such as development and differentiation, maintenance of cellular homeostasis, and growth control. Consequently, the disturbance of cell communication has been associated with pathological conditions. For 30 years, it has been hypothesized that gap junctions play an important role in the regulation of carcinogenesis. In addition, during the last years insights have been gained into the complex regulation of Cx-phosphorylation via certain proteinkinases in cancer cells and consecutive aberrant protein-phosphorylation.[9] As a consequence, gap junctions have emerged as an attractive target for cancer therapy, not only for chemoprevention, but also for chemotherapeutic and gene therapy strategies relying on the bystander effect.[10]

In this study, we investigated for the first time expression of Cx in human malignant pheochromocytoma. We saw a differential expression of connexins in human adrenals. Gene deletion of Cx32 in mice led to the development of nonsecreting malignant adrenomedullary tumors in two experiments.[11] The finding that expression of Cx50 in malignant pheochromocytomas was decreased in comparison to normal adrenal medulla and benign pheochromocytomas is new and seems to support the hypothesis that cancer cells show a decrease of GJIC and/or Cx expression. It has been demonstrated in various cancer cells that restoration of GJIC by transfection of Cx genes may lead to a decrease in malignancy and even growth arrest. Hence, basic knowledge concerning the mechanisms of deficient GJIC in cancer cells is important for establishing advanced anticancer strategies. However, immunohistological testing for expression of Cx does not seem to constitute a helpful tool reliable enough to distinguish benign from malignant pheochromocytomas.

ACKNOWLEDGMENTS

This work was supported by a Grant from the University of Düsseldorf and by the GlaxoSmithKline Stiftung, Goettingen, Germany to H.S.W. and by a DFG grant (SFB 655/1-05) to S.R.B. We would like to acknowledge the valuable contributions by Pauline Patak, M.D., Department of Clinical Neuroscience, St. George's Hospital Medical School, London, UK.

REFERENCES

1. WILLECKE, K., J. EIBERGER, J. DEGEN, *et al.* 2002. Structural and functional diversity of connexin genes in the mouse and human genome. Biol. Chem. **383:** 725–737.
2. MURRAY, S.A., K. DAVIS, L.M. FISHMAN, *et al.* 2000. Alpha1 connexin 43 gap junctions are decreased in human adrenocortical tumors. J. Clin. Endocrinol. Metab. **85:** 890–895.
3. EISENHOFER, G., S.R. BORNSTEIN, F.M. BROUWERS, *et al.* 2004. Malignant pheochromocytoma: current status and initiatives for future progress. Endocr. Relat. Cancer **11:** 423–436.
4. LEHNERT, H., J. MUNDSCHENK & K. HAHN. 2004. Malignant pheochromocytoma. Front. Horm. Res. **31:** 155–162.
5. SCHRÖDER, S., P. KOMMINOTH, B. PADBERG, *et al.* 1995. Morphological typing, evaluation of tumor dignity and prognosis and etiologic classification of adrenomedullary and adrenocortical neoplasias. Pathologe **16:** 307–314.
6. SUWA, T., M. M. CHEN, C.L. HAWKS, *et al.* 2003. Zonal expression of dickkopf-3 and components of the Wnt signalling pathways in the human adrenal cortex. J. Endocrinol. **178:** 149–158.
7. WOLF, A., H.S. WILLENBERG, K. K. CUPISTI, *et al.* 2005. Adrenal pheochromocytoma with contralateral cortisol-producing adrenal adenoma: diagnostic and therapeutic management. Horm. Metab. Res. **37:** 391–395.
8. MARTIN, A.O., M.N. MATHIEU, C. CHEVILLARD, *et al.* 2001. Gap junctions mediate electrical signaling and ensuing cytosolic Ca2+ increases between chromaffin cells in adrenal slices: a role in catecholamine release. J. Neurosci. **21:** 5397–5405.
9. LAMPE, P.D. & A.F. LAU. 2004. The effects of connexin phosphorylation on gap junctional communication. Int. J. Biochem. Cell Biol. **36:** 1171–1186.
10. VRIONIS, F.D., J.K. WU, P. QI, *et al.* 1997. The bystander effect exerted by tumor cells expressing the herpes simplex virus thymidine kinase (HSVtk) gene is dependent on connexin expression and cell communication via gap junctions. Gene Ther. **4:** 577–585.
11. KING, T.J. & P.D. LAMPE. 2004. Mice deficient for the gap junction protein connexin32 exhibit increased radiation-induced tumorigenesis associated with elevated mitogen-activated protein kinase (p44/Erk1, p42/Erk2) activation. Carcinogenesis **25:** 669–680.

Index of Contributors

www.ingramcontent.com/pod-product-compliance
Ingram Content Group UK Ltd.
Pitfield, Milton Keynes, MK11 3LW, UK
UKHW020128290926
15471UKWH00003B/358

9 781573 315975